Advances in Breast Cancer Research

Advances in Breast Cancer Research

Editor: Ava Santiago

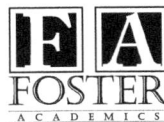

FA
FOSTER
ACADEMICS

www.fosteracademics.com

www.fosteracademics.com

FA FOSTER ACADEMICS

Cataloging-in-Publication Data

Advances in breast cancer research / edited by Ava Santiago.
    p. cm.
Includes bibliographical references and index.
ISBN 978-1-63242-735-9
1. Breast--Cancer. 2. Breast--Cancer--Surgery. 3. Breast--Diseases--Diagnosis.
4. Breast--Diseases--Treatment. I. Santiago, Ava.
RC280.B8 A38 2019
616.994 49--dc23

Foster Academics,
118-35 Queens Blvd., Suite 400,
Forest Hills, NY 11375, USA

ISBN 978-1-63242-735-9 (Hardback)

Contents

Preface

This book has been a concerted effort by a group of academicians, researchers and scientists, who have contributed their research works for the realization of the book. This book has materialized in the wake of emerging advancements and innovations in this field. Therefore, the need of the hour was to compile all the required researches and disseminate the knowledge to a broad spectrum of people comprising of students, researchers and specialists of the field.

Breast cancer is the cancer, which develops in breast tissue. Breast cancers can be of 18 different forms, including ductal carcinoma and lobular carcinoma. The treatment of breast cancer depends on the person's age and the stage of the cancer. It may be approached aggressively if the prognosis is poor or if there is a high chance of recurrence following the treatment. Surgery, chemotherapy and radiotherapy are some treatment options. Surgery involves the physical removal of the tumor. This can be done through a mastectomy, lumpectomy or quadrantectomy. After surgery, breast cancer treatment may include chemotherapy, hormone-blocking therapy and monoclonal antibodies. Radiation therapy may be delivered to a cancer patient in the form of brachytherapy or as external beam therapy. This book aims to elucidate the causes, diagnosis and treatment of breast cancer. It unravels the recent studies in this medical condition. It is an essential guide for clinicians, doctors and medical students.

At the end of the preface, I would like to thank the authors for their brilliant chapters and the publisher for guiding us all-through the making of the book till its final stage. Also, I would like to thank my family for providing the support and encouragement throughout my academic career and research projects.

Editor

The combined effect of mammographic texture and density on breast cancer risk: a cohort study

Johanna O. P. Wanders[1], Carla H. van Gils[1]*, Nico Karssemeijer[2], Katharina Holland[2], Michiel Kallenberg[3,4], Petra H. M. Peeters[1,5], Mads Nielsen[3,4] and Martin Lillholm[3,4]

Abstract

Background: Texture patterns have been shown to improve breast cancer risk segregation in addition to area-based mammographic density. The additional value of texture pattern scores on top of volumetric mammographic density measures in a large screening cohort has never been studied.

Methods: Volumetric mammographic density and texture pattern scores were assessed automatically for the first available digital mammography (DM) screening examination of 51,400 women (50–75 years of age) participating in the Dutch biennial breast cancer screening program between 2003 and 2011. The texture assessment method was developed in a previous study and validated in the current study. Breast cancer information was obtained from the screening registration system and through linkage with the Netherlands Cancer Registry. All screen-detected breast cancers diagnosed at the first available digital screening examination were excluded. During a median follow-up period of 4.2 (interquartile range (IQR) 2.0–6.2) years, 301 women were diagnosed with breast cancer. The associations between texture pattern scores, volumetric breast density measures and breast cancer risk were determined using Cox proportional hazard analyses. Discriminatory performance was assessed using c-indices.

Results: The median age of the women at the time of the first available digital mammography examination was 56 years (IQR 51–63). Texture pattern scores were positively associated with breast cancer risk (hazard ratio (HR) 3.16 (95% CI 2.16–4.62) (p value for trend <0.001), for quartile (Q) 4 compared to Q1). The c-index of texture was 0.61 (95% CI 0.57–0.64). Dense volume and percentage dense volume showed positive associations with breast cancer risk (HR 1.85 (95% CI 1.32–2.59) (p value for trend <0.001) and HR 2.17 (95% CI 1.51–3.12) (p value for trend <0.001), respectively, for Q4 compared to Q1). When adding texture measures to models with dense volume or percentage dense volume, c-indices increased from 0.56 (95% CI 0.53–0.59) to 0.62 (95% CI 0.58–0.65) (p < 0.001) and from 0.58 (95% CI 0.54–0.61) to 0.60 (95% CI 0.57–0.63) (p = 0.054), respectively.

Conclusions: Deep-learning-based texture pattern scores, measured automatically on digital mammograms, are associated with breast cancer risk, independently of volumetric mammographic density, and augment the capacity to discriminate between future breast cancer and non-breast cancer cases.

Keywords: Volumetric mammographic breast density, Texture pattern scores, Breast cancer risk

* Correspondence: C.vanGils@umcutrecht.nl
[1]Julius Center for Health Sciences and Primary Care, University Medical Center Utrecht, P.O. Box 85500, 3508 GA Utrecht, The Netherlands
Full list of author information is available at the end of the article

Background

Many countries have a breast cancer screening program [1]. The intention of these programs is to find breast cancers at an early stage, to increase the chance of successful treatment and to prevent premature mortality [2, 3]. Although most screening programs have been shown to decrease breast cancer mortality [4], the programs do not work equally well for all women. It is well-known that women with more fibroglandular breast tissue (dense tissue) have a lower probability that a cancer, if present, is detected through mammographic screening: the screening sensitivity is lower in women with dense breasts [5–13]. High mammographic density does not only lower mammographic screening sensitivity, it is also a well-known breast cancer risk factor [14, 15]. Therefore, the possibility of developing more personalized screening, taking mammographic density and breast cancer risk into account, is being discussed widely [16, 17]. In the USA, legislation enforces physicians to inform a woman of her mammographic density after mammographic screening. Breast density legislation is now in place in 36 states. Depending on her mammographic density, a woman can choose to be screened with another imaging modality, like ultrasound (US) or magnetic resonance imaging (MRI), in addition to mammography [16].

Besides mammographic density, mammographic texture patterns have also been shown to be associated with breast cancer risk, and also to improve breast cancer risk segregation in addition to area-based mammographic density [18–21]. These texture patterns characterize the spatial distribution of parenchymal tissue in the breast. Examples of radiographic features of texture patterns are, for example, co-occurrence features, which take into account the pixel intensities or gray-levels of neighboring pixels in different directions; run-length features, which characterize the coarseness of the texture patterns by determining the length of consecutive pixels with the same pixel intensity in linear directions; structural features, which characterize the tissue complexity and variations in gray level between a specific pixel and its neighboring pixels; and multi-resolution or spectral features, which use frequency transforms, like Fourier or wavelet, to capture texture structures that are repeatedly found in a mammogram [19].

All these texture features are manually designed and selected and will only capture mammographic, risk-prone patterns to the extent the feature designs were relevant. This problem is normally overcome by initially using large banks of potential features but only maintaining the informative ones in the final classification system [22, 23]. However, more modern texture quantification methods based on deep learning address this challenge in a more principled, domain, and task-specific way [24]. Here, features are not designed but are learned from the domain data as part of training of the overall classification system. In its simplest form, as those features that best describe the domain (e.g., mammographic images) and in a more complex form as the features that best describe the domain and simultaneously contribute optimally to the task at hand (e.g., cancer risk). It has been suggested that the methods developed with deep learning have a better ability to quantify breast cancer risk compared to methods based on manually designed and selected texture features [24].

Therefore, the aim of this study was to determine the association between a previously developed deep-learning-based texture score [24] alone and in combination with automatically measured volumetric mammographic density and breast cancer risk, and their ability to segregate future breast cancer cases from non-breast cancer cases in a "new" dataset. This dataset consists of a consecutive series of unprocessed digital mammograms of a breast cancer screening population in whom mammograms are prospectively collected.

Methods
Study population

In the Netherlands, women aged 50–75 years have been invited for mammographic breast cancer screening every other year from 1989 and onwards. Approximately 80% of the women attend the screening program [25]. Since 2003 the transition from analog to digital mammography gradually took place, starting at one screening unit (Preventicon screening unit, Utrecht, The Netherlands) and in 2010 the transition was complete. For this study, all women were included who had one or more digital mammographic screening examinations at the Preventicon screening unit between 2003 and 2011. There are five screening regions in the Netherlands that follow the exact same procedures. The Preventicon screening unit is part of the Foundation of Population Screening Mid-West region. Women consent to their data being used for evaluation and improvement of the screening, by participating in the Dutch breast cancer screening program, unless they have stated otherwise.

The research ethics committee of the Radboud University Nijmegen Medical Centre declared that this study does not fall within the remit of the Medical Research Involving Human Subjects Act. Therefore, this study could be carried out (in The Netherlands) without approval by an accredited research ethics committee.

Data collection

We selected each woman's first unprocessed (raw) digital mammography examination. All mammograms were taken using Lorad Selenia DM systems (Hologic, Danbury, CT, USA). During the first examination in the screening program, both craniocaudal (CC) and mediolateral oblique

(MLO) views are always acquired. In subsequent rounds the MLO is the standard view and an additional CC view is taken only when indicated (e.g., visible abnormality, high mammographic density). Information during follow up was obtained through the screening registration system and through linkage with the Netherlands Cancer Registry to obtain complete information on both screen-detected and interval breast cancers. Screen-detected breast cancers were defined as breast cancers diagnosed on the basis of diagnostic work-up of an "abnormal" screening examination. Interval breast cancers were defined as breast cancers diagnosed within 24 months after a screening examination that did not lead to recall (negative mammogram), and before the next scheduled screening examination. The median time between the first available digital screening mammogram and breast cancer diagnosis was 3.7 years (IQR 2.0–4.3, minimum 0.1 years, maximum 7.9 years) for screen-detected breast cancers and 2.2 years (IQR 1.1–3.9, minimum 0.1 years, maximum 9.6 years) for interval cancers. Both invasive and ductal carcinoma in situ breast cancers were used for analyses.

We excluded all screen-detected breast cancer cases that were diagnosed based on the first digital screening examination, to minimize the number of breast cancer cases in the study that were diagnosed based on the same mammogram as was used for breast density and texture score assessment.

The texture measure used in this study was previously developed using a selection of women with and without breast cancer who had one or more digital mammographic screening examinations at the Preventicon screening unit between 2003 and 2011 [24]. Therefore, we also excluded all women whose mammograms were used to train the texture measure used in this study, to ensure an independent validation.

The data were obtained through the registry of a breast cancer screening program in which mammograms are routinely collected. Therefore, besides age, no additional information was available about the women.

Volumetric mammographic density assessment

Absolute dense volume (DV) and percentage dense volume (PDV) were automatically assessed from unprocessed mammograms of the left and right breasts, using Volpara Density (version 1.5.0, Volpara Health Technologies, Wellington, New Zealand) [26]. We used the mean of the left and right MLO views, since this is the routinely acquired view and CC views were not available for all women. In this way, we ensured that mammographic density was assessed in the exact same way in all participants.

Mammographic texture assessment

The deep-learning-based mammographic texture-based risk assessment was calculated from unprocessed mammograms

using prototype software by Biomediq A/S as described by Kallenberg et al. [24]. The deep-learning framework was a 5-layer convolutional neural network that maps mammographic patches to a cancer risk score when trained as described below. The first four layers were three convolutional and one pooling layer. These layers learned mammographic features (mammographic structure/texture) of decreasing size and increasing level of abstraction. The initial three layers were trained in an unsupervised fashion: they learn features that describe mammographic structure independent of cancer risk. The final two layers (the last convolution layer and the final 5th Softmax classification layer) were trained in a supervised fashion using the features encoded in the previous layers as the starting point. The weights of these final layers were optimized to distinguish between patches from breasts without cancer diagnosis (at both baseline and follow up) and patches from breasts that were without diagnosis at baseline but were diagnosed with breast cancer at follow up. The implication of this is that the network was trained to score cancer risk realized as the probability that a patch originates from a breast with cancer-prone mammographic texture/structure. Further technical/mathematical details of texture methodology can be found in the article of Kallenberg et al. [24].The training dataset described subsequently corresponds to the dataset named "Dutch Breast Cancer Screening Dataset" in that same article [24]. For the purposes of this study, the deep-learning framework was trained on a subset of the Preventicon data consisting of 394 cancer cases and 1182 healthy controls - 3 controls per case, matched on age and acquisition date. The cancer cases included 285 screen-detected cancers and 109 interval cancers. For screen-detected cancers, the cases were represented by the contralateral view at the time of diagnosis. For interval cancers, the cases were represented by the contralateral view from the screening visit immediately prior to diagnosis. The laterality distribution of the controls was sampled to match that of the cases.

The left and right MLO views in the remaining independent validation subset of the Preventicon cohort were scored for texture-based risk using the framework above. The texture score for a single screening visit was obtained as the average of the left and right MLO texture risk scores. This scoring was performed such that both software and operator were fully blinded to cancer outcome during scoring. For each MLO view, the software extracted 500 randomly sampled patches within the fully compressed part of the breast tissue. To identify the fully compressed part of the breast, the geometry of the uncompressed breast is modelled as a semi-sphere, as has been proposed in the works of Highnam and Brady [27]. According to this model, the boundary between the fully compressed and the uncompressed part of the breast is found at those locations within the breast where the distance to the skin edge equals half the height of the breast.

Each patch was scored for cancer risk using the trained deep-learning framework described above and the resulting texture score for a single view was obtained as the average of the 500 patch-based risk scores.

An example of mammograms from each of the four combinations of high or low texture score with high or low percentage dense volume is given in Fig. 1. The stronger textural properties of mammograms with high texture scores are clear in both density categories.

Statistical analysis

Age and breast measures (mammographic density and mammographic texture scores) were determined for the first available unprocessed digital mammography examination of each woman. In addition, the number of digital screening rounds and follow-up years were determined. We described our study population by the median and interquartile range (IQR) for each of these characteristics and tested whether these characteristics were significantly different in breast cancer and non-breast cancer cases. We used the two-sample t test for normally distributed measures and the Mann-Whitney U test for non-normally distributed measures. Breast density measures were transformed using the natural logarithm (ln) to obtain normal distributions

and Pearson correlation coefficients were determined to test correlation between breast measures and between age and breast measures.

Associations of continuous measures (per standard deviation (SD) increase, using normally distributed measures) and quartiles of density and texture scores with breast cancer risk were determined using Cox proportional hazards analyses. We calculated hazard ratios (HR) and their 95% confidence intervals (95% CI). Age was used as the underlying time scale. The entry time was defined as subject's age at the time of the first available digital mammogram. Exit time was defined as one of the following options: (1) age at breast cancer diagnosis (event), (2) age at death (censoring), or (3) age at 2 years after the last digital mammogram performed before 1 January 2012 (censoring). The age used as the exit time was determined by the option that occurred first.

We aimed to determine whether the previously described texture score is associated with breast cancer risk and has additional value, next to volumetric mammographic density measures, in distinguishing future breast cancer cases from non-breast cancer cases. To study this, we constructed several models. First, three Cox proportional hazard models were developed with dense volume, percentage dense volume, or texture as the determinant (model 1, 2 and 3, respectively). With these models we could determine the ability of a density or texture measure alone to separate breast cancer from non-breast cancer cases. Thereafter, we constructed two additional Cox proportional hazard models. The first contained both dense volume and texture determinants (model 1a). The other model contained both percentage dense volume and texture determinants (model 2a). To determine the ability of the models to discriminate between breast cancer cases and non-cases, concordance indices (c-indices) were obtained for all models. The c-index can be seen as the fraction of "case - non-case" pairs for which the model correctly identified the breast cancer case. Across 2000 bootstrap samples, c-indices of models containing only a breast density measure (model 1 or 2) were compared to models containing both density measures and texture scores (model 1a or 2a) to test whether differences in c-indices were statistically significant.

As the density and texture scores were expected to be strongly correlated, we prevented multicollinearity from occurring in models 1a and 2a by including the residuals of the texture scores regressed on breast density instead of the texture score itself. This "residual method" is often used in the field of nutritional epidemiology [28]. Residuals were obtained by using linear regression analysis. There was no correlation between the residuals and breast density.

Additionally, two extra Cox proportional hazard models were constructed in which the residuals of breast density (dense volume for model 3a and percentage dense volume

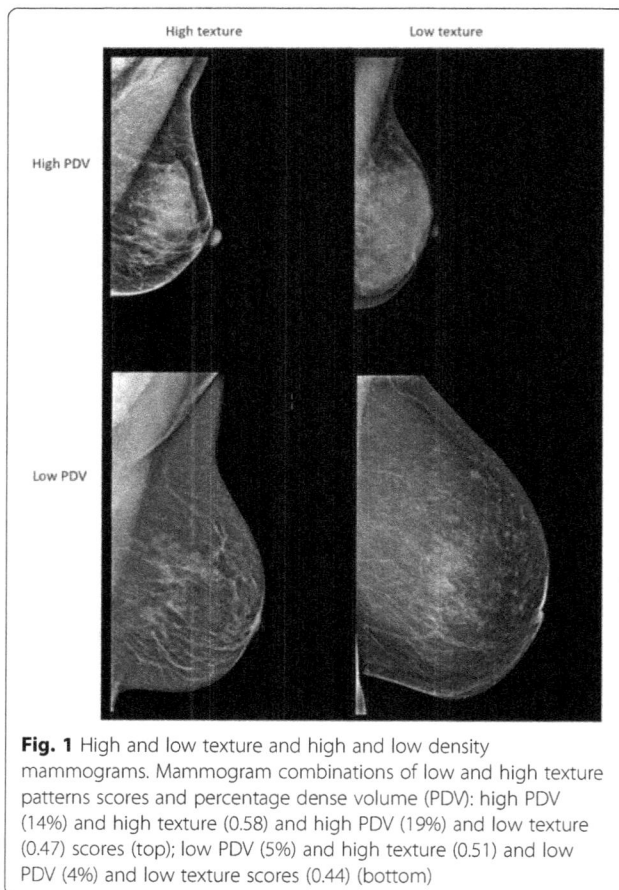

Fig. 1 High and low texture and high and low density mammograms. Mammogram combinations of low and high texture patterns scores and percentage dense volume (PDV): high PDV (14%) and high texture (0.58) and high PDV (19%) and low texture (0.47) scores (top); low PDV (5%) and high texture (0.51) and low PDV (4%) and low texture scores (0.44) (bottom)

for model 3b) regressed on texture were combined with the texture score. Using these models, we could determine whether breast density measures added some distinctive power to the texture score alone.

The proportional hazards assumption was evaluated by Schoenfeld residual plots and log minus log plots, and the assumption was not violated. To examine the presence of a linear trend in HRs over the quartiles of breast measures, quartiles were added to the models as continuous variables.

Finally, in a secondary analysis we also separately determined the associations between breast measures (dense volume, percentage dense volume, and texture) and breast cancer for screen-detected and interval breast cancers. Statistical analyses were performed using SPSS version 22 and R version 3.2.0.

Results

Of the 54,285 women in our screening cohort, 898 were diagnosed with breast cancer within 2 years after their last digital screening mammogram. In the development study of the texture score used in this study, mammograms of 1576 women (both with and without breast cancer) from the aforementioned cohort were used for texture score development and therefore excluded from our analyses [24]. Next, 217 women were excluded as they were diagnosed with breast cancer as a result of their first digital screening examination and for 1062 women the breast density and/or texture scores could not be determined from the first digital screening examinations, therefore the mammograms of these women were also excluded. Finally, women were excluded for whom information on breast cancer outcome was missing ($N = 20$) and for whom the screening examination date came after the date of death (as we only had information on year of death and therefore set the date of death for all women on 1 July in the year they died) ($N = 10$). This resulted in a dataset that was used for data analysis containing 51,400 women, of whom 301 women developed breast cancer and 51,099 women did not (Fig. 2).

Characteristics of the study population are presented in Table 1. At the first available digital screening examination, the median age of women in our cohort ($N = 51,400$) was 56 years (IQR 51–63), the median dense breast volume was 57.8 cm^3 (IQR 42.9–78.9), the percentage breast volume was 6.4% (IQR 4.8–9.8) and the texture score was 0.50 (IQR 0.48–0.53). The median total number of screening examinations (analog and digital combined) that a woman had was 5 (IQR 2–8) of which the median number of digital examinations was 2 (IQR 1–3). The median follow-up time was 4.2 years (IQ: 2.0–6.2).

Table 2 shows that age was negatively correlated with dense volume (Pearson correlation coefficient -0.16, $p < 0.01$), percentage dense volume (-0.29, $p < 0.01$), and texture (-0.35, $p < 0.01$). Percentage dense volume and texture were strongly positively correlated (0.90 ($p < 0.01$)). Finally, dense volume was positively correlated with percentage dense volume (0.27, $p < 0.01$) and texture (0.20, $p < 0.01$).

High mammographic dense volume, percentage dense breast and texture scores were all associated with a higher breast cancer risk (Table 3, model 1, 2, and 3, respectively). Women in the highest compared to the lowest quartile (Q) of dense volume had almost two times higher

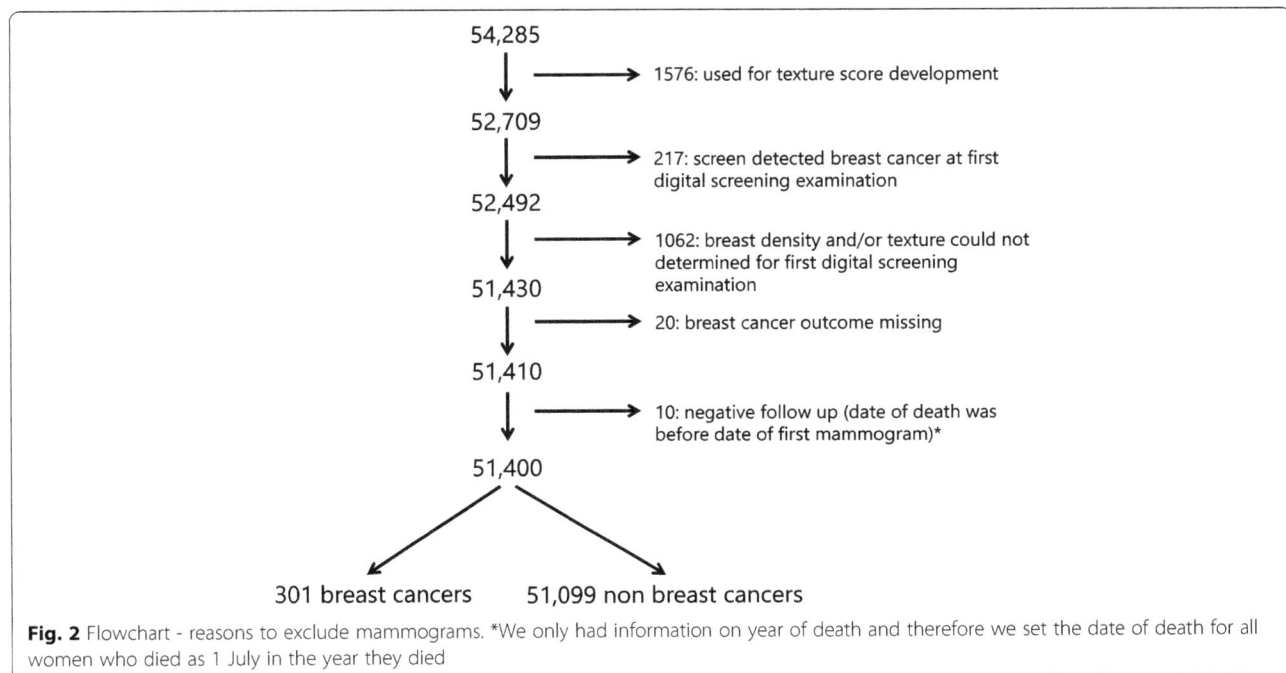

Fig. 2 Flowchart - reasons to exclude mammograms. *We only had information on year of death and therefore we set the date of death for all women who died as 1 July in the year they died

Flowchart content:

54,285 → 1576: used for texture score development

52,709 → 217: screen detected breast cancer at first digital screening examination

52,492 → 1062: breast density and/or texture could not determined for first digital screening examination

51,430 → 20: breast cancer outcome missing

51,410 → 10: negative follow up (date of death was before date of first mammogram)*

51,400 → 301 breast cancers / 51,099 non breast cancers

Table 1 Characteristics of the total study population (N = 51,400) and of women with breast cancer (cases) (N = 301) and without breast cancer (N = 50,099)

Variable	Total study population Median (IQR)		Breast cancer cases Median (IQR)		Non breast cancer cases Median (IQR)		p value
Age (years)[a]	56	(51–63)	58	(51–63)	56	(51–63)	0.21
Digital screening rounds, number	2	(1–3)	2	(2–3)	2	(1–3)	0.05
Follow up (years)[b]	4.2	(2.0–6.2)	2.8	(1.9–4.3)	4.2	(2.0–6.2)	<0.01
Dense volume (cm³)[a]	57.8	(42.9–78.9)	63.9	(48.4–86.9)	57.8	(42.9–78.8)	<0.01
Percent dense volume (%)[a]	6.4	(4.8–9.8)	7.5	(5.5–7.5)	6.4	(4.8–9.8)	<0.01
Non-dense volume (cm³)[a]	804.9	(518.6–1183.9)	825.3	(521.8–1159.1)	804.9	(518.5–1184.0)	0.88
Total breast volume (cm³)[a]	866.9	(573.9–1256.7)	900.8	(592.4–1228.4)	866.8	(573.8–1256.8)	0.88
Texture score[a]	0.50	(0.48–0.53)	0.51	(0.49–0.54)	0.50	(0.48–0.53)	<0.01

[a]At first available digital screening mammogram
[b]Women were followed until breast cancer diagnosis (event), till death or till 2 years after the last available mammogram, whichever came first

breast cancer risk during a median follow up of 4.2 years (Q4 vs Q1 HR 1.85, 95% CI 1.32–2.59, p value for trend <0.001). There were comparable results for percentage dense volume (Q4 vs Q1 HR 2.17, 95% CI 1.51–3.12, p value for trend <0.001). Women with a high texture pattern score had three times higher breast cancer risk than women with a low texture pattern score (Q4 vs Q1 HR 3.16, 95% CI 2.16–4.62, p value for trend < 0.001).

When the residuals of texture scores regressed on dense volume were added to the model with only dense volume (model 1a vs 1 in Table 3) the c-index increased from 0.56 (95% CI 0.53–0.59) to 0.62 (0.58–0.65). This difference was statistically significant (p < 0.001). When both dense volume and texture residuals were included in the model, they were both positively associated with breast cancer risk (Q4 vs Q1 HR 1.98, 95% CI 1.41–2.79, p value for trend <0.001 and Q4 vs Q1 HR 2.69, 95% CI1.87–3.88, p value for trend <0.001, respectively).

When the residuals of texture scores regressed on percentage dense volume were added to the model containing only percentage dense volume (model 2a vs 2 in Table 3) the c-index increased from 0.58 (95% CI 0.54–0.61) to 0.60 (95% CI 0.57–0.63). This difference was borderline significant (p = 0.054). In the model with both

Table 2 Pearson correlation coefficients for tests of correlation between mammographic measures and between mammographic measures and age

	Age	DV	PDV	Texture
Age	1	−0.16	−0.29	−0.35
DV		1	0.27	0.20
PDV			1	0.90
Texture				1

Age, breast density, and texture were assessed at the first digital screening mammogram
DV dense volume (natural logarithm (Ln) transformed), PDV percent dense volume (Ln transformed)
The p values were statistically significant (<0.01) for all correlation coefficients

percentage dense volume and texture residuals (model 2a, Table 3), both breast measures showed an approximately two times higher breast cancer risk for women in the highest compared to lowest quartile (Q4 vs Q1 HR 2.15, 95% CI 1.49–3.10, p value for trend <0.001 and Q4 vs Q1 HR 1.92, 95% CI 1.37–2.70, p value for trend <0.001, respectively).

The results of the models including continuous breast density measures were in line with those including quartiles of breast measures (Table 3).

The results of model 3a (texture score in combination with the residuals of dense volume regressed on texture scores) and model 3b (texture score in combination with the residuals of *percentage* dense volume regressed on texture scores) are presented in Additional file 1: Table S1. Dense volume and percentage dense volume did not significantly improve the discriminative power in addition to the texture score (p = 0.076 and p = 0.760, respectively).

The results of analysis of the associations between breast measures and screen-detected breast cancer are presented in Additional file 2: Table S2 and Additional file 3: Table S3. The corresponding results for interval breast cancers are presented in Additional file 4: Table S4 and Additional file 5: Table S5. The associations between density or texture measures and interval breast cancer were stronger overall than the associations with screen-detected breast cancer. Both for screen-detected and for interval-detected breast cancers, the highest predictive values were for the combination of dense volume and texture models.

Discussion

In this study, we found that the deep-learning-based texture score [24] assessed on digital mammograms was positively associated with breast cancer risk. Women in the highest quartile of texture pattern scores had approximately three times higher breast cancer risk than women in the lowest quartile. In addition, we found that the texture pattern score had additional value for the discriminatory performance

Table 3 The association between breast measures and breast cancer risk

Variables in the model		HR (95% CI) per one SD	HR (95% CI) Q2	HR (95% CI) Q3	HR (95% CI) Q4	p value for trend	c-index (95% CI)
Model 1	DV	1.32 (1.18–1.48)	1.24 (0.87–1.78)	1.53 (1.08–2016)	1.85 (1.32–2.59)	<0.001	0.56 (0.53–0.59)
Model 1a	DV	1.32 (1.18–1.47)	1.40 (0.97–2.01)	1.75 (1.23–2.48)	1.98 (1.41–2.79)	<0.001	0.62 (0.58–0.65)
	Texture residuals (DV)[a]	1.38 (1.23–1.56)	1.68 (1.15–2.44)	2.40 (1.68–3.43)	2.69 (1.87–3.88)	<0.001	
Model 2	PDV	1.34 (1.20–1.50)	1.49 (1.03–2.15)	2.07 (1.46–2.96)	2.17 (1.51–3.12)	<0.001	0.58 (0.54–0.61)
Model 2a	PDV	1.36 (1.21–1.53)	1.50 (1.04–2.17)	2.00 (1.41–2.86)	2.15 (1.49–3.10)	<0.001	0.60 (0.57–0.63)
	Texture residuals (PDV)[b]	1.27 (1.13–1.42)	1.28 (0.90–1.82)	1.69 (1.21–2.37)	1.92 (1.37–2.70)	<0.001	
Model 3	Texture	1.46 (1.30–1.64)	1.69 (1.15–2.50)	2.65 (1.83–3.84)	3.16 (2.16–4.62)	<0.001	0.61 (0.57–0.64)

Difference c-index model 1 and 1a, $p < 0.001$; difference c-index model 2 and 2a, $p = 0.054$
SD standard deviation, Q quartile, DV dense volume, PDV percentage dense volume
[a]Texture residuals (DV): residuals of texture pattern scores regressed on natural logarithm (Ln) transformed DV using a linear regression model
[b]Texture residuals (PDV): residuals of texture pattern scores regressed on Ln transformed PDV using a linear regression model

next to breast density. The highest c-index was observed for the combination of dense volume with the texture score (0.62, 95% CI 0.58–0.65).

This was the first study investigating the combination of a deep-learning-based texture score method and volumetric breast density (both percent density and absolute dense volume) in relation to breast cancer risk. In a review by Gastounioti et al., studies were described in which computerized approaches with manually designed and selected texture features were used for breast cancer risk assessment on both digitized film screen and digital mammograms [19]. In some of these studies the predictive value of these texture measures was studied in combination with area-based percent density. Three of these were on digital mammograms, like our study [29–31]. The first study by Li et al. used a Bayesian artificial neural network (BANN) model and found discriminatory capacities (area under the curve (AUC)) of 0.70, 0.57, and 0.68 for texture, percent density, and the combination of both, respectively [29]. Chen et al. and Zheng et al. both used logistic regression models and found discriminatory capacities (AUC) of 0.71, 0.62, and 0.68 (Chen et al) [30] and 0.85, 0.59, and 0.86 (Zheng et al.) [31] for texture, percent density, and the combination of both, respectively. The discriminatory ability in the last study is remarkably high. As this texture score has not been externally validated, the results should be interpreted with caution. Also the studies of Li et al. and Chen et al. have not been externally validated. Additionally, in all three studies the texture score was trained and tested in the same group of cases and controls, using cross-validation techniques. The texture measure used in the current study was developed and trained in a study sample drawn from the screening cohort used in this study, also using cross-validation techniques. In this study, we, however, validated this texture score in an independent "new" dataset, as we excluded the training sample used for texture development from our cohort data.

The current texture measure was developed in a relatively large population (394 cases and 1182 controls) compared to other studies developing a texture measure [19, 24]. The use of a larger dataset reduces the chance of model overfitting. The comparable discriminative performance for texture found in the development study and the current study suggests that the degree of overfitting was only limited in the development study.

In our study, we used a cohort design, studying mammograms in a breast-cancer-free cohort and then following up for breast cancer diagnosis, for an average period of 4 years. In the previously discussed studies mammograms of the contralateral breast at the time of breast cancer diagnosis were used [29–31]. For personalized breast cancer screening, knowing which women will develop breast cancer in the future is of greater added value compared to predicting it at time of breast cancer diagnosis. In addition, by using cohort data, we were able to determine how well the texture pattern score performs in the "general screening population" instead of in a selected subset, which is the case in case-control studies.

All studies investigating the combination of texture and breast density in relation to breast cancer risk or the ability to separate breast cancer from non-breast cancer cases used area-based percent breast density measures. The most widely used quantitative are-based breast density assessment method is the semi-automatic method, Cumulus [32]. This is a very labor-intensive method to determine breast density. With the advent of digital mammography, fully automatic volumetric breast density assessment methods, like Volpara [26], have been developed. Volpara gives objective and reproducible density measurements, representing the amount of dense tissue rather than the size of the dense tissue projection as measured by area-based methods. We are the first to investigate the additional value of adding texture to both volumetric percent and absolute breast density to separate breast cancer from non-breast cancer cases.

A limitation of our study is that as far as potential confounders are concerned, we only had information about age. We made use of anonymized routinely collected screening data and the Dutch screening program, like many other screening programs, does not collect any information on risk factors. In studies where adjustment for breast cancer risk factors, in particular body mass index, was possible, this usually led to slightly higher risk estimates for percent density [14, 22]. The association between absolute dense volume and breast cancer risk is hardly influenced by adjustment for body mass index (BMI) [33, 34]. Despite the absence of information on BMI or other breast cancer risk factors, we think that our study provides useful information as to the additional value of adding texture characteristics to breast density estimates. In many screening programs there is either no information or no extensive information available on risk factors other than age, and breast tissue characteristics can be relatively easily obtained from the mammograms. Another limitation is the fact that the texture pattern score in this study was trained on mammograms of women from the same screening population. Despite the fact that mammograms that were used for texture training were excluded from our study population, one might expect that the mammograms that were used for texture training were more similar to the mammograms in our study population as compared to other breast cancer screening populations in the world. Therefore, the performance of this texture pattern score should also be externally validated in other screening populations.

Strengths of this study are the automatically measured density and texture scores, as they give objective and reproducible results. In addition, these are high-throughput methods which make them suitable for screening practice. Finally, the ability of breast density and texture to discriminate non-breast cancer from breast cancer cases in a population-based breast cancer screening cohort resembles the performance of these measures in real screening practice, probably better than when using a case-control study.

Conclusions

Deep-learning-based texture pattern scores measured automatically on digital mammograms were shown to be related to breast cancer risk. Additionally, texture pattern scores statistically significantly improved the discriminatory performance in addition to absolute dense volume. Therefore, texture measures in addition to density may be taken into account in the development of more personalized breast cancer screening.

Abbreviations
AUC: Area under the curve; BANN: Bayesian artificial neural network; CC: Craniocaudal; CI: Confidence interval; DM: Digital mammography; DV: Dense volume; HR: Hazard ratio; IQR: Interquartile range; Ln: Natural logarithm; MLO: Mediolateral oblique; MRI: Magnetic resonance imaging; PDV: Percentage dense volume; Q: Quartile; SD: Standard deviation; US: Ultrasound

Acknowledgements
We want to thank the Foundation of Population Screening Mid-West (The Netherlands) for providing data.

Funding
The research leading to these results has received funding from the European Union Seventh Framework Programme FP7 under grant agreement no 306088 and a personal grant of the Dutch Cancer Society (to CG) (grant number KWF UU 2009–4348). The funding bodies were not involved in the design of the study and collection, analysis, and interpretation of data or in writing the manuscript.

Authors' contributions
JW performed the data analysis and wrote the manuscript. KH and NK collected the data used in this study; in addition they critically reviewed the manuscript. MK, PP, and MN were involved in the conception and design of the study and critically reviewed the manuscript. CvG and ML were the project leaders of this research project and were therefore involved in all stages of this study. All authors read and approved the final manuscript and agree to be accountable for all aspects of the work.

Competing interests
CvG reports a grant from Bayer Healthcare, and non-financial support from Volpara Solutions outside the submitted work. NK reports being one of the co-founders of Volpara Solutions, which develops and markets the breast density measurement software, Volpara, used in this study. In addition, NK has a patent pending and is co-founder of two other companies in the field of breast imaging next to his position as professor in the University. The two companies are Qview Medical (Los, Altos, CA, USA), and ScreenPoint Medical (Nijmegen, the Netherlands). These companies develop products for computer-aided detection of breast cancer, in whole breast ultrasound and in mammography respectively. MN and ML both report having shares in Biomediq A/S; this company developed the texture pattern score which is used in this study. The other authors (JW, KH, MK, and PP) declare that they have no competing interests.

Author details
[1]Julius Center for Health Sciences and Primary Care, University Medical Center Utrecht, P.O. Box 85500, 3508 GA Utrecht, The Netherlands. [2]Department of Radiology and Nuclear Medicine, Radboud University Medical Center, Geert Grooteplein 10, 6525 GA Nijmegen, The Netherlands.

[3]Department of Computer Science, University of Copenhagen, Universitetsparken 5, DK-2100 Copenhagen, Denmark. [4]Biomediq A/S, Fruebjergvej 3, 2100 Copenhagen, Denmark. [5]MRC-PHE Centre for Environment and Health, Department of Epidemiology and Biostatistics, School of Public Health, Imperial College London, St. Mary's Campus, Norfolk Place W2 1PG, London, UK.

References

1. International Cancer Screening Network (ICSN) website [http://healthcaredelivery.cancer.gov/icsn/]. Accessed 18 Feb 2018.
2. World Health Organization [http://www.euro.who.int/en/health-topics/noncommunicable-diseases/cancer/policy/screening-and-early-detection]. Accessed 18 Feb 2018.
3. Lauby-Secretan B, Scoccianti C, Loomis D, Benbrahim-Tallaa L, Bouvard V, Bianchini F, Straif K, International Agency for Research on Cancer Handbook Working Group. Breast-cancer screening–viewpoint of the IARC Working Group. N Engl J Med. 2015;372(24):2353–8.
4. Myers ER, Moorman P, Gierisch JM, Havrilesky LJ, Grimm LJ, Ghate S, Davidson B, Montgomery RC, Crowley MJ, McCrory DC, et al. Benefits and harms of breast cancer screening: a systematic review. JAMA. 2015; 314(15):1615–34.
5. Weigel S, Heindel W, Heidrich J, Hense HW, Heidinger O. Digital mammography screening: sensitivity of the programme dependent on breast density. Eur Radiol. 2017;27(7):2744–51. https://doi.org/10.1007/s00330-016-4636-4.
6. Destounis S, Johnston L, Highnam R, Arieno A, Morgan R, Chan A. Using volumetric breast density to quantify the potential masking risk of mammographic density. AJR Am J Roentgenol. 2017p;208(1):222–7. https://doi.org/10.2214/AJR.16.16489.
7. Boyd NF, Guo H, Martin LJ, Sun L, Stone J, Fishell E, Jong RA, Hislop G, Chiarelli A, Minkin S, et al. Mammographic density and the risk and detection of breast cancer. N Engl J Med. 2007;356(3):227–36.
8. Boyd NF, Huszti E, Melnichouk O, Martin LJ, Hislop G, Chiarelli A, Yaffe MJ, Minkin S. Mammographic features associated with interval breast cancers in screening programs. Breast Cancer Res. 2014;16(4):417.
9. Kerlikowske K. The mammogram that cried Wolfe. New Engl J Med. 2007; 356(3):297–300.
10. Pisano ED, Hendrick RE, Yaffe MJ, Baum JK, Acharyya S, Cormack JB, Hanna LA, Conant EF, Fajardo LL, Bassett LW, et al. Diagnostic accuracy of digital versus film mammography: exploratory analysis of selected population subgroups in DMIST. Radiology. 2008;246(2):376–83.
11. Prummel MV, Muradali D, Shumak R, Majpruz V, Brown P, Jiang H, Done SJ, Yaffe MJ, Chiarelli AM. Digital Compared with Screen-Film Mammography: Measures of Diagnostic Accuracy among Women Screened in the Ontario Breast Screening Program. Radiology. 2016;278(2):365-73. https://doi.org/10.1148/radiol.2015150733.
12. Kerlikowske K, Zhu W, Tosteson AN, Sprague BL, Tice JA, Lehman CD, Miglioretti DL. Identifying women with dense breasts at high risk for interval cancer: a cohort study. Ann Intern Med. 2015;162(10):673–81.
13. Wanders JO, Holland K, Veldhuis WB, Mann RM, Pijnappel RM, Peeters PH, van Gils CH, Karssemeijer N. Volumetric breast density affects performance of digital screening mammography. Breast Cancer Res Treat. 2017;162(1):95–103. https://doi.org/10.1007/s10549-016-4090-7.
14. McCormack VA, dos Santos Silva I. Breast density and parenchymal patterns as markers of breast cancer risk: a meta-analysis. Cancer Epidemiol Biomarkers Prev. 2006;15(6):1159–69.
15. Eng A, Gallant Z, Shepherd J, McCormack V, Li J, Dowsett M, Vinnicombe S, Allen S, dos-Santos-Silva I. Digital mammographic density and breast cancer risk: a case-control study of six alternative density assessment methods. Breast Cancer Res. 2014;16(5):439.
16. Are You Dense Advocacy Website [http://www.areyoudenseadvocacy.org]. Accessed 18 Feb 2018.
17. Trentham-Dietz A, Kerlikowske K, Stout NK, Miglioretti DL, Schechter CB, Ergun MA, van den Broek JJ, Alagoz O, Sprague BL, van Ravesteyn NT, et al. Tailoring breast cancer screening intervals by breast density and risk for women aged 50 years or older: collaborative modeling of screening outcomes. Ann Intern Med. 2016;165(10):700–12.
18. Torres-Mejia G, De Stavola B, Allen DS, Perez-Gavilan JJ, Ferreira JM, Fentiman IS, Dos Santos Silva I. Mammographic features and subsequent risk of breast cancer: a comparison of qualitative and quantitative evaluations in the Guernsey prospective studies. Cancer Epidemiol Biomarkers Prev. 2005;14(5):1052–9.
19. Gastounioti A, Conant EF, Kontos D. Beyond breast density: a review on the advancing role of parenchymal texture analysis in breast cancer risk assessment. Breast Cancer Res. 2016;18(1):91.
20. Winkel RR, von Euler-Chelpin M, Nielsen M, Petersen K, Lillholm M, Nielsen MB, Lynge E, Uldall WY, Vejborg I. Mammographic density and structural features can individually and jointly contribute to breast cancer risk assessment in mammography screening: a case-control study. BMC Cancer. 2016;16:414.
21. Malkov S, Shepherd JA, Scott CG, Tamimi RM, Ma L, Bertrand KA, Couch F, Jensen MR, Mahmoudzadeh AP, Fan B, et al. Mammographic texture and risk of breast cancer by tumor type and estrogen receptor status. Breast Cancer Res. 2016;18(1):122.
22. Manduca A, Carston MJ, Heine JJ, Scott CG, Pankratz VS, Brandt KR, Sellers TA, Vachon CM, Cerhan JR. Texture features from mammographic images and risk of breast cancer. Cancer Epidemiol Biomarkers Prev. 2009;18(3):837–45.
23. Haberle L, Wagner F, Fasching PA, Jud SM, Heusinger K, Loehberg CR, Hein A, Bayer CM, Hack CC, Lux MP, et al. Characterizing mammographic images by using generic texture features. Breast Cancer Res. 2012;14(2):R59.
24. Kallenberg M, Petersen K, Nielsen M, Ng A, Diao P, Igel C, Vachon C, Holland K, Karssemeijer N. Lillholm M. IEEE Trans Med Imaging: Unsupervised deep learning applied to breast density segmentation and mammographic risk scoring; 2016;35(5):1322–31. https://doi.org/10.1109/TMI.2016.2532122.
25. (NETB) NETfBcs: National evaluation of breast cancer screening in the Netherlands 1990–2011/2012; 2014. ISBN: 978-94-6169-548-2.
26. Highnam R, Brady M, Yaffe MJ, Karssemeijer N, Harvey J. Robust breast composition measurement - Volpara (TM). Lect Notes Comput Sci. 2010; 6136:342–9.
27. Highnam R, Brady JM: Mammographic image analysis: Kluwer Academic Publishers; 1999.
28. Willett WC, Howe GR, Kushi LH. Adjustment for total energy intake in epidemiologic studies. Am J Clin Nutr. 1997;65(4 Suppl):1220S–8S. discussion 1229S–1231S
29. Li H, Giger ML, Lan L, Janardanan J, Sennett CA. Comparative analysis of image-based phenotypes of mammographic density and parenchymal patterns in distinguishing between BRCA1/2 cases, unilateral cancer cases, and controls. J Med Imaging (Bellingham). 2014;1(3):031009.
30. Chen X, Moschidis E, Taylor C, Astley S. Breast cancer risk analysis based on a novel segmentation framework for digital mammograms. Med Image Comput Comput Assist Interv. 2014;17(Pt 1):536–43.
31. Zheng Y, Keller BM, Ray S, Wang Y, Conant EF, Gee JC, Kontos D. Parenchymal texture analysis in digital mammography: A fully automated pipeline for breast cancer risk assessment. Med Phys. 2015;42(7):4149–60.
32. Byng JW, Boyd NF, Fishell E, Jong RA, Yaffe MJ. The quantitative analysis of mammographic densities. Phys Med Biol. 1994;39(10):1629–38.
33. Kerlikowske K, Ma L, Scott CG, Mahmoudzadeh AP, Jensen MR, Sprague BL, Henderson LM, Pankratz VS, Cummings SR, Miglioretti DL, et al. Combining quantitative and qualitative breast density measures to assess breast cancer risk. Breast Cancer Res. 2017;19(1):97.
34. Brandt KR, Scott CG, Ma L, Mahmoudzadeh AP, Jensen MR, Whaley DH, Wu FF, Malkov S, Hruska CB, Norman AD, et al. Comparison of clinical and automated breast density measurements: implications for risk prediction and supplemental screening. Radiology. 2016;279(3):710–9.

2

Membrane associated collagen XIII promotes cancer metastasis and enhances anoikis resistance

Hui Zhang[1,2], Tricia Fredericks[4], Gaofeng Xiong[2], Yifei Qi[2], Piotr G. Rychahou[5], Jia-Da Li[6], Taina Pihlajaniemi[7], Wei Xu[1*] and Ren Xu[2,3*] (iD)

Abstract

Background: Increased collagen expression and deposition are associated with cancer progression and poor prognosis in breast cancer patients. However, function and regulation of membrane-associated collagen in breast cancer have not been determined. Collagen XIII is a type II transmembrane protein within the collagen superfamily. Experiments in tissue culture and knockout mouse models show that collagen XIII is involved in cell adhesion and differentiation of certain cell types. In the present study, we determined roles of collagen XIII in breast cancer progression and metastasis.

Methods: We analyzed the association of collagen XIII expression with breast cancer development and metastasis using published gene expression profiles generated from human breast cancer tissues. Utilizing gain- and loss- of function approaches and 3D culture assays, we investigated roles of collagen XIII in regulating invasive tumor growth. Using the tumorsphere/mammosphere formation assay and the detachment cell culture assay, we determined whether collagen XIII enhances cancer cell stemness and induces anoikis resistance. We also inhibited collagen XIII signaling with β1 integrin function-blocking antibody. Finally, using the lung colonization assay and the orthotopic mammary tumor model, we investigated roles of collagen XIII in regulating breast cancer colonization and metastasis. Cox proportional hazard (log-rank) test, two-sided Student's t-test (two groups) and one-way ANOVA (three or more groups) analyses were used in this study.

Results: Collagen XIII expression is significantly higher in human breast cancer tissue compared with normal mammary gland. Increased collagen XIII mRNA levels in breast cancer tissue correlated with short distant recurrence free survival. We showed that collagen XIII expression promoted invasive tumor growth in 3D culture, enhanced cancer cell stemness, and induced anoikis resistance. Collagen XIII expression induced β1 integrin activation. Blocking β1 integrin activation significantly reduced collagen XIII-induced invasion and mammosphere formation. Importantly, silencing collagen XIII in MDA-MB-231 cells reduced lung colonization and metastasis.

Conclusions: Our results demonstrate a novel function of collagen XIII in promoting cancer metastasis, cell invasion, and anoikis resistance.

Keywords: Extracellular matrix, Membrane-associated collagen, Stemness, Cell anoikis, Metastasis

---

* Correspondence: ren.xu2010@uky.edu; xu_w@jlu.edu.cn
[1]Department of Laboratory Medicine, The First Hospital of Jilin University, Changchun 130021, Jilin Province, China
[2]UK Markey Cancer Center, University of Kentucky, Lexington, KY 40536, USA
Full list of author information is available at the end of the article

Background

Despite the recent progress in hormone and targeted therapy, breast cancer still remains the second cause of cancer-related death in women. Most of breast cancer death is due to metastasis [1]. Therefore, it is important to determine how the metastasis process is regulated and to identify potential targets for repressing cancer metastasis. Breast cancers can be classified into luminal (A and B), Her2, and basal-like/triple-negative breast cancer (TNBC) based on the expression status of estrogen receptor, progesterone receptor, and Her2/neu [2].

Increased collagen expression and deposition are associated with cancer progression and poor prognosis in breast cancer patients [3]. For instance, type I collagen has been identified as a prognosis marker and is associated with cancer recurrence in human breast cancer patients [4]. Collagen VI knockout mice have reduced primary tumor formation and growth [5]. Importantly, the transgenic mice with increased collagen deposition in mammary tissue have a three-fold increase in tumor formation. These mice also have three times more lung metastases [6]. In addition, aligned collagen fibers can facilitate cell migration and metastasis [7, 8]. These results suggest that increased collagen deposition can transform cells into a malignant phenotype and promote cancer metastasis [9]. Dense breast is a risk factor for breast cancer [10], and the increased breast density is due in part to increased deposition of collagen proteins [11]. In addition, the extracellular matrix (ECM) surrounding a breast tumor is more dense or stiff from increased collagen deposition and crosslink [12]. These researches indicate that increased collagen expression and deposition promotes breast cancer development and progression by enhancing tumor growth and invasion.

The collagen family can be divided into several groups based on the protein structure and localization [13]. One group of collagen, including collagen XIII, collagen XXIII, and collagen XXV, is a type II transmembrane protein [14–17]. Collagen XIII protein is 90 to 100 kDa and folds in an opposite fashion to the fibrillar collagens. It has a membrane spanning region near the NC1 domain, which results in a large extracellular region with a short intracellular portion [17]. The function of collagen XIII at the molecular level has largely remained unclear; however, it is thought to have a role in cell-cell and cell-matrix interactions [18]. The extracellular domain binds integrin [19], and can be cleaved from the cell resulting in possible paracrine activity in the cellular microenvironment. When the ectodomain is shed, the pericellular surrounding is less supportive of cell adhesion, migration and proliferation [20]. The function of the short intracellular portion after cleavage is unclear but has been shown to feedback and increase collagen XIII production [21, 22]. Collagen XIII mRNA has been shown to be expressed in higher levels in epithelial tumors, such as tumors from the colon, cervix, bladder, endometrium and ovary [23, 24]. Increased collagen XIII protein expression is also detected in invasive foci of bladder cancer [24, 25]. However, the function of collagen XIII in breast cancer progression has not been determined.

Integrin is one of the cell membrane receptors that mediate the cell-collagen interaction [26, 27]. Binding of integrin to collagen induces activation of downstream signaling, and subsequently modulates cell proliferation, differentiation, apoptosis and cell migration [28–31]. Expression of $\beta 1$ integrin is required for the epithelial integrity and plays a crucial role in the proliferation of mammary epithelial cells [32]. Treatment with a $\beta 1$ integrin functional blocking antibody can reverse breast cancer cells back to the normal phenotype in 3D culture [33]. It has been shown in a mouse mammary tumor model that disruption of $\beta 1$ integrin function inhibits tumor development at the initial stages of mammary tumor formation [34]. These results suggest that $\beta 1$ integrin is a key mediator of collagen-induced cancer development and progression.

In this study, we showed that expression of collagen XIII is higher in breast cancer tissue compared with normal mammary gland, and that the increased mRNA level of collagen XIII in cancer tissue is associated with poor prognosis and cancer metastasis. We also demonstrate that collagen XIII expression enhanced cancer stemness and invasive tumor growth through $\beta 1$ integrin. Importantly, silencing collagen XIII in breast cancer cells significantly reduced cancer metastasis. These results identified a novel function of membrane associated collagen in breast cancer progression.

Methods

Cell lines and culture conditions

MDA-MB-231 (ATCC) were maintained in DMEM/F12 with 10% FBS and 1% Pen/Strep. BT549 (ATCC) cells were maintained in RPMI-1640 with 10% FBS and 1% Pen/Strep. MCF-10A cells were kind gifts from Michael W. Kilgore, University of Kentucky, Lexington, KY. MCF10A cells were cultured as previously described [35]. Hs-578 T cells (ATCC) were kept as previously described [36]. S1 and T4–2 cells are kind gifts from Dr. Mina J Bissell, and they were cultured as previously described [37]. All the cells were tested for mycoplasma contamination every two months.

Antibodies and reagents

Anti-flag M2 (Sigma, F1804, 1:1000 for WB, 1:500 for IF). Anti-human $\beta 1$ integrins,active (Millipore, MAB2079Z, 1:500 for IF). Anti-human Collagen XIII $\alpha 1$ (R&D systems, AF6346, 1:200 for WB). Anti-smad2/3 (BD Transduction

Laboratories, 610842, 1:1000 for WB). Anti-p-smad2 (cell signaling, 130D4, 1:1000 for WB). Anti-tubulin (Cell Signaling, 2148, 1:5000). Anti-Integrin β1 subunit (AIIB2) (DSHB, 528306, 80 μg/ml for block assay). Anti-rat IgG1 (Santa Cruz Biotechology, sc-3882, 1:1000). Anti-PARP (Cell Signaling, 9542, 1:1000). Bovine Collagen Solution, Type I (Advanced BioMatrix, 5005).

Dual-luciferase reporter assay system (Promega, E1960). Click-It EdU Alexa Fluor 488 Imaging kit (Invitrogen, C10337). Growth Factor Reduced BD Matrigel™ (BD Biosciences, 354230). Annexin V (Thermo, A13201). Lenti-CRISPR v2 (Addgene, 52961), pCDH-EF1-MCS-T2A-Puro (System Biosciences, CD520A-1), p3TP-lux (Addgene, 306281), pGL4.10 (Addgene, 66128).

Plasmid construction
Mouse Collagen XIII (NM_007731.3) were amplified from constructs pCMV-SPORT6-COL13a1 (Transomic, BC034164), and cloned into pCDH-EF1-MCS-T2A-Puro (System Biosciences, CD520A-1) with the primers of

Forward: 5' AATTGAATTCGCCACCATGGTGGC GGAGCGCACCCGC 3';

Reverse: 5'ACTGGCGGCCGCCTTATCGTCGTC ATCCTTGTAATCCTGCCCTCCAGGCCTGCTTCT3'.

Human Collagen XIII (NM_001130103.1) was amplified from an expression construct described by Dennis et al. [38], and cloned into FLAG-tagged pCDH-EF1-MCS-T2A-Puro with the primers of

Forward: 5'AATTGCTAGCGCCACCATGGTAGC GGAGCGCACCCAC 3';

Reverse: 5'ACTGGAATTCCTTGTTCCAGCAGC CTTGGAC 3'.

3D culture
Three-dimensional (3D) IrECM on-top culture was performed as previous described [39]. Briefly, Growth Factor Reduced BD Matrigel™ was plated on the bottom of the cell culture dish. MDA-MB-231 and MCF10A cells were seeded on the top of the matrigel layer, and additional medium containing 10% Matrigel was added on the top.

CRISPR-Cas9 deletion of collagen XIII in MDA-MB-231 and T4–2 cells
CRISPR-Cas9 plasmid for collagen XIII (NM_001130103.1) deletion was constructed with gDNA primers: 5' CACC GCAGCTCGGCCGTCCGAAAGT 3' (Forward) and 5'AAACACTTTCGGACGGCCGAGCTGC 3' (Reverse). MDA-MB-231 cells were infected with the lentivirus containing the CRISPR-Cas9 construct, and monoclones were selected and verified by genomic DNA sequencing and western blot. The collagen XIII-knockout luciferase-expressing or GFP-expressing MDA-MB-231 cells were pooled together for the mouse experiments.

Western blot and luciferase reporter assay
Protein samples were harvested by using 2% SDS in PBS with protease inhibitor cocktail and NaF (2.5 mM), NaVO4 (2 mM). SDS gel electrophoresis, immunoblot and a LI-COR Odyssey Infrared Imaging System were employed for detecting the target protein as previously described [39]. The Image Studio Lite software was used for quantification.

The Dual-luciferase reporter assay was performed as previously described [40]. Briefly, MDA-MB-231cells or MCF10A cells were seeded into a 24-well plate at the density of 0.1×10^6/well. 24 h later the cells will reach 80% confluence. Then 0.5 μg p3TP-lux and 0.025 μg renilla plasmids were transfected into the cells using Fugene HD Transfection Reagent. The cells were starved before 5 ng/ml TGF-β was added. The relative luciferase activity was defined as firefly luciferase activity normalized by renilla luciferase activity. The final results were normalized by the relative luciferase activity of the control vector pGL4.10.

Transwell invasion and single cell migration assay
The Transwell invasion assay was performed as previously described [41]. As for the single cell migration assay, MCF-10A and MDA-MB-231 cells were seeded into a 4 chamber glass bottom dish (Invitro Scientific, D35C4–20-1-N) at the density of 2000 cell/cm². About 4 h after seeding, the single cell migration was monitored by Nikon BioStation (Nikon, IMQ) every 10 min for 10 h [41]. In some experiments, the cells were pre-incubated with β1 integrin blocking antibody AIIB2 with the final concentration of 80 μg/ml for 30 min, and then the Transwell invasion and single cell migration assay were performed in the presence of the blocking antibody.

Mammosphere/Tumorsphere assay
Cells were seeded in poly-HEMA (12 mg/ml in 95% ethanol) pre-coat regular plastic culture dish [42] and cultured in tumorsphere medium [DMEM/F12 medium supplemented with B27 (1:50), EGF (20 ng/ml), bFGF (20 ng/ml), insulin (5 μg/ml), hydrocortisone (0.5 ng/ml), Gentamicin (10 μg/ml)] for 5 days without moving or disturbing the plates. The phase images of mammosphere/tumorsphere were taken by Nikon eclipse 80i microscope. Mammosphere or tumorspheres forming efficiency (%) was calculated as follows: (Number of mammosphere or tumorspheres per well / number of cells seeded per well) × 100.

Flow cytometry analysis apoptosis
Poly-HEMA (12 mg/ml in 95% ethanol) pre-coated dishes were used for detachment cell culture [42]. MCF-10A and MDA-MB-231 cells were cultured in regular media with 0.5% methyl cellulose in suspension at a density of 30,000 cells per cm² [42]. Cells were

cultured in suspended condition for 24 h. And then were collected for annexin V analysis as manufacturer's instructions.

Immunofluorescence staining

For immunofluorescence staining, cells were cultured in a chamber slide (Nalge Nunc International, 154526). The cells were fixed with Methanol/Acetone (1:1) or formalin and permeabilized with 0.5% Triton X-100. The slides were blocked by 10% goat serum at room temperature for 60 min, and incubated with the primary antibodies (anti-flag/anti-active-β1 integrin/anti-caspase 3) at 4 °C overnight. The slides were incubated with secondary antibodies at room temperature for 60 min. Images were taken with Nikon Eclipse 80i fluorescence microscope and Nikon eclipse Ti2 confocal microscope.

Cell proliferation assay

Cell proliferation was performed per the instructions of the Click-It EdU Alexa Fluor 488 Imaging kit and assessed by quantification of the proportion of cells with EdU-positive staining. The number of nuclei positive for EdU was counted and divided by the total number of nuclei (DAPI).

Xenograft experiment and in vivo colonization experiments

For the xenograft experiment, 6-week old female SCID mice were randomly grouped and injected with 2×10^6 control or collagen XIII-silenced MDA-MB-231-luc-D3H2LN cells at 4th mammary fat pad. Tumors were measured with a caliper every other day. Tumor volume (mm^3) was estimated using the formula [volume = π × (width)^2 × (length) / 6]. Twenty five days after tumor cell implantation, the primary tumors are removed by surgery. To detect lung metastasis, bioluminescent images were taken at 3 weeks after primary tumor removal with in vivo imaging system (IVIS).

For lung colonization experiment, 6-week old female SCID mice were randomly grouped and injected with 0.5×10^6 (in 200 µl PBS) control or collagen XIII-silenced MDA-MB-231-luc-D3H2LN cells via tail vein. To detect lung metastasis, bioluminescent images were taken once a week begining 4 weeks after the injection of cancer cells with IVIS. At the experimental endpoint, lung tissues were harvested and fixed with 4% PFA for paraffin-embedded section. H&E staining was performed in lung tissue sections, and images were taken by a Nikon microscope. Metastasized tumors in the lung were quantified by counting three sections per lung sample. For the intracardiac inoculation experiment, 6-week old female nude mice were randomly grouped. 0.2×10^6 (in 100 µl PBS) control, collagen XIII-silenced MDA-MB-231-luc-D3H2LN cells or collagen XIII-silenced MDA-MB-231-GFP cells were injected into left cardiac ventricle. Bioluminescent images were taken once a week to detect lung and bone metastasis.

Illumatool was used to detect GFP labeled cells metastasis.

Statistical analysis

To address the clinical relevance of increased collagen XIII expression, we assessed the association between mRNA levels of Col13A1 and recurrence or distant recurrence free survival using the published microarray dataset generated from 3554 human breast cancer tissue samples [43] (2014 version). Patients were equally grouped into low and high Col13A1 expression based on the mRNA levels. Significant differences in recurrence or distant recurrence survival time were assessed with the Cox proportional hazard (log-rank) test.

All experiments were conducted by three independent experiments. Data were reported as mean ± s.e.m.. Student's t-test (two groups) or one-way ANOVA (three or more groups) were used to determine the significant differences between means. Statistical analysis was performed with Graph Pad Prism 5 and IBM SPSS Statistics 22. $p < 0.05$ represents statistical significance and $p < 0.01$ represents sufficiently statistical significance. All reported p values were from two-sided tests.

Results

Collagen XIII expression is increased during breast cancer development

To determine whether collagen XIII expression is induced during breast cancer development, we analyzed collagen XIII protein levels in a panel of non-malignant and malignant mammary epithelial cells. Triple negative breast cancer cell line MDA-MB-231, Hs578T, BT549, and T4–2 expressed higher levels of collagen XIII protein than luminal type breast cancer cell lines and non-malignant mammary epithelial cell lines (Fig. 1a). By analyzing TCGA and Finak datasets (www.oncomine.com), we found that collagen XIII mRNA levels were significantly increased in human breast cancer tissue compared to normal mammary gland tissue (Fig. 1b, c). Collagen XIII expression in ER negative breast cancer was much higher than the expression in ER positive breast cancer (Fig. 1d). Consistence with cancer cell line data, we also found that triple negative breast cancer tissue had higher level of collagen XIII expression compared with other subtypes (Fig. 1e).

Next, we asked whether collagen XIII expression is associated with clinical outcome in human breast cancer patients. Breast cancer patients were divided into two groups based on collagen XIII mRNA levels (low and high). Kaplan-Meier log rank analysis showed that patients whose tumors had high collagen XIII expression levels had a significantly shorter overall survival period (Fig. 1f). Moreover, the association of collagen XIII expression with poor clinical outcome is stronger in ER

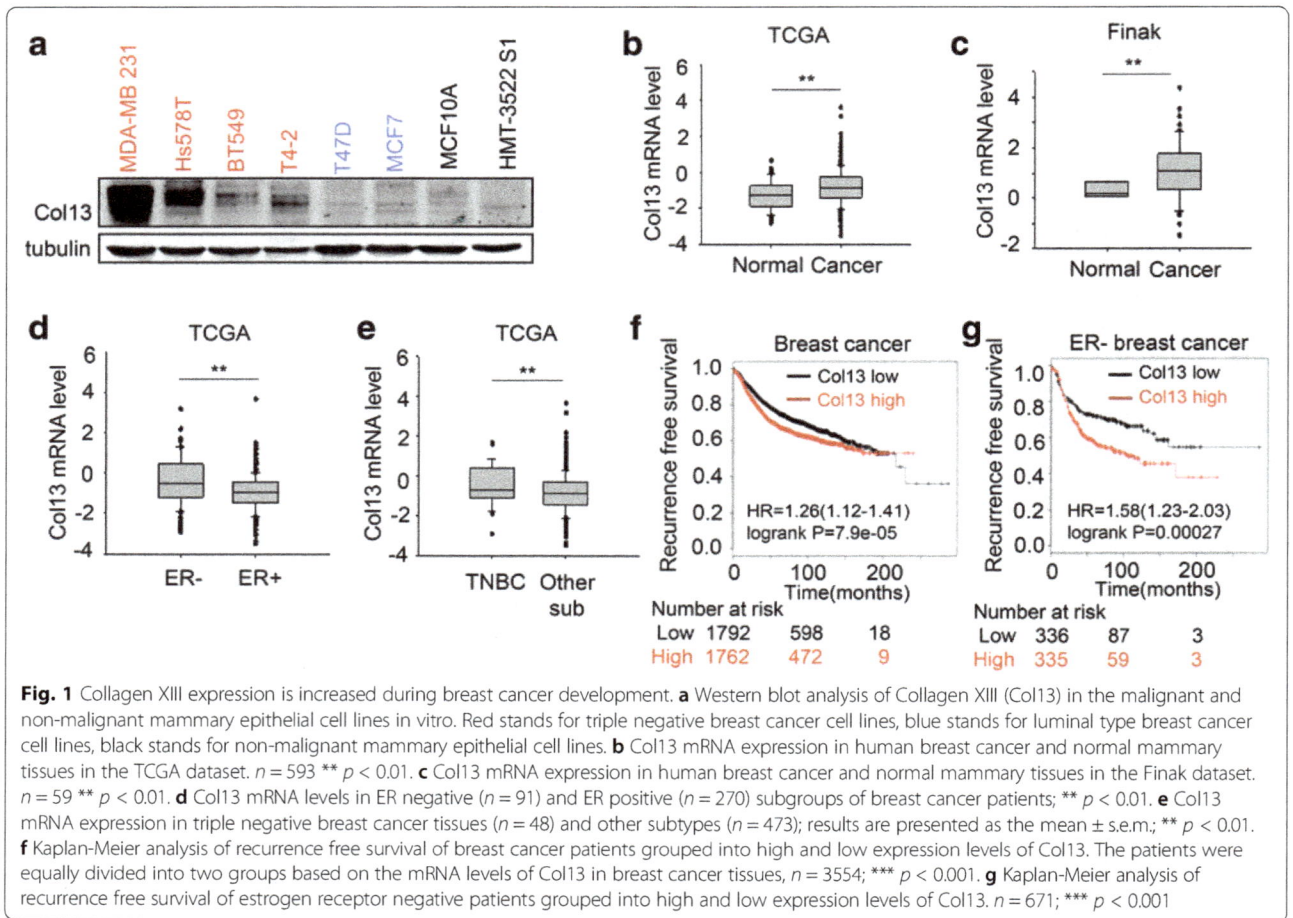

Fig. 1 Collagen XIII expression is increased during breast cancer development. **a** Western blot analysis of Collagen XIII (Col13) in the malignant and non-malignant mammary epithelial cell lines in vitro. Red stands for triple negative breast cancer cell lines, blue stands for luminal type breast cancer cell lines, black stands for non-malignant mammary epithelial cell lines. **b** Col13 mRNA expression in human breast cancer and normal mammary tissues in the TCGA dataset. $n = 593$ ** $p < 0.01$. **c** Col13 mRNA expression in human breast cancer and normal mammary tissues in the Finak dataset. $n = 59$ ** $p < 0.01$. **d** Col13 mRNA levels in ER negative ($n = 91$) and ER positive ($n = 270$) subgroups of breast cancer patients; ** $p < 0.01$. **e** Col13 mRNA expression in triple negative breast cancer tissues ($n = 48$) and other subtypes ($n = 473$); results are presented as the mean ± s.e.m.; ** $p < 0.01$. **f** Kaplan-Meier analysis of recurrence free survival of breast cancer patients grouped into high and low expression levels of Col13. The patients were equally divided into two groups based on the mRNA levels of Col13 in breast cancer tissues, $n = 3554$; *** $p < 0.001$. **g** Kaplan-Meier analysis of recurrence free survival of estrogen receptor negative patients grouped into high and low expression levels of Col13. $n = 671$; *** $p < 0.001$

negative breast cancer (Fig. 1g). Although collagen XIII mRNA levels are lower in ER positive breast cancer compared to ER negative cancer, increased collagen XIII expression in ER positive breast cancer is still associated with poor clinical outcome (Additional file 1: Figure S1). These results indicate that breast cancer development and progression are accompanied by increased expression of collagen XIII.

Collagen XIII promotes invasive 3D malignant phenotypes in MDA-MB 231 cells.

Increased expression of collagen XIII has been detected in several types of cancer [24, 25]. However, function of collagen XIII in cancer progression is not clear. Since collagen XIII protein is highly expressed in MDA-MB-231 cells but non-detectable in MCF-10A cells, these cell lines were used for loss- and gain-of function experiments, respectively, to define roles of collagen XIII in breast cancer progression. Collagen XIII expression was silenced in MDA-MB-231 cell line using CRISPR technology (Fig. 2a, b and Additional file 2: Figure S2). 3D culture models have been widely used to examine the malignant mammary tissue morphogenesis [44, 45]. Invasive branching structure in 3D

culture is associated with cancer invasion and aggressive cancer phenotypes [36, 41]. We showed that silencing collagen XIII in MDA-MB-231 significantly reduced the number of invasive branches and inhibited invasive growth in 3D culture (Fig. 2c). For the gain-of function experiments, MCF10A cells were infected with lentivirus containing the collagen XIII expression construct. The majority of exogenous collagen XIII was detected on cell surface (Fig. 2d, 2e, and Additional file 3: Figure S3a). We found that collagen XIII expression increased 3D colony size in MCF10A cells (Fig. 2f). The ratio of EdU positive cells was significantly higher in the collagen XIII expression group compared with the control group (Fig. 2g, Additional file 3: Figure S3b). A reduction of activated caspase 3 staining was also detected in collagen XIII-expressing cells (Additional file 3: Figure S3c).

Invasive growth of breast cancer in 3D culture depends on cancer cell invasion and migration [46, 47]. Thus, we asked whether collagen XIII regulates invasion and migration of mammary epithelial cells. Silencing collagen XIII significantly reduced invasion of MDA-MB-231 cells in Transwell experiments (Fig. 3a). Using single cell tracking analysis, we showed that knockout of collagen XIII

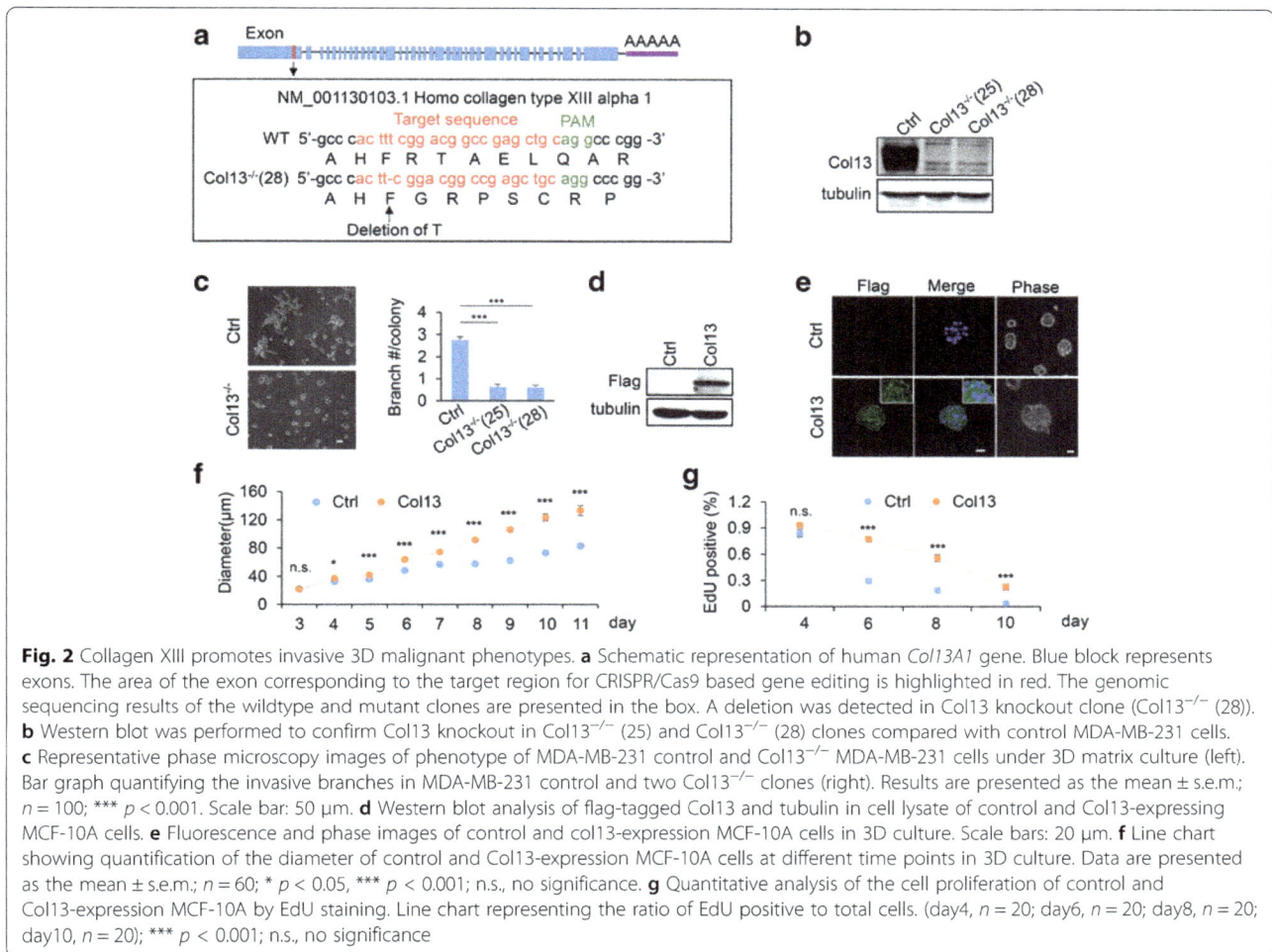

Fig. 2 Collagen XIII promotes invasive 3D malignant phenotypes. **a** Schematic representation of human *Col13A1* gene. Blue block represents exons. The area of the exon corresponding to the target region for CRISPR/Cas9 based gene editing is highlighted in red. The genomic sequencing results of the wildtype and mutant clones are presented in the box. A deletion was detected in Col13 knockout clone (Col13$^{-/-}$ (28)). **b** Western blot was performed to confirm Col13 knockout in Col13$^{-/-}$ (25) and Col13$^{-/-}$ (28) clones compared with control MDA-MB-231 cells. **c** Representative phase microscopy images of phenotype of MDA-MB-231 control and Col13$^{-/-}$ MDA-MB-231 cells under 3D matrix culture (left). Bar graph quantifying the invasive branches in MDA-MB-231 control and two Col13$^{-/-}$ clones (right). Results are presented as the mean ± s.e.m.; $n = 100$; *** $p < 0.001$. Scale bar: 50 μm. **d** Western blot analysis of flag-tagged Col13 and tubulin in cell lysate of control and Col13-expressing MCF-10A cells. **e** Fluorescence and phase images of control and col13-expression MCF-10A cells in 3D culture. Scale bars: 20 μm. **f** Line chart showing quantification of the diameter of control and Col13-expression MCF-10A cells at different time points in 3D culture. Data are presented as the mean ± s.e.m.; $n = 60$; * $p < 0.05$, *** $p < 0.001$; n.s., no significance. **g** Quantitative analysis of the cell proliferation of control and Col13-expression MCF-10A by EdU staining. Line chart representing the ratio of EdU positive to total cells. (day4, $n = 20$; day6, $n = 20$; day8, $n = 20$; day10, $n = 20$); *** $p < 0.001$; n.s., no significance

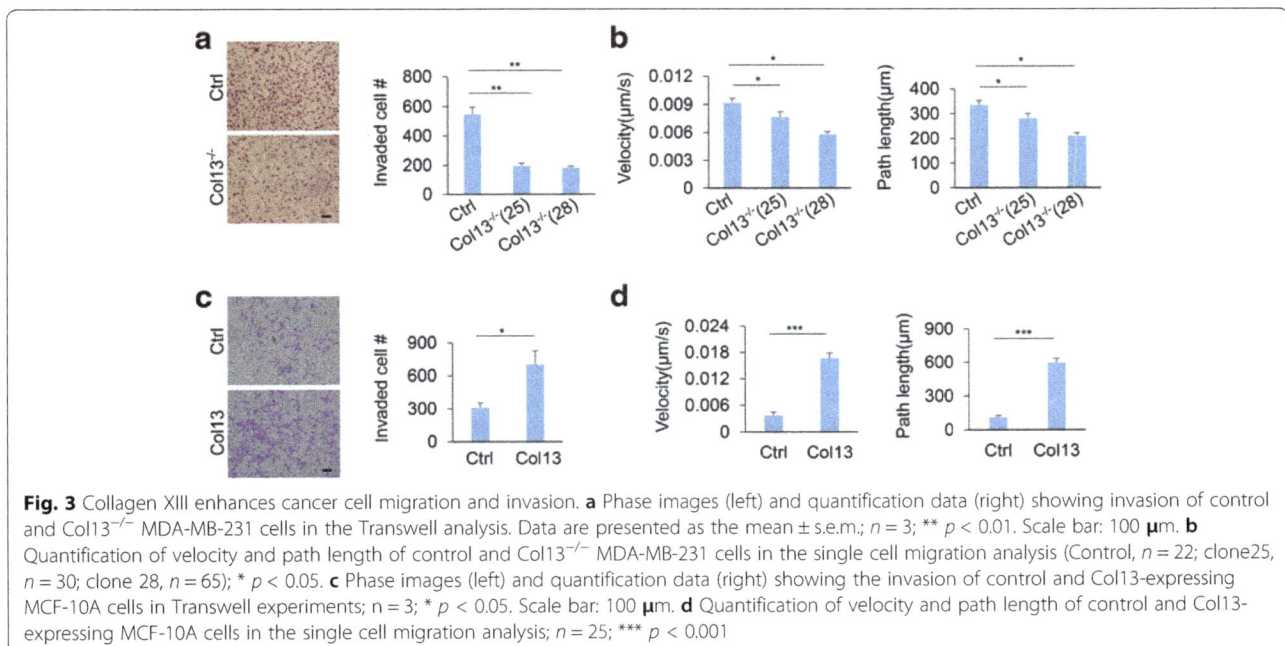

Fig. 3 Collagen XIII enhances cancer cell migration and invasion. **a** Phase images (left) and quantification data (right) showing invasion of control and Col13$^{-/-}$ MDA-MB-231 cells in the Transwell analysis. Data are presented as the mean ± s.e.m.; $n = 3$; ** $p < 0.01$. Scale bar: 100 μm. **b** Quantification of velocity and path length of control and Col13$^{-/-}$ MDA-MB-231 cells in the single cell migration analysis (Control, $n = 22$; clone25, $n = 30$; clone 28, $n = 65$); * $p < 0.05$. **c** Phase images (left) and quantification data (right) showing the invasion of control and Col13-expressing MCF-10A cells in Transwell experiments; n = 3; * $p < 0.05$. Scale bar: 100 μm. **d** Quantification of velocity and path length of control and Col13-expressing MCF-10A cells in the single cell migration analysis; $n = 25$; *** $p < 0.001$

reduced the velocity and the distance of cell migration in MDA-MB-231 cells (Fig. 3b). In contrast, MCF-10A cells with collagen XIII overexpression were more invasive than control cells (Fig. 3c). Collagen XIII expression also significantly increased the cell migration velocity and distance in MCF-10A (Fig. 3d, and Additional file 4: Figure S4a, b). These results indicate that increased expression of collagen XIII in MDA-MB 231 cells promotes malignant phenotypes in 3D culture by enhancing cancer cell migration and invasion. Collagen XIII is expressed at the intermediate level in malignant T4–2 cells (Fig.1a), and we performed both loss- and gain-of-function experiments using this cell line. Silencing collagen XIII reduced T4–2 invasion, while overexpression of collagen XIII did not significantly enhance cell invasion in the Transwell experiments (Additional file 5: Figure S5). Therefore, the moderate expression of collagen XIII may be sufficient to promote cancer invasion. To determine whether collagen XIII regulates cell invasion in a cell-autonomous fashion, we performed co-culture experiments by mixing GFP-labeled collagen XIII-silenced MDA-MB-231 cells with non-labeled wild type MDA-MB-231 cells. We found that wild type MDA-MB-231 cells could not rescue cell invasion in the collagen XIII-silenced cells (Additional file 6: Figure S6). These results suggest that collagen XIII promotes cancer cell invasion through the receptor on the same cells.

Collagen XIII expression enhances cancer cell stemness. Tumor-initiating cells are the driver of cancer relapses and metastasis [48, 49]. The tumorsphere assay has been used to enrich tumor-initiating cells and to study their colony formation activity [50, 51]. By analyzing the published microarray dataset [52], we found that collagen XIII expression was upregulated in tumor spheroids compared to the corresponding primary tumors (Fig. 4a). To determine whether collagen XIII contributes to tumorsphere formation, we cultured control, collagen XIII-silenced MDA-MB-231 and T4–2 cells in non-adhesive plates. We found that silencing collagen XIII significantly reduced tumorsphere formation in both MDA-MB-231 and T4–2 cells (Fig. 4b and Additional file 7: Figure S7a). In contrast, expression of collagen XIII enhanced mammosphere formation in MCF10A cells (Fig. 4c). Interestingly, overexpression of collagen XIII in T4–2 had little effect on tumorsphere formation, suggesting that the moderate expression of collagen XIII is

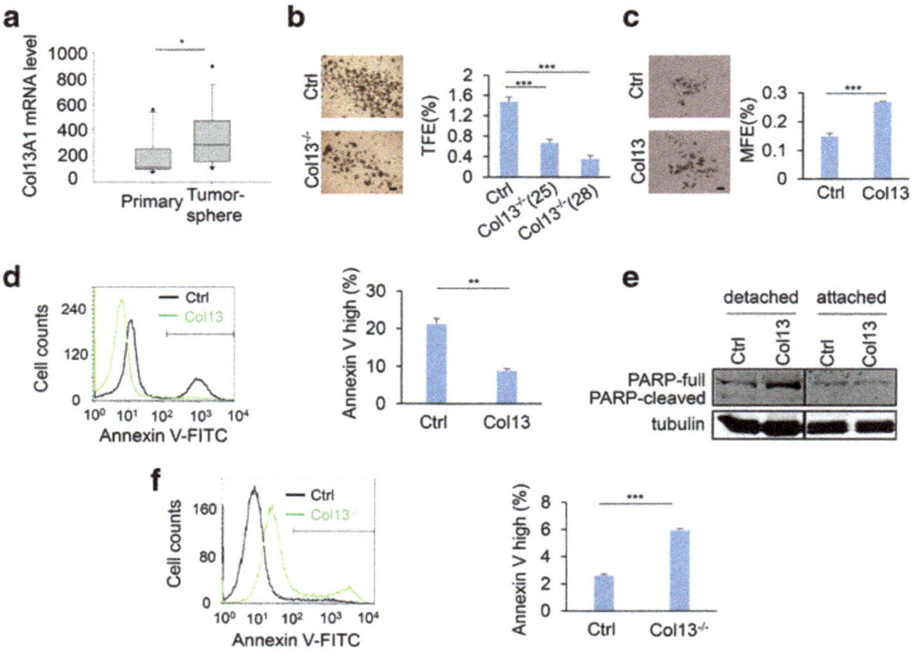

Fig. 4 Collagen XIII expression enhances cancer cell stemness. **a** Quantification of mRNA levels of Col13 in primary tumors ($n = 11$) and tumorsphere ($n = 15$). Data are presented as the mean ± s.e.m.; * $p < 0.05$. **b** Phase images and quantification data showed tumorsphere formation in control and Col13$^{-/-}$ MDA-MB-231 cells; $n = 5$; *** $p < 0.001$. Scale bar: 200 μm. **c** Phase images and quantification data showed mammosphere formation in control and Col13-expressing MCF-10A cells; n = 6; *** $p < 0.001$. Scale bar: 200 μm. **d** Cell detachment induced apoptosis was quantified in control and Col13-expressing cells. Cells were cultured with 0.5% methyl cellulose in suspension for 24 h to induce anoikis before the analysis. Cell surface phosphatidylserine was analyzed by annexin-V and followed by flow cytometry analysis. Early apoptosis was quantified with bar graph; $n = 3$; ** $p < 0.01$. **e** Western blot analyzing PARP-cleavage in control and Col13-expressing MCF-10A cells. Cells were treated as described in d before the analysis. **f** Cell detachment induced apoptosis was quantified in control and Col13$^{-/-}$ MDA-MB-231 as described in d. Data are presented as the mean ± s.e.m.; $n = 3$; *** $p < 0.001$

sufficient to enhance cancer cell stemness (Additional file 7: Figure S7b). Next, we performed another tumorsphere formation experiments by mixing GFP-labeled collagen XIII-silenced MDA-MB-231 cells with non-labeled wild type MDA-MB-231 cells. Wild type MDA-MB-231 cells did not increase the tumorsphere formation efficiency in GFP-labeled collagen XIII-silenced cells (Additional file 8: Figure S8). These results suggest that collagen XIII enhances cancer cell stemness in a cell-autonomous manner.

Tumor initiating cells are more resistant to detachment-induced anoikis, which is crucial for the cancer cell survival during cancer metastasis [53]. To determine whether collagen XIII promotes anoikis resistance, control, collagen XIII-silenced MDA-MB-231, and collagen-expressing MCF10A cells were cultured in methyl cellulose. Cell anoikis was assessed by analyzing PARP cleavage and cell surface-expressed phosphatidylserine with FITC-labeled annexin-V. We found that collagen XIII expression reduced detachment-induced cell

surface-expressed phosphatidylserine and PARP cleavage in MCF-10A cells (Fig. 4d, e), while silencing collagen XIII increased annexin-V staining in MDA-MB-231 cells (Fig. 4f). These results suggest that collagen XIII promotes breast cancer progression by enhancing cancer cell stemness and its associated anoikis resistance.

Collagen XIII enhances tumorsphere formation and TGF-β signaling through β1 integrin

To understand how collagen XIII regulates cancer progression, we determined whether collagen XIII induces β1 integrin activation. Monoclonal antibody HUTS-4 is specific against active human β1 integrin [54]. Activated β1 integrin was analyzed by immune fluorescence staining with HUTS-4 in control, collagen XIII-silenced or collagen XIII-expressing cells. Quantified data showed that silencing collagen XIII reduced the activated β1 integrin foci in MDA-MB-231 cells (Fig. 5a). In contrast, expression of collagen XIII induced β1 integrin

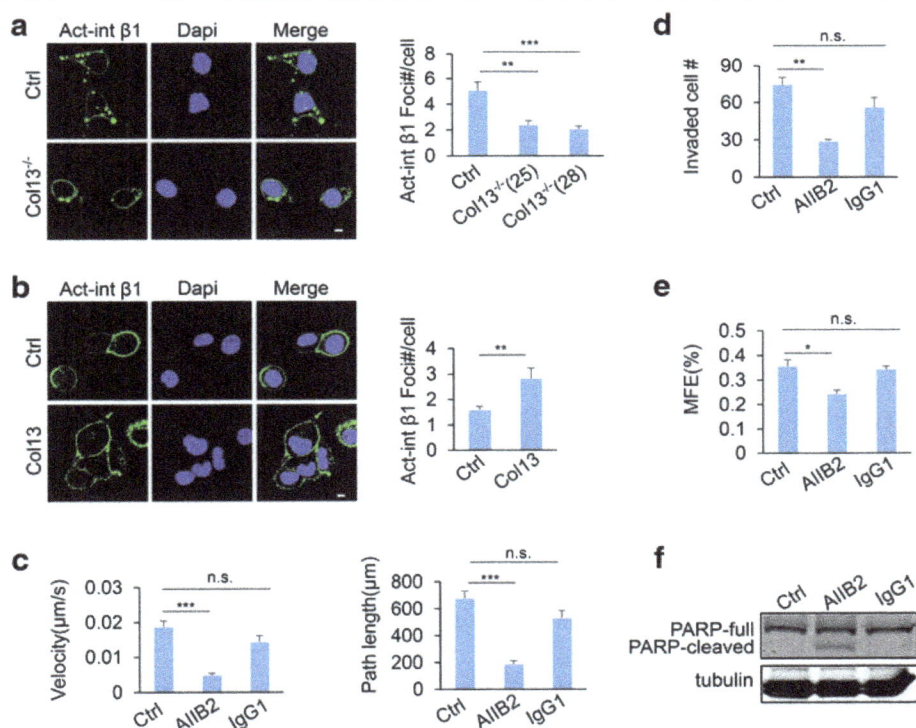

Fig. 5 Collagen XIII enhances cancer cell invasion and stemness through β1 integrin. **a** Immune fluorescence imaging analysis of β1 integrin activation in control and Col13$^{-/-}$ MDA-MB-231 cells (left). Bar graph quantifying the foci number of activated β1 integrin staining on cell membrane in control and Col13$^{-/-}$ MDA-MB-231 cells (right). Data are represented as the mean ± s.e.m.; n = 10 (fields); ** $p < 0.01$, *** $p < 0.001$. Scale bar: 5 μm. **b** Immune fluorescence imaging analyzed β1 integrin activation in control and Col13-expressing MCF-10A cells (left). Bar graph quantifying the foci number of activated β1 integrin staining on cell membrane in control and Col13-expressing MCF-10A cells (right); n = 10 (fields); ** $p < 0.01$. Scale bar: 5 μm. **c** The velocity (left) and path length (right) of single cell migration were quantified in Col13-expressing MCF-10A cells in the presence of β1 integrin functional blocking antibody AIIB2 or control IgG; n = 27; *** $p < 0.001$; n.s., no significance. **d** Bar graph quantifying invasion of Col13-expressing MCF-10A cells in the presence of AIIB2 or IgG; n = 3; ** $p < 0.01$. **e** Bar graph quantifying the mammosphere forming efficiency of Col13-expressing MCF-10A cells in the presence of AIIB2 or IgG; n = 3; * $p < 0.05$. **f** Western blot data showing that AIIB2 treatment enhanced PARP-cleavage in Col13-expressing MCF-10A cells

activation in MCF-10A cells (Fig. 5b). AIIB2 is an antibody that blocks β1 integrin activity [33]. To determine whether β1 integrin activation is crucial for collagen XIII-induced cell function, the collagen XIII-expressing MCF10A cells were treated with the control IgG or AIIB2 antibody in the single cell migration, invasion, and mammosphere formation experiments. We showed that the AIIB2 treatment blocked collagen XIII-induced cell migration (Fig. 5c), invasion (Fig. 5d), and mammosphere formation in MCF10A cells (Fig. 5e), while IgG treatment had little effect. In addition, inhibition of β1 integrin activation enhanced PARP cleavage in collagen-expressing cell (Fig. 5f). These results indicate that collagen XIII enhances cell invasion and mammosphere formation at least partially through the β1 integrin pathway.

Aberrant activation of the TGF-β pathway promotes cancer progression by enhancing cancer cell stemness and invasion [55–57]. It has been shown that β1 integrin contributes to the activation of the TGF-β pathway [58, 59]. We asked whether collagen XIII enhances the TGF-β signaling through β1 integrin. Control and collagen XIII knock-out MDA-MB-231 clones were treated with

TGF-β1. The cell lysates at various time points were analyzed by western blot to determine the ratio of phosphorylated SMAD2/3 compared to total SMAD. The TGF-β-induced SMAD2/3 phosphorylation was decreased in the collagen XIII knockout clones compared to control MDA-MB-231 cells (Fig. 6a). Consistent with western blot data, the TGF-β-induced TPA response elements (TREs)--driven luciferase activities were significantly reduced in collagen XIII-silenced cells (Fig. 6b). These experiments were repeated in the MCF-10A cells. Results showed that the TGF-β-induced SMAD2/3 phosphorylation and reporter activities were enhanced by exogenous collagen XIII expression (Fig. 6c, d). Importantly, AIIB2 treatment significantly reduced the collagen XIII-enhanced SMAD2/3 phosphorylation (Fig. 6e). Therefore, collagen XIII expression may enhance the TGF-β signaling through β1 integrin which subsequently promotes cancer progression.

Silencing collagen XIII inhibits breast cancer metastasis in mice

We showed that expression of collagen XIII was associated with short distant recurrence free survival in

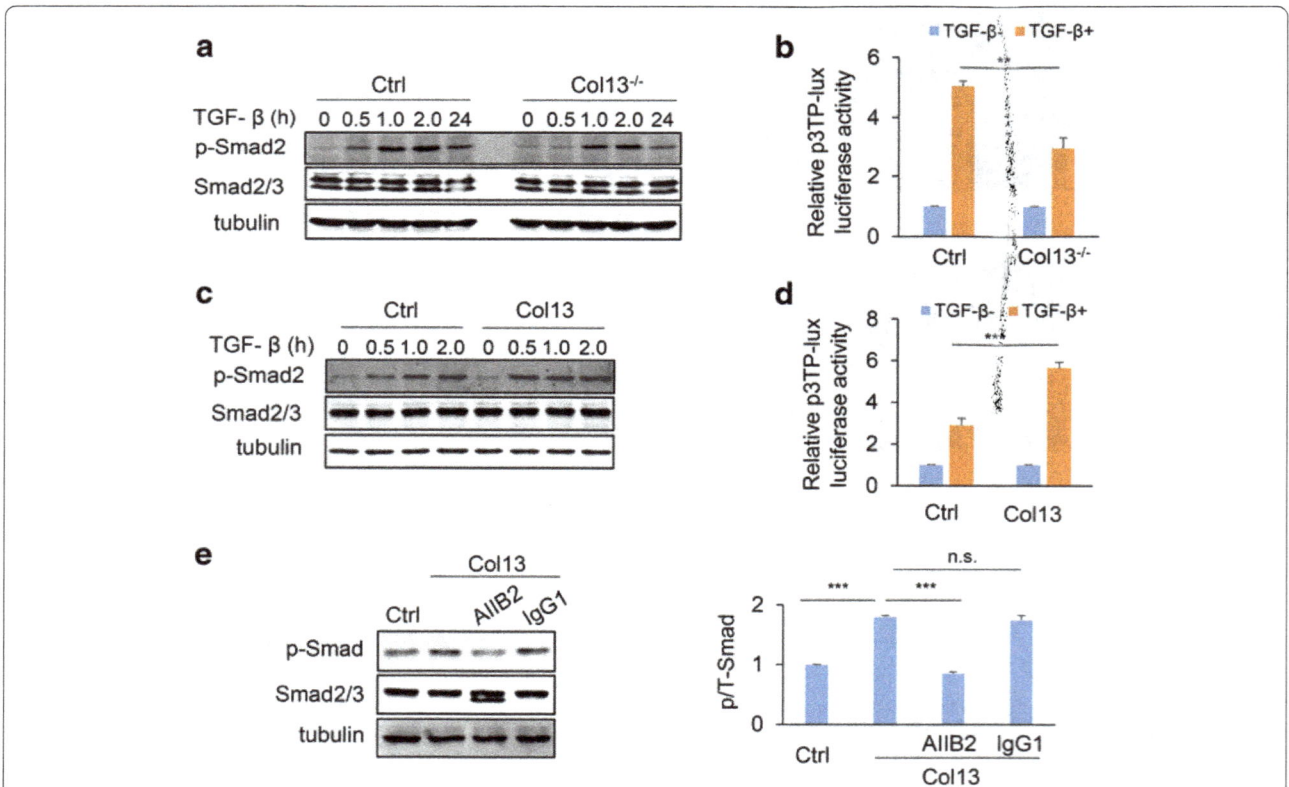

Fig. 6 Collagen XIII enhances activation of the TGF-β pathway. a Western blot analyzed TGF-β-induced Smad phosphorylation in control and Col13⁻/⁻ MDA-MB-231 cells. b Bar graph quantifying TGF-β-induced TPA response elements (TREs)-driven luciferase activity in control and Col13⁻/⁻ MDA-MB-231; n = 3; ** p < 0.01. c Western blot analyzed TGF-β-induced Smad phosphorylation in control and Col13-expressing MCF-10A cells. d Bar graph showing TGF-β-induced TRE-driven luciferase activity in control and Col13-expressing MCF-10A cells; n = 4, *** p < 0.001. e AIIB2 treatment reduced the level of TGF-β-induced Smad2/3 phosphorylation in Col13-expressing MCF-10A cells. Western bolt images (left) and quantification (right); n = 3; *** p <0.001; n.s., no significance

patients with ER negative (Fig. 7a) and ER positive breast cancer (Additional file 9: Figure S9), suggesting that collagen XIII contributes to cancer metastasis. To determine whether collagen XIII expression promotes cancer cell colonization at distant organs, we silenced collagen XIII expression in MDA-MB-231-luc-D3H2LN cells and pooled multiple clones together (Additional file 10: Figure S10). Control and collagen XIII-silenced cells were injected into the tail veins of SCID mice. Lung colonization of the cancer cells was monitored by IVIS imaging. We showed that the mice injected with control cells developed lung metastasis within 5 weeks, while silencing collagen XIII significantly reduced the lung metastasis (Fig. 7b). Haemotoxylin and Eosin (H&E) staining further confirmed that silencing collagen XIII inhibited the lung colonization of cancer cells in SCID mice (Fig. 7c). Intracardiac inoculation of MDA-MB-231 cells has been used as a model to investigate breast cancer bone metastasis. Using this model, we also found that silencing collagen XIII reduced colonization of MDA-MB-231-luc-D3H2LN cells in nude mice (Fig. 7d).

We further analyzed cancer cell colonization in bone using the GFP-labeled MDA-MB-231 cells. Interestingly, bone metastasis was detected in all four mice in the collagen-silenced group, while only three mice had bone metastasis in the control group (Additional file 11: Figure S11). Thus, function of collagen XIII in breast cancer bone metastasis remains for further clarification.

Next we defined roles of collagen XIII in primary tumor growth and cancer metastasis using the MDA-MB-231-luc-D3H2LN orthotopic mammary tumor model [60]. The orthotopic mammary tumor model is a physiologically relevant model to study cancer metastasis. It reproduces the entire metastatic process, including tumor cell dissemination from the mammary fat pad, followed by colonization and outgrowth at distant organs. The same amount of control and collagen XIII-silenced cancer cells were injected into the mammary fat pads of 6-week-old female SCID mice, and tumor growth was monitored twice per week. Then the primary tumors were removed, and mice were maintained for another month before

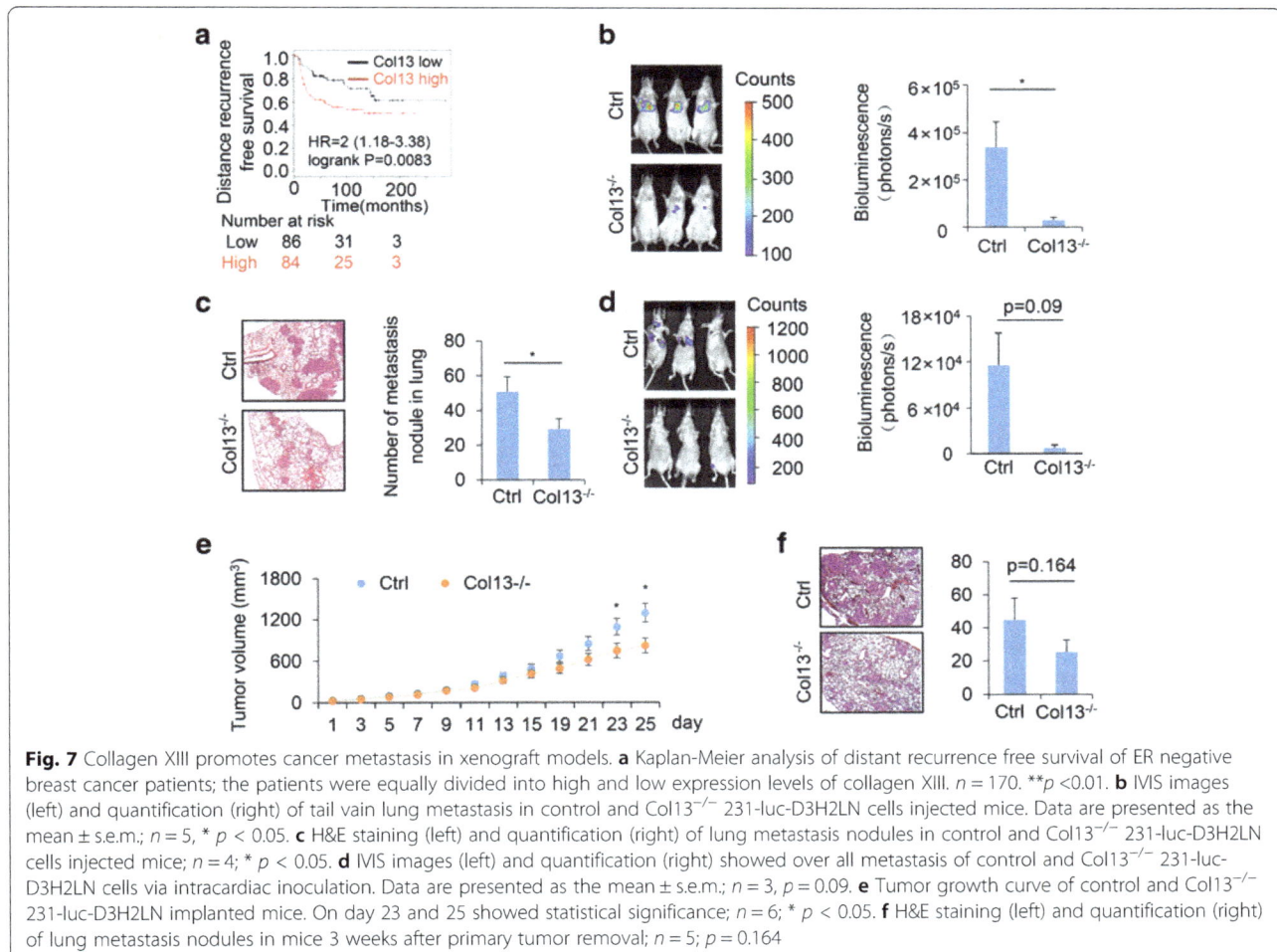

Fig. 7 Collagen XIII promotes cancer metastasis in xenograft models. **a** Kaplan-Meier analysis of distant recurrence free survival of ER negative breast cancer patients; the patients were equally divided into high and low expression levels of collagen XIII. $n = 170$. **$p < 0.01$. **b** IVIS images (left) and quantification (right) of tail vain lung metastasis in control and $Col13^{-/-}$ 231-luc-D3H2LN cells injected mice. Data are presented as the mean ± s.e.m.; $n = 5$, * $p < 0.05$. **c** H&E staining (left) and quantification (right) of lung metastasis nodules in control and $Col13^{-/-}$ 231-luc-D3H2LN cells injected mice; $n = 4$; * $p < 0.05$. **d** IVIS images (left) and quantification (right) showed over all metastasis of control and $Col13^{-/-}$ 231-luc-D3H2LN cells via intracardiac inoculation. Data are presented as the mean ± s.e.m.; $n = 3$, $p = 0.09$. **e** Tumor growth curve of control and $Col13^{-/-}$ 231-luc-D3H2LN implanted mice. On day 23 and 25 showed statistical significance; $n = 6$; * $p < 0.05$. **f** H&E staining (left) and quantification (right) of lung metastasis nodules in mice 3 weeks after primary tumor removal; $n = 5$; $p = 0.164$

analyzing the metastases in the lung. We found that silencing collagen XIII slightly reduced tumor growth (Fig. 7e). We also observed a reduction of lung metastases in collagen XIII-silenced group (Fig. 7f). Therefore, increased collagen XIII expression may promote cancer colonization and metastasis by enhancing cancer cell invasion and stemness.

Discussion

Roles of interstitial collagen and BM collagen in mammary tumor development have been determined [61–63]. However, function of membrane-associated collagens in breast cancer is not well studied. We identified increased collagen XIII expression in breast cancer tissue, especially in triple negative breast cancers. Using the orthotopic mammary tumor model and lung colonization assay, we showed for the first time that collagen XIII expression is required for breast cancer cell metastasis. These results identified a novel function of membrane associated collagen in cancer progression.

Stromal cells, such as cancer-associated fibroblasts, are considered the major source of ECM protein in cancer tissue. It has been shown that collagen XIII is highly expressed in fibroblasts and localizes in the focal adhesion [24]. Interestingly, we found that collagen XIII is expressed in TNBC cell lines and tissues. The metastatic MDA-MB-231 cell line contains the highest level of collagen XIII compared to non-metastatic or non-malignant cell lines. A recent study shows that collagen XIII is expressed in the invasive bladder cancer cell line and the infiltrative bladder cancer tissue. Collagen XIII enhances cancer cell invasion in these cell lines [25]. We further show that the increased expression of collagen XIII promotes cancer cell migration and invasion through β1 integrin. Collagen I, collagen IV, laminin, and fibronectin are also produced by cancer cells and deposited in cancer tissue [36, 64–66]. These results indicate that cancer cells produce a significant amount of ECM proteins. Importantly, we demonstrate that collagen XIII is crucial for cancer cell stemness and metastasis, which provide additional insights about the cancer cell produced ECM.

Results from lung colonization experiments suggest that collagen XIII expression is crucial for cancer cell survival in circulation and colonization at distant organs. It has been shown that tumor initiating cells are the driver of cancer metastasis and initiate the colonization at distal sites [67, 68]. Silencing collagen XIII reduced tumorsphere formation in breast cancer cells, suggesting that the collagen XIII expression enhances cancer cell stemness. Cancer cells also need to acquire anoikis resistance to survive in circulation during cancer metastasis. We found that collagen XIII

induces anoikis resistance in mammary epithelial cells. These results suggest that collagen XIII derived from cancer cells promotes cancer metastasis by enhancing cancer cell stemness and by inducing anoikis resistance.

Collagen XIII expression is detected in the invasion front of bladder cancer [24, 25]. Consistent with these results we show that collagen XIII is required for the invasive growth of MDA-MB-231 cells in 3D culture. Therefore, membrane protein collagen XIII may promote cancer cell metastasis at multiple stages, including dissemination from the primary tumor and colonization at the distant organs. Interestingly, collagen XIII is also involved in the inflammatory process and regulation of the immune system. It has been identified as a favorable prognostic factor in B-cell lymphoma [69]. In addition, mice expressing a mutant collagen XIII develop clonal mature B cell lineage lymphomas [70]. These results suggest that function of collagen XIII in the development of solid tumors and lymphoma may be different.

We found that collagen XIII expression induced the activation of β1 integrin. Inhibition of β1 integrin activation blocks collagen XIII-induced tumorsphere formation and TGF-β signaling, suggesting that β1 integrin is a crucial downstream target of collagen XIII in promoting cancer progression. It has been shown that integrin α1β1 mediates CHO cell spreading on collagen XIII [19]. The solid phase assay confirms the binding of europium-labeled αI domains to the collagen XIII. Our co-culture experiments suggest that collagen XIII binds to the integrin on the same cell and enhance cell invasion and tumorsphere formation in the cell-autonomous manner. Discoidin domain receptors (DDRs) are a family membrane proteins that bind to collagen separated from the integrin-β1 pathway [71, 72]. DDRs are tyrosine kinase receptors that are activated when bound to collagen, subsequently regulating cell proliferation, differentiation, survival, and migration [73]. Therefore, it is important to investigate if collagen XIII also regulates DDR activation in the future.

Conclusions

In summary, this study identified a novel function of collagen XIII in breast cancer metastasis. We demonstrate that collagen XIII enhances breast cancer invasive growth and anoikis resistance through β1 integrin. These findings provide insights in the roles of membrane associated collagen in cancer progression, and suggest that targeting collagen XIII is a potential strategy for suppressing breast cancer progression.

Additional files

Additional file 1: Figure S1. Kaplan-Meier analysis of recurrence free survival in ER positive breast cancer patients; the patients were equally divided into two groups based on the mRNA level of Col13 in breast cancer tissue. $n = 1802$. **$p < 0.01$. (PDF 2061 kb)

Additional file 2: Figure S2. Genomic DNA sequencing results of wild type and Col13 knockout MDA-MB-231 clone 28. There is a T deleted in the Col13 knockout MDA-MB-231 cells. (PDF 3096 kb)

Additional file 3: Figure S3. Immunofluorescence staining analyzes collagen XIII expression, EdU labeling, and caspase 3 activation. **a** 2D culture fluorescent microscopy images of MCF-10A control and Col13 overexpression cells. Flag (green), dapi (blue) and merged images. Scale bar: 20 μm. **b** EdU staining fluorescent microscopy images of MCF-10A control and Col13 overexpression cells. Representative image was on day6 of 3D culture. EdU (green), dapi (blue) and merged images. Scale bar: 20 μm. **c** The images (left) stand for caspase3 3D fluorescent staining and the bar graph (right) shows the ratio of caspase3 positive to total cells. Caspase3 (green), dapi (blue). Scale bar: 20 μm. Data are presented as the mean ± s.e.m. ($n = 20$); $p = 0.098$. (PDF 4348 kb)

Additional file 4: Figure S4. The path of single cell migration in control (left) and Col13-expressing MCF-10A cells (right); $n = 13$. (PDF 1546 kb)

Additional file 5: Figure S5. Transwell analysis of T4–2 cell invasion. **a** Quantification data showing invasion of control and Col13$^{-/-}$ T4–2 cells. Data are presented as the mean ± s.e.m.; $n = 3$; * $p < 0.05$. **b** Quantification data showing invasion of control and Col13-expressing T4–2 cells. Data are presented as the mean ± s.e.m.; $n = 3$; n.s., no significance. (PDF 1423 kb)

Additional file 6: Figure S6. Co-culture invasion analysis in Transwell. Images (upper) and quantification data (lower) showing the invasion of GFP-labeled MDA-MB-231-vector control cells mixed with wild type MDA-MB-231 cells (1:1), GFP-labeled Col13$^{-/-}$ MDA-MB-231 cells alone, and GFP-labeled Col13$^{-/-}$ MDA-MB-231 cells mixed with wild type MDA-MB-231-Control cells (1:1). Each group had same amount of cells plated in the upper chamber; total cell number plated in the upper chamber is 0.1 M. The invaded GFP-labeled cell numbers were counted, and the number of GFP-labeled Col13$^{-/-}$MDA-MB-231 alone group was divided by 2. Data are presented as the mean ± s.e.m. $n = 3$; ** $p < 0.01$. n.s., no significance. Scale bar: 50 μm. (PDF 4617 kb)

Additional file 7: Figure S7. Tumorsphere forming efficiency in T4–2 cells. **a** Phase images (left) and quantification data (right) showed tumorshpere formation efficiency in control and Col13$^{-/-}$T4–2 cells. Data are presented as the mean ± s.e.m. $n = 3$; * $p < 0.05$. Scale bar: 100 μm. **b** Phase images (left) and quantification data (right) showed tumorshpere formation efficiency in control and Col13-expressing T4–2 cells. Data are presented as the mean ± s.e.m. $n = 3$; n.s., no significance. Scale bar: 100 μm. (PDF 5721 kb)

Additional file 8: Figure S8. Co-culture tumorsphere forming efficiency analysis. Quantification data showing tumorsphere forming efficiency of GFP-labeled MDA-MB-231 vector control cells mixed with wild type MDA-MB-231 cells (1:1), GFP-labeled Col13$^{-/-}$ MDA-MB-231 cells alone, and GFP-labeled Col13$^{-/-}$ MDA-MB-231 mixed with wild type MDA-MB-231 cells (1:1). Each group had the same amount of cells plated on poly-HEMA coated dishes, and GFP-labeled tumorsphere was counted, and the tumorsphere number of GFP-labeled Col13$^{-/-}$ MDA-MB-231alone group was divided by 2. Data are presented as the mean ± s.e.m. $n = 3$; * $p < 0.05$, ** $p < 0.01$. n.s., no significance. (PDF 1452 kb)

Additional file 9: Figure S9. Kaplan-Meier analysis of distant recurrence free survival in ER positive breast cancer patients; the patients were equally divided into two groups based on the mRNA level of collagen XIII. $n = 577$. ***$p < 0.001$. (PDF 2351 kb)

Additional file 10: Figure S10. Western blot confirming Col13 knockout in 231-luc-D3H2LN cells. (PDF 1372 kb)

Additional file 11: Figure S11. Bright field and fluorescence images showing bone metastasis of GFP-labeled MDA-MB-231 cells in nude mice. Left two images showed bone metastasis of the control MAD-MB-231 cells on the hind leg after intracardiac inoculation. Right two images showed bone metastasis of Col13$^{-/-}$ MAD-MB-231 cells on the fore leg after intracardiac inoculation. $n = 4$. (PDF 7411 kb)

Abbreviations
CRISPR: Clustered regularly interspaced short palindromic repeats; DDRs: Discoidin domain receptors; ECM: Extracellular matrix; ER: Estrogen receptor; IVIS: in vivo imaging system; NC: Non-collagenous; SCID: Severe combined immun deficiency; TNBC: Triple-negative breast cancer

Acknowledgements
The authors acknowledge the assistance of the following Markey Cancer Center Shared Resource Facilities, all of which are supported by the grant P30 CA177558: the Biospecimen and Tissue Procurement Shared Resource Facility for assistance in tissue fixation and section; the Flow Cytometry and Cell Sorting Core Facility for performing FACS analysis. The authors also thank the First Hospital of Jilin University support an Overseas Research Plan to H.Z..

Funding
This study was supported by start-up funding from Markey Cancer Center and funding support from NCI (1R01CA207772, 1R01CA215095 and 1R21CA209045 to R.X.), Markey Cancer Center CCSG pilot funding (P30 CA177558), and United States Department of Defense (W81XWH-15-1-0052 to R.X.). National Natural Science Foundation of China (81728013 to J.D.L), and the Centre of Excellence Grant 2012–2017 of the Academy of Finland (284605), the Sigrid Jusélius Foundation and the Finnish Cancer Foundation (to T.P.). National Natural Science Foundation of China (81672106 to W.X.).

Authors' contributions
RX and WX conceived the work, designed all experiments, supervised the analysis and edited the manuscript. HZ performed most of experiments and analyzed the data. TF prepared manuscript and conducted some in vitro experiments. GFX performed the in vivo experiments. YFQ carried out some of in vitro experiments. PGR helped with xenograft experiments. JDL helped to revise the manuscript. TP provided the important material of the experiments and revised the manuscript. All authors read and approved the final manuscript.

Competing interests
The authors declare that they have no competing interests.

Author details
[1]Department of Laboratory Medicine, The First Hospital of Jilin University, Changchun 130021, Jilin Province, China. [2]UK Markey Cancer Center, University of Kentucky, Lexington, KY 40536, USA. [3]Department of Pharmacology and Nutritional Sciences, University of Kentucky, Lexington, KY 40536, USA. [4]Division of Gynecologic Oncology, Department of Obstetrics and Gynecology, University of Kentucky, Lexington, KY 40504, USA. [5]Department of Surgery, College of Medicine, University of Kentucky, Lexington, KY 40504, USA. [6]Center for Medical Genetics, School of Life Sciences, Central South University, Changsha 410078, Hunan Province, China. [7]Center for Cell-Matrix Research and Biocenter Oulu, Faculty of Biochemistry and Molecular Medicine, University of Oulu, 90014 Oulu, Finland.

References
1. Lynce F, Blackburn MJ, Cai L, Wang H, Rubinstein L, Harris P, Isaacs C, Pohlmann PR. Characteristics and outcomes of breast cancer patients

enrolled in the National Cancer Institute Cancer Therapy Evaluation Program sponsored phase I clinical trials. Breast Cancer Res Treat. 2018; 168(1):35–41

2. Kumar N, Patni P, Agarwal A, Khan MA, Parashar N. Prevalence of molecular subtypes of invasive breast cancer: a retrospective study. Med J Armed Forces India. 2015;71(3):254–8.

3. Lu P, Weaver VM, Werb Z. The extracellular matrix: a dynamic niche in cancer progression. J Cell Biol. 2012;196(4):395–406.

4. van 't Veer LJ, Dai H, van de Vijver MJ, He YD, Hart AA, Mao M, Peterse HL, van der Kooy K, Marton MJ, Witteveen AT, et al. Gene expression profiling predicts clinical outcome of breast cancer. Nature. 2002;415(6871):530–6.

5. Iyengar P, Espina V, Williams TW, Lin Y, Berry D, Jelicks LA, Lee H, Temple K, Graves R, Pollard J, et al. Adipocyte-derived collagen VI affects early mammary tumor progression in vivo, demonstrating a critical interaction in the tumor/stroma microenvironment. J Clin Invest. 2005;115(5):1163–76.

6. Provenzano PP, Inman DR, Eliceiri KW, Knittel JG, Yan L, Rueden CT, White JG, Keely PJ. Collagen density promotes mammary tumor initiation and progression. BMC Med. 2008;6:11.

7. Shields MA, Dangi-Garimella S, Krantz SB, Bentrem DJ, Munshi HG. Pancreatic cancer cells respond to type I collagen by inducing snail expression to promote membrane type 1 matrix metalloproteinase-dependent collagen invasion. J Biol Chem. 2011;286(12):10495–504.

8. Condeelis J, Segall JE. Intravital imaging of cell movement in tumours. Nat Rev Cancer. 2003;3(12):921–30.

9. Provenzano PP, Inman DR, Eliceiri KW, Keely PJ. Matrix density-induced mechanoregulation of breast cell phenotype, signaling and gene expression through a FAK-ERK linkage. Oncogene. 2009;28(49):4326–43.

10. Boyd NF, Guo H, Martin LJ, Sun L, Stone J, Fishell E, Jong RA, Hislop G, Chiarelli A, Minkin S, et al. Mammographic density and the risk and detection of breast cancer. N Engl J Med. 2007;356(3):227–36.

11. Guo YP, Martin LJ, Hanna W, Banerjee D, Miller N, Fishell E, Khokha R, Boyd NF. Growth factors and stromal matrix proteins associated with mammographic densities. Cancer Epidemiol Biomark Prev. 2001;10(3):243–8.

12. Levental KR, Yu H, Kass L, Lakins JN, Egeblad M, Erler JT, Fong SF, Csiszar K, Giaccia A, Weninger W, et al. Matrix crosslinking forces tumor progression by enhancing integrin signaling. Cell. 2009;139(5):891–906.

13. Myllyharju J, Kivirikko KI. Collagens, modifying enzymes and their mutations in humans, flies and worms. Trends Genet. 2004;20(1):33–43.

14. Hellewell AL, Adams JC. Insider trading: extracellular matrix proteins and their non-canonical intracellular roles. Bioessays. 2016;38(1):77–88.

15. Banyard J, Bao L, Zetter BR. Type XXIII collagen, a new transmembrane collagen identified in metastatic tumor cells. J Biol Chem. 2003;278(23):20989–94.

16. Hashimoto T, Wakabayashi T, Watanabe A, Kowa H, Hosoda R, Nakamura A, Kanazawa I, Arai T, Takio K, Mann DM, et al. CLAC: a novel Alzheimer amyloid plaque component derived from a transmembrane precursor, CLAC-P/collagen type XXV. EMBO J. 2002;21(7):1524–34.

17. Hagg P, Rehn M, Huhtala P, Vaisanen T, Tamminen M, Pihlajaniemi T. Type XIII collagen is identified as a plasma membrane protein. J Biol Chem. 1998; 273(25):15590–7.

18. Maatta M, Vaisanen T, Vaisanen MR, Pihlajaniemi T, Tervo T. Altered expression of type XIII collagen in keratoconus and scarred human cornea: increased expression in scarred cornea is associated with myofibroblast transformation. Cornea. 2006;25(4):448–53.

19. Nykvist P, Tu H, Ivaska J, Kapyla J, Pihlajaniemi T, Heino J. Distinct recognition of collagen subtypes by alpha(1)beta(1) and alpha(2)beta(1) integrins. Alpha(1)beta(1) mediates cell adhesion to type XIII collagen. J Biol Chem. 2000;275(11):8255–61.

20. Vaisanen MR, Vaisanen T, Pihlajaniemi T. The shed ectodomain of type XIII collagen affects cell behaviour in a matrix-dependent manner. Biochem J. 2004;380(Pt 3):685–93.

21. Snellman A, Keranen MR, Hagg PO, Lamberg A, Hiltunen JK, Kivirikko KI, Pihlajaniemi T. Type XIII collagen forms homotrimers with three triple helical collagenous domains and its association into disulfide-bonded trimers is enhanced by prolyl 4-hydroxylase. J Biol Chem. 2000;275(12): 8936–44.

22. Snellman A, Tu H, Vaisanen T, Kvist AP, Huhtala P, Pihlajaniemi T. A short sequence in the N-terminal region is required for the trimerization of type XIII collagen and is conserved in other collagenous transmembrane proteins. EMBO J. 2000;19(19):5051–9.

23. Juvonen M, Sandberg M, Pihlajaniemi T. Patterns of expression of the six alternatively spliced exons affecting the structures of the COL1 and NC2

24. domains of the alpha 1(XIII) collagen chain in human tissues and cell lines. J Biol Chem. 1992;267(34):24700–7.

24. Vaisanen T, Vaisanen MR, Autio-Harmainen H, Pihlajaniemi T. Type XIII collagen expression is induced during malignant transformation in various epithelial and mesenchymal tumours. J Pathol. 2005;207(3):324–35.

25. Miyake M, Hori S, Morizawa Y, Tatsumi Y, Toritsuka M, Ohnishi S, Shimada K, Furuya H, Khadka VS, Deng Y, et al. Collagen type IV alpha 1 (COL4A1) and collagen type XIII alpha 1 (COL13A1) produced in cancer cells promote tumor budding at the invasion front in human urothelial carcinoma of the bladder. Oncotarget. 2017;8(22):36099–114.

26. Plantefaber LC, Hynes RO. Changes in integrin receptors on oncogenically transformed cells. Cell. 1989;56(2):281–90.

27. Cosgrove D, Rodgers K, Meehan D, Miller C, Bovard K, Gilroy A, Gardner H, Kotelianski V, Gotwals P, Amatucci A, et al. Integrin alpha1beta1 and transforming growth factor-beta1 play distinct roles in alport glomerular pathogenesis and serve as dual targets for metabolic therapy. Am J Pathol. 2000;157(5):1649–59.

28. Howe AK, Aplin AE, Juliano RL. Anchorage-dependent ERK signaling--mechanisms and consequences. Curr Opin Genet Dev. 2002;12(1):30–5.

29. George EL, Georges-Labouesse EN, Patel-King RS, Rayburn H, Hynes RO. Defects in mesoderm, neural tube and vascular development in mouse embryos lacking fibronectin. Development. 1993;119(4):1079–91.

30. Hynes RO. Targeted mutations in cell adhesion genes: what have we learned from them? Dev Biol. 1996;180(2):402–12.

31. Persad S, Attwell S, Gray V, Delcommenne M, Troussard A, Sanghera J, Dedhar S. Inhibition of integrin-linked kinase (ILK) suppresses activation of protein kinase B/Akt and induces cell cycle arrest and apoptosis of PTEN-mutant prostate cancer cells. Proc Natl Acad Sci U S A. 2000;97(7):3207–12.

32. Li N, Zhang Y, Naylor MJ, Schatzmann F, Maurer F, Wintermantel T, Schuetz G, Mueller U, Streuli CH, Hynes NE. Beta1 integrins regulate mammary gland proliferation and maintain the integrity of mammary alveoli. EMBO J. 2005; 24(11):1942–53.

33. Weaver VM, Petersen OW, Wang F, Larabell CA, Briand P, Damsky C, Bissell MJ. Reversion of the malignant phenotype of human breast cells in three-dimensional culture and in vivo by integrin blocking antibodies. J Cell Biol. 1997;137(1):231–45.

34. White DE, Kurpios NA, Zuo D, Hassell JA, Blaess S, Mueller U, Muller WJ. Targeted disruption of beta1-integrin in a transgenic mouse model of human breast cancer reveals an essential role in mammary tumor induction. Cancer Cell. 2004;6(2):159–70.

35. Debnath J, Muthuswamy SK, Brugge JS. Morphogenesis and oncogenesis of MCF-10A mammary epithelial acini grown in three-dimensional basement membrane cultures. Methods. 2003;30(3):256–68.

36. Zhu J, Xiong G, Fu H, Evers BM, Zhou BP, Xu R. Chaperone Hsp47 drives malignant growth and invasion by modulating an ECM gene network. Cancer Res. 2015;75(8):1580–91.

37. Anders M, Hansen R, Ding RX, Rauen KA, Bissell MJ, Korn WM. Disruption of 3D tissue integrity facilitates adenovirus infection by deregulating the coxsackievirus and adenovirus receptor. Proc Natl Acad Sci U S A. 2003; 100(4):1943–8.

38. Dennis J, Meehan DT, Delimont D, Zallocchi M, Perry GA, O'Brien S, Tu H, Pihlajaniemi T, Cosgrove D. Collagen XIII induced in vascular endothelium mediates alpha1beta1 integrin-dependent transmigration of monocytes in renal fibrosis. Am J Pathol. 2010;177(5):2527–40.

39. Li L, Chen J, Xiong G, St Clair DK, Xu W, Xu R. Increased ROS production in non-polarized mammary epithelial cells induces monocyte infiltration in 3D culture. J Cell Sci. 2017;130(1):190–202.

40. Alcaraz-Perez F, Mulero V, Cayuela ML. Application of the dual-luciferase reporter assay to the analysis of promoter activity in zebrafish embryos. BMC Biotechnol. 2008;8:81.

41. Xiong G, Wang C, Evers BM, Zhou BP, Xu R. RORalpha suppresses breast tumor invasion by inducing SEMA3F expression. Cancer Res. 2012;72(7): 1728–39.

42. Reginato MJ, Mills KR, Paulus JK, Lynch DK, Sgroi DC, Debnath J, Muthuswamy SK, Brugge JS. Integrins and EGFR coordinately regulate the pro-apoptotic protein Bim to prevent anoikis. Nat Cell Biol. 2003; 5(8):733–40.

43. Gyorffy B, Lanczky A, Eklund AC, Denkert C, Budczies J, Li Q, Szallasi Z. An online survival analysis tool to rapidly assess the effect of 22,277 genes on breast cancer prognosis using microarray data of 1,809 patients. Breast Cancer Res Treat. 2010;123(3):725–31.

44. Mroue R, Bissell MJ. Three-dimensional cultures of mouse mammary epithelial cells. Methods Mol Biol. 2013;945:221–50.
45. Lo AT, Mori H, Mott J, Bissell MJ. Constructing three-dimensional models to study mammary gland branching morphogenesis and functional differentiation. J Mammary Gland Biol Neoplasia. 2012;17(2):103–10.
46. Campbell JJ, Husmann A, Hume RD, Watson CJ, Cameron RE. Development of three-dimensional collagen scaffolds with controlled architecture for cell migration studies using breast cancer cell lines. Biomaterials. 2017;114:34–43.
47. Sundquist E, Renko O, Salo S, Magga J, Cervigne NK, Nyberg P, Risteli J, Sormunen R, Vuolteenaho O, Zandonadi F, et al. Neoplastic extracellular matrix environment promotes cancer invasion in vitro. Exp Cell Res. 2016; 344(2):229–40.
48. Zhou BB, Zhang H, Damelin M, Geles KG, Grindley JC, Dirks PB. Tumour-initiating cells: challenges and opportunities for anticancer drug discovery. Nat Rev Drug Discov. 2009;8(10):806–23.
49. Singh A, Settleman J. EMT, cancer stem cells and drug resistance: an emerging axis of evil in the war on cancer. Oncogene. 2010;29(34):4741–51.
50. Guttilla IK, Phoenix KN, Hong X, Tirnauer JS, Claffey KP, White BA. Prolonged mammosphere culture of MCF-7 cells induces an EMT and repression of the estrogen receptor by microRNAs. Breast Cancer Res Treat. 2012;132(1):75–85.
51. Charafe-Jauffret E, Ginestier C, Iovino F, Wicinski J, Cervera N, Finetti P, Hur MH, Diebel ME, Monville F, Dutcher J, et al. Breast cancer cell lines contain functional cancer stem cells with metastatic capacity and a distinct molecular signature. Cancer Res. 2009;69(4):1302–13.
52. Creighton CJ, Li X, Landis M, Dixon JM, Neumeister VM, Sjolund A, Rimm DL, Wong H, Rodriguez A, Herschkowitz JI, et al. Residual breast cancers after conventional therapy display mesenchymal as well as tumor-initiating features. Proc Natl Acad Sci U S A. 2009;106(33):13820–5.
53. Celia-Terrassa T, Kang Y. Distinctive properties of metastasis-initiating cells. Genes Dev. 2016;30(8):892–908.
54. Du J, Chen X, Liang X, Zhang G, Xu J, He L, Zhan Q, Feng XQ, Chien S, Yang C. Integrin activation and internalization on soft ECM as a mechanism of induction of stem cell differentiation by ECM elasticity. Proc Natl Acad Sci U S A. 2011;108(23):9466–71.
55. Brown JA, Yonekubo Y, Hanson N, Sastre-Perona A, Basin A, Rytlewski JA, Dolgalev I, Meehan S, Tsirigos A, Beronja S, et al. TGF-beta-induced quiescence mediates Chemoresistance of tumor-propagating cells in squamous cell carcinoma. Cell Stem Cell. 2017;21(5):650–64. e658
56. Cammareri P, Rose AM, Vincent DF, Wang J, Nagano A, Libertini S, Ridgway RA, Athineos D, Coates PJ, McHugh A, et al. Inactivation of TGFbeta receptors in stem cells drives cutaneous squamous cell carcinoma. Nat Commun. 2016;7:12493.
57. Jin Y, Chen W, Yang H, Yan Z, Lai Z, Feng J, Peng J, Lin J. Scutellaria barbata D. Don inhibits migration and invasion of colorectal cancer cells via suppression of PI3K/AKT and TGF-beta/Smad signaling pathways. Exp Ther Med. 2017;14(6):5527–34.
58. Zambruno G, Marchisio PC, Marconi A, Vaschieri C, Melchiori A, Giannetti A, De Luca M. Transforming growth factor-beta 1 modulates beta 1 and beta 5 integrin receptors and induces the de novo expression of the alpha v beta 6 heterodimer in normal human keratinocytes: implications for wound healing. J Cell Biol. 1995;129(3):853–65.
59. Heino J, Ignotz RA, Hemler ME, Crouse C, Massague J. Regulation of cell adhesion receptors by transforming growth factor-beta. Concomitant regulation of integrins that share a common beta 1 subunit. J Biol Chem. 1989;264(1):380–8.
60. Shan L, Zhou X, Liu X, Wang Y, Su D, Hou Y, Yu N, Yang C, Liu B, Gao J, et al. FOXK2 elicits massive transcription repression and suppresses the hypoxic response and breast Cancer carcinogenesis. Cancer Cell. 2016;30(5):708–22.
61. Bartel-Friedrich S, Friedrich RE, Arps H, Holzhausen HJ. Distribution of collagens in carcinomas of salivary and mammary gland origin in irradiated rats. Anticancer Res. 2000;20(6D):5007–14.
62. Noel A, Calle A, Emonard H, Nusgens B, Foidart JM, Lapiere CM. Antagonistic effects of laminin and fibronectin in cell-to-cell and cell-to-matrix interactions in MCF-7 cultures. In Vitro Cell Dev Biol. 1988;24(5):373–80.
63. Iizuka D, Sasatani M, Barcellos-Hoff MH, Kamiya K. Hydrogen peroxide enhances TGFbeta-mediated epithelial-to-mesenchymal transition in human mammary epithelial MCF-10A cells. Anticancer Res. 2017;37(3):987–95.
64. Xiong G, Deng L, Zhu J, Rychahou PG, Xu R. Prolyl-4-hydroxylase alpha subunit 2 promotes breast cancer progression and metastasis by regulating collagen deposition. BMC Cancer. 2014;14:1.
65. Hynes RO. The extracellular matrix: not just pretty fibrils. Science. 2009; 326(5957):1216–9.
66. Xiong G-F, Xu R. Function of cancer cell-derived extracellular matrix in tumor progression. J Cancer Metastasis Treat. 2016;2(9):357.
67. Kreso A, Dick JE. Evolution of the cancer stem cell model. Cell Stem Cell. 2014;14(3):275–91.
68. Beck B, Blanpain C. Unravelling cancer stem cell potential. Nat Rev Cancer. 2013;13(10):727–38.
69. Lenz G, Wright G, Dave SS, Xiao W, Powell J, Zhao H, Xu W, Tan B, Goldschmidt N, Iqbal J, et al. Stromal gene signatures in large-B-cell lymphomas. N Engl J Med. 2008;359(22):2313–23.
70. Tuomisto A, Sund M, Tahkola J, Latvanlehto A, Savolainen ER, Autio-Harmainen H, Liakka A, Sormunen R, Vuoristo J, West A, et al. A mutant collagen XIII alters intestinal expression of immune response genes and predisposes transgenic mice to develop B-cell lymphomas. Cancer Res. 2008;68(24):10324–32.
71. Shrivastava A, Radziejewski C, Campbell E, Kovac L, McGlynn M, Ryan TE, Davis S, Goldfarb MP, Glass DJ, Lemke G, et al. An orphan receptor tyrosine kinase family whose members serve as nonintegrin collagen receptors. Mol Cell. 1997;1(1):25–34.
72. Leitinger B. Discoidin domain receptor functions in physiological and pathological conditions. Int Rev Cell Mol Biol. 2014;310:39–87.
73. Lemmon MA, Schlessinger J. Cell signaling by receptor tyrosine kinases. Cell. 2010;141(7):1117–34.

3

ETV4 transcription factor and MMP13 metalloprotease are interplaying actors of breast tumorigenesis

Mandy Dumortier[1], Franck Ladam[2], Isabelle Damour[1], Sophie Vacher[3], Ivan Bièche[3], Nathalie Marchand[1], Yvan de Launoit[1], David Tulasne[1] and Anne Chotteau-Lelièvre[1,4*]

Abstract

Background: The ETS transcription factor ETV4 is involved in the main steps of organogenesis and is also a significant mediator of tumorigenesis and metastasis, such as in breast cancer. Indeed, ETV4 is overexpressed in breast tumors and is associated with distant metastasis and poor prognosis. However, the cellular and molecular events regulated by this factor are still misunderstood. In mammary epithelial cells, ETV4 controls the expression of many genes, *MMP13* among them. The aim of this study was to understand the function of MMP13 during ETV4-driven tumorigenesis.

Methods: Different constructs of the *MMP13* gene promoter were used to study the direct regulation of *MMP13* by ETV4. Moreover, cell proliferation, migration, invasion, anchorage-independent growth, and in vivo tumorigenicity were assayed using models of mammary epithelial and cancer cells in which the expression of MMP13 and/or ETV4 is modulated. Importantly, the expression of *MMP13* and *ETV4* messenger RNA was characterized in 456 breast cancer samples.

Results: Our results revealed that ETV4 promotes proliferation, migration, invasion, and anchorage-independent growth of the MMT mouse mammary tumorigenic cell line. By investigating molecular events downstream of ETV4, we found that MMP13, an extracellular metalloprotease, was an ETV4 target gene. By overexpressing or repressing MMP13, we showed that this metalloprotease contributes to proliferation, migration, and anchorage-independent clonogenicity. Furthermore, we demonstrated that MMP13 inhibition disturbs proliferation, migration, and invasion induced by ETV4 and participates to ETV4-induced tumor formation in immunodeficient mice. Finally, ETV4 and MMP13 co-overexpression is associated with poor prognosis in breast cancer.

Conclusion: MMP13 potentiates the effects of the ETV4 oncogene during breast cancer genesis and progression.

Keywords: ETV4, Transcription factor, MMP13, Tumorigenesis, Breast cancer

Background

ETV4, together with ETV1 and ETV5, constitutes the PEA3 group among the 12 subgroups of the ETS transcription factor family, defined by their conserved DNA binding domain (ETS binding domain) [1, 2]. They control the development of various organs and are involved in the progression of many cancers, including breast cancer [1, 3–8]. ETV4 directly influences the outcome of mammary tumorigenesis induced by the ERBB2, steroid receptor coactivator 1, and Wnt1 oncogenes [9–11]. However, the cellular and molecular mechanisms regulated by the ETV4 factor during mammary cancer progression are still poorly understood.

In most cases, carcinogenesis is associated with an overexpression of ETV4 promoting proliferation, migration, and/or invasion involved in the tumorigenic and/or metastatic process. As a consequence, deregulation of ETV4 target genes has a key role in these processes. Few ETV4 target genes involved in the regulation of these

---

* Correspondence: anne.chotteau@ibl.cnrs.fr
[1]University of Lille, CNRS, Institut Pasteur de Lille, UMR 8161 - M3T – Mechanisms of Tumorigenesis and Targeted Therapies, F-59000 Lille, France
[4]CNRS UMR 8161, Institut de Biologie de Lille - Institut Pasteur de Lille, 1 Rue Pr Calmette, BP447, 59021 Lille, France
Full list of author information is available at the end of the article

biological responses have been described so far, particularly in the mammary cells and tissues. In these latter cases, ETV4 has been shown to regulate the expression of several matrix metalloproteases (MMPs), such as MMP2 or MMP9; transcription factors involved in epithelial-to-mesenchymal transition (EMT), such as Twist1 or Snail; or other cancer-related factors, such as Bax, cyclin D3, or cyclin D2. Therefore, they play an active role during the acquisition of invasive properties by mammary cancer cells [8, 10, 12–15]. A transcriptome-wide identification of ETV4-responsive genes in mammary cells has shown that many more genes are potentially regulated by ETV4, although it is still unclear if they are direct targets and what roles they could play in the context of ETV4-driven tumorigenesis [16]. Therefore, the precise characterization of ETV4 target genes in the context of mammary tumorigenesis will allow a better understanding of the molecular mechanisms involved in this pathology.

MMP13 is one of those genes and was identified as being downregulated following ETV4 knock-down in mammary epithelial cells [16]. MMP13 (collagenase 3) belongs to the collagenase subfamily of MMPs and degrades all fibrillary collagens, particularly the type II collagen [17]. MMP13 has a role in different kind of cancer [18] and is overexpressed in a variety of malignant tumors [19]. It was first identified from overexpressing breast carcinomas [20]. Although the role of MMP13 in mammary tumorigenesis has been reported [18, 21–27], its regulation in the oncogenic process is still misunderstood. Indeed, MMP13 is expressed in the endothelium surrounding breast tumors, suggesting a role in the modulation of extracellular matrix degradation and cell-matrix interactions involved in metastasis [20, 28]. Consistently, functional evidence demonstrates that MMP13 increases the invasive capacities of the malignant cells in breast cancer [29–31]. Yet, the precise role of the MMP13 protein and how the *MMP13* gene is transcriptionally regulated during mammary tumorigenesis remain unclear.

On the basis of the results of this study, we first report that *MMP13* is an ETV4 target gene in various mammary cellular models, and we identify an ETS binding site necessary for the direct regulation of the *MMP13* gene promoter by ETV4. Second, by establishing ETV4- and MMP13-overexpressing and MMP13-repressing MMT cells to assess modification of the phenotypic cellular properties, we show that ETV4 significantly promotes cell proliferation, migration, invasion, and anchorage-independent growth. Moreover, we provide evidence that MMP13, to a lesser extent, presents the same contribution. Next, we assess the consequences of MMP13 knock-down in ETV4-controlled events. Interestingly, MMP13 inhibition disturbs the positive effect of ETV4 on MMT proliferation, migration, and invasion, and we demonstrate that MMP13 acts as a relay of

ETV4 in its functional role in the mammary epithelial tumorigenic cells in vitro as well as in tumor graft assays in vivo. Finally, we investigate the ETV4-MMP13 link in breast cancer samples and describe that the association of both ETV4 and MMP13 overexpression is associated with poor patient outcome. Ultimately, these data shed light on a new ETV4 relay, the extracellular metalloprotease MMP13, which could potentially be targeted in the context of ETV4-controlled mammary tumorigenesis.

Methods
Cell culture and reagents
The TAC murine mammary epithelial cell line [32, 33] was cultured on collagen-coated plates in Gibco high-glucose DMEM (Thermo Fisher Scientific, Waltham, MA, USA) supplemented with 10% FCS, penicillin (110 IU/ml), and streptomycin (110 µg/ml). A wild-type mouse mammary tumor (MMT) cell line (ATCC® CCL-51™; American Type Culture Collection, Manassas, VA, USA) was cultured in DMEM supplemented with 10% (vol/vol) FBS, gentamicin (100 IU/ml), and nonessential amino acids (Gibco; Thermo Fisher Scientific). The MCF10A cell line (ATCC® CRL-10317™; American Type Culture Collection) was propagated in DMEM/F-12 medium (Gibco; Thermo Fisher Scientific) supplemented with 5% horse serum, 20 ng/ml epidermal growth factor, 100 ng/ml cholera toxin, 500 ng/ml hydrocortisone, and 0.01 mg/ml insulin.

Plasmids
pTracer-ETV4 and pLPCX-ETV4-V5 plasmids were described previously [8, 12, 32]. pMX-MMP13 was generated by PCR amplification of the mouse *MMP13* complementary DNA (cDNA) and cloned into the pMX-Puro retroviral vector. pRS-shMMP13 retroviral plasmid was kindly provided by S. Meierjohann [34]. pGL3 constructs containing different parts of the *MMP13* promoter were kindly provided by J. M. Davidson [35]. Mutations to proximal ETS and activator protein (AP)-1 binding site in MMP13 promoter were made using the QuikChange® II XL Site-Directed Mutagenesis Kit (Agilent Technologies, Santa Clara, CA, USA). The proximal ETS site was changed from **GG**AA to **CC**AA, and the proximal AP-1 site was changed from **TG**ACT to **GC**ACT. The sequence of all promoter constructs was verified by DNA sequencing.

Retroviral infections and stable selection
HEK293GP packaging cells (Clontech) (3×10^6) were transfected with pLPCX, pMX, or pRS retroviral constructs, and 1.2×10^6 MMT cells or 1×10^6 MCF-10A cells per 100-mm dish were incubated with supernatant as previously described [16]. The selection procedure was started the next day using puromycin (Life Technologies, Carlsbad, CA, USA).

Stable cell lines

TAC cells overexpressing ETV4 after retroviral infection (ETV4) and control mock-infected TAC cells (ctrl) were previously described [8]. MMT cells infected with pLPCX retroviral vector (Ctrl) were used as a control for MMT cells overexpressing ETV4 after retroviral infection with the pLPCX-ETV4 vector (ETV4). MMT cells infected with pMX retroviral vector (Ctrl) were used as a control for MMT cells overexpressing MMP13 after retroviral infection with the pMX-MMP13 vector (MMP13).

MMT cells infected with pRS retroviral vector (shCtrl) were used as a control for MMT cells overexpressing shMMP13 after retroviral infection with the pRS-shMMP13 vector (shMMP13). MMT-ETV4 cells (overexpressing ETV4) infected with pRS retroviral vector (ETV4 + shCtrl) were used as a control for MMT-ETV4 cells overexpressing shMMP13 after retroviral infection with the pRS-shMMP13 vector (ETV4 + shMMP13).

RNA extraction, reverse transcription, and real-time qPCR

Total RNA was extracted using the RNeasy Mini Kit according to the manufacturer's instructions (Qiagen, Hilden, Germany). Total RNA (1 μg) was reverse-transcribed using the high-capacity cDNA reverse transcription kit (Life Technologies). Specific gene expression was determined by real-time PCR using the Fast SYBR® Green Master Mix (Life Technologies) and the Mx3005P qPCR system (Agilent Technologies). The results were analyzed with the comparative cycle threshold method normalized to cyclophilin A and compared with a comparator sample. The nucleotide sequences of the primers used were as follows: MMP13-F (5′-TCCCTGCCCCTTCCCTATGG-3′) and MMP13-R (5′-CTCGGAGCCTGTCAACTGTGG-3′) for the *MMP13* gene (PCR product of 173 bp), ETV4-F (5′-CCGCTCGCT GCGATACTATT-3′) and ETV4-R (5′-CGGTCAAAC TCAGCCTTCAGA-3′) for the *ETV4* gene (PCR product of 162 bp), and PPIA-F (5′-GGGAACCGTTTGTGTTTGG T-3′) and PPIA-R (5′-TGTGCCAGGGTGGTGACTTT-3′) for *PPIA* gene.

Luciferase reporter assays

TAC cells (3×10^4) were seeded in 12-well plates and transfected with ExGen 500 (Euromedex, Strasbourg, France) and 250 ng of DNA (200 ng of expression vector, 25 ng of firefly luciferase reporter vector, 25 ng of the Renilla luciferase pRL-TK; Promega, Madison, WI, USA), according to a protocol previously described [12].

Chromatin immunoprecipitation

TAC pLNCX, pLNCX-ETV4 and MMT pLPCX, pLPCX ETV4 were fixed, lysed, and used for chromatin immunoprecipitation (ChIP) with an anti-ETV4 immunoglobulin G

(IgG) (sc-113x; Santa Cruz Biotechnology, Dallas, TX, USA) or a nonrelevant antibody normal rabbit IgG (sc-2027), as described in Additional file 1. Detection of specific DNA regions was performed by PCR using the *MMP13* gene promoter region and CCND2 gene promoter region. The nucleotide sequences of the primers used were as follows: MMP13 forward: 5′-TCCATTTCCCTCAGATTCTGCCA C-3′ and MMP13 reverse: 5′- TCTCTCCTTCCCAGGGC AAGCAT-3′ for the *MMP13* gene (PCR product of 164 bp) and CCND2 forward: 5′-GAGAGGGAGGGAAAGATTG AAAGGA-3′ and CCND2 reverse: 5′- AGGTGGGCG AGCGGAGCCTCAAG-3′ for the CCND2 gene (PCR product of 212 bp).

RNA interference

MMP13 and oligonucleotides used for RNA interference were purchased from Dharmacon (SMARTpool ON-TARGET*plus MMP13* J-047459, Dharmacon, Lafayette, CO, USA) and consisted of a mix of four siRNAs: J-047459-12-GGCCCAUACAGUUUGAAUA/J-047459 11-AGACUAUGGACAAAGAUUA/J-047459-10-UCA AAUGGUCCCAAACGAA/J-047459-9-CUGCGACUC UUGCGGGAAU. Control oligonucleotide consisted of ON-TARGET*plus* nontargeting siRNA#1 (D-00181 0-01-UGGUUUACAUGUCGACUAA control siRNA). MMT cells (3.5×10^5) were seeded in six-well plates for reverse transfection with 75 pmol of each siRNA and 5 μl of Lipofectamine® 2000 reagent (Thermo Fisher Scientific) as recommended by the manufacturer. Cells were incubated for another 24 hours under standard conditions before being assayed.

Western blotting

Cells were lysed in buffer made of 150 mM NaCl, 50 mM Tris-HCl, pH 7.5, 1% Nonidet P-40 (vol/vol), 1 mM sodium orthovanadate, 1 mM phenylmethylsulfo-nyl fluoride, 10 g/ml leupeptin, and 10 g/ml aprotinin. After scraping, cellular debris was removed by centrifugation at $10,000 \times g$ for 5 minutes. Protein concentrations were determined by using a Bradford assay. For the supernatant, a subconfluent culture was grown for 24 hours in serum-free medium, then the supernatant was centrifuged at $3000 \times g$ for 3 minutes. Whole-cell extracts (50 μg) or 1:20 of supernatants were separated in precast gels (Mini-PROTEAN® TGX Stain-Free™; Bio-Rad Laboratories, Hercules, CA, USA) gel and transferred onto nitrocellulose membranes (Trans-Blot Turbo Transfer System; Bio-Rad Laboratories). After blocking with Tris-buffered saline, 0.1% Tween, and 3% bovine serum albumin (BSA), the membrane was probed with the primary and secondary antibodies. The enzymatic activity was detected using an Amersham enhanced chemiluminescence kit (GE Healthcare Life Sciences, Marblehead, MA, USA). Equal transfer of proteins from the gel was controlled by using the stain-free system of the gel and the membrane as well as by using an anti-GAPDH antibody. We used anti-ETV4 1:500 (GTX114393; GeneTex, Irvine, CA, USA), anti-MMP13 1:500 (18165-1-AP; Proteintech, Rosemont, IL, USA), anti-GAPDH 1:1000 (6C5-sc-32233; Santa Cruz Biotechnology), and secondary antimouse or antirabbit antibodies coupled to horseradish peroxidase (HRP) (GE Healthcare Life Sciences).

Zymography

Gelatin zymography was used to determine the activity of MMP13. The supernatant from subconfluent serum-free culture medium was collected, and the cells were removed by centrifugation. Then, 40 µl of sample were loaded onto a 10% precast polyacrylamide gel with 0.1% of gelatin (Bio-Rad Laboratories). After electrophoresis, the gels were renatured by soaking for 30 minutes at room temperature in 2.5% Triton X-100. The gels were then incubated in a developing buffer (50 mM Tris, 200 mM NaCl, 5 mM CaCl$_2$, 0.02% Brij-35 [MilliporeSigma], pH 7.5) overnight at 37 °C. The gels were stained with Coomassie Brilliant Blue R-250 and destained in demineralized water. The transparent bands of gelatinolytic activity were visualized as clear bands against the blue-stained gelatin background.

Cell proliferation assays

Stable MMT cells (1.5×10^4; pLPCX/pLPCX-ETV4-pMX/pMX-MMP13-pRS/pRS-shMMP13 and MMT-ETV4-pRS/MMT-ETV4-pRS-shMMP13) were seeded in six-well plates. The cells were trypsinized and counted after 10, 35, 55, 80, and 100 hours using an Invitrogen Tali™ Image-based Cytometer (Thermo Fisher Scientific). Each time point was counted three times.

Anchorage-independent growth

Stable MMT cells (3×10^5; pLPCX/pLPCX-ETV4-pMX/pMX-MMP13-pRS/pRS-shMMP13 and MMT-ETV4-pRS/MMT-ETV4-pRS-shMMP13) were seeded in 500 µl of medium mixed with 1 ml of 0.35% agar in growth medium (DMEM [Thermo Fisher Scientific] with 10% FBS). The cell suspension was cast onto 12-well plates with 500 µl of 0.65% agar in growth medium, which was used as an underlay. Growth medium was added onto the agar layer and changed weekly. Colonies were photographed after 10 days using a light microscope (Axio Vert A.1; Carl Zeiss Microscopy, Jena, Germany).

Cell migration assays

Boyden chamber cell migration was assayed using a cell culture chamber insert system (BD Biosciences, San Jose, CA, USA) with an 8-µm polyethylene terephthalate (PET) membrane. Stable MMT cells (4×10^4;

pLPCX/pLPCX-ETV4-pMX/pMX-MMP13-pRS/pRS-shMMP13 and MMT-ETV4-pRS/MMT-ETV4-pRS-shMMP13) were seeded in the upper chamber in DMEM with 10% FBS. The same medium was added in the lower chamber. After 18 hours, cells that did not cross the membrane were scraped off the upper side of the membrane with a cotton swab. Cells that had migrated to the lower side were fixed with methanol at − 20 °C and stained with Hoechst 33258 (MilliporeSigma). The membrane was excised from its support and mounted on a glass side with Dako Glycergel mounting medium (Agilent Technologies). Cells were photographed using a light microscope (Axio Vert A.1) and counted using ImageJ software (National Institutes of Health, Bethesda, MD, USA).

Cell invasion assays

Boyden chamber cell invasion was assayed using a cell culture chamber insert system (Corning® BioCoat™ Growth Factor Reduced Matrigel® Invasion Chamber; Corning Life Sciences, Corning, NY, USA) with an 8-µm PET membrane coated with Matrigel®. Stable MMT cells (8×10^4; pLPCX/pLPCX-ETV4-pMX/pMX-MMP13-pRS/pRS-shMMP13 and MMT-ETV4-pRS/MMT-ETV4-pRS-shMMP13) were seeded in the upper chamber in DMEM with 0% FBS and 0.1% BSA. DMEM with 5% FBS was added in the lower chamber. After 36 hours, cells that did not cross the membrane were scraped off the upper side of the membrane with a cotton swab. Cells that had migrated to the lower side were fixed with methanol at − 20 °C and stained with Hoechst 33258. The membrane was excised from its support and mounted on a glass side with Dako Glycergel mounting medium. Cells were photographed using a light microscope (Axio Vert A.1) and counted using ImageJ software.

Tumor grafts

MMT pLPCX-ETV4-pRS and MMT pLPCX-ETV4-pRS-shMMP13 cells were trypsinized, then suspended in PBS (5×10^6 cells/ml). Cells (5×10^5) were injected subcutaneously into the inguinal flank of 6–7-week-old female severe combined immunodeficiency (SCID)-deficient mice. A total of six mice per condition were used in three independent experiments. Tumor size was assessed by measuring the length and width of tumors every 3–4 days. Tumor volume was estimated using the formula: (length × width^2)/2. The experiments were stopped when the largest tumors reached the critical size of about 10% of the mouse's weight in accordance with the ethical approval form, thus meaning between 2 and 3 weeks postinjection. At the time the mice were killed, the tumors were removed, fixed in 4% paraformaldehyde, and embedded in paraffin. Results are expressed as the mean tumor volume for each experimental group. All animal procedures were conducted with the approval of and in compliance with the guidelines of the Nord Pas de Calais Regional for Ethical Animal Care and Use Committee (CEEA-003243.01).

IHC

IHC of paraffin-embedded mouse tumor tissue sections was performed using anti-ETV4 (1:100, GTX100812; GeneTex), anti-MMP13 (1:100, 18165-1-AP; Proteintech), anti-Ki67 (1:200, ab15580; Abcam, Cambridge, UK), and anti-cleaved caspase 3 (1:100, Asp175, catalogue no. 9661; Cell Signaling Technology, Danvers, MA, USA). Sections were incubated with secondary HRP-conjugated antibody. Counterstaining was performed using Mayer's hematoxylin (Merck, Darmstadt, Germany). Imaging was carried out using ZEN Blue imaging software (Carl Zeiss Microscopy).

Patients and samples for MMP13 and ETV4 expression

Samples of 456 primary unilateral invasive breast tumors excised from women managed at Curie Institute-René Huguenin Hospital (St. Cloud, France) from 1978 to 2008 were analyzed. Immediately after biopsy or surgery, the tumor samples were stored in liquid nitrogen until messenger RNA (mRNA) extraction. Tumor samples were considered suitable for our study if the proportion of tumor cells exceeded 70%.

All patients (mean age 61.7 years, range 31–91 years) met the following criteria: primary unilateral nonmetastatic breast carcinoma for which complete clinical, histological, and biological data were available; no radiotherapy or chemotherapy before surgery; and full follow-up at Curie Institute-René Huguenin Hospital. Treatment consisted of modified radical mastectomy in 278 cases (63.6%) and breast-conserving surgery plus locoregional radiotherapy in 159 cases (36.4%) (information available for only 437 cases). The patients underwent a physical examination and routine chest radiography every 3 months for 2 years, then annually. Mammograms were done annually. Adjuvant therapy was administered to 369 patients, consisting of chemotherapy alone in 91 cases, hormone therapy alone in 176 cases, and both treatments in 102 cases. The histological type and the number of positive axillary nodes were established at the time of surgery. The malignancy of infiltrating carcinomas was scored according to the Scarff-Bloom-Richardson (SBR) histoprognostic grading system. Hormone receptor (HR) [estrogen receptor (ERα), progesterone receptor (PR)] and human epidermal growth factor receptor 2 (ERBB2) status were determined at the protein level by using biochemical methods (dextran-coated charcoal method, enzyme immunoassay, or IHC) and confirmed by qPCR assays as described in Additional file 1.

The population was divided into four groups according to HR (ERα and PR) and ERBB2 status, as follows: two luminal subtypes [HR+ (ERα + or PR+)/ERBB2+ (n = 54)] and [HR+ (ERα + or PR+)/ERBB2− (n = 289)]; an ERBB2+ subtype [HR− (ERα− and PR−)/ERBB2+ (n = 45)] and a triple-negative subtype [HR− (ERα− and PR−)/ERBB2− (n = 68)]. The median follow-up was 8.9 years (range 130 days to 33.2 years). One hundred eighty-one patients had a metastasis. Clinicopathological characteristics of patients in relation to metastasis-free survival (MFS) are provided in Additional file 2: Table S1. Ten specimens of adjacent normal breast tissue from patients with breast cancer or normal breast tissue from women undergoing cosmetic breast surgery were used as sources of normal mRNA.

Statistical analysis

For in vitro and in vivo analyses, all values are expressed the means of triplicate samples ± SE. Data were analyzed using unpaired t tests.

For human statistical analysis, relationships between mRNA expression of genes and clinical parameters were identified using nonparametric tests, the χ^2 nonparametric test (relationship between two qualitative parameters), and the Kruskal-Wallis H test (relationship between one quantitative parameter and two or more qualitative parameters). Differences were considered significant at confidence levels greater than 95% ($P < 0.05$). MFS was determined as the interval between initial diagnosis and detection of the first metastasis.

To visualize the efficacy of $MMP13$ and $ETV4$ mRNA levels for discriminating between two populations (patients who developed/did not develop metastases) in the absence of an arbitrary cutoff value, data were summarized in an ROC curve. The AUC was calculated as a single measure to discriminate efficacy. The population was divided into four patient subgroups according to $MMP13$ ROC curve value in the series of 456 breast cancer samples and then according to $ETV4$ ROC curve value in the high and low $MMP13$ mRNA expression level subpopulations. Finally, the very small subgroup ($n = 16$) of high $MMP13$/low $ETV4$ mRNA expression level was merged with the subgroup ($n = 66$) of low $MMP13$/low $ETV4$ mRNA expression level to obtain a unique group of 82 patients with low $ETV4$ mRNA expression level. Survival distributions were estimated by the Kaplan-Meier method, and the significance of differences between survival rates was ascertained with the log-rank test. The Cox proportional hazards regression model was used to assess prognostic significance in multivariate analysis [36]. We also analyzed an independent dataset of breast tumors for which microarray data were publicly available (Netherlands Cancer Institute [NKI], $n = 295$; http://ccb.nki.nl/data/).

Results

MMP13 is an ETV4 target gene in mammary epithelial cells

We previously described ETV4-regulated genes in mammary tumorigenic MMT cells following ETV4 inhibition [16]. Among them, MMPs such as MMPs 1, 2, 3, 9, and 14 were shown to be slightly regulated [16]. However, our attention was focused on MMP13, which was identified as a potentially interesting ETV4 target gene through large-scale transcriptomic analysis that we performed on these MMT cells [16], thereafter completed with transcriptomic analysis performed with ETV4-overexpressing and ETV4-repressing TAC cells (unpublished data). In these latter analyses, we found that ETV4 positively modulates *MMP13* gene expression (18.12-fold, $P = 0.0014$ following ETV4 overexpression; 0.16-fold, $P = 0.02$ following ETV4 inhibition). In order to characterize the regulation

of *MMP13* expression by ETV4, we used the mammary epithelial TAC cell line overexpressing ETV4 [8] as well as the mammary cancerous MMT cell line and the breast epithelial MCF10A cell line, engineered to overexpress a V5-tagged ETV4 protein after a retroviral infection (MMT-ETV4 and MCF10A-ETV4) (Fig. 1a and c and Additional file 3: Figure S1a and c). Overexpression of ETV4 upregulates *MMP13* mRNA and protein expression in the mouse TAC, MMT (Fig. 1b and d) and human MCF10A cells (Additional file 3: Figure S1b and d). Moreover, the secretion of the active form of MMP13 is increased in the supernatant of ETV4-overexpressing cells, as shown by Western blotting (Fig. 1e) and zymography (Fig. 1f).

We next completed these data by analyzing the ETV4-regulated *MMP13* promoter. TAC cells were transfected with various *MMP13* gene promoter fragments cloned into a luciferase reporter vector and ETV4 expression vector or control vector. Our results indicate that the *MMP13* promoter (− 1800) is active in TAC

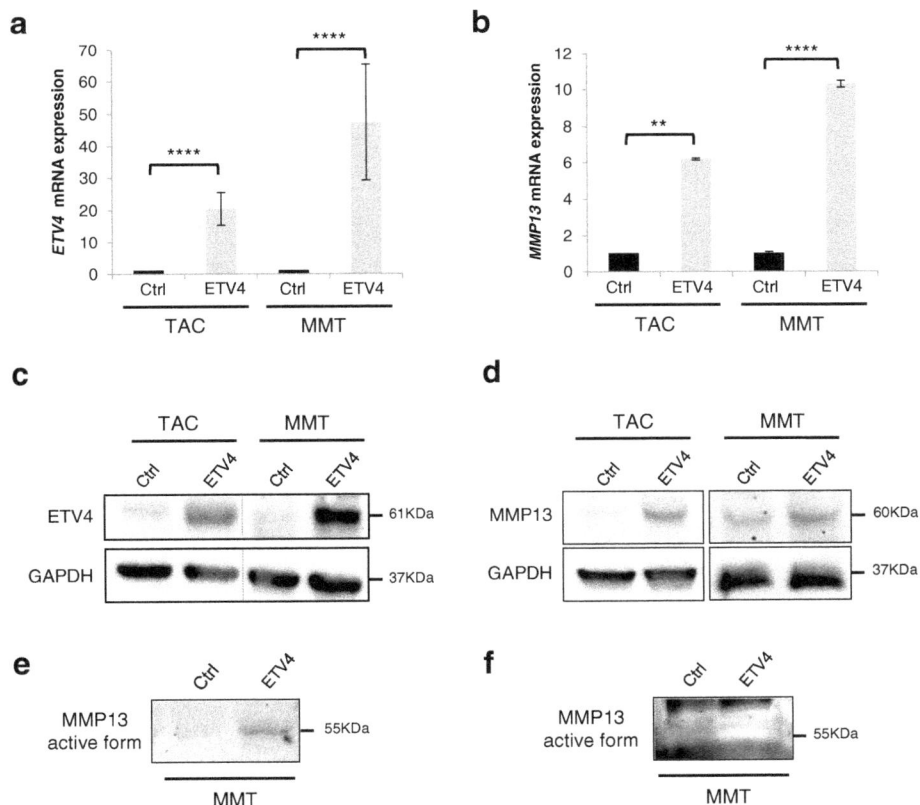

Fig. 1 Expression of ETV4 and MMP13 in TAC-Ctrl/ETV4 and MMT-Ctrl/ETV4 cells. **a** and **b** Relative *ETV4* (**a**) or *MMP13* (**b**) mRNA expression in TAC/MMT-Ctrl and TAC/MMT-ETV4-overexpressing cells determined by real-time PCR and normalized to cyclophilin A levels. mRNA expression in TAC/MMT-Ctrl cells was arbitrarily = 1. Error bars indicate SD. ****$P \leq 0.0001$; **$P \leq 0.01$. **c** and **d** Western blot analysis of ETV4 protein expression (61 kDa) (**c**) or MMP13 protein expression (60 kDa) (**d**) in TAC/MMT-Ctrl and TAC/MMT-ETV4 cells. GAPDH expression served as the loading control. **e** Western blot analysis of the secreted MMP13 protein expression (55 kDa) from the supernatant of MMT-Ctrl and MMT-ETV4-overexpressing cells. **f** Zymographic analysis of MMP13 protein activity (55 kDa) in MMT-Ctrl and MMT-ETV4 cells

cells. Moreover, ETV4 transactivates the *MMP13* gene promoter region spanning 1800 bp downstream from the translation start codon (MMP13; – 1800) (Fig. 2a and b). To delineate the responsive elements driving the promoter activity, we tested various deletion constructs (Fig. 2a) and

identified a region of 91 bp (MMP13–91), which displays an optimal promoter activity as well as induction by ETV4 (Fig. 2b). This region contains a putative ETS binding site (EBS) and a putative AP-1 binding site. These two sites are very highly conserved among mouse, human, and

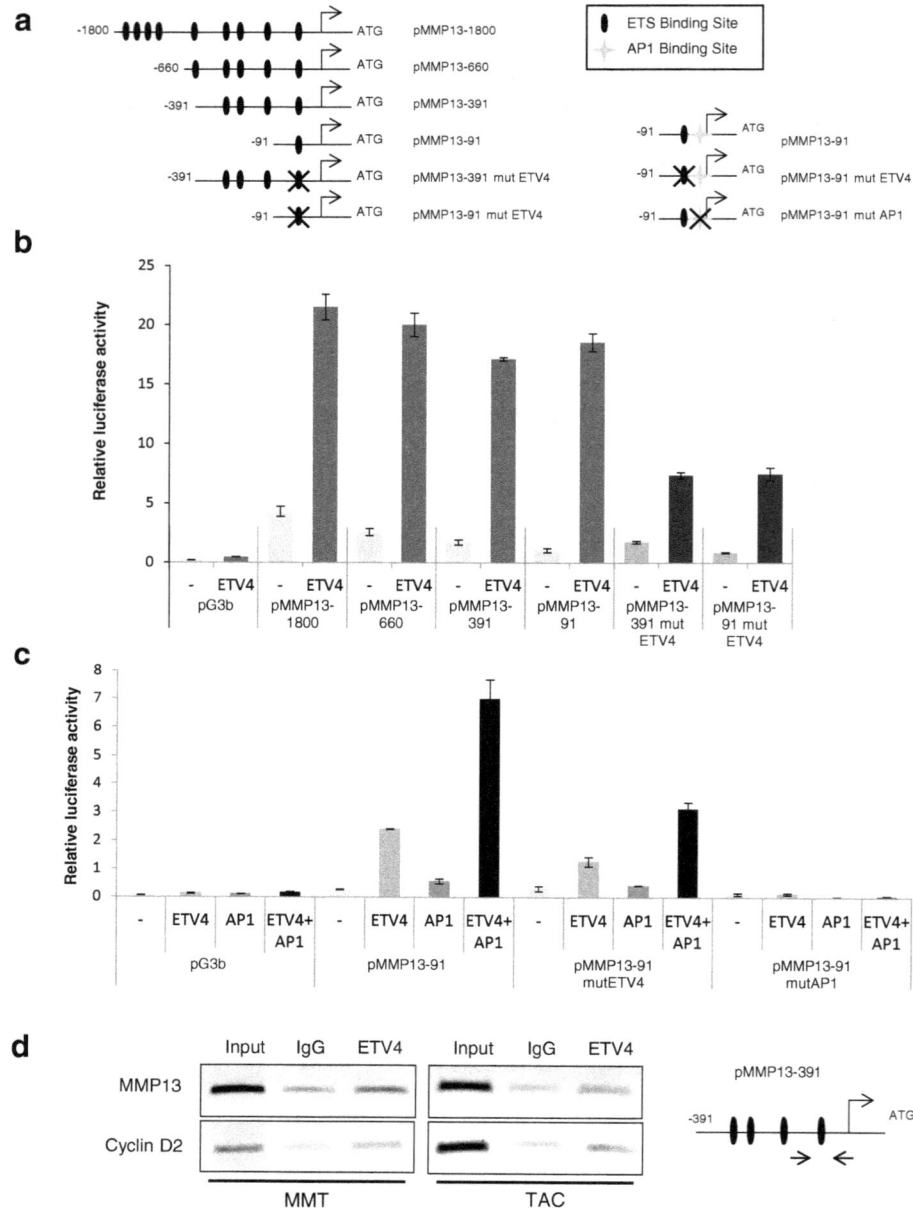

Fig. 2 *MMP13* gene is an ETV4 target gene in mammary epithelial TAC and MMT cells. Effect of ETS/AP1 binding site mutations in the *MMP13* promoter regulation. **a** Schematic representation of the mouse *MMP13* promoter fragments (pMMP13–1800 to pMMP13–91) and AP-1 and/or ETV4 mutant versions cloned into a pG3bLuc reporter vector (pG3b). Position of the conserved ETS binding sites (EBS) is represented by ●. AP-1 binding site is represented by ✦. ➤: Transcription start site. ✖: Mutation of the ETS site. **b** and **c** Histograms representing the relative luciferase activity measured for each promoter construct cotransfected into the TAC cell line with pTracer vector (−) or pTracer-ETV4 expression vector (ETV4) and/or AP-1 expression vector (AP1). Experiments were conducted three times in triplicate. Error bars indicate SD. **d** ChIP experiment. PCR detection of the *MMP13* promoter region after ETV4 immunoprecipitation in MMT (left panel) and TAC (right panel). Primers allowing the amplification of the proximal *MMP13* promoter region containing EBS are schematized in the lower panel. Cyclin D2 was used as a positive control [8]. Immunoprecipitation with a nonrelevant antibody (IgG) was used as a negative control.

rabbit [37, 38] (Additional file 4: Figure S2), and the EBS was previously described to be important in *MMP13* gene promoter activity [38]. In fact, the mutation of the EBS site in the MMP13 – 91 and MMP13 – 391 fragments reduced by half the transactivation by ETV4 (Fig. 2b). Moreover, AP-1 synergized the ETV4-induced transactivation effect, and the AP-1 site is required for this activity (Fig. 2c). We thereafter evidenced ETV4 recruitment to this chromatin region in TAC and MMT cells by ChIP using an antibody directed against ETV4, and, as a positive control, we analyzed the binding of ETV4 at the cyclin D2 promoter, as previously described [8] (Fig. 2d). It is noteworthy that the same results were obtained in TAC and MMT cells that overexpress ETV4 (Additional file 5: Figure S3). Therefore, *MMP13* is an ETV4 target gene in TAC and MMT mammary epithelial cells with AP-1 as a likely coactivator.

ETV4 enhances cell proliferation, migration, invasion, and anchorage-independent growth

Proliferation and migration assays showed that MMT cells overexpressing ETV4 display enhanced proliferation and migration abilities as determined using a Boyden chamber (Fig. 3a and b). Similar results were obtained with or without treatment with Mitomycin C, an inhibitor of proliferation, indicating that the effect on cell migration was not a consequence of an increase in cell number (data not shown). Moreover, invasion assay in a Matrigel®-overlaid Boyden chamber and in a clonogenic assay revealed that ETV4 significantly increases invasion (Fig. 3c) and anchorage-independent growth (Fig. 3d) in vitro. These data confirm that ETV4 is an important actor of the cellular abilities (proliferation, migration, invasion, anchorage-independent growth) involved in the tumorigenic properties of MMT cells.

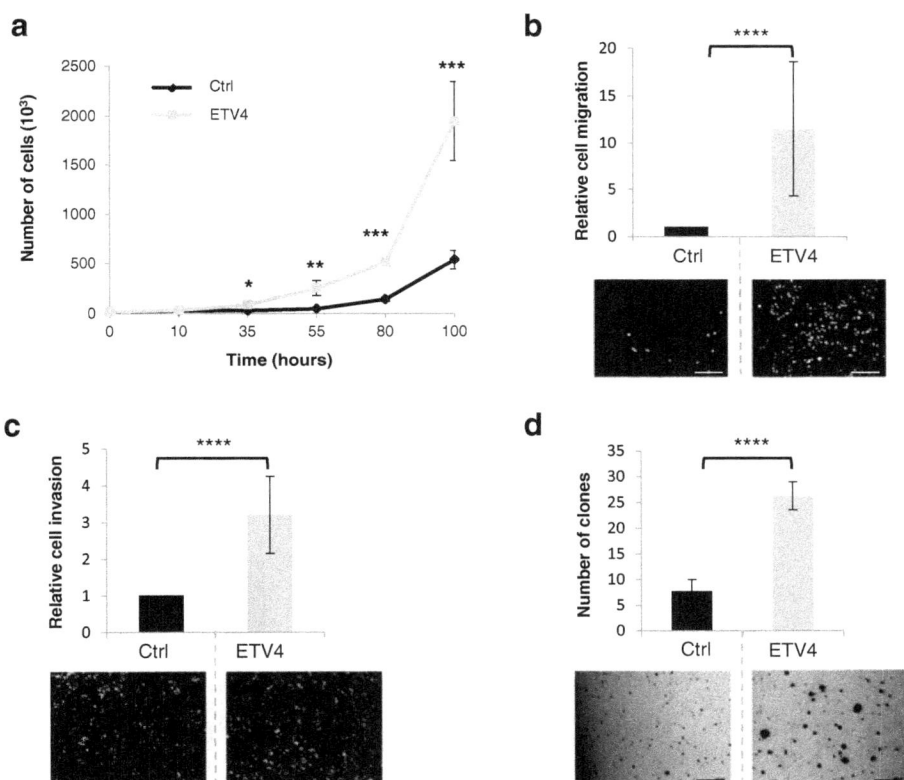

Fig. 3 ETV4 enhances proliferation, migration, invasion, and anchorage-independent growth capacity of MMT mammary cancer cells. **a** MMT-Ctrl and MMT-ETV4 cell proliferation analysis by cell counting. The two charts represent the number of counted cells at 10, 35, 55, 80, and 100 hours. Experiments were conducted three times in triplicate. Error bars indicate SD. ***$P \leq 0.001$; **$P \leq 0.01$; *$P \leq 0.1$. **b** MMT-Ctrl and MMT-ETV4 cell migration analysis using a Boyden chamber culture system. Histograms represent the relative number of counted cells that migrated to the lower side. The number of MMT-Ctrl cells was arbitrarily = 1. Experiments were conducted three times in triplicate. Error bars indicate SD. ****$P \leq 0.0001$. The lower panel depicts a representative picture of each experiment. Scale bar = 100 µm. **c** MMT-Ctrl and MMT-ETV4 cell invasion analysis using a Boyden chamber culture system coated with Matrigel®. Histogram represents the relative number of cells that invaded to the lower side. The number of MMT-Ctrl cells was arbitrarily = 1. Experiments were conducted three times in triplicate. Error bars indicate SD. ****$P \leq 0.0001$. The lower panel depicts a representative picture of each experiment. Scale bar = 100 µm. **d** Anchorage-independent growth. MMT-Ctrl and MMT-ETV4 cells were cultured for 10 days in soft agar. This histogram represents the number of clones counted for experimental time point. Soft agar assays were conducted three times in triplicate. Magnification × 5. Error bars indicate SD. ****$P \leq 0.0001$. The lower panel depicts a representative picture of each experiment. Scale bar = 100 µm

MMP13 is a regulator of ETV4-dependent tumorigenic properties in mammary cancer cells

Next, we evaluated the role of MMP13 during MMT cell migration, invasion, or clonogenicity by using MMT cells in which MMP13 is overexpressed (MMT-MMP13) or knocked down by shRNA (MMT-shMMP13). MMP13 overexpression or repression was confirmed by qPCR (Additional file 6: Figure S4a and b), Western blotting (Additional file 6: Figure S4c) and/or zymography (Additional file 6: Figure S4d). As shown in Fig. 4, MMP13

overexpression increases cell proliferation (Fig. 4a), migration (Fig. 4b), and anchorage-independent growth (Fig. 4c). As expected, MMP13 repression leads to a reduction in cell proliferation (Fig. 4d), cell migration (Fig. 4e), and anchorage-independent cell growth (Fig. 4f). Thus, similarly to ETV4, but with a weaker effect, MMP13 is an inducer of cancer cell proliferation, migration, and invasion.

In order to determine if MMP13 participates in ETV4-regulated cancer cell properties, we repressed MMP13 in the ETV4-overexpressing MMT cell line.

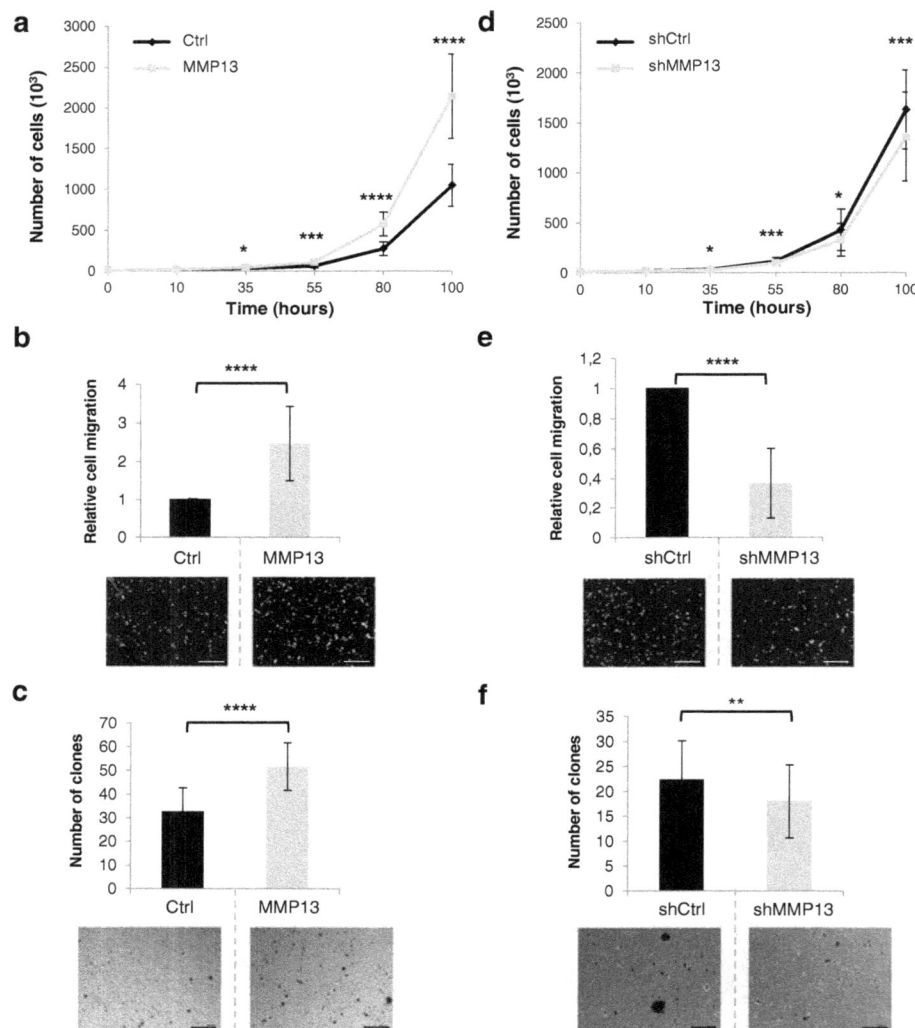

Fig. 4 MMP13 acts as ETV4 in the modification of tumorigenic properties of MMT cells. **a** and **d** MMT-Ctrl and MMT-MMP13 (**a**) or MMT-shCtrl and MMT-shMMP13 (**d**) cell proliferation analysis by cell counting. The two charts represent the number of counted cells at 10, 35, 55, 80, and 100 hours. Experiments were conducted three times in triplicate. Error bars indicate SD. ****$P \leq 0.0001$; ***$P \leq 0.001$; *$P \leq 0.1$. **b** and **e** MMT-Ctrl and MMT-MMP13 (**b**) or MMT-shCtrl and MMT-shMMP13 (**e**) cell migration analysis using a Boyden chamber culture system. Histogram represents the relative number of counted cells that migrated to the lower side. The number of MMT-Ctrl (**b**) and MMT-shCtrl (**e**) cells was arbitrarily = 1. Experiments were conducted three times in triplicate. Error bars indicate SD. ****$P \leq 0.0001$. The lower panel depicts a representative picture of each experiment. Scale bar = 100 μm. **c** and **f** Anchorage-independent growth. MMT-Ctrl and MMT-MMP13 (**c**) or MMT-shCtrl and MMT-shMMP13 (**f**) cells were cultured for 10 days in soft agar. This histogram represents the number of clones counted for experimental time points. Soft agar assays were conducted three times in triplicate. Magnification × 5. Error bars indicate SD. ****$P \leq 0.0001$; **$P \leq 0.01$. The lower panel depicts a representative picture of each experiment. Scale bar = 100 μm

To that end, we established the MMT-ETV4 + shMMP13 cell line, which expresses an MMP13-shRNA construct allowing for a significant reduction in *MMP13* mRNA expression and subsequently a reduction in MMP13 metalloprotease activity (Fig. 5a and b). Importantly, as determined by qPCR and Western blotting, ETV4 mRNA and protein expression remains unchanged in these cells (Additional file 7: Figure S5a and b). The repression of MMP13 in the ETV4-overexpressing MMT cells drastically decreases their proliferation (by 60% at 100 hours after the beginning of the experiment) (Fig. 5c) and significantly reduces cell migration (twofold decrease compared with ETV4 + shCtrl) (Fig. 5d), cell invasion (twofold decrease compared with ETV4 + shCtrl) (Fig. 5e), and anchorage-independent growth (2.5-fold increase compared with ETV4 + shCtrl) (Fig. 5f). This was confirmed by transient transfection of a siRNA directed against MMP13 in the MMT-ETV4-overexpressing cells, which led to a 60% decrease in MMP13 expression (Additional file 8: Figure S6a) and a significant reduction in anchorage-independent cell growth (Additional file 8: Figure S6b). Altogether, these results show that MMP13 acts as a relay of ETV4 to control mammary cancer cells' tumorigenic abilities.

MMP13 silencing inhibits the tumorigenic activity of ETV4 in vivo

To investigate whether MMP13 expression is necessary for the induction of tumors by ETV4 in vivo, MMT-ETV4 + shCtrl and MMT-ETV4 + shMMP13 cells were injected into the inguinal flanks of immunocompromised mice, and tumor growth was evaluated every 3–4 days (Fig. 6). Three days postinjection, all of the mice that received an injection of MMT-ETV4 + shCtrl cells showed a palpable tumor, whereas none could be detected at this stage in the group that received an injection of MMT-ETV4 + shMMP13 cells. By day 6 postinjection, all MMT-injected mice developed palpable tumors. However, a 3–4-day measurement of tumor size over the course of 10 more days (until animals were killed) indicated that MMP13 expression was required for optimal tumor growth because MMP13-shRNA-expressing ETV4 cells are, on average, twofold smaller than controls. Immunocytochemistry performed on paraffin-embedded mouse tumor tissue sections showed an equivalent Ki-67 expression in tumors from ETV4 + shCtrl and ETV4 + shMMP13 cells, which all show proliferative activity. Cleaved caspase 3 expression showed that apoptosis events are present in both conditions, to a slightly greater extent in the ETV4 + shMMP13 tumors, according to their slow growth. ETV4 expression is, as expected, equivalent in both ETV4-expressing cell-derived tumors. In contrast, MMP13 expression decreased in ETV4 + shMMP13-derived tumors, thus confirming the suitable

MMP13 regulation (here a repression) in these in vivo assays (Fig. 6b). Therefore, these data bring out that MMP13 is a mediator of ETV4 tumorigenic activity in MMT cancer cells.

MMP13 and ETV4 expression in breast tumors is associated with a poor prognosis

In order to corroborate the relevance of the phenotypic and mouse in vivo data and to explore the link between ETV4 and MMP13 in human breast cancer, we assessed *MMP13* and *ETV4* mRNA expression levels in a series of 456 primary unilateral invasive primary breast tumors from patients with known clinical and pathological status and long-term outcome. We used a log-rank test to identify relationships between MFS and *MMP13* and/or *ETV4* expression. Tumors with the highest levels of *MMP13* mRNA ($n = 135$ [29.6%]) were significantly associated with poor MFS ($P = 0.00016$), which was not the case for ETV4-expressing tumors (Additional file 9: Figure S7a and b). This result was confirmed in the NKI breast cancer cohort (Additional file 10: Figure S8b and c). Combined analysis (as described in the "Patients and samples for MMP13 and ETV4 expression" subsection of the Methods section above) of *MMP13* and *ETV4* mRNA expression levels defined three separate prognostic groups of 82 (Low-ETV4), 255 (High-ETV4/Low-MMP13), and 119 (High-ETV4/High-MMP13) patients with significantly different survival ($P = 0.000041$) (Fig. 7). The patients with the poorest prognosis were observed in the subgroup of 119 of 456 (26.1%) patients characterized by association of high *MMP13* and high *ETV4* mRNA expression levels. These data were also confirmed in the NKI breast cancer cohort ($P = 0.0013$) (Additional file 10: Figure S8a). Multivariate analysis using a Cox proportional hazards model was performed to assess the prognostic value for MFS of the parameters found to be significant in univariate analysis (i.e., SBR histological grade, lymph node status, macroscopic tumor size, PR status [Additional file 2: Table S1] and combined *MMP13* and *ETV4* mRNA levels). The prognostic significance of the lymph node status ($P = 0.000016$), macroscopic tumor size ($P = 0.0028$), and combined *MMP13* and *ETV4* mRNA level was maintained (Additional file 11: Table S2).

We sought links between the three prognostic groups and classical clinicopathological parameters in breast cancer (Table 1). Using HR (ERα and PR) and ERBB2 status, we also subdivided the total population ($n = 456$) into four breast cancer molecular subtypes: HR+/ERBB2+ ($n = 54$), HR+/ERBB2– ($n = 289$), HR–/ERBB2+ ($n = 45$) and HR–/ERBB2– ($n = 68$). High *MMP13* and *ETV4* mRNA expression levels were associated with negative ER status ($P = 0.00067$) and the HR–/ERBB2+ subtype ($P = 0.0015$), two parameters associated with breast

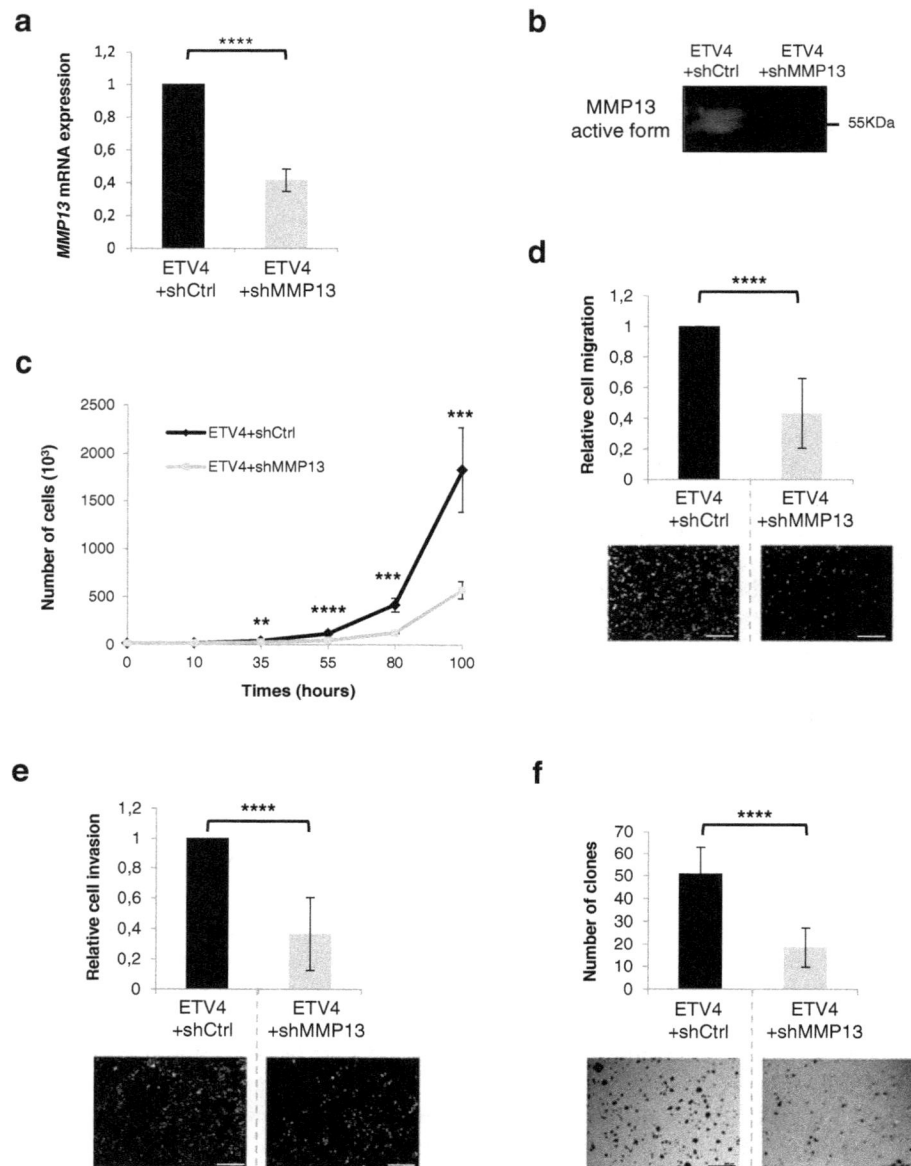

Fig. 5 MMP13 acts as a regulator of ETV4 tumorigenic-induced response in mammary epithelial MMT cells. **a** Relative *MMP13* mRNA expression in the MMT-ETV4 + shCtrl and MMT-ETV4 + shMMP13 cells determined by real-time PCR and normalized to cyclophilin A levels. mRNA expression in MMT-ETV4 + shCtrl cells was arbitrarily = 1. Error bars indicate SD. ****$P \leq 0.0001$. **b** Zymographic analysis of MMP13 protein activity (55 kDa) from the supernatant of MMT-ETV4 + shCtrl and MMT-ETV4 + shMMP13 cells. **c** MMT-ETV4 + shCtrl and MMT-ETV4 + shMMP13 cell proliferation analysis by cell counting. The two charts represent the number of counted cells at 10, 35, 55, 80, and 100 hours. Experiments were conducted three times in triplicate. Error bars indicate SD. ****$P \leq 0.0001$; ***$P \leq 0.001$; **$P \leq 0.01$. **d** MMT-ETV4 + shCtrl and MMT-ETV4 + shMMP13 cell migration analysis using a Boyden chamber culture system. Histogram represents the relative number of counted cells that migrated to the lower side. The number of MMT-ETV4 + shCtrl cells was arbitrarily = 1. Experiments were conducted three times in triplicate. Error bars indicate SD. ****$P \leq 0.0001$. The lower panel depicts a representative picture of each experiment. Scale bar = 100 μm. **e** MMT-ETV4 + shCtrl and MMT-ETV4 + shMMP13 cell invasion analysis using a Boyden chamber culture system coated with Matrigel®. Histograms represent the relative number of counted cells that invaded to the lower side. The number of MMT-ETV4 + shCtrl cells was arbitrarily = 1. Experiments were conducted three times in triplicate. Error bars indicate SD. ****$P \leq 0.0001$. The lower panel depicts a representative picture of each experiment. Scale bar = 100 μm. **f** Anchorage-independent growth. MMT-ETV4 + shCtrl and MMT-ETV4 + shMMP13 cells were cultured for 10 days in soft agar. This histogram represents the number of clones counted for experimental time points. Soft agar assays were conducted three times in triplicate. Magnification × 5. Error bars indicate SD. ****$P \leq 0.0001$. The lower panel depicts a representative picture of each experiment. Scale bar = 100 μm

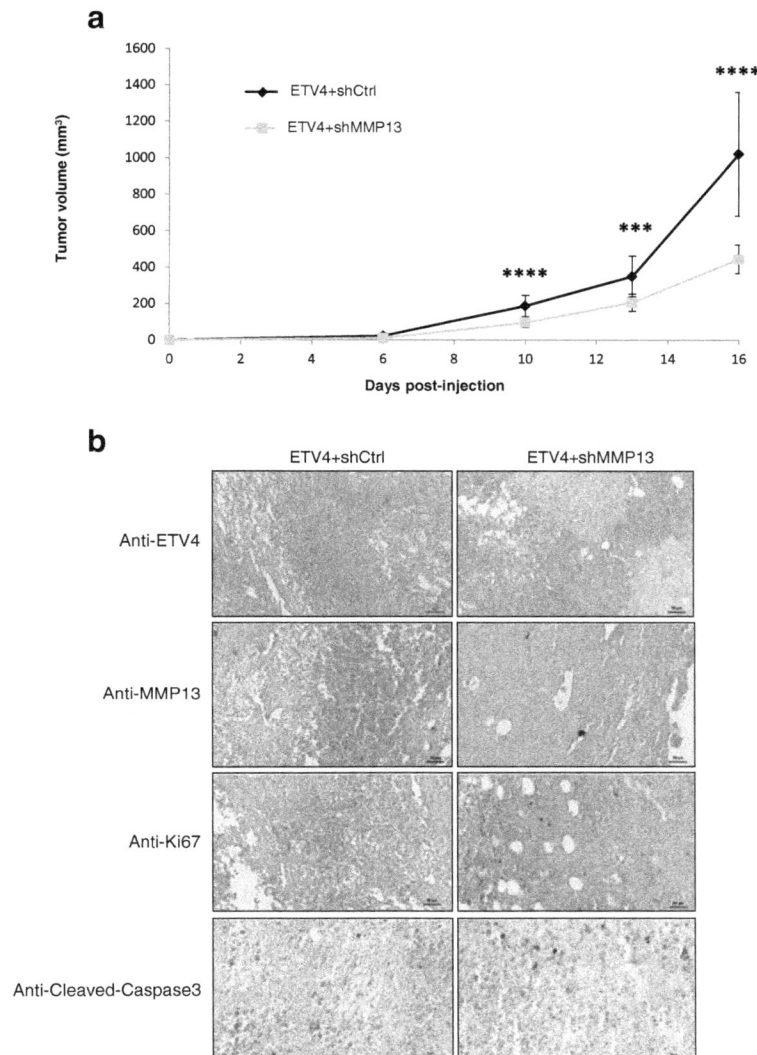

Fig. 6 MMP13 reinforces the tumorigenic activity of ETV4 in vivo. **a** In vivo tumor growth assay. Tumor presence was determined by palpation of the mammary gland every 3–4 days. The graph represents the volume of tumor (mm³) versus time in weeks after graft of MMT-ETV4 + shCtrl ($n = 14$) and MMT-ETV4 + shMMP13 ($n = 15$) cells into the fat pad of the mammary gland of SCID-deficient mice. Three independent experiments were conducted. ***$P \leq 0.001$ and ****$P \leq 0.0001$. **b** Histologic analysis of ETV4 + shCtrl MMT cell-derived tumors (left panel) and ETV4 + shMMP13 MMT cell-derived tumors (right panel) with anti-ETV4 antibody, anti-MMP13 antibody, anti-Ki67 antibody, and anti-cleaved caspase 3 antibody. Representative staining is shown for each experiment. Scale bar = 50 μm

cancer aggressiveness (Table 1). We did not observe a correlation between the three prognostic groups and mutations of *PIK3CA*, which is the most frequently mutated oncogene in breast cancer ($P = 0.96$), as well as mRNA level of the *MKI67* gene, which encodes for the proliferation-related Ki-67 antigen ($P = 0.073$).

Discussion

ETV4 is an ETS transcription factor involved in important steps of organ development, such as in mammary gland morphogenesis. ETV4 is also a significant mediator of tumorigenesis through the activation of several downstream pathways that are associated with migration and invasion. ETV4 is overexpressed in breast tumors and is associated with distant metastasis and poor prognosis [1, 5, 39, 40]. However, the cellular and molecular events regulated by this factor remain poorly understood. We previously identified target genes implicated in phenotypic cellular modulation induced in mammary tumorigenesis as Bax or cyclin D2. We have described cyclin D2 to act as a negative regulator of the ETV4-induced responses in mammary cancer cells [8, 12]. We also described that ETV4 overexpression in a mammary epithelial cell line confers tumorigenesis-like properties as well as an

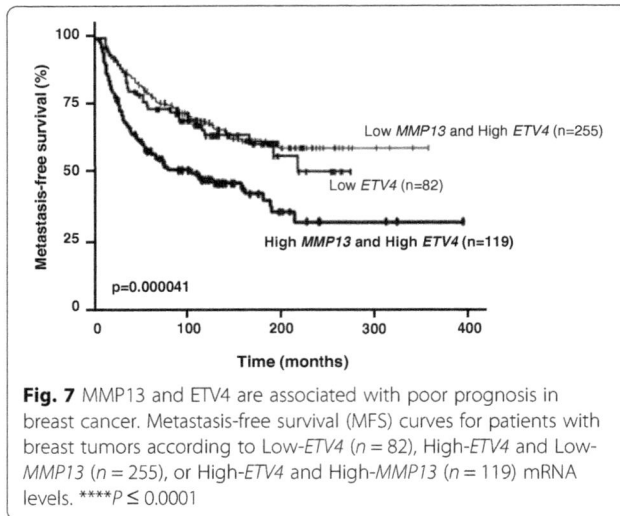

Fig. 7 MMP13 and ETV4 are associated with poor prognosis in breast cancer. Metastasis-free survival (MFS) curves for patients with breast tumors according to Low-*ETV4* (*n* = 82), High-*ETV4* and Low-*MMP13* (*n* = 255), or High-*ETV4* and High-*MMP13* (*n* = 119) mRNA levels. ****$P \leq 0.0001$

increased ability to grow [32] and that ETV4 repression reduces tumorigenesis in mammary cancer cells [16].

In this work, we demonstrate that ETV4 enhances tumorigenic properties of mammary epithelial cancer cells (MMT cells) and that MMP13, as an ETV4 target gene, relays these effects. ETV4 is now well known to be involved in events participating in tumor development and progression. For example, repression of ETV4 in colorectal carcinoma cells significantly impairs their invasive capacity [41], and several EMT markers and MMPs were downregulated in shETV4-expressing cells. In the same way, in gastric adenocarcinoma cell lines, ETV4 increases MMP1 and MMP7 expression and stimulates invasion in vitro [42]. Ectopic overexpression of ETV4 in nonmetastatic human breast cancer cells increases their invasiveness and their metastatic potential in nude mice [43]. Therefore, deregulated metalloprotease expression and/or activity have often been associated with ETV4 tumorigenic properties [1, 44]. However, the precise molecular mechanism by which they act during mammary tumorigenesis is currently unknown.

MMT cells, a mammary tumorigenic cell model, have previously been used to explore the functional involvement of ETV4 in their tumorigenic properties [16]. ETV4 downregulation in MMT cells leads to a decrease in their tumor-forming abilities. Similarly, we show that ETV4 overexpression in MMT cells promotes cell proliferation, migration, invasion, and anchorage-independent growth, demonstrating that ETV4 is an actor of tumorigenic development, as previously described.

Among the well-known MMPs associated with tumorigenic occurrences, MMP13 is a metalloprotease playing an important role in tissue remodeling during fetal and subsequent postnatal bone development [45, 46]. Nevertheless, MMP13 was first identified in a breast tumor library [17], and an increasing amount of data demonstrates its role in

tumorigenesis and particularly in breast cancer [22, 24, 27, 47]. In accordance with this, on the basis of transcriptomic analysis, we initially described regulation of MMP13 expression by ETV4 in a mammary epithelial cell line [16].

To shed light on the functional relevance of the ETV4-MMP13 interplay, we explored MMP13 expression in different contexts of murine (TAC, MMT) or human (MCF10A) ETV4-expressing cells and analyzed the regulation of the *MMP13* gene by ETV4. MMP13 expression and activity are positively correlated with ETV4 expression. Moreover, ETV4 is a transactivator of the *MMP13* gene promoter because we identified a 91-bp minimal promoter that contains putative ETS and AP-1 binding sites. We detected the binding of ETV4 to this chromatin region, the cooperation between ETV4 and AP-1 to enhance the transactivation effect of ETV4 and the importance of the proximal EBS, and the requirement of the AP-1 binding motif, a known cofactor of various ETS proteins [43, 48–51]. This synergistic action between AP-1 and ETV4 in MMP13 regulation could emphasize the role of MMP13 in the ETV4-dependent tumorigenic effects and serve as a potential target to treat ETV4-driven diseases.

Given that MMPs are key actors of the tumorigenic and metastatic processes, we evaluated the influence of MMP13 on phenotypic modification of mammary cancer cells and in a context of ETV4 overexpression. On the one hand, MMP13 overexpression is able to slightly increase cell proliferation, migration, and anchorage-independent growth, and on the other hand, MMP13 repression has the reverse effect. In fact, MMP13 has the same behavior as ETV4 in these cancer cells but is less potent. These are relevant findings, considering that MMP13 is overexpressed in a variety of malignant tumors, such as in breast carcinomas [20, 52, 53], and is implicated in bone metastasis in breast cancer [23, 54, 55].

In order to determine if MMP13 is a relay of ETV4 tumorigenic activity, we compared the behavior of MMT cells overexpressing ETV4 and at the same time have a downregulation of MMP13 expression and activity. These ETV4-overexpressing/MMP13-silencing cells show a significant decrease of their proliferation, migration, and anchorage-independent growth rate. Furthermore, we provide evidence that the silencing of MMP13 inhibits ETV4-induced tumor formation in mice, confirming the in vitro data and highlighting the importance of MMP13 activity in ETV4 tumorigenic functions.

Even though numerous studies suggested the importance of MMP13 in tumor progression and metastasis development, by describing its up- or downregulation, very few of them analyzed the impact of these modulations. One of them, by using a similar approach to studying the role of Pit1, a POU class 1 homeobox 1 transcription factor, revealed that it regulates MMP13 expression in

Table 1 Relationship between *MMP13* and *ETV4* transcripts levels and classical clinical biological parameters in 456 breast cancer samples

	Total population (%)	Number of patients (%)			P value[a]
		Low *ETV4*	High *ETV4*-Low *MMP13*	High *ETV4*-High *MMP13*	
Total	456 (100.0)	82 (18.0)	255 (55.9)	119 (26.1)	
Age, yr					
≤ 50	98 (21.5)	10 (12.2)	60 (23.5)	28 (23.5)	0.075 (NS)
> 50	358 (78.5)	72 (87.8)	195 (76.5)	91 (76.5)	
SBR histological grade[b, c]					
I	58 (13.0)	10 (12.3)	37 (15.0)	11 (9.2)	0.24 (NS)
II	229 (51.2)	48 (59.3)	122 (49.4)	59 (49.6)	
III	160 (35.8)	23 (28.4)	88 (35.6)	49 (41.2)	
Lymph node status[d]					
0	119 (26.1)	21 (25.9)	67 (26.5)	31 (26.3)	0.085 (NS)
1–3	237 (52.1)	37 (45.7)	144 (56.9)	56 (47.5)	
> 3	96 (21.8)	23 (28.4)	42 (16.6)	31 (26.3)	
Macroscopic tumor size[e]					
≤ 25 mm	223 (49.8)	40 (50.0)	132 (52.4)	51 (44.0)	0.32 (NS)
> 25 mm	225 (50.2)	40 (50.0)	120 (47.6)	65 (56.0)	
ERα status					
Negative	118 (25.9)	9 (11.0)	67 (26.3)	42 (35.3)	**0.00067**
Positive	338 (74.1)	73 (89.0)	188 (73.7)	77 (64.7)	
PR status					
Negative	194 (42.5)	31 (37.8)	103 (40.4)	60 (50.4)	0.12 (NS)
Positive	262 (57.5)	51 (62.2)	152 (59.6)	59 (49.6)	
ERBB2 status					
Negative	357 (78.3)	71 (86.6)	200 (78.4)	86 (72.3)	0.052 (NS)
Positive	99 (21.7)	11 (13.4)	55 (21.6)	33 (27.7)	
Molecular subtypes					
HR−ERBB2−	68 (14.9)	8 (9.8)	41 (16.1)	19 (16.0)	**0.0015**
HR−ERBB2+	45 (9.9)	1 (1.2)	22 (8.6)	22 (18.5)	
HR+ERBB2−	289 (63.4)	63 (76.8)	159 (62.4)	67 (56.3)	
HR+ERBB2+	54 (11.8)	10 (12.2)	33 (12.9)	11 (9.2)	
PIK3CA mutation status					
Wild type	307 (67.3)	56 (68.3)	172 (67.5)	79 (66.4)	0.96 (NS)
Mutated	149 (32.7)	26 (31.7)	83 (32.5)	40 (33.6)	
MKI67 mRNA expression					
Median	12.5 (0.80–117)	11.7 (1.74–117)	12.1 (0.80–94.5)	13.6 (2.1–58.5)	0.073 (NS)

Abbreviations: ERa Estrogen receptor alpha, *PR* Progesterone receptor, *ERBB2* Human epidermal growth factor receptor 2, *HR* Hormone receptor, *PIK3CA* Phosphatidylinositol-4,5-bisphosphate 3-kinase catalytic subunit alpha, *MKI67* Marker of proliferation Ki-67
The bold values are statistically significant ($P < 0.05$)
Numbers represent the part of the 456 patients in each condition (e.g., age, SBR histological grade) and in regard to the expression level group (Low *ETV4*/High *ETV4*-Low *MMP13*/High *ETV4*-High *MMP13*). For these three groups, percentages in brackets correspond to the proportion of patients in the group (82 for Low *ETV4*; 255 for High *ETV4*-Low *MMP13*; 119 for High *ETV4*-High *MMP13*)
[a] χ^2 test
[b] Scarff Bloom Richardson classification
[c] Information available for 447 patients
[d] Information available for 452 patients
[e] Information available for 448 patients

human breast cancer cells and that MMP13 knock-down blocks cancer cell invasion into the lungs, suggesting that MMP13 is a mediator of Pit1 induction of breast cancer lung metastasis [56]. These data underline the importance of MMP13 in the mediation of tumorigenesis and invasiveness and corroborate our findings.

The MMT cell model was considered to be a useful model in which to perform the in vitro and in vivo phenotypic assays according to the previously published data and characterization we obtained regarding their ability to form tumors in immunodeficient mice [8, 16]. Indeed, to decipher the relevance of ETV4 and MMP13 association in breast cancer, we assessed *MMP13* and *ETV4* mRNA expression levels in a series of 456 breast cancer samples. Even if high *ETV4* mRNA expression was not shown to be associated with poor MFS, the group with a high *MMP13* mRNA expression level was significantly associated with a bad prognosis ($P = 0.00016$). Nevertheless, by combining *MMP13* and *ETV4* mRNA expression status, we identified three distinct prognostic groups with significantly different MFS curves ($P = 0.000041$). These data revealed that the tumor group overexpressing both *ETV4* and *MMP13* is correlated with the poorest prognosis, much more significant than that of *MMP13* alone. These results were confirmed in the NKI breast cancer cohort ($P = 0.0013$), reinforcing the high prognostic value of *ETV4*- and *MMP13*-associated high expression. Moreover, this correlation was strengthened by the independent prognostic value shown for combined high expression levels of *ETV4* and *MMP13* ($P = 0.000041$). Indeed, our study suggests an important interplay of ETV4 and MMP13 in human breast cancers that could, together, be assessed for their possible signature for guiding diagnosis or therapeutics.

ETV4 overexpression is associated with increased metastatic risk and poor patient survival in triple-negative breast cancer distant metastasis and poor patient survival [57]. Similarly, high levels of *MMP13* expression are associated with high tumor aggressiveness and poor survival rate [58]. Thus, these data corroborate our findings, and in combination, they underline the importance of these two factors, ETV4 and its relay MMP13, in mammary tumorigenesis. Nevertheless, the real way by which they interplay needs to be deciphered, and further investigations should be done to evaluate their potential as prognostic and diagnostic markers as well as potential therapeutic targets to prevent or treat the disease.

Conclusions

The ETV4 transcription factor is involved in tumorigenesis and metastatic processes, particularly in breast cancer, a heterogeneous illness with different subtypes. In the present study, we showed that ETV4 promotes proliferation,

migration, invasion, and anchorage-independent growth of mammary tumorigenic MMT cells. In parallel, we identified MMP13, an extracellular metalloprotease, as an ETV4 target gene. We showed that, by overexpressing or repressing MMP13 expression, this metalloprotease contributes to ETV4-induced proliferation, migration, and clonogenicity capacity. Thus, MMP13 acts as a relay of ETV4 in its functional role in the mammary epithelial tumorigenic cells in vitro as well as in tumor development in animal models. Finally, we showed that ETV4 and MMP13 co-overexpression is correlated with poor prognosis in breast cancer. Taken together, these data highlight the role of these actors in mammary tumorigenesis and breast cancer progression and underline the potential prognostic value of their combined expression in breast cancer.

Additional files

Additional file 1: Supplementary methods. (PDF 40 kb)

Additional file 2: Table S1. Pathological and clinical characteristics of patients in relation to metastasis-free survival (MFS). (PDF 33 kb)

Additional file 3: Figure S1. Validation of the overexpression of ETV4 and MMP13 in MCF10A cells. a and b Relative *ETV4* mRNA (a) and *MMP13* mRNA (b) expression in the MCF10A-Ctrl and MCF10A-ETV4 cells determined by real-time PCR and normalized to cyclophilin A levels. mRNA expression in MCF10A-Ctrl cells was arbitrarily = 1. Error bars indicate SD. *$P \leq 0.1$. c and d Western blot analysis of ETV4 protein expression (61 kDa) (c) and MMP13 protein expression (60 kDa) (d) in the MCF10A-Ctrl and MCF10A-ETV4 cells. GAPDH expression served as the loading control. (PDF 100 kb)

Additional file 4: Figure S2. ETS and AP-1 binding sites are highly conserved among mouse, human, and rabbit. Nucleotide sequence comparison of mouse, human, and rat proximal *MMP13* promoters. Shaded boxes indicate the conserved ETS and AP-1 binding site sequences. (PDF 46 kb)

Additional file 5: Figure S3. ChIP experiment for ETV4 and MMP13 in MMT and TAC cells. PCR detection of the *MMP13* promoter region after ETV4 immunoprecipitation in MMT-ETV4 (left panel) and TAC-ETV4 (right panel). Primers allowing the amplification of the proximal *MMP13* promoter region containing EBS are schematized in the lower panel of Fig. 2. Cyclin D2 was used as a positive control [8]. Immunoprecipitation with a nonrelevant antibody (IgG) was used as negative control. (PDF 60 kb)

Additional file 6: Figure S4. Expression of MMP13 in MMT cells overexpressing or repressing MMP13. a and b Relative *MMP13* mRNA expression in the MMT-Ctrl and MMT-MMP13 (a) or MMT-shCtrl and MMT-shMMP13 cells (b) determined by real-time PCR and normalized to cyclophilin A levels. mRNA expression in MMT-Ctrl cells was arbitrarily = 1. Error bars indicate SD. ****$P \leq 0.0001$. c Western blot analysis of MMP13 protein expression (60 kDa) in the MMT-Ctrl and MMT-MMP13 cells. GAPDH expression served as the loading control. d Zymographic analysis of MMP13 protein activity (55 kDa) from the supernatant of MMT-Ctrl and MMT-MMP13 cells. (PDF 72 kb)

Additional file 7: Figure S5. Expression of ETV4 in MMT-shMMP13-repressing cells. a Relative *ETV4* mRNA expression in the MMT-ETV4 + shCtrl and MMT-ETV4 + shMMP13 cells determined by real-time PCR and normalized to cyclophilin A levels. mRNA expression in MMT-Ctrl + shCtrl cells was arbitrarily = 1. Error bars indicate SD. The results were not statistically significant. b Western blot analysis of ETV4 protein expression (61 kDa) in the MMT-ETV4 + shCtrl and MMT-ETV4 + shMMP13 cells. GAPDH expression served as the loading control. (PDF 71 kb)

Additional file 8: Figure S6. The repression of MMP13 reduces the anchorage-independent growth capacity of MMT-ETV4-overexpressing cells. a Relative *MMP13* mRNA expression in the transiently transfected

MMT-siCtrl and MMT-siMMP13 cells determined by real-time PCR and normalized to cyclophilin A levels. mRNA expression in MMT-siCtrl cells was arbitrarily = 1. Error bars indicate SD. ****$P \leq 0.0001$. b Anchorage-independent growth. MMT-ETV4-siCtrl and MMT-ETV4-siMMP13 cells were cultured for 10 days in soft agar. This histogram represents the number of clones counted for experimental time points. Soft agar assays were conducted three times in triplicate. Magnification × 5. Error bars indicate SD. ****$P \leq 0.0001$. (PDF 45 kb)

Additional file 9: Figure S7. High *MMP13* mRNA expression level is associated with a poor prognosis in breast cancer. a Metastasis-free survival (MFS) curves for patients with breast tumors according to Low-*MMP13* ($n = 321$) or High-*MMP13* ($n = 135$) mRNA levels. ***$P \leq 0.001$. b Metastasis-free survival (MFS) curves for patients with breast tumors according to Low-*ETV4* ($n = 82$) and High-*ETV4* ($n = 374$) mRNA levels. The results were not statistically significant. (PDF 14 kb)

Additional file 10: Figure S8. Metastasis-free survival analysis from the publicly available NKI datasets of breast tumors. a Metastasis-free survival (MFS) curves for patients with breast tumors according to Low-*ETV4* ($n = 12$), High-*ETV4* and Low-*MMP13* ($n = 243$), or High-*ETV4* and High-*MMP13* ($n = 9$) mRNA levels. ****$P \leq 0.0001$. b Metastasis-free survival (MFS) curves for breast tumor patients according to Low-*MMP13* ($n = 255$) or High-*MMP13* ($n = 9$) mRNA levels. ****$P \leq 0.0001$. c Metastasis-free survival (MFS) curves for patients with breast tumors according to Low-*ETV4* ($n = 13$) and High-*ETV4* ($n = 251$) mRNA levels. ****$P \leq 0.0001$. (PDF 19 kb)

Additional file 11: Table S2. Multivariate Cox proportional hazards analysis of MFS for *MMP13* and *ETV4* expression levels in the series of 456 breast tumors. (PDF 42 kb)

Abbreviations
AP-1: Activator protein 1; bp: base pair; BSA: Bovine serum albumin; cDNA: Complementary DNA; ChIP: Chromatin immunoprecipitation; EBS: ETS binding site; EMT: Epithelial-mesenchymal transition; ERBB2: human epidermal growth factor receptor 2; ERα: Estrogen receptor alpha; ETV-4: ETS translocation variant 4; GAPDH: Glyceraldehyde 3-phosphate dehydrogenase; HEK-293: Human embryonic kidney 293 cells; HR: Hormone receptor; HRP: Horseradish peroxidase; IgG: Immunoglobulin G; MFS: Metastasis-free survival; MMP: Matrix metalloproteinase; MMT: Mouse mammary tumor; mRNA: Messenger RNA; PET: Polyethylene terephthalate; PIK3CA: Phosphatidylinositol 3-kinase catalytic; PR: Progesterone receptor; SBR: Scarff-Bloom-Richardson histoprognostic grading system; SCID: Severe combined immunodeficiency; shRNA: Short hairpin RNA; siRNA: Small interfering RNA; TNBC: Triple-negative breast cancer

Acknowledgements
We thank Martine Duterque-Coquillaud, Anne Flourens, and Antonino Bongiovanni for their precious help in IHC experiments. We thank the Microscopy-Imaging-Cytometry Facility of the BioImaging Center Lille Nord-de-France for access to instruments and technical advice.

Funding
This work was supported by the Centre national de la recherche scientifique (CNRS), the Institut Pasteur de Lille, and Institut National de la Santé et de la Recherche Médicale (INSERM), as well as by grants from the Ligue contre le Cancer, comité Aisne and the Association pour la Recherche sur le Cancer.

Authors' contributions
MD, YdL, DT, FL, and ACL participated in the design of the study. MD and ID performed all the in vitro experiments and molecular biology studies. NM and ACL contributed to the animal manipulations and analysis of in vivo results. IB and SV performed the experiments and the analysis concerning the breast cancer samples. MD helped to write the manuscript, and IB wrote the breast cancer patient portion. ACL supervised the project, the results, and the experimental procedures and drafted the manuscript. All authors read and approved the final manuscript.

Competing interests
The authors declare that they have no competing interests.

Author details
[1]University of Lille, CNRS, Institut Pasteur de Lille, UMR 8161 - M3T – Mechanisms of Tumorigenesis and Targeted Therapies, F-59000 Lille, France. [2]Department of Biochemistry and Molecular Pharmacology, University of Massachusetts Medical School, Worcester, MA 01605-2324, USA. [3]Unit of Pharmacogenomics, Department of Genetics, Institut Curie, Paris, France. [4]CNRS UMR 8161, Institut de Biologie de Lille - Institut Pasteur de Lille, 1 Rue Pr Calmette, BP447, 59021 Lille, France.

References
1. de Launoit Y, Baert JL, Chotteau-Lelièvre A, Monte D, Coutte L, Mauen S, Firlej V, Degerny C, Verreman K. The Ets transcription factors of the PEA3 group: transcriptional regulators in metastasis. Biochim Biophys Acta. 2006; 1766:79–87.
2. Laudet V, Hanni C, Stehelin D, Duterque-Coquillaud M. Molecular phylogeny of the ETS gene family. Oncogene. 1999;18(6):1351–9.
3. Chotteau-Lelièvre A, Desbiens X, Pelczar H, Defossez PA, De Launoit Y. Differential expression patterns of the PEA3 group transcription factors through murine embryonic development. Oncogene. 1997;15(8):937–52.
4. Chotteau-Lelièvre A, Dolle P, Peronne V, Coutte L, De Launoit Y, Desbiens X. Expression patterns of the Ets transcription factors from the PEA3 group during early stages of mouse development. Mech Dev. 2001;108(1–2):191–5.
5. Kurpios NA, Sabolic NA, Shepherd TG, Fidalgo GM, Hassell JA. Function of PEA3 Ets transcription factors in mammary gland development and oncogenesis. J Mammary Gland Biol Neoplasia. 2003;8:177–90.
6. Oh S, Shin S, Janknecht R. ETV1, 4 and 5: an oncogenic subfamily of ETS transcription factors. Biochim Biophys Acta. 2012;1826(1):1–12.
7. Shepherd T, Hassell JA. Role of Ets transcription factors in mammary gland development and oncogenesis. J Mammary Gland Biol Neoplasia. 2001;6: 129–40.
8. Ladam F, Damour I, Dumont P, Kherrouche Z, de Launoit Y, Tulasne D, Chotteau-Lelièvre A. Loss of a negative feedback loop involving Pea3 and cyclin D2 is required for Pea3-induced migration in transformed mammary epithelial cells. Mol Cancer Res. 2013;11:1412–24.
9. Baker R, Kent CV, Silbermann RA, Hassell JA, Young LJT, Howe LR. Pea3 transcription factors and Wnt1-induced mouse mammary neoplasia. PLoS One. 2010;5:e8854.
10. Qin L, Liu Z, Chen H, Xu J. The steroid receptor coactivator-1 regulates twist expression and promotes breast cancer metastasis. Cancer Res. 2009;69: 3819–27.
11. Shepherd TG, Kockeritz L, Szrajber MR, Muller WJ, Hassell JA. The *pea3* subfamily *ets* genes are required for HER2/Neu-mediated mammary oncogenesis. Curr Biol. 2001;11:1739–48.
12. Firlej V, Bocquet B, Desbiens X, de Launoit Y, Chotteau-Lelièvre A. Pea3 transcription factor cooperates with USF-1 in regulation of the murine bax transcription without binding to an Ets-binding site. J Biol Chem. 2005;280: 887–98.
13. Jiang J, Wei Y, Liu D, Zhou J, Shen J, Chen X, Zhang S, Kong X, Gu J. E1AF promotes breast cancer cell cycle progression via upregulation of cyclin D3 transcription. Biochem Biophys Res Commun. 2007;358:53–8.

14. Qin L, Liao L, Redmond A, Young L, Yuan Y, Chen H, O'Malley BW, Xu J. The AIB1 oncogene promotes breast cancer metastasis by activation of PEA3-mediated matrix metalloproteinase 2 (MMP2) and MMP9 expression. Mol Cell Biol. 2008;28:5937–50.

15. Yuen HF, Chan YK, Grills C, McCrudden CM, Gunasekharan V, Shi Z, Wong AS, Lappin TR, Chan KW, Fennell DA, Khoo US, Johnston PG, El-Tanani M. Polyomavirus enhancer activator 3 protein promotes breast cancer metastatic progression through Snail-induced epithelial-mesenchymal transition. J Pathol. 2011;224:78–89.

16. Firlej V, Ladam F, Brysbaert G, Dumont P, Fuks F, de Launoit Y, Benecke A, Chotteau-Lelièvre A. Reduced tumorigenesis in mouse mammary cancer cells following inhibition of Pea3- or Erm-dependent transcription. J Cell Sci. 2008;121:3393–402.

17. Knäuper V, López-Otin C, Smith B, Knight G, Murphy G. Biochemical characterization of human collagenase-3. J Biol Chem. 1996;271:1544–50.

18. Nielsen BS, Rank F, López JM, Balbin M, Vizoso F, Lund LR, Danø K, López-Otín C. Collagenase-3 expression in breast myofibroblasts as a molecular marker of transition of ductal carcinoma in situ lesions to invasive ductal carcinomas. Cancer Res. 2001;61:7091–100.

19. Martin MD, Matrisian LM. The other side of MMPs: protective roles in tumor progression. Cancer Metastasis Rev. 2007;26:717–24.

20. Freije JM, Díez-Itza I, Balbín M, Sánchez LM, Blasco R, Tolivia J, López-Otín C. Molecular cloning and expression of collagenase-3, a novel human matrix metalloproteinase produced by breast carcinomas. J Biol Chem. 1994;269: 16766–73.

21. Leeman MF, Curran S, Murray GI. The structure, regulation, and function of human matrix metalloproteinase-13. Crit Rev Biochem Mol Biol. 2002;37:149–66.

22. Rizki A, Weaver VM, Lee SY, Rozenberg GI, Chin K, Myers CA, Bascom JL, Mott JD, Semeiks JR, Grate LR, Mian IS, Borowsky AD, Jensen RA, Idowu MO, Chen F, Chen DJ, Petersen OW, Gray JW, Bissell MJ. A human breast cell model of preinvasive to invasive transition. Cancer Res. 2008;68:1378–87.

23. Nannuru KC, Futakuchi M, Varney ML, Vincent TM, Marcusson EG, Singh RK. Matrix metalloproteinase (MMP)-13 regulates mammary tumor-induced osteolysis by activating MMP9 and transforming growth factor-beta signaling at the tumor-bone interface. Cancer Res. 2010;70:3494–504.

24. Vargas AC, McCart Reed AE, Waddell N, Lane A, Reid LE, Smart CE, Cocciardi S, da Silva L, Song S, Chenevix-Trench G, Simpson PT, Lakhani SR. Gene expression profiling of tumour epithelial and stromal compartments during breast cancer progression. Breast Cancer Res Treat. 2012;135:153–65.

25. Nielsen BS, Egeblad M, Rank F, Askautrud HA, Pennington CJ, Pedersen TX, Christensen IJ, Edwards DR, Werb Z, Lund LR. Matrix metalloproteinase 13 is induced in fibroblasts in polyomavirus middle T antigen-driven mammary carcinoma without influencing tumor progression. PLoS One. 2008;3:e2959.

26. Chang HJ, Yang MJ, Yang YH, Hou MF, Hsueh EJ, Lin SR. MMP13 is potentially a new tumor marker for breast cancer diagnosis. Oncol Rep. 2009;22:1119–27.

27. Wang L, Wang X, Liang Y, Diao X, Chen Q. S100A4 promotes invasion and angiogenesis in breast cancer MDA-MB-231 cells by upregulating matrix metalloproteinase-13. Acta Biochim Pol. 2012;59:593–8.

28. Balduyck M, Zerimech F, Gouyer V, Lemaire R, Hemon B, Grard G, Thiebaut C, Lemaire V, Dacquembronne E, Duhem T, Lebrun A, Dejonghe MJ, Huet G. Specific expression of matrix metalloproteinases 1, 3, 9 and 13 associated with invasiveness of breast cancer cells in vitro. Clin Exp Metastasis. 2000;18:171–8.

29. Jiang W, Crossman DK, Mitchell EH, Sohn P, Crowley MR, Serra R. WNT5A inhibits metastasis and alters splicing of Cd44 in breast cancer cells. PLoS One. 2013;8:e58329.

30. Li H, Huang F, Fan L, Jiang Y, Wang X, Li J, Wang Q, Pan H, Sun J, Cao X, Wang X. Phosphatidylethanolamine-binding protein 4 is associated with breast cancer metastasis through Src-mediated Akt tyrosine phosphorylation. Oncogene. 2014;33:4589–98.

31. Datar I, Feng J, Qiu X, Lewandowski J, Yeung M, Ren G, Aras S, Al-Mulla F, Cui H, Trumbly R, Arudra SK, De Las Casas LE, de la Serna I, Bitar MS, Yeung KC. RKIP inhibits local breast Cancer invasion by antagonizing the transcriptional activation of MMP13. PLoS One. 2015;10:e0134494.

32. Chotteau-Lelièvre A, Montesano R, Soriano J, Soulie P, Desbiens X, de Launoit Y. PEA3 transcription factors are expressed in tissues undergoing branching morphogenesis and promote formation of duct-like structures by mammary epithelial cells in vitro. Dev Biol. 2003;259:241–57.

33. Soriano JV, Pepper MS, Nakamura T, Orci L, Montesano R. Hepatocyte growth factor stimulates extensive development of branching duct-like structures by cloned mammary gland epithelial cells. J Cell Sci. 1995;108: 413–30.

34. Meierjohann S, Hufnagel A, Wende E, Kleinschmidt MA, Wolf K, Friedl P, Friedl P, Gaubatz S, Schartl M. MMP13 mediates cell cycle progression in melanocytes and melanoma cells: in vitro studies of migration and proliferation. Mol Cancer. 2010;9:201.

35. Wu N, Opalenik S, Liu J, Jansen ED, Giro MG, Davidson JM. Real-time visualization of MMP-13 promoter activity in transgenic mice. Matrix Biol. 2002;21:149–61.

36. Cox DR. Regression Models and Life-Tables. JR Stat Soc Series B Methodol. 1972;34(2):187–220.

37. Mengshol JA, Vincenti MP, Brinckerhoff CE. IL-1 induces collagenase-3 (MMP-13) promoter activity in stably transfected chondrocytic cells: requirement for Runx-2 and activation by p38 MAPK and JNK pathways. Nucleic Acids Res. 2001;29:4361–72.

38. Otero M, Plumb DA, Tsuchimochi K, Dragomir CL, Hashimoto K, Peng H, Olivotto E, Bevilacqua M, Tan L, Yang Z, Zhan Y, Oettgen P, Li Y, Marcu KB, Goldring MB. E74-like factor 3 (ELF3) impacts on matrix metalloproteinase 13 (MMP13) transcriptional control in articular chondrocytes under proinflammatory stress. J Biol Chem. 2012;287:3559–72.

39. Kurpios NA, MacNeil L, Shepherd TG, Gludish DW, Giacomelli AO, Hassell JA. The Pea3 Ets transcription factor regulates differentiation of multipotent progenitor cells during mammary gland development. Dev Biol. 2009;325(1):106–21.

40. de Launoit Y, Chotteau-Lelièvre A, Beaudoin C, Coutte L, Netzer S, Brenner C, Huvent I, Baert JL. The PEA3 group of ETS-related transcription factors: role in breast cancer metastasis. Adv Exp Med Biol. 2000;480:107–16.

41. Mesci A, Taeb S, Huang X, Jairath R, Sivaloganathan D, Liu SK. Pea3 expression promotes the invasive and metastatic potential of colorectal carcinoma. World J Gastroenterol. 2014;20:17376.

42. Yamamoto H, Horiuchi S, Adachi Y, Taniguchi H, Nosho K, Min Y, Imai K. Expression of ets-related transcriptional factor E1AF is associated with tumor progression and over-expression of matrilysin in human gastric cancer. Carcinogenesis. 2004;25:325–32.

43. Kaya M, Yoshida K, Higashino F, Mitaka T, Ishii S. Fujinaga K. A single ets-related transcription factor, E1AF, confers invasive phenotype on human cancer cells. Oncogene. 1996;12:221–7.

44. Verger A, Duterque-Coquillaud M. When Ets transcription factors meet their partners. Bioessays. 2002;24:362–70.

45. Ståhle-Bäckdahl M, Sandstedt B, Bruce K, Lindahl A, Jiménez MG, Vega JA, López-Otín C. Collagenase-3 (MMP-13) is expressed during human fetal ossification and re-expressed in postnatal bone remodeling and in rheumatoid arthritis. Lab Investig. 1997;76:717–28.

46. Johansson N, Saarialho-Kere U, Airola K, Herva R, Nissinen L, Westermarck J, Vuorio E, Heino J, Kähäri VM. Collagenase-3 (MMP-13) is expressed by hypertrophic chondrocytes, periosteal cells, and osteoblasts during human fetal bone development. Dev Dyn. 1997;208:387–97.

47. Culhaci N, Metin K, Copcu E, Dikicioglu E. Elevated expression of MMP-13 and TIMP-1 in head and neck squamous cell carcinomas may reflect increased tumor invasiveness. BMC Cancer. 2004;4:42.

48. Majérus MA, Bibollet-Ruche F, Telliez JB, Wasylyk B, Bailleul B. Serum, AP-1 and Ets-1 stimulate the human ets-1 promoter. Nucleic Acids Res. 1992;20: 2699–703.

49. Zhang M, Maass N, Magit D, Sager R. Transactivation through Ets and Ap1 transcription sites determines the expression of the tumor-suppressing gene maspin. Cell Growth Differ. 1997;8:179–86.

50. Li Z, Tognon CE, Godinho FJ, Yasaitis L, Hock H, Herschkowitz JI, Lannon CL, Cho E, Kim SJ, Bronson RT, Perou CM, Sorensen PH, Orkin SH. ETV6-NTRK3 fusion oncogene initiates breast cancer from committed mammary progenitors via activation of AP1 complex. Cancer Cell. 2007;12:542–58.

51. Newberry EP, Willis D, Latifi T, Boudreaux JM, Towler DA. Fibroblast growth factor receptor signaling activates the human interstitial collagenase promoter via the bipartite Ets-AP1 element. Mol Endocrinol. 1997;11:1129–44.

52. Yamada T, Oshima T, Yoshihara K, Tamura S, Kanazawa A, Inagaki D, Yamamoto N, Sato T, Fujii S, Numata K, Kunisaki C, Shiozawa M, Morinaga S, Akaike M, Rino Y, Tanaka K, Masuda M, Imada T. Overexpression of MMP-13 gene in colorectal cancer with liver metastasis. Anticancer Res. 2010;30:2693–9.

53. Kominsky SL, Doucet M, Thorpe M, Weber KL. MMP-13 is over-expressed in renal cell carcinoma bone metastasis and is induced by TGF-β1. Clin Exp Metastasis. 2008;25:865–70.

54. Ibaragi S, Shimo T, Hassan NMM, Isowa S, Kurio N, Mandai H, Kodama S, Sasaki A. Induction of MMP-13 expression in bone-metastasizing cancer cells by type I collagen through integrin $\alpha_1\beta_1$ and $\alpha_2\beta_1$-p38 MAPK signaling. Anticancer Res. 2011;31:1307–13.

55. Shah M, Huang D, Blick T, Connor A, Reiter LA, Hardink JR, Lynch CC, Waltham M, Thompson EW. An MMP13-selective inhibitor delays primary tumor growth and the onset of tumor-associated osteolytic lesions in experimental models of breast cancer. PLoS One. 2012;7:e29615.

56. Sendon-Lago J, Seoane S, Eiro N, Bermudez MA, Macia M, Garcia-Caballero T, Vizoso FJ, Perez-Fernandez R. Cancer progression by breast tumors with Pit-1-overexpression is blocked by inhibition of metalloproteinase (MMP)-13. Breast Cancer Res. 2014;16:505.

57. Yuan ZY, Dai T, Wang SS, Peng RJ, Li XH, Qin T, Song LB, Wang X. Overexpression of ETV4 protein in triple-negative breast cancer is associated with a higher risk of distant metastasis. Onco Targets Ther. 2014;7:1733–42.

58. Zhang B, Cao X, Liu Y, Cao W, Zhang F, Zhang S, Li H, Ning L, Fu L, Niu Y, Niu R, Sun B, Hao X. Tumor-derived matrix metalloproteinase-13 (MMP-13) correlates with poor prognoses of invasive breast cancer. BMC Cancer. 2008;8:83.

4

Breast cancer patients suggestive of Li-Fraumeni syndrome: mutational spectrum, candidate genes, and unexplained heredity

Judith Penkert[1]* (iD), Gunnar Schmidt[1], Winfried Hofmann[1], Stephanie Schubert[1], Maximilian Schieck[1], Bernd Auber[1], Tim Ripperger[1], Karl Hackmann[2,3,4], Marc Sturm[5], Holger Prokisch[6], Ursula Hille-Betz[7], Dorothea Mark[8], Thomas Illig[1], Brigitte Schlegelberger[1] and Doris Steinemann[1]

Abstract

Background: Breast cancer is the most prevalent tumor entity in Li-Fraumeni syndrome. Up to 80% of individuals with a Li-Fraumeni-like phenotype do not harbor detectable causative germline *TP53* variants. Yet, no systematic panel analyses for a wide range of cancer predisposition genes have been conducted on cohorts of women with breast cancer fulfilling Li-Fraumeni(-like) clinical diagnostic criteria.

Methods: To specifically help explain the diagnostic gap of *TP53* wild-type Li-Fraumeni(-like) breast cancer cases, we performed array-based CGH (comparative genomic hybridization) and panel-based sequencing of 94 cancer predisposition genes on 83 breast cancer patients suggestive of Li-Fraumeni syndrome who had previously had negative test results for causative *BRCA1*, *BRCA2*, and *TP53* germline variants.

Results: We identified 13 pathogenic or likely pathogenic germline variants in ten patients and in nine genes, including four copy number aberrations and nine single-nucleotide variants or small indels. Three patients presented as double-mutation carriers involving two different genes each. In five patients (5 of 83; 6% of cohort), we detected causative pathogenic variants in established hereditary breast cancer susceptibility genes (i.e., *PALB2, CHEK2, ATM*). Five further patients (5 of 83; 6% of cohort) were found to harbor pathogenic variants in genes lacking a firm association with breast cancer susceptibility to date (i.e., Fanconi pathway genes, RECQ family genes, *CDKN2A*/p14^ARF, and *RUNX1*).

Conclusions: Our study details the mutational spectrum in breast cancer patients suggestive of Li-Fraumeni syndrome and indicates the need for intensified research on monoallelic variants in Fanconi pathway and RECQ family genes. Notably, this study further reveals a large portion of still unexplained Li-Fraumeni(-like) cases, warranting comprehensive investigation of recently described candidate genes as well as noncoding regions of the *TP53* gene in patients with Li-Fraumeni(-like) syndrome lacking *TP53* variants in coding regions.

Keywords: Breast cancer, HBOC, Li-Fraumeni syndrome, Li-Fraumeni-like syndrome, *TP53*, Fanconi pathway, RECQ family, *CDKN2A, FANCA*

* Correspondence: penkert.judith@mh-hannover.de
[1]Department of Human Genetics, Hannover Medical School,
Carl-Neuberg-Strasse 1, 30625 Hannover, Germany
Full list of author information is available at the end of the article

Background

Li-Fraumeni syndrome (LFS) is a rare but highly penetrant cancer predisposition syndrome characterized by the early onset and familial aggregation of a variety of malignant neoplasms [1]. Germline pathogenic variants (PVs) in the tumor suppressor gene *TP53* are primarily responsible for this autosomal dominantly inherited disease [2]; however, because *TP53* PVs can be confirmed in only about 70% of suspected families [3], diagnosis of LFS is usually based on clinical evaluation and conformance to stringent criteria independent of mutational status. Different diagnostic criteria with varying stringency in terms of tumor abundance, age of onset, and spectrum of malignancies are in use, including classic LFS criteria, Birch's and Eeles' Li-Fraumeni-like syndrome (LFL) criteria, and several versions of the Chompret criteria [1, 4–9]. Although in principle any type of neoplasm may occur, a set of core cancers, namely breast cancer (BC), sarcomas, brain tumors, adrenocortical carcinomas, and leukemia, are expected to account for up to 77% of all tumor types occurring in patients with LFS [10].

Penetrance is remarkably high in carriers of germline *TP53* PVs, with 84% of female carriers and 41% of male carriers developing a tumor by age 45 years [11]. The gender difference is due to BC being one of the most predominating factors in this syndrome, representing up to 80% of all cancer cases in the age class of 16–45 years in females with LFS [10, 11]. However, because the syndrome itself is rare, the contribution of *TP53* germline alterations to hereditary BC overall is estimated to be less than 1% [12]. Because patients with BC harboring germline *TP53* PVs typically present with very early age of onset, routine *TP53* testing has been suggested for women who develop BC before the age of 30 years, independent of family history, and *TP53* detection rates within cohorts of patients with early-onset BC have been reported to be between 4% and 8% [8, 13, 14]. The 2008 and 2015 versions of the revised Chompret criteria [7, 9] are the sole criteria incorporating this important factor into their diagnostics, allowing for patients with early-onset BC (< 36 years) or very early-onset BC (< 31 years), respectively, to be included in LFS/LFL diagnostic procedures. Yet, two recent studies focused on cohorts of women meeting hereditary breast and ovarian cancer (HBOC) criteria clearly illustrate that a large percentage of germline *TP53* mutation carriers may still be missed by current criteria; the two studies reported *TP53* PVs in 13 patients overall, half of whom did not clinically meet either classic LFS or Chompret criteria, nor did they present with very early-onset disease [15, 16].

While not all germline *TP53* mutation carriers may be covered by LFS/LFL criteria, many families who do clinically conform to LFS/LFL criteria lack detectable germline *TP53* PVs, which is demonstrated by *TP53* mutation detection rates ranging from ~ 55% to 70% in classic LFS criteria, ~ 25% to 30% in LFL criteria, and ~ 20% to 35% in Chompret criteria [3, 6, 13]. This means that up to 45% of patients meeting classical LFS criteria and up to 80% of patients meeting Chompret or LFL criteria are left unexplained in a genetic sense. Few other candidate genes in the *TP53* pathway have been investigated in this context, one of them being *CDKN2A*, which was recently found to be mutated on a germline level in several LFL families in which the index case had a sarcoma [17]. Moreover, germline PVs in *CHEK2* have continuously but controversially been implicated in LFL phenotypes.

To the best of our knowledge, no systematic panel analyses for a wide range of known and suspected cancer predisposition genes have been conducted on cohorts of women with BC fulfilling LFL clinical diagnostic criteria. To further address this issue, as well as to elucidate the mutational spectrum in German population subjects with BC suggestive of LFS/LFL, we conducted both massive parallel sequencing and copy number analyses for a set of 94 cancer predisposition genes in a cohort of 83 *TP53*-negative and *BRCA1/2*-negative BC patients from the German population who met at least one of the hitherto suggested Li-Fraumeni-related criteria (LFS/LFL/Chompret criteria).

Methods
Study cohort
Patient selection

Eighty-three unrelated study subjects were selected from among a pool of female patients with BC who conformed to the German consortium criteria for HBOC [18] and whose pedigree had been established during genetic counseling in the tumor genetics outpatient clinic at Hannover Medical School, Germany, between 2002 and 2015. Prior to study inclusion, all patients had a negative test result for pathogenic single-nucleotide variants or small indels (Sanger sequencing) as well as gross genomic rearrangements (multiplex ligation-dependent probe amplification [MLPA], SALSA MLPA kits [MRC Holland, Amsterdam, The Netherlands], P002B/P087 for *BRCA1*, P045-B3/P077 for *BRCA2*, and P056-C1 for *TP53*) within the genes *BRCA1*, *BRCA2*, and *TP53*. Final inclusion of study participants was based on personal medical or family history characteristics suggestive of Li-Fraumeni-like traits and conformance to at least one of the hitherto existing Li-Fraumeni-related criteria (LFS/LFL/Chompret criteria). Classification into LFS/LFL and Chompret criteria was performed either on the particular proband undergoing mutation analysis or on another index case within the same family. The majority of patients were assumed to be of European-Caucasian ancestry. All patients signed informed consent forms, and the project was approved by the research ethics committee of Hannover Medical School (approval number 3528).

Cohort characteristics

Among our cohort of 83 patients with BC, 50 unrelated women had early-onset BC (age at diagnosis ranging from 19 to 34 years, median age 29 years), 9 index cases were diagnosed with bilateral BC or two primary independent breast carcinomas, 4 individuals harbored at least one independent neoplasm besides BC, in 10 families either the index patient or one of her relatives had a sarcoma, and in 16 families either the index patient or a relative was diagnosed with a brain tumor (multiple entries being possible).

Next-generation sequencing and bioinformatics analysis

Germline DNA was isolated from peripheral blood leukocytes according to standard procedures. For library preparation, the Illumina TruSight Cancer Panel (Illumina, San Diego, CA, USA) was used (see Additional file 1 for the entire list of the 94 included genes and SNPs). All samples were processed according to the manufacturer's recommendations and sequenced on an Illumina NextSeq 500 platform. Mean sequence depth was at least 100 × for each sample. A minimum sequence depth of 20 × for at least 97% of the region of interest (ROI) (i.e., coding regions and the first two base pairs [bp] of flanking intronic regions) could be obtained for 81 of 83 samples; 2 samples failed to confer to these quality parameters. The majority of samples (68 of 83; 82%) reached 20 × coverage for at least 99% of the target region. All 94 panel genes were analyzed using the megSAP analysis pipeline [19], filtering for variants with a minimum variant allele frequency (VAF) of 15%, a relatively low VAF that was chosen for the eventuality of constitutional TP53 mosaicism [20]. Yet, all detected PVs exhibited a VAF of > 40% (range, 43–56%). Reported nucleotide positions refer to GRCh37/hg19.

Integrative Genomics Viewer (IGV) [21, 22] was employed to visualize sequencing results. Variants were further filtered with the software GSvar (part of ngs-bits [23]) to identify frameshift, nonsense, splice site, missense, inframe insertion/deletion, and 3′/5′ untranslated region (UTR) variants that had a minor allele frequency (MAF) at or below 0.1% in the 1000 Genomes Project [24], ExAC [25], and Kaviar [26] databases and were located in the ROI as defined above. As a second measure, via GSvar analysis, we filtered all variants that were predicted to be pathogenic by at least 2 of 4 in silico prediction tools (i.e., MetaLR [27], Sift [28], PolyPhen-2 HVAR, and PolyPhen-2 HDIV [29]) or that were documented as pathogenic in either the ClinVar [30] or HGMD [31] database, as long as they were neither listed $n > 2$ in the FLOSSIES database of healthy older women [32], nor classified as class 1–2 variants according to a consented expert decision within the German HBOC Consortium, nor reported as predominantly benign or likely benign in ClinVar [30]. Variants were classified

according to American College of Medical Genetics and Genomics (ACMG) guidelines [33]. For splicing prediction, in silico splicing tools (i.e., SSF, MaxEnt, NNSplice, GeneSplicer, and HSF) included in Alamut software version 2.8 rev. 1 (interactive biosoftware, Rouen, France) were used. In addition, and with particular relevance to potential TP53 variants of reduced penetrance or hypomorphic alleles, all variants detected within the TP53 gene (including synonymous and intronic variants) were analyzed. Regarding TP53's UTRs, the Illumina gene panel used captures approximately 70 bp of both 5′ and 3′ UTRs with adequate depth, resulting in only a small fraction of the 3′ UTR being covered.

Array CGH and copy number evaluation

For detection of copy number changes, a custom-made eArray covering the identical set of genes targeted by Illumina's TruSight Cancer Panel was used (SureDesign 069100, 8x60K; Agilent Technologies, Santa Clara, CA, USA) [34]. All samples were processed according to the manufacturer's instructions. Microarray slides were scanned using an Agilent microarray scanner system, and standard settings of the Feature Extraction Software (version 11.0.1.1) were applied for data normalization. Data analysis was subsequently performed via Agilent's Genomic Workbench (version 7.0.4.0). Nucleotide positions refer to GRCh37/hg19. Annotation of alterations was computed under different settings dependent on data quality. Verification of detected copy number variations with a second independent method was performed either via MLPA, if probe sets were commercially available for the relevant region (SALSA MLPA kits [MRC Holland], P042-B1 for *ATM*; P056 for *CHEK2*; P008-C1 for *PMS2*), and/or via next-generation sequencing (NGS)-based copy number evaluation using CnvHunter, which is part of ngs-bits [23].

Results

LFS/LFL classification details and performance of classification systems

Of the 83 families in our cohort, 48 met Eeles' LFL criteria [5]; 23 met the original stringent Chompret criteria [6]; 75 were consistent with the temporarily suggested 2008 version of Chompret criteria, which loosened age restrictions and included all *BRCA1/2*-negative patients with BC before age 36 years, regardless of family history [7]; 43 met the 2009 version of Chompret criteria, which again reversed the latter point [8]; 53 met the current Chompret 2015 version criteria, which by definition include all *BRCA1/2*-negative patients with BC before age 31 years, regardless of family history [9]; 12 families met Birch's LFL criteria [4]; and 1 family met classic LFS criteria [1] (multiple entries being possible). Considering mutation carriers' families only (10 of 83 families), all 10 families were consistent with the 2008 version of Chompret criteria, whereas 6 of 10 could be classified into Eeles' LFL and Chompret's 2009 version criteria. When we examined the mutation detection rate for each classification system separately, we found that the majority of the applied criteria performed similarly, with the highest detection rate observed within members of both Eeles' LFL criteria and Chompret's original/2008/2009 criteria (13–14%).

For an overview of the classification results and phenotypic characteristics of the cohort, see Table 1. Information about LFS and LFL criteria definitions is given in Additional file 2.

Variant detection in patients with LFL personal or family history

Within the cohort of 83 subjects with BC, we detected 13 pathogenic or likely pathogenic heterozygous germline variants (ACMG class 4–5; i.e., nonsense, frameshift, missense, [consensus] splice site variants, or copy number aberrations) in 10 unrelated patients and 9 genes [ATM (n = 3), CDKN2A (n = 1), CHEK2 (n = 1), FANCI (n = 1), PALB2 (n = 2), PMS2 (n = 1), RECQL4 (n = 2), RUNX1 (n = 1), and WRN (n = 1)]. These 13 deleterious variants include 4 gross genomic deletions/insertions and 9 truncating NGS-detected variants. Altogether, 3 patients presented as double-mutation carriers, harboring 2 (likely) PVs each (i.e., PMS2 and FANCI, CDKN2A and RECQL4, as well as ATM and CHEK2). Half of the 10 mutation carriers (5 of 83; 6% of the entire cohort) were found to harbor PVs in widely accepted BC susceptibility genes (i.e., PALB2, ATM, and CHEK2), whereas the remaining half (5 of 83; 6% of the entire cohort) carried PVs in candidate genes for which no firm association with BC incidence has yet been established in

a heterozygous germline setting (CDKN2A, RUNX1, FANCI, WRN, and RECQL4). Four variants detected via NGS and 2 of the 4 copy number aberrations detected via array-based CGH (comparative genomic hybridization) have not previously been described in the literature. For an overview of all identified classes 4 and 5 variants, see Table 2. An overview of all index patients carrying (likely) pathogenic germline variants, including their personal and family histories as well as available clinical data and LFS/LFL classification, is given in Table 3, and respective pedigrees can be accessed in Additional file 3.

Besides classes 4–5 variants, we detected 49 variants of unknown significance (VUS, ACMG class 3) within our collective for the parameters detailed above. Via array-based CGH, we identified a duplication of exons 1–21 of the BLM gene, which currently ranks as a class 3 variant owing to a lack of more precise breakpoint information. Via NGS-based sequencing, we detected 46 missense or disruptive inframe deletion and 2 splice region VUS with an MAF ≤ 0.1% occurring in 35 of the 94 investigated genes. Among this list of VUS, we observed an unexpected frequency of very rare FANCA missense variants that were linked to either very early-onset BC or exceptionally Li-Fraumeni-suggestive family/personal history. For a summary of all VUS with an MAF ≤ 0.1% detected via NGS-based sequencing, see Table 4. Neither of the identified VUS was included in the statistical analysis of this work.

Regarding the detection of unconventional, potentially harmful aberrations in TP53 itself, we did not identify any variants other than commonly known polymorphisms in our cohort. A list of all detected TP53 variants is accessible in Additional file 4.

Table 1 Classification and cohort characteristics

	Total sample, n (%)	Mutation carriers, n (%)	Mutation carriers per group, n (%)
Eeles' LFL criteria	48/83 (58%)	6/10 (60%)	6/48 (13%)
Birch's LFL criteria	12/83 (15%)	1/10 (10%)	1/12 (8%)
Original Chompret criteria	23/83 (28%)	3/10 (30%)	3/23 (13%)
Chompret 2008 version criteria	75/83 (90%)	10/10 (100%)	10/75 (13%)
Chompret 2009 version criteria	43/83 (52%)	6/10 (60%)	6/43 (14%)
Chompret 2015 version criteria	53/83 (64%)	5/10 (50%)	5/53 (9%)
Classic LFS criteria	1/83 (1%)	0/10	0/1
Early-onset BC (i.e., ≤ 34 years)	50/83 (60%)	7/10 (70%)	7/50 (14%)
Bilateral BC/two primary BCs	9/83 (11%)	2/10 (20%)	2/9 (22%)
Additional neoplasms besides BC	4/83 (5%)	0/10	0/4
Sarcoma in family or self	10/83 (12%)	0/10	0/10
Brain tumor in family or self	16/83 (20%)	2/10 (20%)	2/16 (13%)

Abbreviations: BC Breast cancer, LFL Li-Fraumeni-like syndrome, LFS Li-Fraumeni syndrome
See Additional file 2 regarding LFS/LFL criteria

Table 2 Detected pathogenic and likely pathogenic single-nucleotide variants, small indels, and copy number alterations

Index patient identifier	Gene (transcript GRCh37/hg19)	Variant type	dbSNP	Exons/total no. of exons	cDNA change	Predicted amino acid change	Aberration array CGH	ACMG class	Previously reported[a]
7	PALB2 (NM_024675.3)	Frameshift	rs515726124	4/13	c.509_510delGA	p.(Arg170Ilefs*14)		5	Yes
30	RUNX1 (NM_001754.4)	Splice donor	rs375131372	3/8	c.97+1G>A			4	No
32	ATM (NM_000051.3)	Deletion		62-63/63			arr [GRCh37]11q22.3 (108233779_108240057)×1	5	Yes
40	ATM (NM_000051.3)	Nonsense		61/63	c.8793T>A	p.(Cys2931*)		5	Yes
	CHEK2 (NM_007194.3)	Deletion		9-10/15			arr [GRCh37]22q12.1 (29092709_29097723)×1	5	Yes
58	CDKN2A (NM_058195.3)	Nonsense		2/3	c.292C>T	p.(Arg98*)		4	No
	RECQL4 (NM_004260.3)	Splice donor		7/21	c.1390+1G>C			4	No
59	WRN (NM_000553.4)	Deletion		15-16/35			arr [GRCh37]8p12 (30948138_30949422)×1	4	No
60	ATM (NM_000051.3)	Nonsense	rs587779852	40/63	c.5932G>T	p.(Glu1978*)		5	Yes
65	FANCI (NM_001113378.1)	Nonsense	rs121918164	37/38	c.3853C>T	p.(Arg1285*)		5	Yes
	PMS2 (NM_000535.5)	Deletion		3-8/15			arr [GRCh37]7p22.1 (6035238_6042593)×1	5	No
76	PALB2 (NM_024675.3)	Frameshift	rs180177143	3/13	c.172_175delTTGT	p.(Gln60Argfs*7)		5	Yes
79	RECQL4 (NM_004260.3)	Missense and splice region	rs186739072	16/22	c.2755G>A	p.(Ala919Thr)		4	No

Abbreviations: ACMG American College of Medical Genetics and Genomics, *cDNA* Complementary DNA, *CGH* Comparative genomic hybridization, *dbSNP* Single Nucleotide Polymorphism database
[a]Based on reports in the literature, ClinVar, Decipher, and gene-specific databases

Table 3 Clinical information and summary of personal and family histories of mutation carriers

Index patient identifier	Variant	Personal history (age at diagnosis in years)	Immunohistochemistry (if available)	Family history of cancer (age at diagnosis in years)	Conformance to LFS/LFL criteria[a]
7	PALB2:p.(Arg170Ilefs*14)	BC (40)	1. TNBC	Mat. – M: BC (40)	Eeles
				Pat. – F: leukemia (< 50), GM: esophagus (60)	Chompret 2008
					Chompret 2009
30	RUNX1:c.97+1G>A	BC (33)	N/A	Mat. – M: BC (56), GM: BC (60)	Chompret 2008
32	ATM exon 62–63 del	BC bilateral (30 + 40)	1. Triple-positive 2. Triple-positive	Mat. – M: OvCa (51), half-S: BC (41) + lung (46), U: leukemia (45), GM: cancer, GF: cancer	Eeles
					orig. Chompret
					Chompret 2008
					Chompret 2009
					Chompret 2015
40	ATM:p.(Cys2931*)	BC (39)	N/A	Mat. – M: OvCa (40), A: leukemia (20)	Eeles
	CHEK2 exon 9–10 del				Chompret 2008
					Chompret 2009
58	CDKN2A:p.(Arg98*)	BC (32)	HER2+	Mat. – GM: ureter (64)	Chompret 2008
	RECQL4:c.1390+1G>C			Pat. – GF: hypopharynx (62)	
59	WRN exon 15–16 del	BC (32)	N/A	Mat. – half-S: melanoma (46), GF: lung (64), GM: CRC (50), GGM: CRC (59), U: kidney (60), this U's sons: melanoma (45), basalioma (36)	Eeles
					orig. Chompret
					Chompret 2008
				Pat. – U: brain (25), 10 Us/As: all died of cancer at a young age	Chompret 2009
					Chompret 2015
					Birch
60	ATM:p.(Glu1978*)	BC (40)	HR+	Mat. – M: BC (51), GM: BC (73)	Eeles
				Pat. – F: glioblastoma (42)	Chompret 2008
					Chompret 2009
					Chompret 2015
65	FANCI:p.(Arg1285*)	BC (30)	HER2+	Mat. – U: CRC (37), GF: CRC (70), GGM: cancer	Chompret 2008
	PMS2 exon 3–8 del			Pat. – GF: esophagus (74)	Chompret 2015
76	PALB2:p.(Gln60Argfs*7)	BC bilateral (33 + 39)	1. HR+ lobular 2. HR+ (HER2+ in metastases)	B: lung (43)	Eeles
				Mat. – M: pancreas (58), A: melanoma (67)	orig. Chompret
					Chompret 2008
					Chompret 2009
79	RECQL4:p.(Ala919Thr)	BC (27)	HR+	Mat. – M: NHL (42), GF: bladder (54)	Chompret 2008
				Pat. – GM: BC (53), GU: lymphoma (52), GA: BC (57), this GA's daughter: BC (47)	Chompret 2015

Abbreviations: A Aunt, *B* Brother, *BC* Breast cancer, *CRC* Colorectal cancer, *del* Deletion, *F* Father, *GA* Grand aunt, *GF* Grandfather, *GGM* Great grandmother, *GM* Grandmother, *GU* Grand uncle, *HER2+* HER2 *(ERBB2)* overexpression/amplification, *HR+* Hormone receptor-positive, *M* Mother, *Mat.* Maternal, *N/A* Not accessible, *Ne* Nephew, *NHL* Non-Hodgkin lymphoma, *Ni* Niece, *OvCa* Ovarian cancer, *Pat.* Paternal, *S* Sister, *TNBC* Triple-negative breast cancer, *U* Uncle
[a]Information about Li-Fraumeni and Li-Fraumeni-like criteria definition are given in Additional file 2

Discussion

In this study, we approached the question whether breast cancer patients with an LFS/LFL-suggestive phenotype may harbor germline aberrations in known or proposed cancer susceptibility genes beyond *TP53* and *BRCA1/2*. Investigating the spectrum of germline mutations in a cohort of 83 BC patients suggestive of LFS/LFL, we identified 10 patients carrying (likely) PVs in the analyzed genes. 3 of these 10 patients carried 2 (likely) PVs each.

Table 4 Missense and splice variants of unknown significance detected by NGS-based sequencing

Gene (transcript GRCh37/hg19)	Index patient identifier	Variant type	Exons/total no. of exons	cDNA change	Predicted amino acid change	dbSNP	Total allele frequency, gnomAD; population with highest AF[a]	In silico prediction[b]	Splicing predictions at nearest natural junction
ALK (NM_004304.4)	52	Splice region and synonymous	17/29	c.2817C>T	p.(Gly939Gly)	rs112022466	0.0001840; SA: 0.0006173		Native acceptor site: MaxEnt: + 23.7% NNSPLICE: + 9.5% HSF: + 0.9% GeneSplicer: + 32.0%
APC (NM_001127510.2)	83	Missense	17/17	c.4918C>T	p.(Arg1640Trp)	rs373440614	0.00007223; O: 0.0001548	C	
ATM (NM_000051.3)	20	Missense	10/63	c.1271C>A	p.(Pro424His)	rs147472613	0.00002188; A: 0.00004189	D	
ATM (NM_000051.3)	20	Missense	50/63	c.7357C>T	p.(Arg2453Cys)	rs755418571	0.00001219; EA: 0.00005807	C	
BRCA2 (NM_000059.3)	36	Missense	10/27	c.831T>G	p.(Asn277Lys)	rs2897705	0.00006632; NFE: 0.0001440	B	
BRCA2 (NM_000059.3)	30	Missense	11/27	c.6101G>A	p.(Arg2034His)	rs80358849	0.000004069; NFE: 0.000008973	B	
BRCA2 (NM_000059.3)	80	Missense	14/27	c.7021C>T	p.(Arg2341Cys)	rs41293505	0.00002439; EA: 0.00005798	D	
BRIP1 (NM_032043.2)	68	Missense	15/20	c.2220G>T	p.(Gln740His)	rs45589637	0.0005198; L: 0.001395	B	
CHEK2 (NM_007194.3)	79	Missense	4/15	c.539G>A	p.(Arg180His)	rs137853009	0.00006494; L: 0.0002615	C	
CHEK2 (NM_007194.3)	83	Missense	6/15	c.688G>C	p.(Ala230Pro)	rs74636216	0.000004063; NFE: 0.000008956	D	
DDB2 (NM_000107.2)	23	Missense	7/10	c.947C>T	p.(Ser316Phe)	rs375788966	0.00001218; SA: 0.00003249	C	
DICER1 (NM_030621.4)	8	Missense	25/29	c.4228A>T	p.(Asn1410Tyr)		not found	D	
DIS3L2 (NM_152383.4)	65	Missense	20/21	c.2450C>T	p.(Thr817Met)	rs376816858	0.00006697; SA: 0.0003505	C	

Table 4 Missense and splice variants of unknown significance detected by NGS-based sequencing (Continued)

Gene (transcript GRCh37/hg19)	Index patient identifier	Variant type	cDNA change	Exons/total no. of exons	Predicted amino acid change	dbSNP	Total allele frequency, gnomAD; population with highest AF[a]	In silico prediction[b]	Splicing predictions at nearest natural junction
EGFR (NM_005228.3)	54	Missense	c.2039G>A	17/28	p.(Arg680Gln)	rs373336251	0.00009084; FE: 0.0003912	D	
ERCC2 (NM_000400.3)	24	Disruptive inframe deletion	c.1857_1859delCAT	20/23	p.(Ile619del)		0.000008127; EA: 0.00005800		
ERCC2 (NM_000400.3)	55	Missense	c.2083C>T	22/23	p.(Arg695Cys)	rs201392911	0.0001372; A: 0.0003331	D	
ERCC4 (NM_005236.2)	23	Missense	c.2395C>T	11/11	p.(Arg799Trp)	rs121913049	0.0004476; NFE: 0.0008138	D	
ERCC5 (NM_000123.3)	23	Missense	c.56C>T	1/15	p.(Pro19Leu)	rs34291397	0.0005702; NFE: 0.001092	C	
ERCC5 (NM_000123.3)	76	Missense	c.2818G>A	13/15	p.(Val940Met)	rs146344855	0.0009378; AJ: 0.005122	C	
EXT2 (NM_000401.3)	13	Missense	c.1064G>A	6/14	p.(Arg355His)	rs149727518	0.0006422; AJ: 0.003448	D	
EXT2 (NM_000401.3)	54	Missense	c.1186G>A	7/14	p.(Val396Met)	rs138943091	0.0004148; NFE: 0.0007261	D	
FANCA (NM_000135.2)	41, 73	Missense	c.64T>G	1/43	p.(Trp22Gly)		not found	D	
FANCA (NM_000135.2)	8	Missense	c.1489C>G	16/43	p.(Pro497Ala)		not found	D	
FANCA (NM_000135.2)	27	Missense	c.2000C > G	22/43	p.(Pro667Arg)	rs755293596	0.00002230; SA: 0.00004382	D	
FANCA (NM_000135.2)	49	Missense	c.3430C>T	35/43	p.(Arg1144Trp)	rs143671872	0.0005269; NFE: 0.0009237	D	
FANCA (NM_000135.2)	54	Missense	c.3688C>G	37/43	p.(Leu1230Val)	rs576401459	0.00002030; A: 0.00006535	D	
FANCD2 (NM_033084.3)	57	Missense	c.1933G>T	21/43	p.(Asp645Tyr)	rs146496253	0.0001371; NFE: 0.0002288	C	
FANCI (NM_001113378.1)	35	Missense	c.1589T>C	17/38	p.(Leu530Pro)	rs766346156	0.000008122; SA: 0.00006497	D	
GPC3 (NM_001164617.1)	19	Missense	c.1630C>T	8/9	p.(Arg544Cys)	rs759543703	0.0009270; A: 0.0001707	D	

Table 4 Missense and splice variants of unknown significance detected by NGS-based sequencing (Continued)

Gene (transcript GRCh37/hg19)	Index patient identifier	Variant type	Exons/ total no. of exons	cDNA change	Predicted amino acid change	dbSNP	Total allele frequency, gnomAD; population with highest AF[a]	In silico prediction[b]	Splicing predictions at nearest natural junction
HNF1A (NM_000545.6)	48	Missense	5/10	c.1061C>T	p.(Thr354Met)	rs757068809	0.00006495; L: 0.0001743	D	
KIT (NM_000222.2)	39	Missense	3/21	c.391G>A	p.(Asp131Asn)		0.00001807; A: 0.00004164	C	
MET (NM_001127500.1)	13	Missense	2/21	c.1076G>A	p.(Arg359Gln)	rs201274041	0.0002347; NFE: 0.0004298	D	
MET (NM_001127500.1)	75	Missense	14/21	c.3023G>A	p.(Ser1008Asn)		not found	D	
MLH1 (NM_000249.3)	51	Missense	13/19	c.1457C>T	p.(Ser486Phe)	rs532873141	0.000004061; EA: 0.00005798	C	
NF1 (NM_001042492)	28	Missense	5/58	c.575G>A	p.(Arg192Gln)	rs587781670	0.00005294; EA: 0.0005803	C	
NSD1 (NM_022455.4)	10	Missense	23/23	c.7352G>A	p.(Arg2451Lys)	rs200115665	0.0001119; NFE: 0.0002212	D	
PALB2 (NM_024675.3)	56	Missense	8/13	c.2792T>G	p.(Leu931Arg)	rs773831304	0.00001221; NFE: 0.00002694	D	
PMS1 (NM_000534.4)	67	Missense	2/13	c.118G>C	p.(Val40Leu)		not found	B	
PMS1 (NM_000534.4)	12	Missense	3/13	c.287C>A	p.(Ala96Asp)	rs139414606	0.000004063; NFE: 0.000008962	D	
PTCH1 (NM_001083602.1)	4	Missense	23/24	c.3749A>G	p.(Tyr1250Cys)	rs147067171	0.0005463; AJ: 0.001098	D	
RAD51C (NM_058216.2)	42	Splice region	8/8	c.1026+5_1026+7 delGTA		rs747311993	0.00001219; NFE: 0.00002687		Native donor site: SSF: −100.0% MaxEnt: −100.0% NNSPLICE: −99.6% HSF: −14.8%
RAD51D (NM_002878.3)	52	Missense	5/10	c.355T>C	p.(Cys119Arg)	rs201313861	0.00005413; L: 0.00008716	B	
RHBDF2 (NM_024599.5)	3, 75	Missense	8/19	c.940G>A	p.(Ala314Thr)	rs140433374	0.0007812; FE: 0.001173	C	
SDHB (NM_003000.2)	81	Missense	2/8	c.178A>G	p.(Thr60Ala)	rs34599281	0.00006095; NFE: 0.0001165	D	

Table 4 Missense and splice variants of unknown significance detected by NGS-based sequencing *(Continued)*

Gene (transcript GRCh37/hg19)	Index patient identifier	Variant type	Exons/ total no. of exons	cDNA change	Predicted amino acid change	dbSNP	Total allele frequency, gnomAD; population with highest AF[a]	In silico prediction[b]	Splicing predictions at nearest natural junction
SLX4 (NM_032444.2)	14	Missense	14/15	c.4831G>A	p.(Glu1611Lys)	rs766110479	0.00002847; EA: 0.00005798	D	
TSC1 (NM_000368.4)	51	Missense	12/23	c.1178C>T	p.(Thr393Ile)	rs201452238	0.00002170; A: 0.00004165	D	
TSC2 (NM_000548.4)	32	Missense	36/42	c.4582G>C	p.(Glu1528Gln)		not found	D	
WRN (NM_000553.4)	55	Missense	19/35	c.2131C>T	p.(Arg711Trp)	rs34560788	0.0002057; NFE: 0.0003948	D	

Abbreviations: HSF Human Splicing Finder, *SSF* Splice Site Finder

[a]*NFE* European (non-Finnish), *FE* European (Finnish), *A* African, *L* Latino, *EA* East Asian, *SA* South Asian, *AJ* Ashkenazi Jewish, *O* Other

[b]Based on in silico prediction tools Align GVGD, MetaLR, SIFT, and Polymorphism Phenotyping version 2 (PolyPhen-2) (HDIV), as well as phyloP basewise conservation scores; rated as probably damaging (D) with at least 3 of 5 tools predicting damage; rated as probably benign (B) with at least 4 of 5 tools predicting tolerance; or rated as contradictory (C) with 2 of 5 tools predicting damage or conflicting results

Variants in established BC susceptibility genes (*PALB2, ATM, CHEK2*)

As anticipated beforehand, we detected several PVs in established BC-associated genes. Two women (subjects 7, 76) carry previously described, protein-truncating, heterozygous *PALB2* frameshift variants. The variant PALB2:p.(Gln60Argfs*7), occurring in patient 76, has previously been detected in several unrelated patients with BC [35, 36], whereas the variant PALB2:p.(Arg170Ilefs*14) in patient 7 is a known Polish founder mutation [37]. Notably, patient 76 developed hormone receptor-positive BC disease at the age of 33 years and contralateral BC at age 39 years, whereas patient 7 presented with triple-negative BC, which is in line with studies reporting breast tumors of *PALB2* mutation carriers to be triple-negative in about 34% of these patients [38].

Furthermore, 3 women of our cohort carry heterozygous PVs in *ATM*, one of whom additionally harbors a PV in *CHEK2*. A deletion of the last 2 exons of *ATM* (62–63) was detected in patient 32. Deletions of exon 63 or exons 62–63 of the *ATM* gene have previously been reported in patients with ataxia telangiectasia and are considered to be functionally relevant [39, 40]. In two further patients (60, 40), we detected previously described *ATM* nonsense variants; the variant ATM:p.(Glu1978*) has been reported in BC cases before [41], whereas the variant ATM:p.(Cys2931*) has been described as a class 5 variant in a patient with ataxia telangiectasia [42]. The latter index person (40) additionally harbors a *CHEK2* exon 9–10 deletion, which is a known pathogenic Slavic founder mutation [43]. Remarkably, 2 of the 3 *ATM* mutation carriers of our cohort have first-degree relatives presenting with ovarian cancer, one of whom harbors the additional *CHEK2* exon 9–10 deletion. While monoallelic *ATM* germline PVs have been described in patients with ovarian cancer, heterozygous *ATM* variants have been associated predominantly with elevated BC incidence rather than other cancer types [44, 45].

Variants in candidate BC susceptibility genes
Variants in genes associated with BC in a somatic context (*CDKN2A, RUNX1*)

One woman (patient 58), who is additionally affected by the class 4 splice donor site variant RECQL4:c.1390 +1G>C, was identified to carry a *CDKN2A*/p14^{ARF} nonsense variant in exon 2 of 3 total exons [CDKN2A:-p.(Arg98*)]. The *CDKN2A* locus encodes two distinct proteins, p14^{ARF} and p16$^{\text{INK4}}$, that are defined by translating the common second exon in alternate reading frames. The variant we detected is not predicted to affect expression or function of p16$^{\text{INK4}}$, a tumor suppressor implicated in the CDK4/CDK6-RB1 pathway; instead, p14^{ARF} expression is expected to be abolished via nonsense-mediated RNA decay (NMD). The protein

p14^{ARF} acts upstream of TP53 by binding directly to MDM2, an E3 ubiquitin ligase controlling the activity and stability of TP53. Because p14^{ARF} promotes MDM2's degradation, TP53 is stabilized and accumulates, and a TP53 response manifests in elevated levels of p21$^{\text{CIP1}}$, inducing cell cycle arrest [46]. PVs in human p14^{ARF} exon 2 have been reported to disrupt its nucleolar localization and impair its ability to block nuclear export of MDM2 and TP53 [47]. The exon 2 variant in our cohort was identified in an index patient whose grandfather was diagnosed with hypopharyngeal carcinoma, which is in line with *CDKN2A* PVs predisposing to tobacco-related cancers such as orolaryngeal cancer, next to its predominant role in hereditary melanoma, pancreatic cancer, and further tumor entities [MIM:600160]. Of note and with particular relevance to LFS and LFL, germline *CDKN2A* PVs have recently been demonstrated to account for a subset (8 of 190) of hereditary sarcoma cases negative for germline *TP53* PVs [17]. Conversely, however, sarcomas are rare in *CDKN2A* mutation carriers, and the affected family of our cohort also does not present with sarcoma cases. In a somatic context, *CDKN2A* PVs have previously been associated with the mutational landscape of BC [48].

In index patient 30, we detected a splice donor site variant in *RUNX1* (RUNX1:c.97+1G>A) predicted deleterious by 4 of 5 splice prediction programs owing to complete loss of the native splice site. As of yet, this variant has not been described in the literature and was classified by us as a class 4 variant on the basis of in silico prediction. *RUNX1* is a gene well known for its crucial role in the hematopoietic system and for its association with sporadic and familial leukemia [49]. The above-mentioned variant was identified in a family exclusively struck by BC. Of note, no hematologic abnormalities were reported in this family at the time of consultation. Even though the variant was detected in 43% of the sequencing reads (VAF 43%, depth 400 ×), we cannot exclude the possibility that this variant might be due to clonal hematopoiesis (i.e., undiagnosed hematologic disorder). In the case of a confirmed germline event, functional splicing assays would be needed to confirm the disruptive nature of the variant. In regard to BC pathology, *RUNX1* has been suggested to be largely understudied [50], and genome-wide sequencing of cohorts of patients with BC have subsequently exposed *RUNX1* as one of the most frequently mutated and/or deleted genes in BC in a somatic setting [51, 52]. Its role in BC progression has been related to estrogen signaling but remains elusive, likely including oncogenic rather than tumor-suppressive functions in mammary epithelial cells [53–55]. A conclusive role for *RUNX1* germline variations in BC pathogenesis cannot be assessed currently and needs further clarification.

Variants in Fanconi pathway genes (FANCI, FANCA)

The nonsense *FANCI* variant FANCI:p.(Arg1285*) in exon 37 of 38 total exons, located within the last 72 bp of the second to last exon and therefore imprecise in regard to NMD, was detected in patient 65, who was additionally found to carry a deletion of exons 3–8 of the *PMS2* gene, which was verified by MLPA analysis. Because the maternal lineage includes two colorectal carcinomas in two of the index person's second-degree relatives, diagnosed at 37 and 70 years of age, the *PMS2* variant is primarily suggestive of being responsible for the familial cancer phenotypes. Nonetheless, the *FANCI* variant concerns a highly conserved arginine, has previously been described in patients with Fanconi anemia (FA), and has been found to impair DNA binding and ubiquitination of the ID2 complex, a dimeric complex formed by FANCI and FANCD2, which is relevant for DNA crosslink repair [56, 57]. Because the paternal lineage also shows incidence of malignant disease, it is conceivable that the *FANCI* and *PMS2* variants may jointly combine in the index person's genome, leading to a more severe phenotype, such as earlier age of onset of disease.

Furthermore, 6 patients of our cohort were identified to carry 5 very rare *FANCA* VUS: FANCA:p.(Trp22Gly) twice, FANCA:p.(Pro497Ala), FANCA:p.(Pro667Arg), FANCA:p.(Arg1144Trp), and FANCA:p.(Leu1230Val). All but one of these rare *FANCA* VUS were absent in a large cohort of 11,000 exome-sequenced individuals of HMGU (Helmholtz Zentrum München – Deutsches Forschungszentrum für Gesundheit und Umwelt) and are either not or very rarely found in datasets from the Genome Aggregation Database [58] (*see* Table 4 for details). Interestingly, clinical presentation of these heterozygous *FANCA* missense VUS carriers comprises some of the most striking LFL features, involving either very early-onset BC or exceptionally Li-Fraumeni-suggestive personal and family traits, such as a woman with triple primaries (malignant hemangiopericytoma at age 12 years, BC at age 28 years, and contralateral BC at age 47 years) or a woman whose sister and half-brother were diagnosed with two liposarcomas and a melanoma, respectively. The median age of onset of BC disease for these 6 *FANCA* VUS carriers was 29.5 years (27, 27, 28, 31, 35, and 44 years), whereas the median age of onset for the entire cohort was 33 years. In a biallelic context, the Fanconi family genes are associated with FA, a condition characterized by congenital abnormalities, bone marrow failure, and cancer predisposition already during childhood. *FANCA* gene PVs are by far the most common in FA, responsible for at least 60% of all cases of FA [59]. Heterozygous parents and siblings of patients with FA have not been found to exhibit an elevated incidence of malignant disease [60]; however, monoallelic *FANCA* variants have been investigated only sparsely in a

disease context, and with inconsistent results [61–63]. Considering the rarity of each *FANCA* VUS detected in the present study, and given the possibility of differing *FANCA* missense variants conferring vastly diverse effects on protein function, the disproportionate occurrence of these rare variants appears to be worthy of further investigation.

Variants in RECQ helicases (WRN, RECQL4)

Two class 4–5 aberrations (patients 59 and 79) and one class 3 copy number change (patient 63) were identified in *WRN*, *RECQL4*, and *BLM* — 3 of 5 genes belonging to the human family of RecQ helicases, comprising enzymes that drive the unwinding of DNA in an ATP- and Mg^{2+}-dependent manner and which are essential for genome maintenance and stability. In an autosomal recessive setting, each of these genes confers very rare and complex syndromes, namely Werner syndrome (*WRN*), Bloom syndrome (*BLM*), and Rothmund-Thomson syndrome or RAPADILINO syndrome (*RECQL4*). In regard to LFS, in which sarcoma incidence is being considered somewhat of a hallmark within the tumor spectrum, a particularly striking fact about the above-mentioned syndromes is that the spectrum of malignancies conferred by them is dominated by sarcomas as well [64, 65]. Moreover, for all three proteins, a firm association with TP53 has been described [65, 66]. Whereas biallelic impairment is considered mandatory for the full spectrum of the syndromes to develop, *WRN* and *BLM* have additionally been suggested as BC susceptibility genes in a monoallelic setting [67–69], and dominant-negative effects or gain-of-function processes have previously been proposed for specific missense mutant WRN or BLM proteins [70].

To our knowledge, this is the first study focusing on a German population-based cohort of familial BC patients suggestive of LFL but negative for causative *TP53* as well as *BRCA1/2* germline PVs to be systematically panel-tested for aberrations in further cancer susceptibility genes. One hypothesis for the emergence of an LFL phenotype without detectable *TP53* PV is the simultaneous and additive occurrence of dual or multiple clearly pathogenic aberrations in more than one cancer susceptibility gene. Our study design was able to confirm double heterozygosity in 3 cases. In regard to patients with BC, double heterozygosity for germline PVs in BC predisposition genes has been detected and discussed before [67]. This type of oligogenic or polygenic model might explain the fact that often the index patients of our cohort happen to be burdened by cancer incidences from both family lineages. The model would also explain why the family mode may not follow a strict autosomal dominant inheritance pattern, which is usually considered a hallmark of classic LFS.

With the current state of knowledge and excluding all VUS, the presently described aberrations, occurring in 10 (12%) of our cohort's individuals, may in part explain or contribute to some of the corresponding phenotypes. However, the gravity and the spectrum of malignant disease in many of our cohort's families seem to suggest that additional PVs in modifying genes or as yet unknown cancer predisposition genes may play a role in some of them. Importantly, these results indicate that even after testing a fairly extensive number of cancer susceptibility genes with a panel design covering both sequence alterations and copy number changes, a large number of LFL BC cases remain unexplained. Few studies have approached the quest for further susceptibility genes in individual *TP53*-negative LFS/LFL cases, either by specifically testing single genes associated with the spectrum of tumors appearing in LFS or by performing whole-exome sequencing. Associations have been suggested for LFS-associated brain tumors with nonsense PVs in *CASP9* (caspase-9) [71], for a *POT1* (protection of telomeres 1) missense variant with cardiac and breast angiosarcomas [72], and, as mentioned above, for *CDKN2A* PVs with hereditary sarcoma cases [17].

Apart from the idea of aberrations in additional susceptibility genes being responsible for *TP53*-negative LFL cases, novel mechanisms for *TP53* impairment are also emerging. These include structural variants that cannot easily be detected by conventional approaches such as intron 1 rearrangements [73], variants in the far-off 3′ UTR affecting microRNA binding [74] (a region not covered by the Illumina gene panel used in our study), and novel splicing PVs [75]. Whereas the severe phenotype known for LFS is expected to result predominantly from missense or isoform-specific variants conferring a dominant-negative effect of the mutated over the wild-type proteins, *TP53* haploinsufficiency (e.g., loss of function or gene dosage effects due to splice variants or 3′ UTR variants and deletions, respectively) is emerging as a likely mechanism for a more subtle phenotype, one that may in fact be described as LFL, as has previously been suggested [75]. Testing patients without variants in coding *TP53* regions, such as the ones in our cohort, for the above-mentioned variants would constitute a crucial future undertaking.

The strengths of this study include a well-characterized cohort of LFL BC patients and the dual-method study design of NGS and array-based CGH to cover a larger number of aberrations. Limitations include the following:

1. Segregation analyses would be mandatory in order to characterize the impact of the detected variants in affected and unaffected family members and to predict the penetrance associated with these variants; unfortunately, DNA was not available for any of the family members of affected germline mutation carriers.

2. Breakpoint analysis and, if applicable, translocation details are urgently needed for the *BLM* duplication.

3. Functional assays would be helpful in determining the consequences of the detected VUS and novel aberrations.

Conclusions

Our study helps define the mutational spectrum in breast cancer patients suggestive of LFS, contributes to a potential relevance of *CDKN2A*/p14^{ARF} in LFS/LFL settings, and points out the need for intensified research on monoallelic variants in Fanconi pathway and RECQ family genes. Notably, our study further reveals that there remains a large portion of unexplained LFS/LFL cases and emphasizes the necessity of advanced research on novel susceptibility genes as well as noncoding *TP53* variants in patients with negative test results for *TP53* variants in coding regions.

Abbreviations
ACMG: American College of Medical Genetics and Genomics; BC: Breast cancer; bp: Base pair(s); CGH: Comparative genomic hybridization; FA: Fanconi anemia; HBOC: Hereditary breast and ovarian cancer; HMGU: Helmholtz Zentrum München – Deutsches Forschungszentrum für Gesundheit und Umwelt; IGV: Integrative Genomics Viewer; LFL: Li-Fraumeni-like syndrome; LFS: Li-Fraumeni syndrome; MAF: Minor allele frequency; MLPA: Multiplex ligation-dependent probe amplification; NGS: Next-generation sequencing; NMD: Nonsense-mediated RNA decay; PV: Pathogenic variant; ROI: Region of interest; UTR: Untranslated region; VAF: Variant allele frequency; VUS: Variant of unknown significance

Acknowledgements
The authors gratefully acknowledge Christian Blumenberg, Marcel Tauscher, Michael Griese, Bernd Haermeyer, and Michaela Losch for extensive laboratory work.

Funding
This work was funded by the Claudia von Schilling Foundation for Breast Cancer Research (to DS and BS).

Authors' contributions
JP contributed to conception and design, data generation, data interpretation and statistical analysis, critical review and discussion, and the writing of the manuscript. GS contributed to data generation, data

interpretation and statistical analysis, and critical review and discussion. WH contributed to data generation, data interpretation, and statistical analysis. SS contributed to data interpretation, statistical analysis, and critical review and discussion. MS contributed to data interpretation, statistical analysis, and critical review and discussion. BA contributed to data generation and critical review and discussion. TR contributed to data interpretation, statistical analysis, and critical review and discussion. KH contributed to conception and design and to eArray design. MS contributed to conception and design and to NGS pipeline design. HP contributed to data interpretation and statistical analysis. UHB contributed to recruitment of patients and collection of clinical data. DM contributed to recruitment of patients and collection of clinical data. TI contributed to conception and design and to critical review and discussion. BS contributed to conception and design and to critical review and discussion. DS contributed to conception and design and to critical review and discussion. All authors read and approved the final manuscript.

Competing interests

The authors declare that they have no competing interests.

Author details

[1]Department of Human Genetics, Hannover Medical School, Carl-Neuberg-Strasse 1, 30625 Hannover, Germany. [2]Institute for Clinical Genetics, Faculty of Medicine Carl Gustav Carus, TU Dresden, Dresden, Germany. [3]German Cancer Research Center (DKFZ), Heidelberg, Germany. [4]National Center for Tumor Diseases (NCT) Partner Site Dresden, Dresden, Germany. [5]Institute of Medical Genetics and Applied Genomics, University of Tübingen, Tübingen, Germany. [6]Institute of Human Genetics, Helmholtz Zentrum München, Neuherberg, Germany. [7]Department of Gynecology and Obstetrics, Hannover Medical School, Hannover, Germany. [8]Department of Internal Medicine, Hematology/Oncology, University Hospital Frankfurt, Frankfurt, Germany.

References

1. Li FP, Fraumeni JF Jr, Mulvihill JJ, Blattner WA, Dreyfus MG, Tucker MA. Miller RW. A cancer family syndrome in twenty-four kindreds. Cancer Res. 1988; 48(18):5358–62.
2. Malkin D, Li FP, Strong LC, Fraumeni JF Jr, Nelson CE, Kim DH, Kassel J, Gryka MA, Bischoff FZ, Tainsky MA, et al. Germ line p53 mutations in a familial syndrome of breast cancer, sarcomas, and other neoplasms. Science. 1990;250(4985):1233–8.
3. Evans DG, Birch JM, Thorneycroft M, McGown G, Lalloo F, Varley JM. Low rate of TP53 germline mutations in breast cancer/sarcoma families not fulfilling classical criteria for Li-Fraumeni syndrome. J Med Genet. 2002; 39(12):941–4.
4. Birch JM, Hartley AL, Tricker KJ, Prosser J, Condie A, Kelsey AM, Harris M, Jones PH, Binchy A, Crowther D, et al. Prevalence and diversity of constitutional mutations in the p53 gene among 21 Li-Fraumeni families. Cancer Res. 1994;54(5):1298–304.
5. Eeles RA. Germline mutations in the TP53 gene. Cancer Surv. 1995;25: 101–24.
6. Chompret A, Abel A, Stoppa-Lyonnet D, Brugieres L, Pages S, Feunteun J, Bonaiti-Pellie C. Sensitivity and predictive value of criteria for p53 germline mutation screening. J Med Genet. 2001;38(1):43–7.
7. Bougeard G, Sesboue R, Baert-Desurmont S, Vasseur S, Martin C, Tinat J, Brugieres L, Chompret A, de Paillerets BB, Stoppa-Lyonnet D, et al. Molecular basis of the Li-Fraumeni syndrome: an update from the French LFS families. J Med Genet. 2008;45(8):535–8.
8. Tinat J, Bougeard G, Baert-Desurmont S, Vasseur S, Martin C, Bouvignies E, Caron O, Bressac-de Paillerets B, Berthet P, Dugast C, et al. 2009 Version of the Chompret criteria for Li Fraumeni syndrome. J Clin Oncol. 2009;27(26): e108–9. author reply e10
9. Bougeard G, Renaux-Petel M, Flaman JM, Charbonnier C, Fermey P, Belotti M, Gauthier-Villars M, Stoppa-Lyonnet D, Consolino E, Brugieres L, et al. Revisiting Li-Fraumeni syndrome from TP53 mutation carriers. J Clin Oncol. 2015;33(21):2345–52.
10. Nichols KE, Malkin D, Garber JE, Fraumeni JF Jr, Li FP. Germ-line p53 mutations predispose to a wide spectrum of early-onset cancers. Cancer Epidemiol Biomark Prev. 2001;10(2):83–7.
11. Chompret A, Brugieres L, Ronsin M, Gardes M, Dessarps-Freichey F, Abel A, Hua D, Ligot L, Dondon MG, Bressac-de Paillerets B, et al. P53 germline mutations in childhood cancers and cancer risk for carrier individuals. Br J Cancer. 2000;82(12):1932–7.
12. Wooster R, Weber BL. Breast and ovarian cancer. N Engl J Med. 2003; 348(23):2339–47.
13. Gonzalez KD, Noltner KA, Buzin CH, Gu D, Wen-Fong CY, Nguyen VQ, Han JH, Lowstuter K, Longmate J, Sommer SS, et al. Beyond Li Fraumeni syndrome: clinical characteristics of families with p53 germline mutations. J Clin Oncol. 2009;27(8):1250–6.
14. McCuaig JM, Armel SR, Novokmet A, Ginsburg OM, Demsky R, Narod SA, Malkin D. Routine TP53 testing for breast cancer under age 30: ready for prime time? Fam Cancer. 2012;11(4):607–13.
15. Kraus C, Hoyer J, Vasileiou G, Wunderle M, Lux MP, Fasching PA, Krumbiegel M, Uebe S, Reuter M, Beckmann MW, et al. Gene panel sequencing in familial breast/ovarian cancer patients identifies multiple novel mutations also in genes others than BRCA1/2. Int J Cancer. 2017;140(1):95–102.
16. Slavin TP, Maxwell KN, Lilyquist J, Vijai J, Neuhausen SL, Hart SN, Ravichandran V, Thomas T, Maria A, Villano D, et al. The contribution of pathogenic variants in breast cancer susceptibility genes to familial breast cancer risk. NPJ Breast Cancer. 2017;3:22.
17. Jouenne F, Chauvot de Beauchene I, Bollaert E, Avril MF, Caron O, Ingster O, Lecesne A, Benusiglio P, Terrier P, Caumette V, et al. Germline CDKN2A/P16^{INK4A} mutations contribute to genetic determinism of sarcoma. J Med Genet. 2017;54(9):607–12.
18. Meindl A, Ditsch N, Kast K, Rhiem K, Schmutzler RK. Hereditary breast and ovarian cancer: new genes, new treatments, new concepts. Dtsch Arztebl Int. 2011;108(19):323–30.
19. megSAP – Medical Genetics Sequence Analysis Pipeline. https://github.com/imgag/megSAP.
20. Prochazkova K, Pavlikova K, Minarik M, Sumerauer D, Kodet R, Sedlacek Z. Somatic TP53 mutation mosaicism in a patient with Li-Fraumeni syndrome. Am J Med Genet A. 2009;149A(2):206–11.
21. Robinson JT, Thorvaldsdottir H, Winckler W, Guttman M, Lander ES, Getz G, Mesirov JP. Integrative genomics viewer. Nat Biotechnol. 2011;29(1):24–6.
22. Thorvaldsdottir H, Robinson JT, Mesirov JP. Integrative Genomics Viewer (IGV): high-performance genomics data visualization and exploration. Brief Bioinform. 2013;14(2):178–92.
23. ngs-bits – Short-read sequencing tools: GSvar. https://github.com/imgag/ngs-bits.
24. Auton A, Brooks LD, Durbin RM, Garrison EP, Kang HM, Korbel JO, Marchini JL, McCarthy S, McVean GA. Abecasis GR. A global reference for human genetic variation. Nature. 2015;526(7571):68–74.
25. Lek M, Karczewski KJ, Minikel EV, Samocha KE, Banks E, Fennell T, O'Donnell-Luria AH, Ware JS, Hill AJ, Cummings BB, et al. Analysis of protein-coding genetic variation in 60,706 humans. Nature. 2016; 536(7616):285–91.
26. Glusman G, Caballero J, Mauldin DE, Hood L, Roach JC. Kaviar: an accessible system for testing SNV novelty. Bioinformatics. 2011;27(22):3216–7.
27. Dong C, Wei P, Jian X, Gibbs R, Boerwinkle E, Wang K, Liu X. Comparison and integration of deleteriousness prediction methods for nonsynonymous SNVs in whole exome sequencing studies. Hum Mol Genet. 2015;24(8):2125–37.
28. Kumar P, Henikoff S, Ng PC. Predicting the effects of coding non-synonymous variants on protein function using the SIFT algorithm. Nat Protoc. 2009;4(7):1073–81.

29. Adzhubei IA, Schmidt S, Peshkin L, Ramensky VE, Gerasimova A, Bork P, Kondrashov AS, Sunyaev SR. A method and server for predicting damaging missense mutations. Nat Methods. 2010;7(4):248–9.

30. Landrum MJ, Lee JM, Benson M, Brown G, Chao C, Chitipiralla S, Gu B, Hart J, Hoffman D, Hoover J, et al. ClinVar: public archive of interpretations of clinically relevant variants. Nucleic Acids Res. 2016;44(D1):D862–8.

31. Stenson PD, Ball EV, Mort M, Phillips AD, Shiel JA, Thomas NS, Abeysinghe S, Krawczak M, Cooper DN. Human Gene Mutation Database (HGMD): 2003 update. Hum Mutat. 2003;21(6):577–81.

32. FLOSSIES: a database of germline genomic variation in healthy older women. https://whi.color.com/.

33. Richards S, Aziz N, Bale S, Bick D, Das S, Gastier-Foster J, Grody WW, Hegde M, Lyon E, Spector E, et al. Standards and guidelines for the interpretation of sequence variants: a joint consensus recommendation of the American College of Medical Genetics and Genomics and the Association for Molecular Pathology. Genet Med. 2015;17(5):405–24.

34. Hackmann K, Kuhlee F, Betcheva-Krajcir E, Kahlert AK, Mackenroth L, Klink B, Di Donato N, Tzschach A, Kast K, Wimberger P, et al. Ready to clone: CNV detection and breakpoint fine-mapping in breast and ovarian cancer susceptibility genes by high-resolution array CGH. Breast Cancer Res Treat. 2016;159(3):585–90.

35. Janatova M, Kleibl Z, Stribrna J, Panczak A, Vesela K, Zimovjanova M, Kleiblova P, Dundr P, Soukupova J, Pohlreich P. The *PALB2* gene is a strong candidate for clinical testing in *BRCA1*- and *BRCA2*-negative hereditary breast cancer. Cancer Epidemiol Biomark Prev. 2013;22(12):2323–32.

36. Thompson ER, Gorringe KL, Rowley SM, Wong-Brown MW, McInerny S, Li N, Trainer AH, Devereux L, Doyle MA, Li J, et al. Prevalence of *PALB2* mutations in Australian familial breast cancer cases and controls. Breast Cancer Res. 2015;17:111.

37. Dansonka-Mieszkowska A, Kluska A, Moes J, Dabrowska M, Nowakowska D, Niwinska A, Derlatka P, Cendrowski K, Kupryjanczyk J. A novel germline *PALB2* deletion in Polish breast and ovarian cancer patients. BMC Med Genet. 2010;11:20.

38. Cybulski C, Kluzniak W, Huzarski T, Wokolorczyk D, Kashyap A, Jakubowska A, Szwiec M, Byrski T, Debniak T, Gorski B, et al. Clinical outcomes in women with breast cancer and a *PALB2* mutation: a prospective cohort analysis. Lancet Oncol. 2015;16(6):638–44.

39. Huang Y, Yang L, Wang J, Yang F, Xiao Y, Xia R, Yuan X, Yan M. Twelve novel *Atm* mutations identified in Chinese ataxia telangiectasia patients. Neuromolecular Med. 2013;15(3):536–40.

40. Podralska MJ, Stembalska A, Slezak R, Lewandowicz-Uszynska A, Pietrucha B, Koltan S, Wigowska-Sowinska J, Pilch J, Mosor M, Ziolkowska-Suchanek I, et al. Ten new *ATM* alterations in Polish patients with ataxia-telangiectasia. Mol Genet Genomic Med. 2014;2(6):504–11.

41. Bogdanova N, Cybulski C, Bermisheva M, Datsyuk I, Yamini P, Hillemanns P, Antonenkova NN, Khusnutdinova E, Lubinski J, Dork T. A nonsense mutation (E1978X) in the *ATM* gene is associated with breast cancer. Breast Cancer Res Treat. 2009;118(1):207–11.

42. Sandoval N, Platzer M, Rosenthal A, Dork T, Bendix R, Skawran B, Stuhrmann M, Wegner RD, Sperling K, Banin S, et al. Characterization of *ATM* gene mutations in 66 ataxia telangiectasia families. Hum Mol Genet. 1999;8(1):69–79.

43. Cybulski C, Wokolorczyk D, Huzarski T, Byrski T, Gronwald J, Gorski B, Debniak T, Masojc B, Jakubowska A, Gliniewicz B, et al. A large germline deletion in the Chek2 kinase gene is associated with an increased risk of prostate cancer. J Med Genet. 2006;43(11):863–6.

44. Minion LE, Dolinsky JS, Chase DM, Dunlop CL, Chao EC, Monk BJ. Hereditary predisposition to ovarian cancer, looking beyond BRCA1/BRCA2. Gynecol Oncol. 2015;137(1):86–92.

45. Thompson D, Duedal S, Kirner J, McGuffog L, Last J, Reiman A, Byrd P, Taylor M, Easton DF. Cancer risks and mortality in heterozygous *ATM* mutation carriers. J Natl Cancer Inst. 2005;97(11):813–22.

46. Zhang Y, Xiong Y, Yarbrough WG. ARF promotes MDM2 degradation and stabilizes p53: *ARF-INK4a* locus deletion impairs both the Rb and p53 tumor suppression pathways. Cell. 1998;92(6):725–34.

47. Zhang Y, Xiong Y. Mutations in human ARF exon 2 disrupt its nucleolar localization and impair its ability to block nuclear export of MDM2 and p53. Mol Cell. 1999;3(5):579–91.

48. Pereira B, Chin SF, Rueda OM, Vollan HK, Provenzano E, Bardwell HA, Pugh M, Jones L, Russell R, Sammut SJ, et al. The somatic mutation profiles of 2,433 breast cancers refines their genomic and transcriptomic landscapes. Nat Commun. 2016;7:11479.

49. Schlegelberger B, Heller PG. RUNX1 deficiency (familial platelet disorder with predisposition to myeloid leukemia, FPDMM). Semin Hematol. 2017; 54(2):75–80.

50. Janes KA. RUNX1 and its understudied role in breast cancer. Cell Cycle. 2011;10(20):3461–5.

51. Ellis MJ, Ding L, Shen D, Luo J, Suman VJ, Wallis JW, Van Tine BA, Hoog J, Goiffon RJ, Goldstein TC, et al. Whole-genome analysis informs breast cancer response to aromatase inhibition. Nature. 2012;486(7403):353–60.

52. Banerji S, Cibulskis K, Rangel-Escareno C, Brown KK, Carter SL, Frederick AM, Lawrence MS, Sivachenko AY, Sougnez C, Zou L, et al. Sequence analysis of mutations and translocations across breast cancer subtypes. Nature. 2012; 486(7403):405–9.

53. Browne G, Taipaleenmaki H, Bishop NM, Madasu SC, Shaw LM, van Wijnen AJ, Stein JL, Stein GS, Lian JB. Runx1 is associated with breast cancer progression in MMTV-PyMT transgenic mice and its depletion in vitro inhibits migration and invasion. J Cell Physiol. 2015;230(10):2522–32.

54. Chimge NO, Frenkel B. The RUNX family in breast cancer: relationships with estrogen signaling. Oncogene. 2013;32(17):2121–30.

55. Ferrari N, Mohammed ZM, Nixon C, Mason SM, Mallon E, McMillan DC, Morris JS, Cameron ER, Edwards J, Blyth K. Expression of RUNX1 correlates with poor patient prognosis in triple negative breast cancer. PLoS One. 2014;9(6):e100759.

56. Smogorzewska A, Matsuoka S, Vinciguerra P, McDonald ER 3rd, Hurov KE, Luo J, Ballif BA, Gygi SP, Hofmann K, D'Andrea AD, et al. Identification of the FANCI protein, a monoubiquitinated FANCD2 paralog required for DNA repair. Cell. 2007;129(2):289–301.

57. Longerich S, Kwon Y, Tsai MS, Hlaing AS, Kupfer GM, Sung P. Regulation of FANCD2 and FANCI monoubiquitination by their interaction and by DNA. Nucleic Acids Res. 2014;42(9):5657–70.

58. gnomAD – genome Aggregation Database. http://gnomad.broadinstitute.org/.

59. Shimamura A, Alter BP. Pathophysiology and management of inherited bone marrow failure syndromes. Blood Rev. 2010;24(3):101–22.

60. Tischkowitz M, Easton DF, Ball J, Hodgson SV, Mathew CG. Cancer incidence in relatives of British Fanconi anaemia patients. BMC Cancer. 2008;8:257.

61. Solyom S, Winqvist R, Nikkila J, Rapakko K, Hirvikoski P, Kokkonen H, Pylkas K. Screening for large genomic rearrangements in the FANCA gene reveals extensive deletion in a Finnish breast cancer family. Cancer Lett. 2011; 302(2):113–8.

62. Litim N, Labrie Y, Desjardins S, Ouellette G, Plourde K, Belleau P, Durocher F. Polymorphic variations in the FANCA gene in high-risk non-BRCA1/2 breast cancer individuals from the French Canadian population. Mol Oncol. 2013; 7(1):85–100.

63. Abbasi S, Rasouli M. A rare FANCA gene variation as a breast cancer susceptibility allele in an Iranian population. Mol Med Rep. 2017;15(6):3983–8.

64. Calvert GT, Randall RL, Jones KB, Cannon-Albright L, Lessnick S, Schiffman JD. At-risk populations for osteosarcoma: the syndromes and beyond. Sarcoma. 2012;2012:152382.

65. Nakayama H. RecQ family helicases: roles as tumor suppressor proteins. Oncogene. 2002;21(58):9008–21.

66. De S, Kumari J, Mudgal R, Modi P, Gupta S, Futami K, Goto H, Lindor NM, Furuichi Y, Mohanty D, et al. RECQL4 is essential for the transport of p53 to mitochondria in normal human cells in the absence of exogenous stress. J Cell Sci. 2012;125(Pt 10):2509–22.

67. Sokolenko AP, Bogdanova N, Kluzniak W, Preobrazhenskaya EV, Kuligina ES, Iyevleva AG, Aleksakhina SN, Mitiushkina NV, Gorodnova TV, Bessonov AA, et al. Double heterozygotes among breast cancer patients analyzed for BRCA1, CHEK2, ATM, NBN/NBS1, and BLM germ-line mutations. Breast Cancer Res Treat. 2014;145(2):553–62.

68. Prokofyeva D, Bogdanova N, Dubrowinskaja N, Bermisheva M, Takhirova Z, Antonenkova N, Turmanov N, Datsyuk I, Gantsev S, Christiansen H, et al. Nonsense mutation p.Q548X in BLM, the gene mutated in Bloom's syndrome, is associated with breast cancer in Slavic populations. Breast Cancer Res Treat. 2013;137(2):533–9.

69. Wang Z, Xu Y, Tang J, Ma H, Qin J, Lu C, Wang X, Hu Z, Shen H. A polymorphism in Werner syndrome gene is associated with breast cancer susceptibility in Chinese women. Breast Cancer Res Treat. 2009; 118(1):169–75.

Breast cancer patients suggestive of Li-Fraumeni syndrome: mutational spectrum, candidate genes...

57

70. Wu Y, Brosh RM Jr. Helicase-inactivating mutations as a basis for dominant negative phenotypes. Cell Cycle. 2010;9(20):4080–90.

71. Ronellenfitsch MW, Oh JE, Satomi K, Sumi K, Harter PN, Steinbach JP, Felsberg J, Capper D, Voegele C, Durand G, et al. *CASP9* germline mutation in a family with multiple brain tumors. Brain Pathol. 2018;28(1):94–102.

72. Calvete O, Martinez P, Garcia-Pavia P, Benitez-Buelga C, Paumard-Hernandez B, Fernandez V, Dominguez F, Salas C, Romero-Laorden N, Garcia-Donas J, et al. A mutation in the *POT1* gene is responsible for cardiac angiosarcoma in TP53-negative Li-Fraumeni-like families. Nat Commun. 2015;6:8383.

73. Ribi S, Baumhoer D, Lee K, Edison, Teo AS, Madan B, Zhang K, Kohlmann WK, Yao F, Lee WH, et al. TP53 intron 1 hotspot rearrangements are specific to sporadic osteosarcoma and can cause Li-Fraumeni syndrome. Oncotarget. 2015;6(10):7727–40.

74. Macedo GS, Araujo Vieira I, Brandalize AP, Giacomazzi J, Inez Palmero E, Volc S, Rodrigues Paixao-Cortes V, Caleffi M, Silva Alves M, Achatz MI, et al. Rare germline variant (rs78378222) in the TP53 3′ UTR: evidence for a new mechanism of cancer predisposition in Li-Fraumeni syndrome. Cancer Genet. 2016;209(3):97–106.

75. Piao J, Sakurai N, Iwamoto S, Nishioka J, Nakatani K, Komada Y, Mizutani S, Takagi M. Functional studies of a novel germline p53 splicing mutation identified in a patient with Li-Fraumeni-like syndrome. Mol Carcinog. 2013;52(10):770–6.

5

Tricho-rhino-phalangeal syndrome 1 protein functions as a scaffold required for ubiquitin-specific protease 4-directed histone deacetylase 2 de-ubiquitination and tumor growth

Yuzhi Wang[1,2†], Jun Zhang[2†], Lele Wu[1,2], Weiguang Liu[2], Guanyun Wei[2], Xue Gong[1,2], Yan Liu[1,2], Zhifang Ma[2], Fei Ma[2], Jean Paul Thiery[3,4,5] and Liming Chen[1,2*] (ID)

Abstract

Background: Although numerous studies have reported that tricho-rhino-phalangeal syndrome type I (TRPS1) protein, the only reported atypical GATA transcription factor, is overexpressed in various carcinomas, the underlying mechanism(s) by which it contributes to cancer remain unknown.

Methods: Both overexpression and knockdown of TRPS1 assays were performed to examine the effect of TRPS1 on histone deacetylase 2 (HDAC2) protein level and luminal breast cancer cell proliferation. Also, RT-qRCR, luciferase reporter assay and RNA-sequencing were used for transcription detection. Chromatin immunoprecipitation (ChIP) using H4K16ac antibody in conjunction with qPCR was used for determining H4K16ac levels in targeted genes. Furthermore, in vitro cell proliferation assay and in vivo tumor xenografts were used to detect the effect of TRPS1 on tumor growth.

Results: We found that TRPS1 scaffolding recruits and enhances interaction between USP4 and HDAC2 leading to HDAC2 de-ubiquitination and H4K16 deacetylation. We detected repression of a set of cellular growth-related genes by the TRPS1-USP4-HDAC2 axis indicating it is essential in tumor growth. In vitro and in vivo experiments confirmed that silencing *TRPS1* reduced tumor growth, whereas overexpression of HDAC2 restored tumor growth.

Conclusion: Our study deciphered the TRPS1-USP4-HDAC2 axis as a novel mechanism that contributes to tumor growth. Significantly, our results revealed the scaffolding function of TPRS1 in USP4-directed HDAC2 de-ubiquitination and provided new mechanistic insights into the crosstalk between TRPS1, ubiquitin, and histone modification systems leading to tumor growth.

Keywords: TRPS1, HDAC2, USP4, De-ubiquitination, Tumor growth

* Correspondence: chenliming1981@njnu.edu.cn
†Yuzhi Wang and Jun Zhang contributed equally to this work.
[1]The Key Laboratory of Developmental Genes and Human Disease, Ministry of Education, Institute of Life Science, Southeast University, Nanjing 210096, People's Republic of China
[2]Jiangsu Key Laboratory for Molecular and Medical Biotechnology, College of Life Science, Nanjing Normal University, Nanjing 210023, People's Republic of China
Full list of author information is available at the end of the article

Background

TRPS1 transcription factor, the only known atypical member of GATA transcriptional factor family, contains a GATA DNA binding domain like other typical GATAs 1–6 [1]. TRPS1 is important both in development and in carcinogenesis. Mutations in TRPS1 have been documented to cause tricho-rhino-phalangeal syndrome, an autosomal-dominant disorder characterized by craniofacial and skeletal malformations [2]. Elevated TRPS1 expression has been observed in human cancers, including osteosarcoma [3], colon cancer [4], and breast cancer [5]. Recently, *TRPS1* was identified by in vivo transposon-based forward genetic screening as a potential breast cancer driver gene by our group and others [6, 7]. However, the mechanism by which TRPS1 contributes to cancer is not clear.

Histone deacetylases (HDACs) and histone acetyltranferases (HATs) are important in acetylation of histones and non-histone substrates to control and maintain a balance in the transcriptomic landscape of the normal and tumor cells [8–10]. HDACs regulate the expression and activity of numerous proteins involved in both cancer initiation and progression [10]. Eighteen mammalian HDACs have been identified and divided into four classes based on phylogenetic analysis and homology to *Saccharomyces cerevisiae* HDACs [11]. HDAC2, a member of the mammalian class I deacetylases, has been extensively studied. A decrease in HDAC2 markedly inhibits tumor growth, suggesting HDAC2 acts as an oncogene in tumorigenesis [12, 13]. Overexpression of HDAC2 protein was detected in human cancers, including gastric, prostate, and breast cancers [14, 15]. HDAC2 represses gene expression via deacetylating H4K16ac [16], determines the transcription repression program, and acts as a member of nucleosome remodeling deacetylase (NURD) complex [17].

The ubiquitin system plays a significant role in determining the fate of a protein. De-ubiquitinases (DUBs) also have fundamental roles in the ubiquitin system through deconjugating ubiquitin from the targeted proteins [18]. The ubiquitin-specific peptidase 4 (USP4) is proposed to be a potential oncogene, which can transform NIH3T3 cells [19], and USP4-deficient murine embryonic fibroblasts exhibit retarded growth [20]. Previous studies indicate that, compared to normal cells, USP4 is overexpressed in malignant cells [21]. Recently, USP4 was reported to de-ubiquitinate and stabilize HDAC2, which then inhibits p53 and NF-kB [22]. However, the mechanism by which USP4 mediates HDAC2 de-ubiquitination contributing to cancer remains unclear.

In this study, we show that the TRPS1-USP4-HDAC2 regulatory axis is involved in tumor cell proliferation. We provide a novel mechanistic insight into the growth-regulatory role of this axis by providing evidence that TRPS1 recruits USP4 to de-ubiquitinate and stabilize HDAC2. We also illustrate the scaffolding function of TRPS1 as the first example of the non-transcription factor function of GATA transcription factor which affects the ubiquitination and transcription repressive function of HDAC2, acetylation of H4K16, and the de-ubiquitinase function of USP4.

Methods

Cell culture

T47D, BT474, MCF7, MDA-MB-231, and HEK293T cell lines were purchased from American Type Culture Collection (ATCC) and were authenticated by the short tandem repeat (STR) typing. The cell lines were used for the current study within 6 months after cell authentication. BT474 and HEK293T cell lines were cultured in Dulbecco's modified Eagle's medium (DMEM) (Life Technologies, Carlsbad, CA, USA) supplemented with 10% fetal bovine serum (FBS) (HyClone, NY, USA) and 1% penicillin-streptomycin solution (Life Technologies). T47D and MCF7 were maintained in Roswell Park Memorial Institute (RPMI) 1640 medium (Corning Cellgro) supplemented with 10% FBS and 1% penicillin-streptomycin solution. To generate TRPS1 overexpression system in MDA-MB-231, the open reading frame (ORF) of TRPS1 was cloned into the lentivirus vector pCDH-CMV-MCS-EF1-copGFP (System Bioscience, CA, USA) and then transfected into HEK293T cells. The virus-containing supernatant was collected 48 h after transfection, and passed through the 0.45 μm filter to infect MDA-MB-231 cells.

Plasmids

The following plasmids were used in this study: pCDNA3.1-Flag-USP4, pCDNA3.1-Myc-HDAC2, pCDNA 3.1-His-Ub, p3 × Flag-TRPS1, p3 × Flag-TRPS1-N(1–2640), p3 × Flag-TRPS1-ΔC(1–2940), p3 × Flag-TRPS1-C(2941–3885), p3 × Flag-TRPS1-ΔN(2641–3885), p3 × Flag-TRPS1-GATA(2641–2940), 4 × UAS-TK-luciferase, GAL4-HDAC2, and Renilla luciferase (pRL-SV40).

Antibodies

Antibodies used in this study and their sources are as follows: anti-TRPS1 (R&D Systems#AF4838), anti-HDAC2 (Cell Signaling Technology#5113), anti-H4K16ac (Millipore#39929), anti-H4 (Millipore#04–858), anti-USP4 (Cell Signaling Technology#2651), anti-actin (proteintech#60008–1-Ig), anti-HA (Biotool#B23402), anti-Flag (Sigma#F7425), anti-Myc (Biotool#B23402), anti-His (Cell Signaling Technology#12698), and anti-Gal4 (Santa Cruz#510).

Immunoprecipitation and immunoblotting

Cells were collected and lysed for 15 min on ice in the lysis buffer (Beyotime) supplemented with a protease inhibitor. The cell lysates were incubated with antibodies and protein A/G agarose overnight at 4 °C. Unbound proteins were removed by washing three times with wash buffer. The immunoprecipitates from agarose beads were removed using the elution buffer (50 mM Tris–HCl (pH 7.4), 900 mM NaCl, 1 mM EDTA, 1% Triton X-100) for sequential co-immunoprecipitation (Co-IP). For immunoblotting following SDS-PAGE, immunoprecipitated proteins were transferred to polyvinylidene fluoride (PVDF) membranes (Millipore) and probed with various antibodies. The ECL detection system (ImageQuant LAS4000) was used for detection.

Ubiquitination assay

To examine the ubiquitin-modified proteins, cells were lysed in the denaturing buffer (50 mM Tris-HCl pH 7.5, 150 mM NaCl, 4%SDS, 1 mM EDTA, 8% glycerol, 1 mM DTT, 1 mM PMSF and protein inhibitors) supplemented with 20 mM NEM and heated at 90 °C for 10 min. For immunoprecipitation, the lysates were further diluted to 0.1% SDS and immunoprecipitated with anti-Myc antibody at 4 °C overnight and then the ubiquitinated proteins were tested by western blotting.

RT-qPCR analysis

For RT-qPCR analysis, total RNAs were extracted from various cell lines using the RNeasy kit (Qiagen, Hilden, Germany) and reverse transcription of RNA was performed using PrimeScript RT reagent kit (TaKaRa, Otsu, Shiga, Japan) according to the manufacturer's instructions. The primers used for RT-qPCR are listed in Additional file 1: Table S1.

RNA interference (RNAi)

Small interfering RNAs (siRNAs) targeting TRPS1, HDAC2, USP4 or the non-targeting control siRNA (Genepharm, Shanghai, China) were transfected into MCF7, BT474, and T47D cells using Lipofectamine RNAi MAX (Invitrogen; Carlsbad, CA, USA) according to the manufacturer's instructions. All plasmids were transfected using Lipofectamine®2000 (Invitrogen; Carlsbad, CA, USA). An MCF7 cell line with stable depletion of TRPS1 was generated using a lentivirus short hairpin RNA (shRNA) system. The sequences for siRNAs and shRNA are listed in Additional file 2: Table S2.

Luciferase reporter assay

HEK-293 T cells were transfected with 4 × UAS-TK-luc, Gal4-HDAC2, pRL-SV40, and Flag-TRPS1/truncations or control vector as indicated. Cells were subjected to luciferase reporter assay according to instructions provided in the Promega dual luciferase reporter assay kit.

Cell proliferation assay

Cell proliferation was measured using the CCK-8 kit according to the protocol recommended by the manufacturer (Dojindo Laboratories, Kumamoto, Japan). Cells were seeded into 96-well plates. After treatment with siRNA, cells were grown for 24 h or 48 h. Absorbance was read at 450 nm using a Bio-Rad iMark plate reader.

RNA-sequencing (RNA-Seq) analysis

MCF7 cells were transfected with non-targeting siRNAs (control siRNAs), TRPS1 siRNAs, and HDAC2 siRNAs. At 48 h later, total RNA was extracted from the same number of cells from each group with the RNeasy kit (OMEGA). Analysis of RNA-Seq data was performed using a standard TopHat-Cufflinks workflow.

ChIP-qPCR

Formaldehyde was added to the cell culture medium at a final concentration of 1%, then incubated at room temperature (RT) with shaking to create protein-DNA crosslinks. After 10 min, glycine was added to the cell culture medium to stop fixation. Subsequently, the cells were washed with ice-cold PBS, harvested in SDS lysis buffer containing the protease inhibitor, and sheared by sonication. Sheared chromatin was used for immunoprecipitation with IgG and anti-H4K14Ac antibodies. The immunoprecipitates were washed, reverse crosslinked, and eluted to obtain the purified DNA for q-PCR. Primer sequences used for ChIP-qPCR experiments are listed in Additional file 1: Table S1.

Tumor xenografts

Four-to-six-week-old female athymic nude (Foxn/nu/nu) mice were purchased from the Model Animal Research Center of Nanjing University. MCF-7 cells (5×10^6) suspended in 200 µl of the PBS–Matrigel mixture were injected into the mammary fat pads. A 0.72-mg E2 60-day release pellet (Innovative Research of America, Sarasota, FL, USA) was implanted subcutaneously on the dorsal side of each mouse a day before tumor cells injection. The length and width of tumors were examined weekly using a Vernier caliper and the volume was calculated by the formula:

$$\pi/6 \times length \times width^2.$$

Results

TRPS1 regulates HDAC2 protein level by stabilizing HDAC2 in ubiquitin-dependent proteasomal degradation (UDPD)

Analysis of TRPS1 interactome had indicated that TRPS1 is associated with HDAC1 and HDAC2 [23], which belong to class I HDACs. To explore the function of TRPS1, we used luminal breast cancer cells MCF7, T47D, and BT474 with elevated TRPS1 as model cell lines. Silencing *TRPS1* with two different siRNAs in all three cell lines consistently showed decreased HDAC2 but not HDAC1 protein levels indicating TRPS1 positively regulates HDAC2 and not HDAC1 (Fig. 1a–c and Additional file 3: Figure S1A–C). To further confirm this observation, we overexpressed *TRPS1* in MDA-MB-231 cells with no

detectable endogenous TRPS1 expression and detected increased HDAC2 protein levels with ectopic overexpression of *TRPS1* (Additional file 3: Figure S1D). Since TRPS1, a member of the GATA transcription factor family, is a well-documented transcription factor, we first investigated whether TRPS1 transcriptionally regulated the expression of *HDAC2*. We found that neither knockdown nor overexpression of *TRPS1* was able to significantly change *HDAC2* mRNA levels (Fig. 1d–f and Additional file 3: Figure S1E).

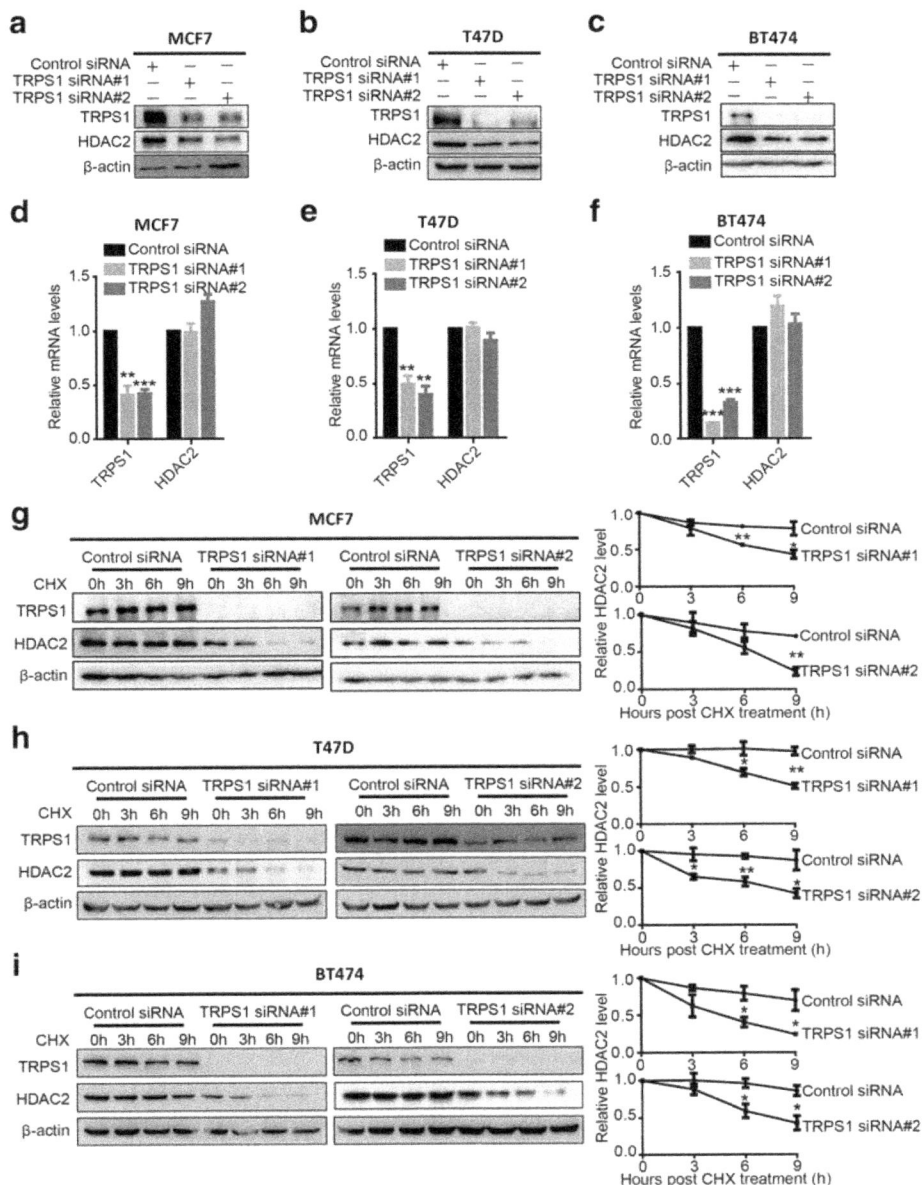

Fig. 1 Tricho-rhino-phalangeal syndrome 1 (TRPS1) transcription factor negatively regulates histone deacetylase 2 (HDAC2) protein level by stabilizing the HDAC2 protein. MCF7 (**a**), T47D (**b**), and BT474 (**c**) exhibit decreased HDAC2 protein levels upon silencing *TRPS1*. MCF7 (**d**), T47D (**e**), and BT474 (**f**) exhibit insignificant alterations in *HDAC2* messenger RNA levels upon silencing *TRPS1*. MCF7 (**g**), T47D (**h**), and BT474 (**i**) show decreased HDAC2 protein stability upon silencing *TRPS1*. The *t* test was used for statistical quantification: *$p < 0.05$, **$p < 0.01$, ***$p < 0.001$, respectively. siRNA, small interfering RNA; CHX, cycloheximide

These observations suggested that TRPS1 regulated HDAC2 protein level independent of its transcription factor function. We then hypothesized that TRPS1 regulates HDAC2 protein level by affecting its protein stability. To test this idea, we first treated cells with cycloheximide (CHX), a eukaryotic protein synthesis inhibitor, and found that in the presence of CHX, silencing of *TRPS1* significantly reduced HDAC2 protein stability (Fig. 1g–i). Conversely, overexpression of *TRPS1* in cells increased HDAC2 stability (Additional file 3: Figure S1F). These results suggested that TRPS1 positively regulated and stabilized HDAC2 protein level.

It is well-known that the majority of intracellular proteins are degraded by UDPD [24]. To test whether TRPS1 stabilized HDAC2 levels by modulating UDPD, we used MG132, a specific 26-s proteasome inhibitor with the ability to reduce the degradation of ubiquitin-conjugated proteins in mammalian cells. Fig. 2a–c shows that HDAC2 protein levels were sustainable in the presence of MG132 if we silenced *TRPS1*. To further confirm if TRPS1 inhibited HDAC2 in a UDPD-dependent manner, we performed ubiquitination assay by co-transfecting HEK293T cells with Myc-HDAC2 vector plus His and Flag-empty vectors, or His-Ubiquitin and Flag empty vectors, or His-Ubiquitin and Flag-TRPS1 vector and compared these with Myc-empty vector plus His and Flag empty vectors. At 24 h later, we immunoprecipitated HDAC2 from whole cell lysates using an anti-Myc antibody, and evaluated HDAC2 ubiquitination (Ub-HDAC2) using anti-His antibody. We found that TRPS1 overexpression reduced HDAC2 ubiquitination level (Fig. 2d). Taken together, these results suggested that TRPS1 stabilized HDAC2 protein levels by reducing the UDPD of HDAC2.

TRPS1 functions as a scaffold protein to recruit UPS4 and HDAC2 to de-ubiquitinate and stabilize HDAC2

To test whether TRPS1 inhibits UDPD of HDAC2 through directly binding to HDAC2, we performed Co-IP using anti-TRPS1 antibody. As displayed in Fig. 3a, b, the results confirmed that TRPS1 physically associated with HDAC2. Since TRPS1 is not a ubiquitin-specific peptidase that could directly de-ubiquitinate and stabilize its interacting partner HDAC2, we hypothesized that TRPS1 reduced HDAC2 ubiquitin level by a ubiquitin-specific peptidase to de-ubiquitinate HDAC2 by reducing UDPD of HDAC2. It has recently been reported that USP4 directly interacts and de-ubiquitinates HDAC2 resulting in its stability in colon cancer cells [22]. To test whether USP4 was responsible for TRPS1-mediated HDAC2 de-ubiquitination and stabilization, we first tested whether, like TRSP1, USP4 had a stabilizing effect on HDAC2. By silencing *USP4* in T47D and MCF7 cells, we detected decreased HDAC2 protein levels as was the case with TRPS1 (Fig. 3c, d).

Since TRPS1 is well-documented as a transcription factor, we examined whether *USP4* is transcriptionally regulated by TRPS1. We investigated USP4 expression upon silencing TRPS1 and found no change in either USP4 mRNA or protein levels (Additional file 4: Figure S2A, B). It appeared that both TRPS1 and USP4 interacted with and stabilized HDAC2 in a UDPD-dependent fashion. We hypothesized that TRPS1, USP4, and HDAC2 formed a complex, used Co-IP to test this notion, and found that TRPS1 co-immunoprecipitated with USP4 and HDAC2 (Fig. 3a, b). To further validate this point, we co-transfected Flag-USP4, Myc-HDAC2, and Flag-TRPS1 in HEK293T cells and performed Co-IP using anti-Myc antibody and found that TRPS1, USP4, and HDAC2 were co-purified as a complex (Fig. 3e).

To further confirm the interaction between TRPS1, USP4, and HDAC2, we generated serial TRPS1 truncates based on the domain structure of TRPS1 consisting of an N-terminal domain and GATA and C-terminal domains (Fig. 3f). We performed Co-IP experiments in HEK293T cells with ectopic overexpression of TRPS1 or TRPS1 truncation mutants. The results indicated that N-terminal or C-terminal domains of TRPS1 together with the GATA domain were sufficient to interact with HDAC2 and USP4 while neither TRPS1 N-terminal or C-terminal domain alone interacted with HDAC2 and USP4 (Fig. 3g). These observations indicated that GATA-zinc finger domain of TRPS1 was essential for its interactions with HDAC2 and USP4. To test whether the TRPS1 GATA domain alone was sufficient to interact with USP4 or HDAC2 or both, we carried out Co-IP experiments in HEK293T cells with ectopic overexpression of TRPS1-GATA truncate containing only the GATA-zinc finger domain. Our results indicated that the GATA domain of TRPS1 alone was unable to interact with HDAC2 and USP4 (Fig. 3h). These observations suggested that the GATA-zinc finger domain of TRPS1 was necessary but not sufficient for TRPS1, USP4, and HDAC2 complex formation. Interestingly, although ectopically overexpressed Flag-UPS4 could be co-immunoprecipitated with overexpressed Myc-HDAC2 using anti-Myc antibodies, overexpression of TRPS1 could increase the co-immunoprecipitated UPS4 levels in this experiment (Fig. 3e). These findings raised the possibility that TRPS1 functions as a scaffold protein to facilitate the UPS4 and HDAC2 interaction. To test this notion, we first performed a sequential immunoprecipitation assay and confirmed that TRPS1, USP4, and HDAC2 formed a ternary complex (Fig. 3i). Furthermore, when we silenced *TRPS1* in cells and carried out Co-IP using anti-HDAC2 antibodies, the co-immunoprecipitated USP4 level with HDAC2 decreased significantly (Fig. 3j, k). We further verified that TRPS1 functioned as a scaffold protein for the complex

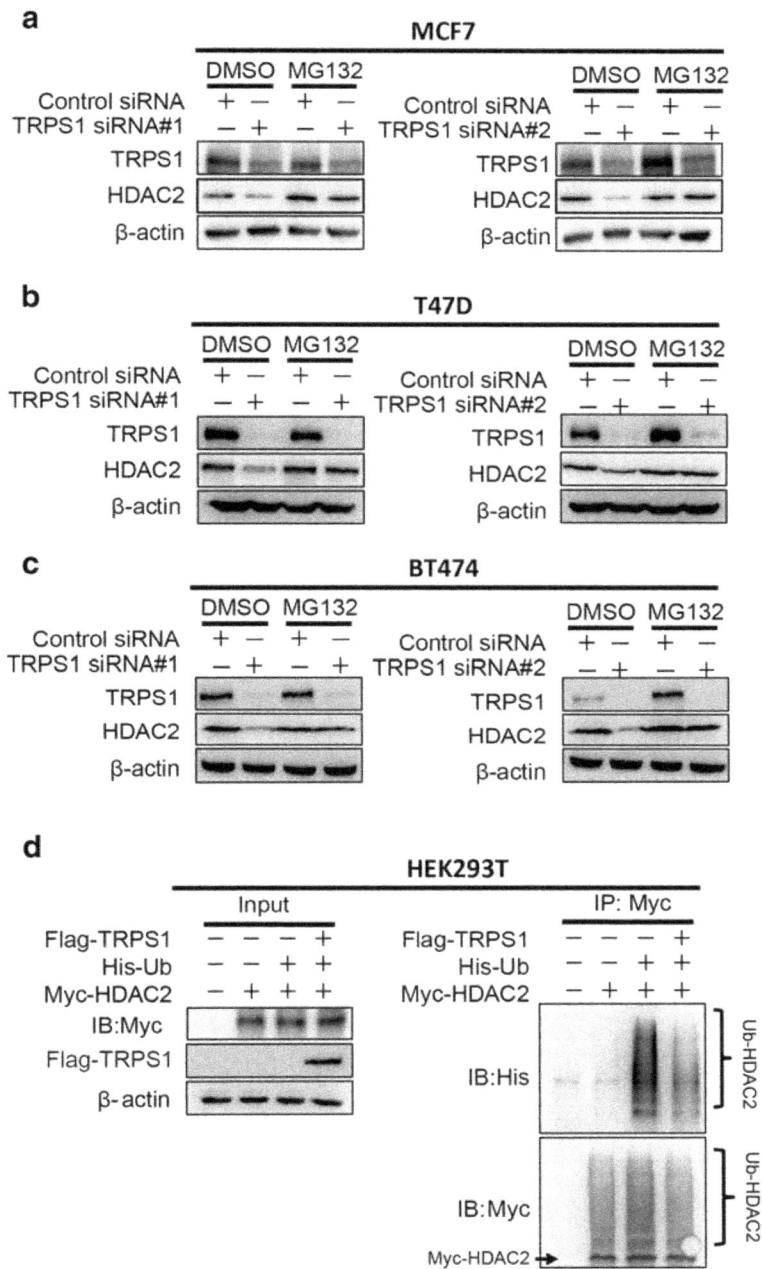

Fig. 2 Tricho-rhino-phalangeal syndrome 1 (TRPS1) transcription factor stabilizes histone deacetylase 2 (HDAC2) through ubiquitin-dependent proteasomal degradation (UDPD). MCF7 (**a**), T47D (**b**), and BT474 (**c**) show decreased HDAC2 protein levels upon MG132 treatment in cells with silencing of *TRPS1*. **d** Ectopic overexpression of TRPS1 reduced HDAC2 ubiquitination level in HEK293T. DMSO, dimethyl sulfoxide; siRNA, small interfering RNA

formation of TRPS1-USP4-HDAC2 and was responsible for the reduction of HDAC2 ubiquitination level by facilitating interaction between USP4 and HDAC2. We carried out ubiquitination assays by co-transfecting HEK293T cells with a Myc-HDAC2 expression plasmid plus His and Flag empty vectors, His-Ubiquitin and Flag empty vectors, His-Ubiquitin, Flag-USP4 and Flag empty vectors,or His-Ubiquitin, Flag-USP4 and Flag-

TRPS1 vectors and compared them with cells transfected with Myc plus His vector and Flag-empty vectors. Although USP4 alone could reduce HDAC2 ubiquitination level, additional overexpression of TRPS1 significantly enhanced the reduction of HDAC2 ubiquitination (Fig. 3l). Taken together, our results suggested that TRPS1 stabilized HDAC2 by functioning as a scaffold protein to bring UPS4 and HDAC2 together forming the TRPS1-UPS4-

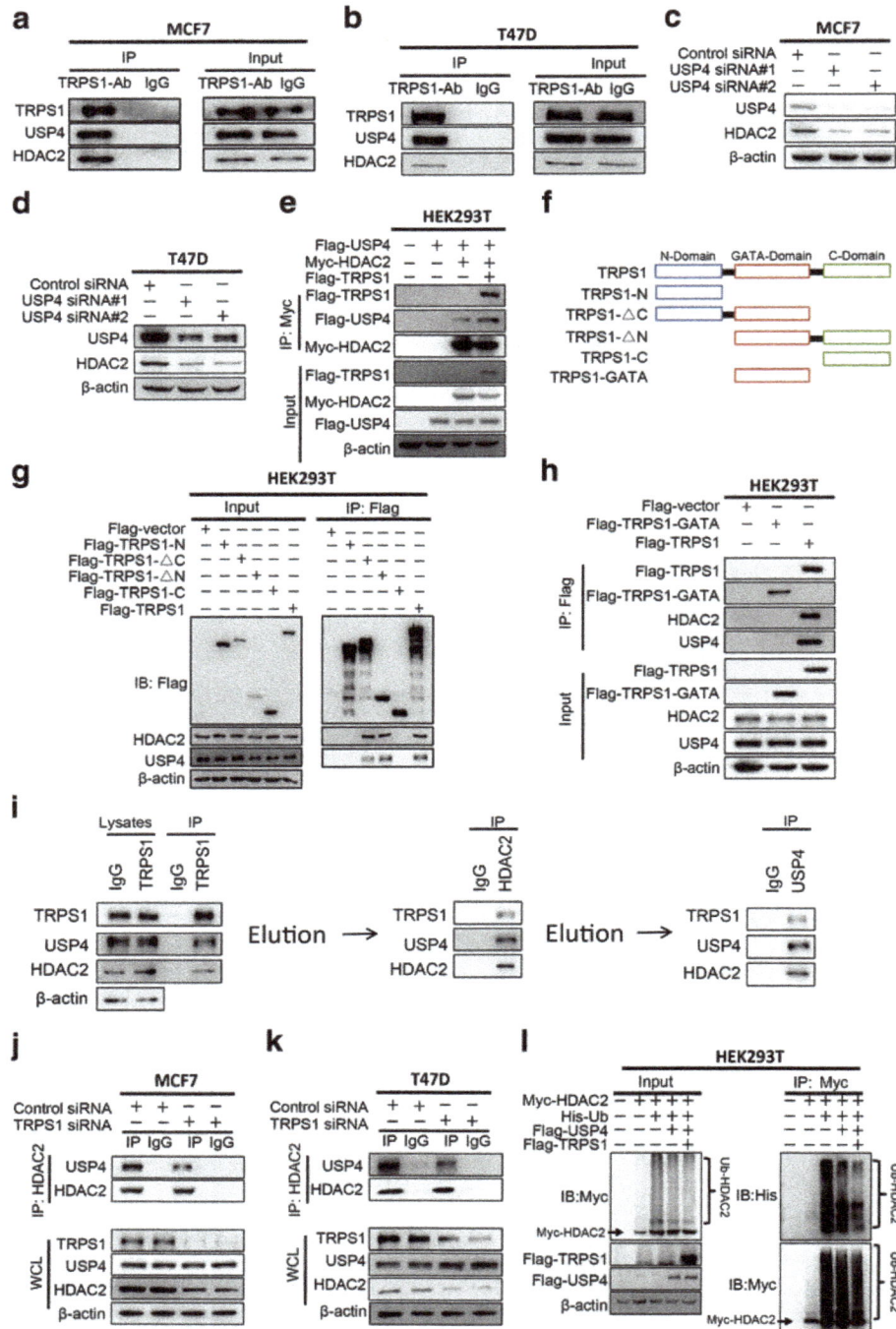

Fig. 3 (See legend on next page.)

(See figure on previous page.)

Fig. 3 Tricho-rhino-phalangeal syndrome 1 (TRPS1) transcription factor recruits ubiquitin-specific protease 4 (USP4) and histone deacetylase 2 (HDAC2) to form a complex in which HDAC2 is de-ubiquitinated by USP4. MCF7 (**a**) and T47D (**b**) show co-immunoprecipitation (Co-IP) of TRPS1, USP4 and HDAC2. MCF7 (**c**) and T47D (**d**) exhibit decreased HDAC2 protein levels upon silencing of *USP4*. **e** Co-IP analysis of the interaction between TRPS1, USP4, and HDAC2 in HEK293T cells with ectopic overexpression of Flag-TRPS1, Flag-USP4, and Myc-HDAC2 using anti-Myc antibody. **f** Domain structures of TRPS1 and its truncation mutants. **g** Co-IP analysis of the interaction between truncation mutants of TRPS1 and USP4 and HDAC2 in HEK293T cells with ectopic overexpression of TRPS1 and its truncation mutants. **h** Co-IP analysis of the interaction between the GATA domain of TRPS1 and USP4 and HDAC2 in HEK293T cells with ectopic overexpression of TRPS1 GATA domain truncation mutant. **i** MCF7 cell lysates were subjected to immunoprecipitation with control IgG or anti-TRPS1 antibody. The immunoprecipitates bound to agarose beads were eluted by elution buffer and sequential immunoprecipitation was performed with the indicated antibodies. **j** MCF7 and **k** T47D show reduced interaction between USP4 and HDAC2 upon silencing TRPS1 in Co-IP assay using anti-HDAC2 antibody. **l** Overexpression of USP4 decreased HDAC2 ubiquitination level and additional overexpression of TRPS1 enhanced reduction of HDAC2 ubiquitination level in HEK293T cells

HDAC2 complex to enhance USP4-directed HDAC2 de-ubiquitination.

TRPS1-UPS4-HDAC2 axis regulates transcriptional repression activity of HDAC2

HDAC2, as a histone deacetylase, exerts its transcriptional repression activity by deacetylating histones [25]. H4K16ac, which is a key epigenetic marker and is necessary for transcriptional regulation [26], has been shown to be a major deacetylation target of HDAC2 [16]. Consistent with these notions, we observed that silencing of *HDAC2* in T47D and MCF7 cells led to increased H4K16ac levels (Additional file 5: Figure S3A, B). Furthermore, silencing *TRPS1* increased H4K16ac level as did silencing *HDAC2* (Additional file 5: Figure S3C–E). These observations indicated that TRPS1-UPS4-HDAC2 formed a functional axis in controlling the acetylation status of H4K16 via HDAC2. To further confirm this notion, we first tested whether TRPS1 controlled the acetylation status of H4K16 via HDAC2. We silenced *TRPS1* with siRNAs with or without rescuing overexpression of HDAC2 in MCF7 and found that silencing *TRPS1* led to decreased HDAC2 and increased H4K16ac, whereas HDAC2 overexpression restored the H4K16ac level (Fig. 4a, b). Furthermore, when we silenced *USP4* with siRNAs with or without HDAC2 overexpression in MCF7, we consistently found that USP4 silencing led to decreased HDAC2 and increased H4K16ac, whereas additional HDAC2 overexpression restored the H4K16ac level (Fig. 4c, d). Reduced H4K16ac has been shown to be an indicator of transcription repression [27–29]. Gal4-TK-luciferase reporter assay is generally used to test HDAC2 transcriptional repression activity [30–33]. To further investigate whether TRPS1 could affect HDAC2 transcriptional repression activity, we co-transfected the Gal4-TK-luciferase plasmid with Gal4-HDAC2 with or without Flag-TRPS1 and TRPS1 domain truncates. As shown in Fig. 4e–i, ectopic overexpression of full-length TRPS1 and TRPS1-△N truncate exhibited strong repression activity of luciferase expression while TRPS1-N, TRPS1-△C, and TRPS1-C truncates did not show significant effects. These

observations indicated that TRPS1 regulated transcriptional repression activity of HDAC2. Furthermore, the C-terminal domain of TRPS1 was necessary but not sufficient for transcriptional repression activity of HDAC2. This could be due to the fact that C-terminal and GATA domains of TRPS1 were required for binding of TRPS1 to HDAC2 (Fig. 3). As we proposed, TRPS1 recruited UPS4 to mediate HDAC2 stability, and regulated its transcriptional repression activity (Additional file 5: Figure S3F).

To further identify the transcriptional output of HDAC2 mediated by TRPS1, we first investigated transcriptional alterations by RNA sequencing in MCF7 cells. Upon silencing of *TRPS1* in MCF7 cells, 66 and 33 genes were up- and down-regulated, respectively (fold change ≥ 2 and $q < 0.05$), and upon silencing *HDAC2* in MCF7 cells, 23 and 44 genes were up-regulated and down-regulated, respectively (fold change ≥ 2 and $q < 0.05$) (Additional file 6: Table S3A, B). There were 10 genes, *ADAMTS7P1*, *AES*, *CASP7*, *GS1-44D20.1*, *IFT27*, *PCDH19*, *PERP*, *SHISA2*, *TPM4*, and *ZW10*, that were consistently upregulated upon silencing either *TRPS1* or *HDAC2*, while 8 genes, *CC2D1B*, *CCDC146*, *CCT6P3*, *GAPDHP1*, *LINC01659*, *RORA*, *SMOX*, and *U1* were consistently down-regulated upon silencing either *TRPS1* or *HDAC2* (Fig. 5a). The genes with consistently up-regulated expression upon silencing either *TRPS1* or *HDAC2* were considered as candidate targets for *TRPS1* transcriptional repressive function over *HDAC2*. RT-qPCR validated that *AES*, *CASP7*, *IFT27*, *PERP*, *SHISA2*, *TPM4*, and *ZW10* were consistently up-regulated upon silencing either *TRPS1* or *HDAC2* (Fig. 5b, c). Furthermore, additional overexpression *HDAC2* in cells with *TRPS1* silencing restored the expression levels of these genes (Fig. 5d). Considering the function of the regulatory axis of TRPS1, USP4, and HDAC2 on transcriptional regulation, we further confirmed that silencing USP4 led to consistent up-regulation of *AES*, *CASP7*, *IFT27*, *PERP*, *SHISA2*, *TPM4*, and *ZW10*, and additional overexpression of HDAC2 restored the expression levels of these genes (Fig. 5e, f). To determine the H4K16ac level at the affected genes, we carried out ChIP-qPCR using H4K16ac antibody upon silencing

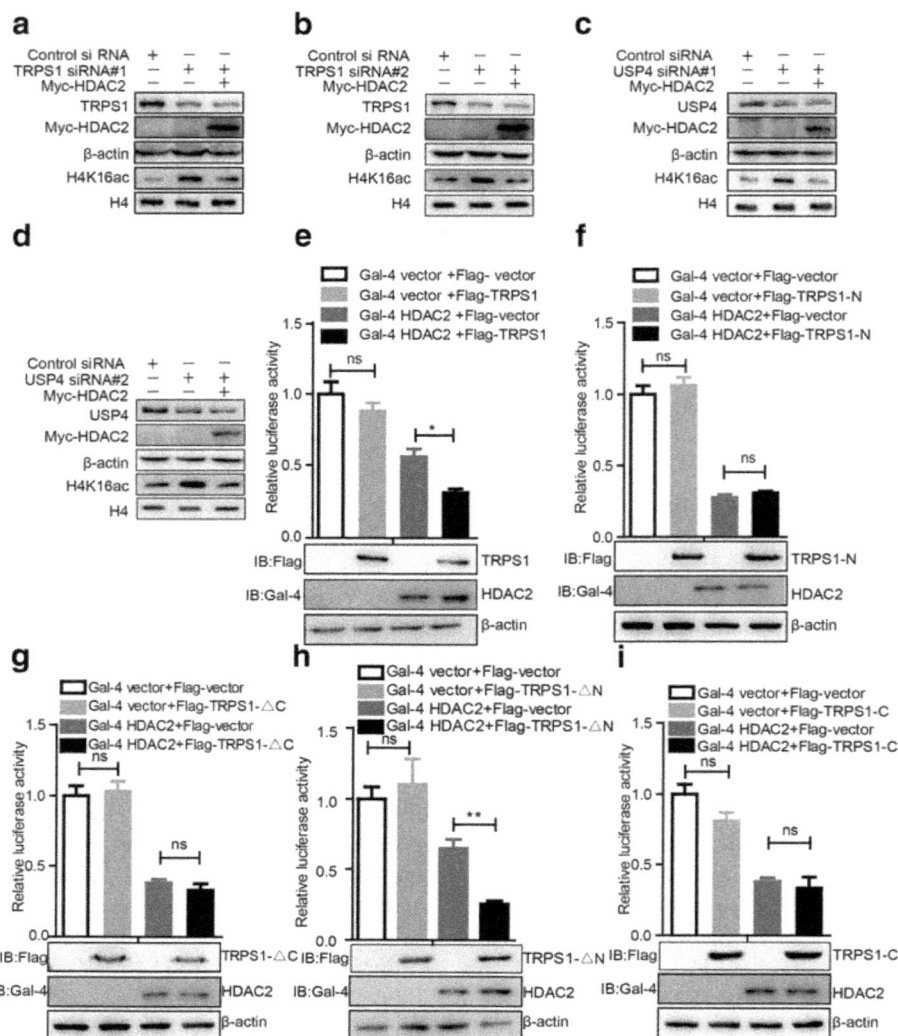

Fig. 4 Tricho-rhino-phalangeal syndrome 1 (TRPS1) transcription factor regulates the transcription repressive activity of histone deacetylase 2 (HDAC2). **a, b** MCF7 shows increased H4K16ac level upon silencing of *TRPS1*, and overexpression of HDAC2 restored H4K16ac level. **c, d** MCF7 shows increased H4K16ac level upon silencing *USP4*, and overexpression of HDAC2 restored H4K16ac level. **e–i** Effects of TRPS1 and its truncation mutants over the transcriptional repression activity of HDAC2. The *t* test was used for statistical analysis: *$p < 0.05$; ns, not significant. Ab, antibody; siRNA, small interfering RNA; USP4, ubiquitin-specific protease 4

TRPS1 or *USP4* and found that silencing either TRPS1 or USP4 alone increased the H4K16ac level at these target genes (Fig. 5g, h). Taken together, these results support our claim that the TRPS1-UPS4-HDAC2 axis regulates transcriptional repression activity of HDAC2.

TRPS1-UPS4-HDAC2 axis confers tumor growth

The set of genes consisting of *AES, CASP7, IFT27, PERP, SHISA2, TPM4,* and *ZW10,* repressed by the TRPS1-USP4-HDAC2 axis were implicated in cell proliferation [34–40]. Thus, we postulated that the TRPS1-USP4-HDAC2 axis contributes to tumor growth. To test this idea, we first performed in vitro cell culture experiments. Silencing of *TRPS1* reduced proliferation of MCF7 cells

while overexpression of HDAC2 in cells with TRPS1 silencing rescued this phenotype (Fig. 6a). Similarly, silencing of *USP4* also reduced proliferation of MCF7 while overexpression of HDAC2 in cells with *USP4* silencing rescued this phenotype (Fig. 6b).

Consistent with the in vitro experiments, in xenograft mouse models, silencing *TRPS1* significantly reduced both tumor volume and weight, and additional overexpression of HDAC2 rescued this phenotype of xenograft tumors (Fig. 6c–e). Thus, both in vitro and in vivo results demonstrated that the TPRS1-USP4-HDAC2 regulatory axis confers tumor growth.

Taken together these results led to a mechanistic scheme in which TRPS1 scaffolding recruits USP4 to

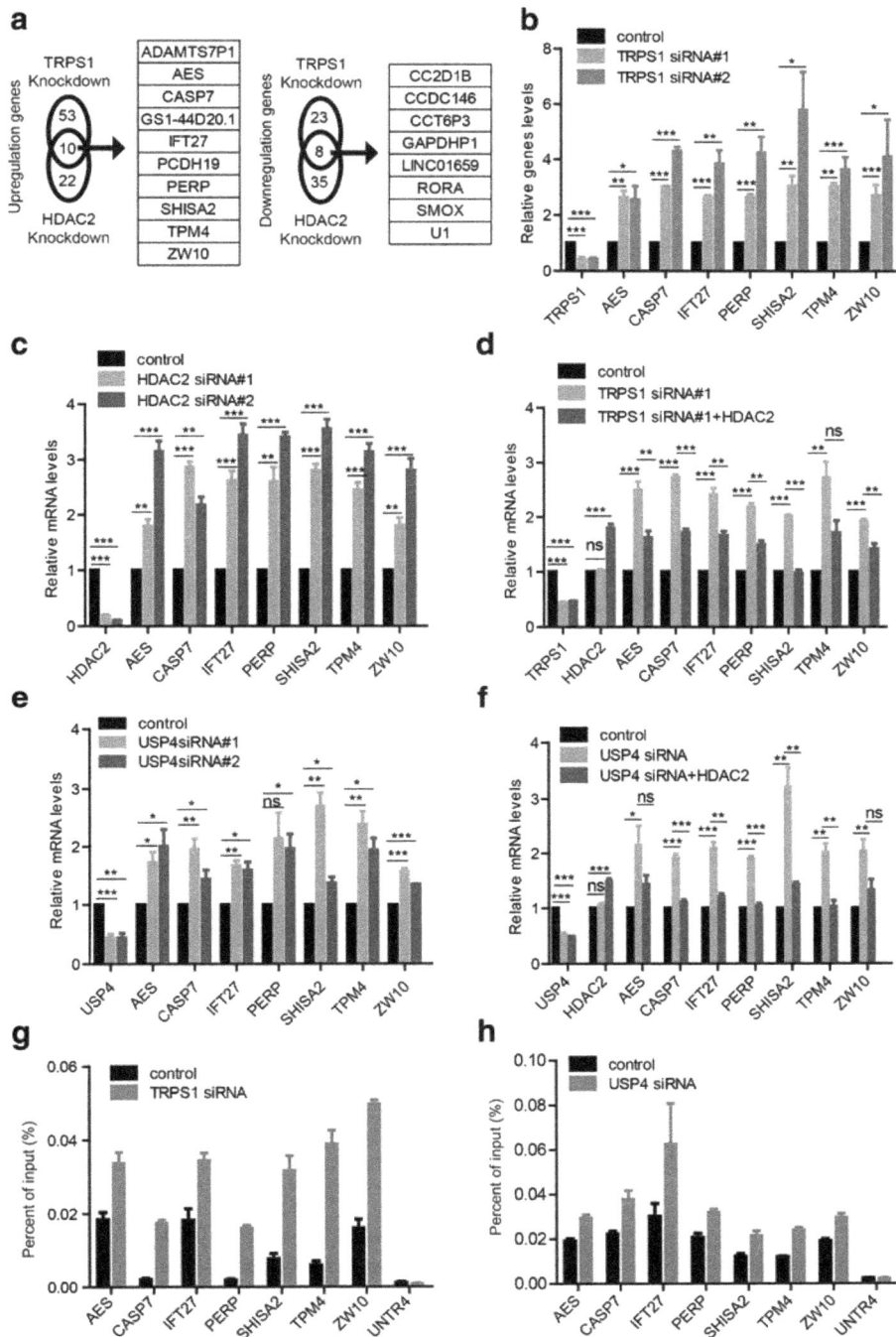

Fig. 5 Transcription output analysis of the tricho-rhino-phalangeal syndrome 1 (TRPSI)-ubiquitin-specific protease 4 (USP4)-histone deacetylase 2 (HDAC2) regulatory axis. **a** Analysis and comparison of transcriptomes of MCF7 upon silencing *TRPS1* or *HDAC2* using RNA sequencing. **b** Validation of the selected TRPS1 target genes using RT-qPCR. **c** Validation the selected HDAC2 target genes using RT-qPCR. **d** Expression levels of genes up-regulated upon silencing of *TRPS1* were restored with overexpression of HDAC2. **e** Selected genes upon silencing of *TRPS1* or *HDAC2* show consistent up-regulation by RT-qPCR upon silencing of *USP4* in MCF7. **f** Expression levels of genes up-regulated upon silencing of *USP4* were restored with additional overexpression of HDAC2. **g, h** Chromatin immunoprecipitation (ChIP)-qPCR using H4K16AC antibodies on selected target genes upon silencing of *TRPS1* or *USP4* in MCF7 cells. The *t* test was used for statistical quantifications: *$p < 0.05$, **$p < 0.01$, ***$p < 0.001$, respectively. SiRNA, small interfering RNA

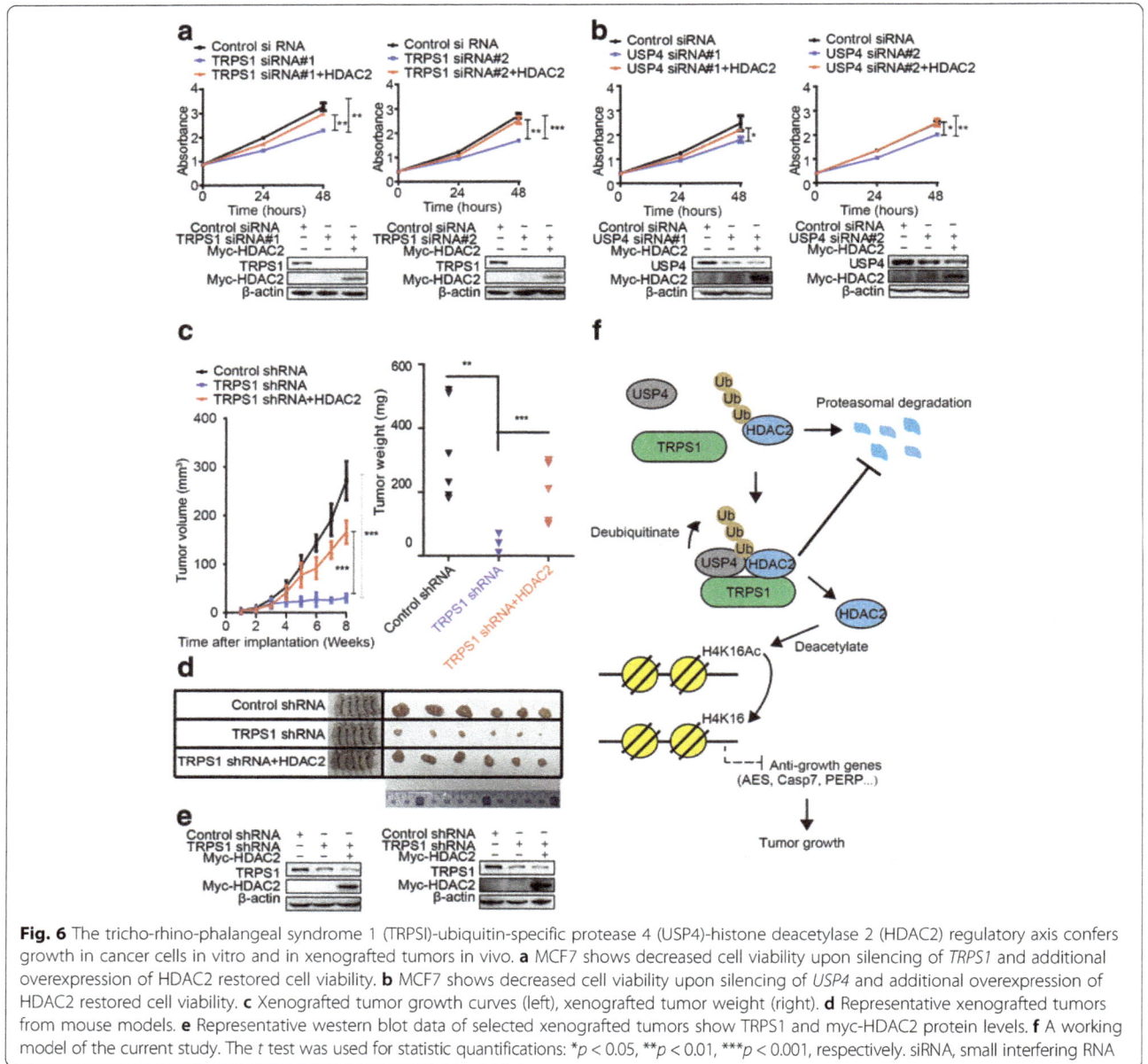

Fig. 6 The tricho-rhino-phalangeal syndrome 1 (TRPSI)-ubiquitin-specific protease 4 (USP4)-histone deacetylase 2 (HDAC2) regulatory axis confers growth in cancer cells in vitro and in xenografted tumors in vivo. **a** MCF7 shows decreased cell viability upon silencing of *TRPS1* and additional overexpression of HDAC2 restored cell viability. **b** MCF7 shows decreased cell viability upon silencing of *USP4* and additional overexpression of HDAC2 restored cell viability. **c** Xenografted tumor growth curves (left), xenografted tumor weight (right). **d** Representative xenografted tumors from mouse models. **e** Representative western blot data of selected xenografted tumors show TRPS1 and myc-HDAC2 protein levels. **f** A working model of the current study. The *t* test was used for statistic quantifications: *$p < 0.05$, **$p < 0.01$, ***$p < 0.001$, respectively. siRNA, small interfering RNA

de-ubiquitinate and stabilize HDAC2, leading to repression of a set of anti-growth genes and acceleration of tumor growth (Fig. 6f).

Discussion

In this study, we report that TRPS1, USP4, and HDAC2 form a regulatory axis to confer tumor growth. TRPS1 acts as a scaffold protein in this axis and recruits USP4 and HDAC2 leading to de-ubiquitination and stabilization of HDAC2, deacetylation of H4K16, and transcriptional repression of anti-proliferative genes.

TRPS1, the only reported atypical GATA transcription factor, had been characterized as the first example of a GATA protein with intrinsic transcriptional

repression activity [1]. Our results provide insight into the non-transcription factor function of GATA transcription factors by discovering the scaffolding effect of TRPS1 in USP4-mediated HDAC2 de-ubiquitination and, for the first time, furnish evidence of the physical association and functional link between TRPS1, USP4, and HDAC2.

TRPS1 is co-amplified with *MYC* in breast carcinomas with an increased proliferation rate [41], and silencing *TRPS1* reduces proliferation of BT474 cells [23]. Also, HDAC2 knockdown in breast cancer cells leads to inhibition of proliferation [42] and USP4 knockout results in the retarded growth of mouse embryonic fibroblasts (MEF) [20]. Our working model suggests that TRPS1 recruits USP4 to stabilize HDAC2 repressing the expression of *AES*, *Casp7*, *PERP*, and *ZW10* to confer tumor growth. Exogenous expression of *AES* suppresses the growth of LNCaP prostate cancer cells, while knockdown of *AES* promotes cell growth [43]. Inhibition or knockdown of *CASP7* impairs the growth of breast cancer cells [40]. Deficiency of *PERP* has been shown to promote tumor growth [44], whereas *ZW10* is essential in mitotic checkpoint control [45]. These scenarios fit well with our working model that TRPS1 recruits USP4 to stabilize HDAC2 and represses expression of *AES*, *Casp7*, *PERP*, and *ZW10* to confer tumor growth. It has been reported that TRPS1 represses the expression of RUNX2 [46] and ZEB2 [47]. Furthermore, reduced metastatic spread of triple negative breast cancer cells by TRPS1 has also been described [7]. How TRPS1 contributes to cancer metastasis needs to be further investigated. Nevertheless, our observations extend current knowledge of the importance of TRPS1 function in carcinogenesis by deciphering the TRPS1-UPS4-HDAC2 regulatory axis and uncovering how TRPS1 contributes to tumor growth.

Global loss of H4K16ac and H4K20me3 is a common marker of human cancer [48]. H4K16ac plays a critical role in the maintenance of active gene transcription, and its loss is important in the epigenetic silencing of some tumor suppressor genes in cancer [49]. H4K16ac has been shown to be a specific target of HDAC2 [16]. Our study has provided evidence that TRPS1, USP4, and HDAC2 are functionally connected through complex formation and that HDAC2 regulates gene transcription by deacetylating H4K16ac.

The ubiquitin system is critical in maintaining protein stability and level. So far, E3 ubiquitin ligase RLIM [50], Mcl-1 ubiquitin ligase E3 (MULE, also named ARF-BP-1) [51], and recently reported de-ubiquitinase USP4 [22] were documented to be involved in regulation of HDAC2 stability by the ubiquitin-proteasome system. However, we found that silencing of neither *RLIM29* nor *MULE* affected HDAC2 protein levels (data not shown). The specific mechanism of HDAC2 ubiquitination by ubiquitin ligases needs to be further investigated. Nevertheless, our observation that TRPS1 recruits USP4 to de-ubiquitinate HDAC2 extends the current knowledge on the regulation of HDAC2 stability by the ubiquitin system, contributing to tumor growth. An important regulatory step to counter the outcome of ubiquitination is by removing ubiquitin from ubiquitinated proteins by de-ubiquitinases [52]. Several studies have reported the importance of de-ubiquitination in stabilizing oncoproteins. For example, USP1 de-ubiquitinates and stabilizes two critical DNA repair proteins, FANCD2 and PCNA, and is involved in Fanconi leukemia [52, 53]; USP9x de-ubiquitates and stabilizes the pro-survival protein MCL1 [54]; USP37 is a de-ubiquitinase that regulates the cell cycle by de-

ubiquitinating cyclin A [55] and c-MYC [56]. Thus, de-ubiquitinases are believed to represent alternative targets in the ubiquitin system for cancer therapies [57]. USP4, a ubiquitin-specific protease, was proposed to be a potential oncogene for decades [19]. Our observation that USP4 is recruited by TRPS1 to de-ubiquitinate HDAC2 and silence USP4, resulting in inhibition of tumor cell growth by TRPS1, is consistent with these notions elucidating the underlying molecular details of the oncogenic function of the TRPS1/HDAC2/USP4 axis in tumor growth.

Conclusions

Our results suggest that the TRPS1-USP4-HDAC2 regulatory axis is implicated in carcinogenesis. HDAC2 implements the transcription repression program by deacetylating H4K16ac and contributes to tumor growth. Our data provide a mechanistic link between TRPS1, the ubiquitin system, and the histone modification system in cancer by revealing the TRPS1-USP4-HDAC2 regulatory axis that is involved in tumor growth. Furthermore, our results identified the novel non-transcription factor scaffolding function of the GATA family member TRPS1 in USP4-directed HDAC2 de-ubiquitination. Our findings suggest GATA transcription factors, ubiquitination regulators, and histone modifiers can serve as potential prognostic indicators and/or therapeutic targets of cancer.

Additional files

Additional file 1: Table S1. RT-qPCR and ChIP-qPCR primer sequences. (DOCX 19 kb)

Additional file 2: Table S2. Sequences of siRNAs and shRNAs. (DOCX 16 kb)

Additional file 3: Figure S1. (**A**) MCF7, (**B**) T47D, and (**C**) BT474 exhibit insignificant alterations of HDAC1 protein level upon silencing of *TRPS1*. (**D**) MDA-MB-231 exhibits increased HDAC2 protein level upon overexpression of *TRPS1*. (**E**) MDA-MB-231 shows insignificant alterations in *HDAC2* mRNA level upon overexpression of *TRPS1*. (**F**) MDA-MB-231 shows increased HDAC2 protein stability upon overexpression of *TRPS1*. (JPG 2596 kb)

Additional file 4: Figure S2. (**A** and **B**) USP4 protein and mRNA levels were unaffected upon silencing of TRPS1 in T47D cell line. (JPG 1408 kb)

Additional file 5: Figure S3. (**A** and **B**) Silencing of *HDAC2* in T47D and MCF7 cells led to increased H4K16ac levels. (**C-E**) Silencing of *TRPS1* increased H4K16ac levels in BT474, T47D and MCF7. (**F**) USP4 could increase transcriptional repression activity of HDAC2. (JPG 3480 kb)

Additional file 6: Table S3. A, B Differential expressed genes upon silencing of *TRPS1* or *HDAC2* in MCF7 by RNA-sequencing. (XLSX 2609 kb)

Abbreviations
ChIP: Chromatin immunoprecipitation; CHX: Cycloheximide; Co-IP: Co-immunoprecipitation; DMEM: Dulbecco's modified Eagle's medium; DMSO: Dimethylsulfoxide; HATs: Histone acetyltranferases; HDAC2: Histone deacetylase 2; KD: Knockdown; NURD: Nucleosome remodeling deacetylase; PBS: Phosphate-buffered saline; RT-PCR: Real-time polymerase chain reaction; siRNA: Small interfering RNA; TRPS1: Tricho-rhino-phalangeal syndrome 1; UDPD: Ubiquitin-dependent proteasomal degradation; USP4: Ubiquitin-specific protease 4

Acknowledgements

We thank all members of Prof. Chen's laboratory for valuable discussions.

Funding

Financial support: this work was funded by the National Natural Science Foundation of China (grant numbers 81572712 and 81772956 to L Chen), the National Basic Research Program of China (973 Program) (grant number 2015CB965000 to L Chen), the Key University Science Research Project of Jiangsu Province (grant number 17KJA320002 to L Chen), grants from the Natural Science Foundation of Jiangsu Province (grant number SBK2016030027 to L Chen), the Six talent peaks project in Jiangsu Province (grant number 2015-JY-002 to L Chen), Jiangsu Shuangchuang talent program to L Chen, and the Priority Academic Program Development of Jiangsu Higher Education Institutions.

Authors' contributions

LMC and YZW conceived the idea for this project; YZW, JZ, LLW, WGL, GYW, XG, YL, ZFM, and FM performed the experiments; LMC and YZW wrote the manuscript; WGL performed bioinformatic analysis of RNA-Seq and ChIP-Seq data. All authors read and approved the final manuscript.

Competing interests

The authors declare that they have no competing interests.

Author details

[1]The Key Laboratory of Developmental Genes and Human Disease, Ministry of Education, Institute of Life Science, Southeast University, Nanjing 210096, People's Republic of China. [2]Jiangsu Key Laboratory for Molecular and Medical Biotechnology, College of Life Science, Nanjing Normal University, Nanjing 210023, People's Republic of China. [3]Cancer Science Institute, National University of Singapore, 14 Medical Drive, Singapore, Singapore. [4]Institute of Molecular and Cell Biology, A*STAR, 61 Biopolis Drive, Singapore, Singapore. [5]Department of Biochemistry, Yong Loo Lin School of Medicine, National University of Singapore, 8 Medical Drive, Singapore, Singapore.

References

1. Malik TH, Shoichet SA, Latham P, Kroll TG, Peters LL, Shivdasani RA. Transcriptional repression and developmental functions of the atypical vertebrate GATA protein TRPS1. EMBO J. 2001;20(7):1715–25.
2. Momeni P, Glockner G, Schmidt O, von Holtum D, Albrecht B, Gillessen-Kaesbach G, Hennekam R, Meinecke P, Zabel B, Rosenthal A, et al. Mutations in a new gene, encoding a zinc-finger protein, cause tricho-rhino-phalangeal syndrome type I. Nat Genet. 2000;24(1):71–4.
3. Li Z, Jia M, Wu X, Cui J, Pan A, Li L. Overexpression of Trps1 contributes to tumor angiogenesis and poor prognosis of human osteosarcoma. Diagn Pathol. 2015;10:167.
4. Hong J, Sun J, Huang T. Increased expression of TRPS1 affects tumor progression and correlates with patients' prognosis of colon cancer. Biomed Res Int. 2013;2013:454085.
5. Radvanyi L, Singh-Sandhu D, Gallichan S, Lovitt C, Pedyczak A, Mallo G, Gish K, Kwok K, Hanna W, Zubovits J, et al. The gene associated with trichorhinophalangeal syndrome in humans is overexpressed in breast cancer. Proc Natl Acad Sci U S A. 2005;102(31):11005–10.
6. Chen L, Jenjaroenpun P, Pillai AM, Ivshina AV, Ow GS, Efthimios M, Zhiqun T, Tan TZ, Lee SC, Rogers K, et al. Transposon insertional mutagenesis in mice identifies human breast cancer susceptibility genes and signatures for stratification. Proc Natl Acad Sci U S A. 2017;114(11):E2215–24.
7. Rangel R, Lee SC, Hon-Kim Ban K, Guzman-Rojas L, Mann MB, Newberg JY, Kodama T, McNoe LA, Selvanesan L, Ward JM, et al. Transposon mutagenesis identifies genes that cooperate with mutant Pten in breast cancer progression. Proc Natl Acad Sci U S A. 2016;113(48):E7749–58.
8. Ropero S, Esteller M. The role of histone deacetylases (HDACs) in human cancer. Mol Oncol. 2007;1(1):19–25.
9. Mottet D, Castronovo V. Histone deacetylases: target enzymes for cancer therapy. Clin ExpMetastasis. 2008;25(2):183–9.
10. Glozak MA, Seto E. Histone deacetylases and cancer. Oncogene. 2007;26(37): 5420–32.
11. Gregoretti IV, Lee YM, Goodson HV. Molecular evolution of the histone deacetylase family: functional implications of phylogenetic analysis. J Mol Biol. 2004;338(1):17–31.
12. Zhu P, Martin E, Mengwasser J, Schlag P, Janssen KP, Gottlicher M. Induction of HDAC2 expression upon loss of APC in colorectal tumorigenesis. Cancer Cell. 2004;5(5):455–63.
13. Huang BH, Laban M, Leung CH, Lee L, Lee CK, Salto-Tellez M, Raju GC, Hooi SC. Inhibition of histone deacetylase 2 increases apoptosis and p21Cip1/WAF1 expression, independent of histone deacetylase 1. Cell Death Differ. 2005;12(4):395–404.
14. Nakagawa M, Oda Y, Eguchi T, Aishima S, Yao T, Hosoi F, Basaki Y, Ono M, Kuwano M, Tanaka M, et al. Expression profile of class I histone deacetylases in human cancer tissues. Oncol Rep. 2007;18(4):769–74.
15. Seo J, Min SK, Park HR, Kim DH, Kwon MJ, Kim LS, Ju YS. Expression of histone deacetylases HDAC1, HDAC2, HDAC3, and HDAC6 in invasive ductal carcinomas of the breast. J Breast Cancer. 2014;17(4):323–31.
16. Ma P, Schultz RM. Histone deacetylase 2 (HDAC2) regulates chromosome segregation and kinetochore function via H4K16 deacetylation during oocyte maturation in mouse. PLoS Genet. 2013;9(3):e1003377.
17. Nitarska J, Smith JG, Sherlock WT, Hillege MMG, Nott A, Barshop WD, Vashisht AA, Wohlschlegel JA, Mitter R, Riccio A. A functional switch of NuRD chromatin remodeling complex subunits regulates mouse cortical development. Cell Rep. 2016;17(6):1683–98.
18. Fraile JM, Quesada V, Rodriguez D, Freije JM, Lopez-Otin C. Deubiquitinases in cancer: new functions and therapeutic options. Oncogene. 2012;31(19): 2373–88.
19. Gupta K, Chevrette M, Gray DA. The Unp proto-oncogene encodes a nuclear protein. Oncogene. 1994;9(6):1729–31.
20. Zhang XN, Berger FG, Yang JH, Lu XB. USP4 inhibits p53 through deubiquitinating and stabilizing ARF-BP1. EMBO J. 2011;30(11):2177–89.
21. Mehic M, de Sa VK, Hebestreit S, Heldin CH, Heldin P. The deubiquitinating enzymes USP4 and USP17 target hyaluronan synthase 2 and differentially affect its function. Oncogenesis. 2017;6(6):e348.
22. Li Z, Hao Q, Luo J, Xiong J, Zhang S, Wang T, Bai L, Wang W, Chen M, Wang W, et al. USP4 inhibits p53 and NF-kappaB through deubiquitinating and stabilizing HDAC2. Oncogene. 2016;35(22):2902–12.
23. Wu LL, Wang YZ, Liu Y, Yu SY, Xie H, Shi XJ, Qin S, Ma F, Tan TZ, Thiery JP, et al. A central role for TRPS1 in the control of cell cycle and cancer development. Oncotarget. 2014;5(17):7677–90.
24. Lecker SH, Goldberg AL, Mitch WE. Protein degradation by the ubiquitin-proteasome pathway in normal and disease states. J Am Soc Nephrol. 2006; 17(7):1807–19.
25. Gonzalez-Zuniga M, Contreras PS, Estrada LD, Chamorro D, Villagra A, Zanlungo S, Seto E, Alvarez AR. C-Abl stabilizes HDAC2 levels by tyrosine phosphorylation repressing neuronal gene expression in Alzheimer's disease. Mol Cell. 2014;56(1):163–73.
26. Klein BJ, Wang XY, Cui GF, Yuan C, Botuyan MV, Lin KV, Lu Y, Wang XL, Zhao Y, Bruns CJ, et al. PHF20 readers link methylation of histone H3K4 and p53 with H4K16 acetylation. Cell Rep. 2016;17(4):1158–70.
27. Shogren-Knaak M, Peterson CL. Switching on chromatin: mechanistic role of histone H4-K16 acetylation. Cell Cycle. 2006;5(13):1361–5.
28. Hajji N, Wallenborg K, Vlachos P, Fullgrabe J, Hermanson O, Joseph B. Opposing effects of hMOF and SIRT1 on H4K16 acetylation and the sensitivity to the topoisomerase II inhibitor etoposide. Oncogene. 2010; 29(15):2192–204.
29. Jo WJ, Ren X, Chu F, Aleshin M, Wintz H, Burlingame A, Smith MT, Vulpe CD, Zhang L. Acetylated H4K16 by MYST1 protects UROtsa cells from arsenic

toxicity and is decreased following chronic arsenic exposure. Toxicol Appl Pharmacol. 2009;241(3):294–302.

30. David G, Neptune MA, DePinho RA. SUMO-1 modification of histone deacetylase 1 (HDAC1) modulates its biological activities. J Biol Chem. 2002; 277(26):23658–63.

31. Colombo R, Boggio R, Seiser C, Draetta GF, Chiocca S. The adenovirus protein Gam1 interferes with sumoylation of histone deacetylase 1. EMBO Rep. 2002;3(11):1062–8.

32. Kirsh O, Seeler JS, Pichler A, Gast A, Muller S, Miska E, Mathieu M, Harel-Bellan A, Kouzarides T, Melchior F, et al. The SUMO E3 ligase RanBP2 promotes modification of the HDAC4 deacetylase. EMBO J. 2002;21(11):2682–91.

33. Brandl A, Wagner T, Uhlig KM, Knauer SK, Stauber RH, Melchior F, Schneider G, Heinzel T, Kramer OH. Dynamically regulated sumoylation of HDAC2 controls p53 deacetylation and restricts apoptosis following genotoxic stress. J Mol Cell Biol. 2012;4(5):284–93.

34. Xia H, Li M, Chen L, Leng W, Yuan D, Pang X, Chen L, Li R, Tang Q, Bi F. Suppression of RND3 activity by AES downregulation promotes cancer cell proliferation and invasion. Int J Mol Med. 2013;31(5):1081–6.

35. Yang N, Li L, Eguether T, Sundberg JP, Pazour GJ, Chen J. Intraflagellar transport 27 is essential for hedgehog signaling but dispensable for ciliogenesis during hair follicle morphogenesis (vol 142, pg 2194, 2015). Development. 2015;142(16):2860.

36. Attardi LD, Reczek EE, Cosmas C, Demicco EG, McCurrach ME, Lowe SW, Jacks T. PERP, an apoptosis-associated target of p53, is a novel member of the PMP-22/gas3 family. Genes Dev. 2000;14(6):704–18.

37. Tamura K, Furihata M, Satake H, Anchi T, Kamei M, Fukuhara H, Shimamoto T, Ashida S, Karashima T, Yamasaki I, et al. Identification and functional analysis of SHISA2 overexpressed in prostate cancer. [abstract] In: Proceedings of the 103rd Annual Meeting of the American Association for Cancer Research; 2012 Mar 31-Apr 4; Chicago, IL. Philadelphia (PA): AACR. Cancer Res. 2012;72(8 Suppl):Abstract nr 1849. https://doi.org/10.1158/1538-7445.AM2012-1849

38. Gunning PW, Hardeman EC, Lappalainen P, Mulvihill DP. Tropomyosin - master regulator of actin filament function in the cytoskeleton. J Cell Sci. 2015;128(16):2965–74.

39. Endo H, Ikeda K, Urano T, Horie-Inoue K, Inoue S. Terf/TRIM17 stimulates degradation of kinetochore protein ZWINT and regulates cell proliferation. J Biochem. 2012;151(2):139–44.

40. Chaudhary S, Madhukrishna B, Adhya AK, Keshari S, Mishra SK. Overexpression of caspase 7 is ER alpha dependent to affect proliferation and cell growth in breast cancer cells by targeting p21(Cip). Oncogenesis. 2016;5:e219.

41. Savinainen KJ, Linja MJ, Saramaki OR, Tammela TL, Chang GT, Brinkmann AO, Visakorpi T. Expression and copy number analysis of TRPS1, EIF3S3 and MYC genes in breast and prostate cancer. Br J Cancer. 2004;90(5):1041–6.

42. Harms KL, Chen XB. Histone deacetylase 2 modulates p53 transcriptional activities through regulation of p53-DNA binding activity. Cancer Res. 2007; 67(7):3145–52.

43. Okada Y, Sonoshita M, Kakizaki F, Aoyama N, Itatani Y, Uegaki M, Sakamoto H, Kobayashi T, Inoue T, Kamba T, et al. Amino-terminal enhancer of split gene AES encodes a tumor and metastasis suppressor of prostate cancer. Cancer Sci. 2017;108(4):744–52.

44. Beaudry VG, Jiang D, Dusek RL, Park EJ, Knezevich S, Ridd K, Vogel H, Bastian BC, Attardi LD. Loss of the p53/p63 regulated desmosomal protein Perp promotes tumorigenesis. PLoS Genet. 2010;6(10):e1001168.

45. Vallee RB, Varma D, Dujardin DL. ZW10 function in mitotic checkpoint control, dynein targeting and membrane trafficking: is dynein the unifying theme? Cell Cycle. 2006;5(21):2447–51.

46. Napierala D, Garcia-Rojas X, Sam K, Wakui K, Chen C, Mendoza-Londono R, Zhou G, Zheng Q, Lee B. Mutations and promoter SNPs in RUNX2, a transcriptional regulator of bone formation. Mol Genet Metab. 2005;86(1–2): 257–68.

47. Stinson S, Lackner MR, Adai AT, Yu N, Kim HJ, O'Brien C, Spoerke J, Jhunjhunwala S, Boyd Z, Januario T, et al. TRPS1 targeting by miR-221/222 promotes the epithelial-to-mesenchymal transition in breast cancer. Sci Signal. 2011;4(177):ra41.

48. Fraga MF, Ballestar E, Villar-Garea A, Boix-Chornet M, Espada J, Schotta G, Bonaldi T, Haydon C, Ropero S, Petrie K, et al. Loss of acetylation at Lys16 and trimethylation at Lys20 of histone H4 is a common hallmark of human cancer. Nat Genet. 2005;37(4):391–400.

49. Kapoor-Vazirani P, Kagey JD, Powell DR, Vertino PM. Role of hMOF-dependent histone H4 lysine 16 acetylation in the maintenance of TMS1/ASC gene activity. Cancer Res. 2008;68(16):6810–21.

50. Kramer OH, Zhu P, Ostendorff HP, Golebiewski M, Tiefenbach J, Peters MA, Brill B, Groner B, Bach I, Heinzel T, et al. The histone deacetylase inhibitor valproic acid selectively induces proteasomal degradation of HDAC2. EMBO J. 2003;22(13):3411–20.

51. Zhang J, Kan S, Huang B, Hao ZY, Mak TW, Zhong Q. Mule determines the apoptotic response to HDAC inhibitors by targeted ubiquitination and destruction of HDAC2. Genes Dev. 2011;25(24):2610–8.

52. Nijman SM, Luna-Vargas MP, Velds A, Brummelkamp TR, Dirac AM, Sixma TK, Bernards R. A genomic and functional inventory of deubiquitinating enzymes. Cell. 2005;123(5):773–86.

53. Kim JM, Parmar K, Huang M, Weinstock DM, Ruit CA, Kutok JL, D'Andrea AD. Inactivation of murine Usp1 results in genomic instability and a Fanconi anemia phenotype. Dev Cell. 2009;16(2):314–20.

54. Schwickart M, Huang X, Lill JR, Liu J, Ferrando R, French DM, Maecker H, O'Rourke K, Bazan F, Eastham-Anderson J, et al. Deubiquitinase USP9X stabilizes MCL1 and promotes tumour cell survival. Nature. 2010;463(7277):103–7.

55. Huang XD, Summers MK, Pham V, Lill JR, Lee G, Kirkpatrick DS, Jackson PK, Fang GW, Dixit VM. Deubiquitinase USP37 is activated by CDK2 to antagonize APC(CDH1) and promote S phase entry. Mol Cell. 2011;42(4):511–23.

56. Pan J, Deng Q, Jiang C, Wang X, Niu T, Li H, Chen T, Jin J, Pan W, Cai X, et al. USP37 directly deubiquitinates and stabilizes c-Myc in lung cancer. Oncogene. 2015;34(30):3957–67.

57. Huang X, Dixit VM. Drugging the undruggables: exploring the ubiquitin system for drug development. Cell Res. 2016;26(4):484–98.

6

Quantitative background parenchymal uptake on molecular breast imaging and breast cancer risk: a case-control study

Carrie B. Hruska[1*], Jennifer R. Geske[2], Tiffinee N. Swanson[1], Alyssa N. Mammel[1], David S. Lake[1], Armando Manduca[1], Amy Lynn Conners[1], Dana H. Whaley[1], Christopher G. Scott[2], Rickey E. Carter[2], Deborah J. Rhodes[3], Michael K. O'Connor[1] and Celine M. Vachon[2]

Abstract

Background: Background parenchymal uptake (BPU), which refers to the level of Tc-99m sestamibi uptake within normal fibroglandular tissue on molecular breast imaging (MBI), has been identified as a breast cancer risk factor, independent of mammographic density. Prior analyses have used subjective categories to describe BPU. We evaluate a new quantitative method for assessing BPU by testing its reproducibility, comparing quantitative results with previously established subjective BPU categories, and determining the association of quantitative BPU with breast cancer risk.

Methods: Two nonradiologist operators independently performed region-of-interest analysis on MBI images viewed in conjunction with corresponding digital mammograms. Quantitative BPU was defined as a unitless ratio of the average pixel intensity (counts/pixel) within the fibroglandular tissue versus the average pixel intensity in fat. Operator agreement and the correlation of quantitative BPU measures with subjective BPU categories assessed by expert radiologists were determined. Percent density on mammograms was estimated using Cumulus. The association of quantitative BPU with breast cancer (per one unit BPU) was examined within an established case-control study of 62 incident breast cancer cases and 177 matched controls.

Results: Quantitative BPU ranged from 0.4 to 3.2 across all subjects and was on average higher in cases compared to controls (1.4 versus 1.2, $p < 0.007$ for both operators). Quantitative BPU was strongly correlated with subjective BPU categories (Spearman's $r = 0.59$ to 0.69, $p < 0.0001$, for each paired combination of two operators and two radiologists). Interoperator and intraoperator agreement in the quantitative BPU measure, assessed by intraclass correlation, was 0.92 and 0.98, respectively. Quantitative BPU measures showed either no correlation or weak negative correlation with mammographic percent density. In a model adjusted for body mass index and percent density, higher quantitative BPU was associated with increased risk of breast cancer for both operators (OR = 4.0, 95% confidence interval (CI) 1.6–10.1, and 2.4, 95% CI 1.2–4.7).

Conclusion: Quantitative measurement of BPU, defined as the ratio of average counts in fibroglandular tissue relative to that in fat, can be reliably performed by nonradiologist operators with a simple region-of-interest analysis tool. Similar to results obtained with subjective BPU categories, quantitative BPU is a functional imaging biomarker of breast cancer risk, independent of mammographic density and hormonal factors.

Keywords: Breast density, Breast cancer risk, Molecular breast imaging, Tc-99m sestamibi, Mammography

* Correspondence: hruska.carrie@mayo.edu
[1]Department of Physiology and Biomedical Engineering, Mayo Clinic, 200 First Street SW, Rochester, MN 55905, USA
Full list of author information is available at the end of the article

Background

Mammographic density, or the amount of fibroglandular tissue in the breast as depicted on a mammogram, is known to reduce the accuracy of mammography in detecting cancer [1–3]. Density is also independently associated with breast cancer risk as established by numerous analyses conducted over the last 40 years, consistently showing women with the densest breasts to be four- to six-times more likely to be diagnosed with breast cancer compared with those with low density [4, 5]. However, because breast density is highly prevalent (approximately 40 to 50% of screening-eligible women have heterogeneously or extremely dense breasts according to American College of Radiology (ACR) Breast Imaging-Reporting and Data System (BI-RADS) categories [6, 7]), it is impractical for clinicians to consider all women with dense breasts to be at elevated risk since doing so would warrant consideration of supplemental screening or preventive options in nearly half the screening population. To identify the subset of women with dense breasts at greatest risk of breast cancer, and those most likely to benefit from these strategies, improved risk stratification tools are needed.

Molecular breast imaging (MBI) is a nuclear medicine test that uses dedicated gamma cameras and injection of a radiotracer, typically Tc-99m sestamibi, to detect breast cancer. As MBI is a functional imaging technique that relies on the preferential uptake of radiotracer in metabolically active cells, it is able to reveal cancers obscured by breast density on mammography. MBI can also depict the functional uptake of radiotracer in benign fibroglandular tissue, which has been termed background parenchymal uptake (BPU). High levels of BPU are hypothesized to represent breast tissue with elevated metabolic activity due to a combination of factors such as abundant mitochondria, cellular proliferation, and blood flow [8, 9]. Among women with similar mammographic density, BPU has been observed to vary substantially from

a lack of uptake in fibroglandular tissue (photopenic) to very high intensity uptake (marked), as shown in Fig. 1. Importantly, subjective categories of high BPU were found to be associated with risk of incident breast cancer relative to those with low BPU in a case-control analysis (odds ratio (OR) range from 3 to 5) after adjustment for mammographic density and exogenous hormone use [10]. These results suggest that BPU is a functional imaging biomarker that depicts risk-related aspects of fibroglandular tissue not observed through measures of mammographic density alone.

Prior investigations of BPU on MBI have used a subjective measure which includes the following four categories: photopenic, minimal to mild, moderate, and marked [11, 12]. While expert readers were observed to have substantial agreement using this subjective classification (κ = 0.84) [13], only fair agreement was observed among nonexpert readers (κ = 0.31) [12]. A quantitative tool for BPU assessment may improve reproducibility of the measure. Additionally, a quantitative measure of BPU on a continuous scale would provide a more precise measurement and could therefore more accurately monitor changes in BPU over serial MBI examinations.

The objective of this work was to develop and evaluate a new quantitative method for assessing BPU by assessing its reproducibility, comparing quantitative to categorical BPU measures, and determining the association of quantitative BPU with breast cancer risk.

Methods
Study population

This retrospective analysis was compliant with the US Health Insurance Portability and Accountability Act and approved by the Mayo Clinic Institutional Review Board, which issued a waiver of informed consent. A case-control study previously established to evaluate the association of subjective BPU categories with breast cancer risk was used

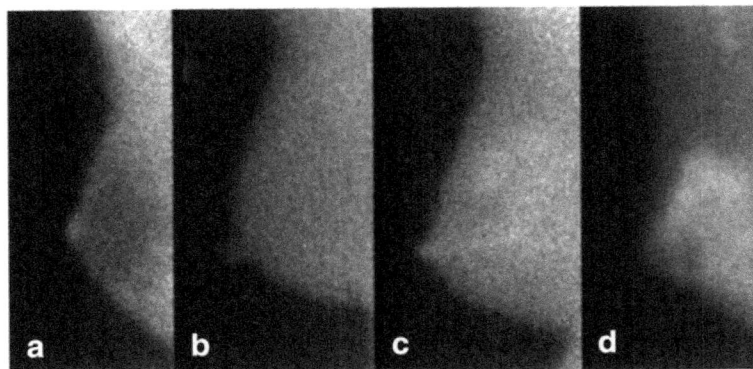

Fig. 1 BPU subjective categories. Example MBI images from four women, all acquired in right mediolateral oblique projection, showing the range of BPU observed: **a** photopenic BPU, **b** minimal to mild BPU, **c** moderate BPU, and **d** marked BPU

in the current analysis [10]. As previously described, we established this case-control group within a cohort of patients who underwent MBI between 1 February 2005 and 28 February 2014 ($n = 3202$) and who were followed for breast cancer diagnoses through 31 December 2014. A total of 3027 patients were eligible for study inclusion as they had provided general authorization to use medical records in research, did not have breast implants at the time of MBI, and did not have a prior history of breast cancer or were diagnosed at the time of MBI (within 180 days).

Any subject with a diagnosis of invasive breast cancer or ductal carcinoma in situ (DCIS) 180 days or more following the MBI was considered a case. Sixty-two cases were identified; the median time from MBI to diagnosis was 3.1 years. Control subjects were matched to cases on age (within 5 years), menopausal status, year of MBI, and follow-up interval (at least as long as matched case); the median follow-up time was 6.1 years. Up to three controls per case were originally selected ($n = 179$). Two controls were excluded as their mammograms were unavailable for use in the quantitative BPU software program (described below) leaving 177 controls for the current analysis.

Patient information at the time of MBI, including body mass index (BMI), menopausal status, postmenopausal hormone use, breast biopsy history, and family history of breast cancer, was obtained from research study questionnaires and medical record review.

Images

MBI examinations were performed as previously described [10]. Briefly, MBI was performed using a dedicated dual-head gamma camera system equipped with semiconductor-based detectors (cadmium zinc telluride). Following injection of Tc-99m sestamibi, two-view acquisitions (craniocaudal (CC) and mediolateral oblique (MLO)) of each breast were made. Thus, the entire MBI dataset comprised of eight images: a CC and MLO projection of left and right breasts acquired with two detector heads of the dual head system (Fig. 2).

Mammograms performed closest to the time of MBI were used for density analysis. The median time from mammogram to MBI was 0 days (interquartile range (IQR) 0–1 days). Mammographic density was classified according to the ACR BI-RADS breast composition categories (4th edition) at the time of clinical interpretation [14]. Density was also quantitatively measured as percent density (PD) by a trained operator using a semi-automated software tool (Cumulus; University of Toronto, Toronto, ON, Canada [15]), as previously described [16].

Quantitative BPU measurement

The subjective BPU categories, as defined in a validated lexicon for gamma imaging of the breast [11, 12], are intended to describe the relative intensity of radiotracer uptake in normal breast parenchyma (or fibroglandular tissue)

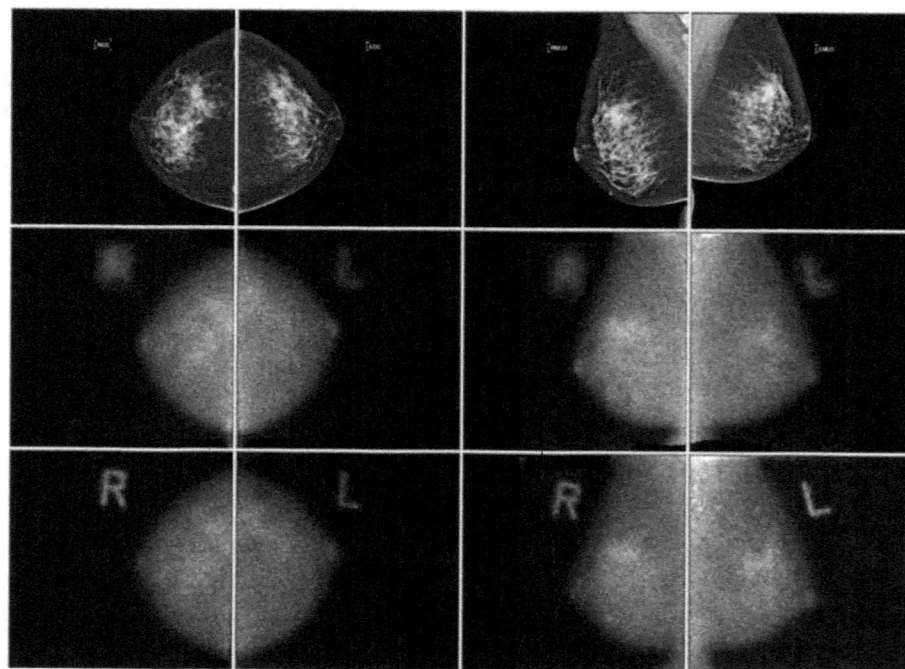

Fig. 2 Example layout of images for quantitative BPU region-of-interest analysis. Bilateral mammogram and MBI views in CC and MLO projections are displayed. Mammogram in top row (from left to right) comprises right CC, left CC, right MLO, and left MLO projections. The same projections acquired by MBI are shown for the upper detector (middle row) and for the lower detector (bottom row)

compared with intensity of uptake in subcutaneous fat. These categories and their definitions are as follows: 1) photopenic BPU, fibroglandular intensity less than fat intensity; 2) minimal to mild BPU, fibroglandular intensity equal to or slightly greater than fat intensity; 3) moderate BPU, fibroglandular intensity greater than mild but less than twice as intense as fat; and 4) marked BPU, fibroglandular intensity greater than twice fat intensity. The quantitative BPU tool was designed to provide values that reflect these definitions, such that it measures the ratio of average image counts (counts per pixel) in fibroglandular tissue versus fat.

As MBI examinations create functional images of radiotracer localization, they do not provide distinct anatomic landmarks of the breast from which to distinguish fibroglandular tissue and fat. However, as MBI is acquired in positions analogous to mammography (CC and MLO), a mammogram viewed in conjunction with MBI may be used to generally determine fibroglandular and fat locations. In this first approach to develop a quantitative tool for BPU, we used a corresponding mammogram to identify fibroglandular and fat regions, applied these regions to the MBI images, and determined the fibroglandular-to-fat count ratio on MBI as a quantitative BPU value, described in more detail as follows.

An in-house software program was created to allow simultaneous display of MBI examinations with mammograms, as shown in Fig. 2. Using this program, each mammogram and its corresponding MBI images were processed as follows. First, a region of interest (ROI) outlining the entire breast visible on the mammogram was automatically drawn, based on a manually adjustable intensity threshold. Next, two other ROIs were drawn by the operator on the mammogram view—one to encompass an

area predominantly made of fat and one to include predominantly fibroglandular tissue. The operator then manually adjusted the fibroglandular ROI using an intensity threshold to reject less-dense tissue, thereby reducing the overall size of the ROI and making it more specific to dense tissue. Finally, the three mammogram ROIs were copied to the corresponding MBI views and manually scaled and rotated as needed (all three as a single object) to register the outer outline of the mammogram to the MBI breast outline. This process was done to account for differences in breast position and compression force between the mammogram and MBI images. Example ROIs are shown in Fig. 3. The ratio of average counts (counts per pixel) in the fibroglandular ROI versus fat ROI was taken as a measure of quantitative BPU.

Two operators used this program to perform quantitative BPU measurements on each of the eight MBI views for all subjects. Each operator independently performed each step in the ROI process as described above, while blinded to the other operator's results and blinded to patient identity and case status. One operator was a novice to medical imaging and image processing tools and the other operator was a nuclear medicine technologist familiar with mammography, MBI, and image processing software. To determine intraoperator agreement, one operator performed quantitative BPU measurements a second time on a sample of 48 subjects.

Statistical analysis

Case and control characteristics are summarized using frequencies for categorical variables or mean and standard deviation (SD) with range for continuous variables. Conditional logistic regression was used to evaluate the

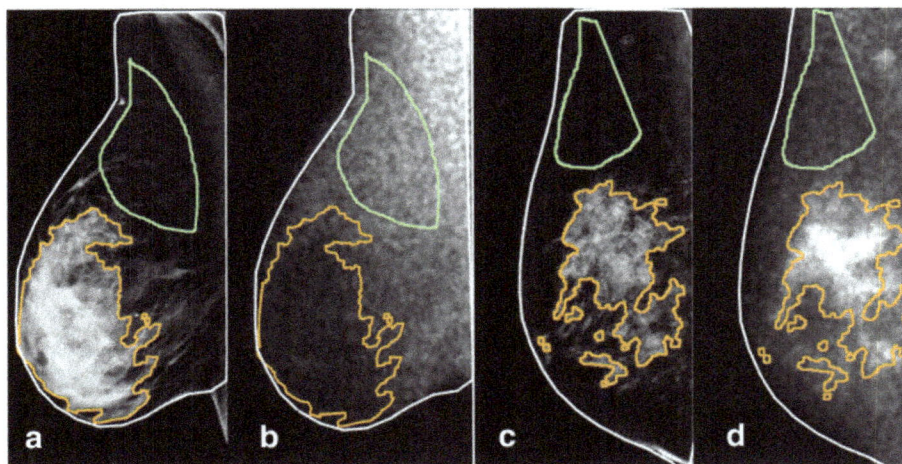

Fig. 3 Example ROIs for quantitative BPU assessment. Breast images acquired in the mediolateral oblique position for two patients. Fibroglandular tissue is defined by the orange ROI and fat is defined by the green ROI. In panels **a** and **b**, the mammogram (**a**) and MBI (**b**) are shown for a patient classified as having photopenic BPU, measured quantitatively as 0.4. In panels **c** and **d**, the mammogram (**c**) and MBI (**d**) are shown for a patient with marked BPU, measured quantitatively as 2.4

primary hypothesis that quantitative BPU is associated with breast cancer. Models were adjusted for BMI and PD and postmenopausal hormone use. All ORs reported are for a one-unit change in quantitative BPU measurement. Analyses were repeated within premenopausal and postmenopausal subgroups.

Agreement in quantitative BPU across eight MBI views was assessed using several methods including intraclass correlation (ICC), principal component (PC) analysis, and a nested random effects model to inform the summary quantitative measure. ICC for each of the eight views was calculated and ranged from 0.74 to 0.92. PC analysis revealed a lack of multidimensionality among the eight views, as the first and second PCs explained 0.83 and 0.09 of the variation in all eight measures. Lastly, a nested random effects model demonstrated that only 2% of the variation in quantitative BPU was due to the eight views within a subject and 83% was intersubject variation, leaving 15% of variation due to random error. Therefore, with low dimensionality and limited variation across the eight images, we used an average of the quantitative BPU values from the eight views as the quantitative BPU measure for each subject herein. Analyses of individual views and other combinations (averages by breast side and view) along with their p values and area under the curves (AUCs) are summarized by operator in Additional file 1 (Table S1).

Interoperator and intraoperator agreement in quantitative BPU measures were summarized by ICC. Agreement between quantitative BPU and subjective BPU categories and PD measured on mammography was determined by Spearman and Pearson correlations, respectively. For all comparisons, $p < 0.05$ was considered statistically significant. Analyses were performed within SAS (Cary, NC; version 9.4).

Results

Subject characteristics

A total of 239 subjects, including 62 cases and 177 controls, were included in the study, with their characteristics presented in Table 1. Cases and controls were similar on matched variables of age and menopausal status, as expected. Cases and controls were not significantly different in any other characteristic examined, including BI-RADs density and PD. Quantitative BPU measures ranged from 0.41 to 3.18, with mean (IQR) values of 1.36 (1.09–1.54) for cases versus 1.18 (0.97–1.31) for controls for operator 1 ($p = 0.002$) and 1.36 (1.04–1.56) for cases and 1.19 (0.93–1.33) for controls for operator 2 ($p = 0.007$) (Table 2).

BPU agreement

The two operators showed good agreement in assessing quantitative BPU; the interoperator ICC for the average of the eight views was 0.92 (95% confidence interval (CI)

0.90–0.94) and ICCs ranged from 0.75 (95% CI 0.68–0.80) to 0.92 (95% CI 0.86–0.95) across the eight views. Intraoperator agreement in quantitative BPU was 0.98 (0.96–0.99) for the average of the eight views and ICCs ranged from 0.80 (95% CI 0.67–0.88) to 0.91 (95% CI 0.84–0.95) across the eight views.

Quantitative BPU measurements correlated well with subjective BPU categories previously assessed by radiologists [10], as shown in Fig. 4. Spearman correlations ranged from 0.59 to 0.69 (all p values < 0.0001) for the four combinations of two categorical BPU readers and two quantitative BPU operators.

Quantitative BPU measures and PD showed weak or no correlation (all p values > 0.05 unless specified) in the total sample (operator 1: $r = -0.11$, operator 2: $r = -0.07$) (Fig. 5), or separately in cases (operator 1: $r = 0.12$, operator 2: $r = 0.14$), or controls (operator 1: $r = -0.20$, $p = 0.009$; operator 2: $r = -0.13$).

Breast cancer cases versus controls

Quantitative BPU was associated with breast cancer risk in models adjusted for BMI, with odds ratios per 1 unit BPU of 3.70 (95% CI 1.54–8.92) and 2.37 (95% CI 1.19–4.70) for the two operators, respectively (Table 3). Results were similar for models including PD or postmenopausal hormone use.

In analyses limited to postmenopausal women, quantitative BPU remained associated with breast cancer risk (BMI-adjusted OR per 1 unit BPU = 5.57, 95% CI 1.62–19.08, for operator 1, and 2.91, 95% CI 1.15–7.35, for operator 2); however, the BPU measure was not a statistically significant predictor for breast cancer in the premenopausal subset for either operator in a small sample of 13 cases.

Analysis of the eight MBI views separately by operator, as well as averages of right breast, left breast, MLO views, CC views, upper detector views, and lower detector views were considered (Additional file 1: Table S1). All models concluded that higher quantitative BPU was significantly associated with breast cancer risk with the exception of one view under operator 2 (OR = 1.5, $p = 0.18$). ORs ranged 2.0 to 4.5 for operator 1 and from 1.5 to 2.6 for operator 2, but reliably showed consistent overall model performance with AUCs from 0.57 to 0.62.

Discussion

In this first evaluation of a simple region-of-interest tool for obtaining quantitative measurements of BPU on MBI, we found an association of quantitative BPU measurements with breast cancer risk, similar to that observed in a prior analysis of subjective BPU categories. This association was independent of mammographic density. In fact, in line with our previous observation that BPU can vary widely among women with similar

Table 1 Characteristics of breast cancer cases and controls, matched on age and menopausal status

Characteristic	Breast cancer cases ($n = 62$)	Controls ($n = 177$)	P
Age at MBI (years)[a]	60.3 ± 10.6 (38–88)	60.2 ± 10.4 (38–86)	NA
Menopausal status			NA
Premenopausal	13 (21)	38 (22)	
Postmenopausal	49 (79)	138 (78)	
Body mass index (kg/m^2)[a]	27.7 ± 6.4 (18.8–55.5)	26.2 ± 4.7 (18.6–44.3)	0.06
Postmenopausal systemic hormone therapy[b]			0.57
Current use at MBI	13 (27)	44 (31)	
No current use at MBI	36 (73)	97 (69)	
BI-RADS density			0.81
Almost entirely fat	1 (2)	3 (2)	
Scattered fibroglandular densities	10 (16)	34 (19)	
Heterogeneously dense	44 (71)	113 (64)	
Extremely dense	7 (11)	26 (15)	
Percent density[a]	24.8 ± 8.3 (3.5–48.0)	24.6 ± 10.2 (1.8–53.8)	0.93
Tumor invasiveness			
Invasive	45 (73)	NA	
DCIS	17 (27)	NA	
Gail model 5-year risk[a]	2.7 ± 1.5 (0.6–7.2)	2.4 ± 1.5 (0.5–9.5)	0.23
BCSC model 5-year risk[a]	2.6 ± 1.2 (0.7–5.4)	2.3 ± 1.5 (0.4–13.2)	0.29
Family history of breast cancer			0.45
One or more first-degree relatives	33 (53)	86 (48)	
No first-degree relatives	29 (47)	93 (52)	
Personal history of biopsy showing atypia or LCIS			0.07
Yes	6 (10)	6 (3)	
No	56 (90)	173 (97)	

Unless otherwise noted, data are number of patients and data in parentheses are percentages
[a]Data are mean ± standard deviation; data in parentheses are the range
[b]Data are among postmenopausal women only (49 breast cancer cases; 138 controls)
BCSC, Breast Cancer Surveillance Consortium; *BI-RADS*, Breast Imaging-Reporting and Data System; *DCIS*, ductal carcinoma in situ; *LCIS*, lobular carcinoma in situ; *MBI*, molecular breast imaging; *NA*, not available

mammographic density [10, 13], we saw no association between quantitative BPU and quantitative percent density in the current analysis.

The lack of relationship between BPU and mammographic density is not unexpected since BPU and density are fundamentally different imaging features. While density measures describe the amount of fibroglandular tissue in the breast by its anatomic appearance, BPU describes the functional radiotracer uptake within that fibroglandular tissue relative to the uptake in fat. Furthermore, density assessment tools, such as Cumulus, use a binary decision to categorize image pixels of a mammogram as "dense" or

Table 2 Molecular breast imaging (MBI) quantitative background parencymal uptake (BPU) components by case status

Characteristic	Operator	Breast cancer cases $n = 62$	Controls $n = 176$	P
Average counts in fibroglandular tissue, mean ± SD (range)	1	41.5 ± 20.7 (6.8–116.6)	37.6 ± 23.2 (7.3–218.4)	0.08
	2	41.2 ± 21.1 (7.2–194.9)	36.5 ± 21.7 (6.5–114.6)	0.08
Average counts in fat, mean ± SD (range)	1	31.5 ± 14.3 (5.9–87.4)	32.7 ± 17.2 (6.2–95.7)	0.99
	2	32.6 ± 16.0 (5.7–90.7)	32.5 ± 17.0 (7.2–98.9)	0.78
Quantitative BPU (fibroglandular/fat), mean ± SD (range)	1	1.4 ± 0.4 (0.8, 2.8)	1.2 ± 0.3 (0.4, 2.9)	0.002
	2	1.4 ± 0.5 (0.8, 2.9)	1.2 ± 0.4 (0.5, 3.2)	0.007

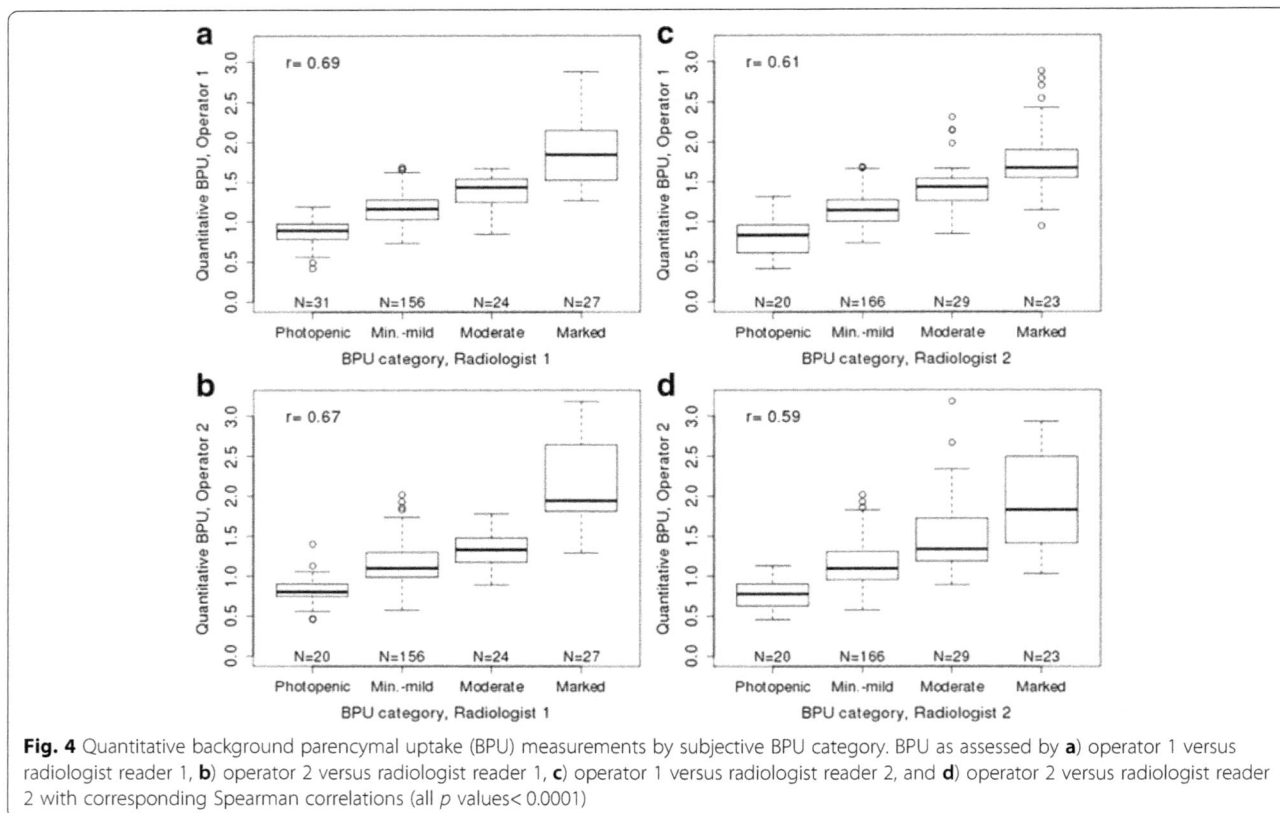

Fig. 4 Quantitative background parencymal uptake (BPU) measurements by subjective BPU category. BPU as assessed by **a**) operator 1 versus radiologist reader 1, **b**) operator 2 versus radiologist reader 1, **c**) operator 1 versus radiologist reader 2, and **d**) operator 2 versus radiologist reader 2 with corresponding Spearman correlations (all p values< 0.0001)

"non-dense", and output the proportion of dense pixels, but do not take into account the intensity of those dense pixels. In contrast, BPU as measured on MBI is determined by the average intensity of the pixels in fibroglandular tissue relative to the intensity of pixels in fat. Therefore, it is possible for a breast to have a small amount of dense tissue and yet have high uptake within that dense tissue on MBI, resulting in high BPU. It is also possible for a breast to be very dense and have low BPU. The quantitative BPU value can vary substantially, even when percent density is similar. For instance, as seen in Fig. 5, women with percent density of about 40% were found to vary in quantitative BPU values from 0.4 to 3.2.

The underlying etiology relating BPU of Tc-99m sestamibi and risk of breast cancer is not yet known. In fact, the mechanism of Tc-99m sestamibi uptake in the breast

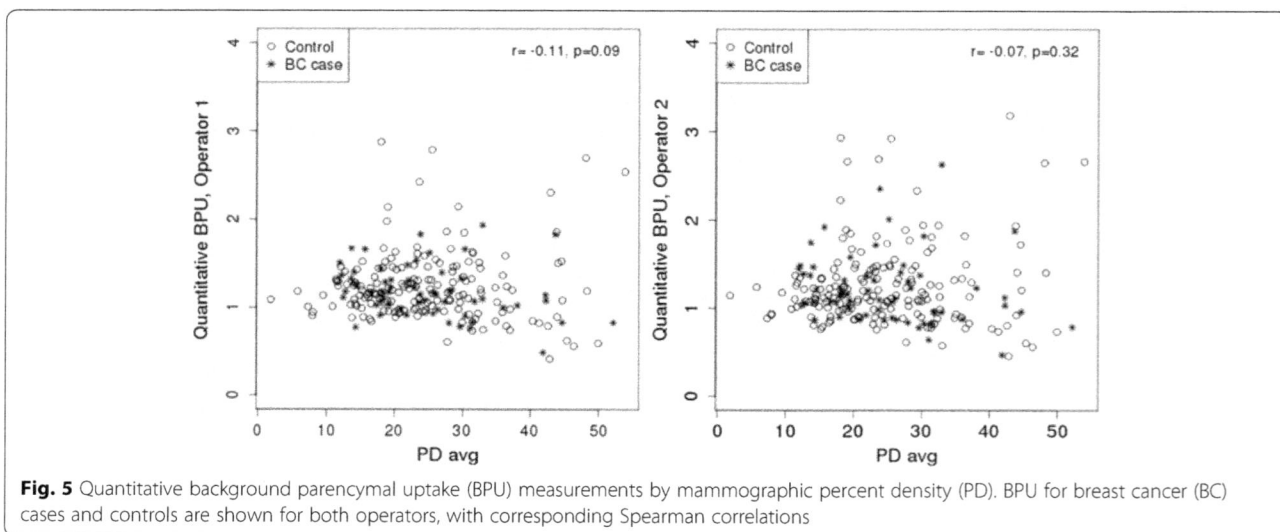

Fig. 5 Quantitative background parencymal uptake (BPU) measurements by mammographic percent density (PD). BPU for breast cancer (BC) cases and controls are shown for both operators, with corresponding Spearman correlations

Table 3 Association of quantitative background parencymal uptake (BPU) (per 1 unit BPU) with breast cancer

	OR (95% CI), adjusted for BMI	OR (95% CI), adjusted for BMI and PD	OR (95% CI), adjusted for BMI and postmenopausal hormones
Overall			
Operator 1	3.70 (1.54–8.92)	3.98 (1.58–10.05)	3.85 (1.58–9.38)
p value	0.0036	0.0034	0.0030
AUC (95% CI)	0.63 (0.56–0.71)	0.66 (0.59–0.73)	0.63 (0.56–0.70)
Operator 2	2.37 (1.19–4.70)	2.35 (1.17–4.71)	2.31 (1.17–4.55)
p value	0.0136	0.0163	0.0154
AUC (95% CI)	0.58 (0.51–0.66)	0.61 (0.54–0.69)	0.61 (0.54–0.69)
Postmenopausal women ($n = 187$: 49 cases, 138 controls)			
Operator 1	5.57 (1.62–19.08)	8.39 (2.10–33.55)	5.87 (1.69–20.36)
p value	0.0063	0.0026	0.0053
AUC (95% CI)	0.65 (0.57–0.73)	0.70 (0.62–0.78)	0.65 (0.57–0.73)
Operator 2	2.91 (1.15–7.35)	3.62 (1.34–9.79)	2.99 (1.18–7.57)
p value	0.0239	0.0113	0.0212
AUC (95% CI)	0.57 (0.48–0.65)	0.66 (0.58–0.74)	0.61 (0.53–0.69)
Premenopausal women ($n = 51$: 13 cases, 38 controls)			
Operator 1	2.42 (0.73–8.04)	2.09 (0.64–6.79)	NA
p value	0.1492	0.2224	
AUC (95% CI)	0.57 (0.41–0.73)	0.58 (0.42–0.73)	
Operator 2	1.70 (0.63–4.58)	1.47 (0.54–3.98)	NA
p value	0.2922	0.4468	
AUC (95% CI)	0.62 (0.47–0.78)	0.61 (0.45–0.76)	

AUC, area under the curve; *BMI*, body mass index; *CI*, confidence interval; *NA*, not applicable; *OR*, odds ratio; *PD*, percent density by Cumulus software

in general is not well understood. Tc-99m sestamibi was developed as a tracer for imaging myocardial perfusion and was only incidentally discovered to accumulate in breast lesions in women undergoing cardiac testing [17]. Tc-99m sestamibi is known to be mostly sequestered in cellular mitochondria [8]. In breast cancer, its uptake is thought to reflect both blood flow to the tumor and mitochondrial status, which is affected by the cellular proliferation rate and apoptotic index [8, 9]. Benign breast lesions that are highly proliferative, such as atypical lesions and fibroadenomas, can also demonstrate high uptake of Tc-99m sestamibi that mimics breast cancer [18]. Although the etiology of variations in BPU among women has not been established, it can be hypothesized that breast fibroglandular tissue with higher blood flow and more proliferative cells would also exhibit higher BPU, and thus may represent tissue that is primed for breast cancer development.

Hormonal factors which are known to impact tissue perfusion and proliferation have been found to impact BPU. We have previously shown that high (moderate or marked) BPU is more prevalent among premenopausal women compared with postmenopausal women [13]. In postmenopausal women, those using exogenous hormonal therapy are more likely to have high BPU [13]. In the

current study, quantitative BPU was strongly associated with breast cancer in postmenopausal women, but this association was somewhat attenuated with adjustment for hormone therapy use. In premenopausal women, BPU can fluctuate with the menstrual cycle, with higher levels of BPU observed in the luteal phase compared with the follicular phase [19]. When we restricted analysis to postmenopausal women in the current work, the association of quantitative BPU with breast cancer remained, suggesting that the association is not merely reflecting changes in BPU with the menstrual cycle. We did not observe a significant association in premenopausal women; however, the analysis was limited in power due to smaller numbers ($n = 13$ cases).

This study found that quantitative BPU assessed by operators correlates well with subjective BPU categories assessed by expert radiologists. We also found good agreement in quantitative BPU measurements between the two operators, one of whom was a novice to medical imaging, indicating that the quantitative method is robust and generalizable to other operators. Importantly, our results on the evaluation of eight views showed that the quantitative BPU obtained from any of the eight MBI views or any of the reported averages of multiple views is a reliable predictor of increased breast cancer risk, shown under two different operators with varying experience. Thus, future investigations could use a single view or combination of views for quantitative BPU assessment.

MBI is indicated for women with dense breasts, as reflected in our study population here where a majority of cases (82%) and controls (79%) were considered mammographically dense. In our institution's practice, MBI is primarily used as a screening tool and is offered to women with dense breasts who seek supplemental screening but either do not wish to undergo or do not meet the high-risk criteria (20% lifetime risk by familial models) for screening breast magnetic resonance (MR) imaging. Supplemental screening MBI, performed with reduced administered doses of 300 MBq (8 mCi) Tc-99m sestamibi, offers a reported incremental cancer detection rate of 7.7 to 8.8 cancers per 1000 women screened [20, 21]. Although breast density is well-established as a breast cancer risk factor, for women with dense breasts included in this study there was no association between breast cancer and mammographic density assessed by mammographic categories or quantitative percent density. Thus, BPU will be an important risk factor for the dense breast population and may offer additional image-based risk information beyond density alone. Further work is needed to determine the impact of incorporating BPU into existing risk models.

Although our quantitative BPU method is relatively simple and easy to implement with minimal operator training, the method does have some limitations. First, given this was the first study relating the quantitative BPU to breast cancer, our estimates for the strength of the association were imprecise. This can be evidenced by the differential estimates of risk between operators (e.g., OR = 5.87 versus 2.99). These confidence intervals for the estimates are wide and overlapping. Further work is needed to develop a comprehensive model on a larger set of patients to ensure the risk estimates are properly calibrated.

Second, our method for measuring quantitative BPU currently requires user interaction to manually segment and align regions from the mammogram to the MBI. Best results are expected when the breast is similarly positioned on the mammogram and MBI, which is not always possible as they are acquired under separate examinations with the MBI performed under substantially less breast compression. Also, our current quantitative measure is based on the ratio of average pixel intensities in fibroglandular and fat regions obtained in two-dimensional planar images. Similar to findings from studies of mammographic density and breast cancer risk, a more precise or more reproducible risk association may be obtained if the BPU area is considered or volumetric BPU estimates are made. Future iterations of this method are anticipated to be automated and to evaluate additional factors such as BPU volume.

Conclusions

Quantitative measurement of BPU, which can be reliably assessed by nonradiologist operators with a simple region-of-interest analysis tool, correlates well with subjective BPU categories assessed by expert radiologists. Similar to findings with subjective BPU categories, quantitative BPU measurement is associated with breast cancer risk, independent of mammographic density and hormonal factors. These results suggest that quantitative measures of BPU could serve as an additional tool for identifying a subset of women with mammographically dense breasts who are at greatest risk of breast cancer.

Abbreviations

ACR: American College of Radiology; AUC: Area under the curve; BI-RADS: Breast Imaging-Reporting and Data System; BMI: Body mass index; BPU: Background parenchymal uptake; CC: Craniocaudal; CI: Confidence interval; DCIS: Ductal carcinoma in situ; ICC: Intraclass correlation; IQR: Interquartile range; MBI: Molecular breast imaging; MLO: Mediolateral oblique; OR: Odds ratio; PC: Principal component; PD: Percent density; ROI: Region of interest

Funding

This work was supported by grants from the National Cancer Institute (R21 CA 197752), National Center for Advancing Translational Sciences (UL1 TR000135), the Mayo Clinic Cancer Center, Fraternal Order of Eagles Cancer Research Fund, and the Mayo Clinic Department of Radiology.

Authors' contributions

CBH, CGS, and CMV conceived and designed the study. JRG, CGS, and REC performed statistical analysis and interpretation of the data. ALC and DHW performed the reading of molecular breast imaging examinations and mammograms. CBH, TNS, ANM, DSL, and AM developed and tested the quantitative BPU tool. DJR and MKO provided image and questionnaire data from molecular breast imaging research trials. All authors contributed to drafting and revising the manuscript, and all read and approved the final manuscript.

Competing interests

CBH and MKO receive royalties for licensed technologies per agreement between Mayo Clinic and Gamma Medica, a manufacturer of molecular breast imaging systems. The remaining authors declare that they have no competing interests.

Author details

[1]Department of Physiology and Biomedical Engineering, Mayo Clinic, 200 First Street SW, Rochester, MN 55905, USA. [2]Department of Health Sciences Research, Mayo Clinic, 200 First Street SW, Rochester, MN 55905, USA. [3]Department Medicine, Mayo Clinic, 200 First Street SW, Rochester, MN 55905, USA.

References

1. Carney PA, Miglioretti DL, Yankaskas BC, Kerlikowske K, Rosenberg R, Rutter CM, Geller BM, Abraham LA, Taplin SH, Dignan M, et al. Individual and combined effects of age, breast density, and hormone replacement therapy use on the accuracy of screening mammography. Ann Intern Med. 2003; 138(3):168–75.

2. Mandelson MT, Oestreicher N, Porter PL, White D, Finder CA, Taplin SH, White E. Breast density as a predictor of mammographic detection: comparison of interval- and screen-detected cancers. J Natl Cancer Inst. 2000;92(13):1081–7.

3. Buist DS, Porter PL, Lehman C, Taplin SH, White E. Factors contributing to mammography failure in women aged 40-49 years. J Natl Cancer Inst. 2004; 96(19):1432–40.

4. Vachon CM, Gils CH, Sellers TA, Ghosh K, Pruthi S, Brandt KR. Mammographic density, breast cancer risk and risk prediction. Breast Cancer Res. 2007;9(6):217.

5. McCormack VA. Breast density and parenchymal patterns as markers of breast cancer risk: a meta-analysis. Cancer Epidemiol Biomark Prev. 2006; 15(6):1159–69.

6. Brandt KR, Scott CG, Ma L, Mahmoudzadeh AP, Jensen MR, Whaley DH, Wu FF, Malkov S, Hruska CB, Norman AD, et al. Comparison of clinical and automated breast density measurements: implications for risk prediction and supplemental screening. Radiology. 2016;279(3):710–9.

7. Sprague BL, Gangnon RE, Burt V, Trentham-Dietz A, Hampton JM, Wellman RD, Kerlikowske K, Miglioretti DL. Prevalence of mammographically dense breasts in the United States. J Natl Cancer Inst. 2014;106(10)

8. Arbab AS, Koizumi K, Toyama K, Araki T. Uptake of technetium-99m-tetrofosmin, technetium-99m-MIBI and thallium-201 in tumor cell lines. J Nucl Med. 1996;37(9):1551–6.

9. Del Vecchio S, Salvatore M. 99mTc-MIBI in the evaluation of breast cancer biology. Eur J Nucl Med Mol Imaging. 2004;31(1):S88–96.

10. Hruska CB, Scott CG, Conners AL, Whaley DH, Rhodes DJ, Carter RE, O'Connor MK, Hunt KN, Brandt KR, Vachon CM. Background parenchymal uptake on molecular breast imaging as a breast cancer risk factor: a case-control study. Breast Cancer Res. 2016;18(1):42.

11. Conners AL, Maxwell RW, Tortorelli CL, Hruska CB, Rhodes DJ, Boughey JC, Berg WA. Gamma camera breast imaging lexicon. AJR Am J Roentgenol. 2012;199(6):W767–74.

12. Conners AL, Hruska CB, Tortorelli CL, Maxwell RW, Rhodes DJ, Boughey JC, Berg WA. Lexicon for standardized interpretation of gamma camera molecular breast imaging: observer agreement and diagnostic accuracy. Eur J Nucl Med Mol Imaging. 2012;39(6):971–82.

13. Hruska CB, Rhodes DJ, Conners AL, Jones KN, Carter RE, Lingineni RK, Vachon CM. Background parenchymal uptake during molecular breast imaging and associated clinical factors. Am J Roentgenol. 2015;204(3):W363–70.

14. D'Orsi CJ, Bassett LW, Berg WA. Breast imaging reporting and data system, BI-RADS: mammography. 4th ed. American College of Radiology: Reston; 2003.

15. Byng JW, Boyd NF, Fishell E, Jong RA, Yaffe MJ. Automated analysis of mammographic densities. Phys Med Biol. 1996;41(5):909.

16. Vachon CM, Pankratz VS, Scott CG, Maloney SD, Ghosh K, Brandt KR, Milanese T, Carston MJ, Sellers TA. Longitudinal trends in mammographic percent density and breast cancer risk. Cancer Epidemiol Biomark Prev. 2007;16(5):921–8.

17. Campeau RJ, Kronemer KA, Sutherland CM. Concordant uptake of Tc-99m sestamibi and Tl-201 in unsuspected breast tumor. Clin Nucl Med. 1992; 17(12):936–7.

18. Rhodes DJ, Hruska CB, Phillips SW, Whaley DH, O'Connor MK. Dedicated dual-head gamma imaging for breast cancer screening in women with mammographically dense breasts. Radiology. 2011;258(1):106–18.

19. Hruska CB, Conners AL, Vachon CM, O'Connor MK, Shuster LT, Bartley AC, Rhodes DJ. Effect of menstrual cycle phase on background parenchymal uptake at molecular breast imaging. Acad Radiol. 2015;22(9):1147–56.

20. Rhodes DJ, Hruska CB, Conners AL, Tortorelli CL, Maxwell RW, Jones KN, Toledano AY, O'Connor MK. Journal club: molecular breast imaging at reduced radiation dose for supplemental screening in mammographically dense breasts. Am J Roentgenol. 2015;204(2):241–51.

21. Shermis RB, Wilson KD, Doyle MT, Martin TS, Merryman D, Kudrolli H, Brenner RJ. Supplemental breast cancer screening with molecular breast imaging for women with dense breast tissue. Am J Roentgenol. 2016;207:1–8.

7

Breast cancer risk factors, survival and recurrence, and tumor molecular subtype: analysis of 3012 women from an indigenous Asian population

Mustapha Abubakar[1], Hyuna Sung[1,2], Devi BCR[3], Jennifer Guida[4], Tieng Swee Tang[3], Ruth M. Pfeiffer[1] and Xiaohong R. Yang[1]* [ID]

Abstract

Background: Limited evidence, mostly from studies in Western populations, suggests that the prognostic effects of lifestyle-related risk factors may be molecular subtype-dependent. Here, we examined whether pre-diagnostic lifestyle-related risk factors for breast cancer are associated with clinical outcomes by molecular subtype among patients from an understudied Asian population.

Methods: In this population-based case series, we evaluated breast cancer risk factors in relation to 10-year all-cause mortality (ACM) and 5-year recurrence by molecular subtype among 3012 women with invasive breast cancer in Sarawak, Malaysia. A total of 579 deaths and 314 recurrence events occurred during a median follow-up period of ~ 24 months. Subtypes (luminal A-like, luminal B-like, HER2-enriched, triple-negative) were defined using immunohistochemical markers for hormone receptors and human epidermal growth factor receptor 2 (HER2) in conjunction with histologic grade. Hazard ratios (HRs) and 95% confidence intervals (CIs) for the associations between risk factors and ACM/recurrence were estimated in subtype-specific Cox regression models.

Results: We observed heterogeneity in the relationships between parity/breastfeeding, age at first full-term pregnancy (FFP), family history, body mass index (BMI), and tumor subtype (p value < 0.05). Among luminal A-like patients only, older age at menarche [HR (95% CI) $_{\geq 15 \text{ vs} \leq 12 \text{ years}}$ = 2.28 (1.05, 4.95)] and being underweight [HR$_{\text{BMI} < 18.5 \text{kg/m}^2 \text{ vs. } 18.5-24.9 \text{kg/m}^2}$ = 3.46 (1.21, 9.89)] or overweight [HR$_{25-29.9 \text{kg/m}^2 \text{ vs. } 18.5-24.9 \text{kg/m}^2}$ = 3.14 (1.04, 9.50)] were associated with adverse prognosis, while parity/breastfeeding [HR$_{\text{breastfeeding vs nulliparity}}$ = 0.48 (0.27, 0.85)] and older age at FFP [HR $_{> 30 \text{ vs} < 21 \text{ years}}$ = 0.20 (0.04, 0.90)] were associated with good prognosis. For these women, the addition of age at menarche, parity/breastfeeding, and BMI, provided significantly better fit to a prognostic model containing standard clinicopathological factors alone [LRχ^2 (8df) = 21.78; p value = 0.005]. Overall, the results were similar in relation to recurrence.

Conclusions: Our finding that breastfeeding and BMI were associated with prognosis only among women with luminal A-like breast cancer is consistent with those from previously published data in Western populations. Further prospective studies will be needed to clarify the role of lifestyle modification, especially changes in BMI, in improving clinical outcomes for women with luminal A-like breast cancer.

Keywords: Breast cancer, Risk factors, Survival, Recurrence, Molecular subtype

* Correspondence: royang@mail.nih.gov
[1]Integrative Tumor Epidemiology Branch, Division of Cancer Epidemiology and Genetics, National Cancer Institute (NCI), National Institutes of Health, 9609 Medical Center Drive, Rockville, MD 20850, USA
Full list of author information is available at the end of the article

Background

In addition to impacting incidence, lifestyle and environmental risk factors for breast cancer may influence disease progression. Several studies have previously evaluated this question, with mixed results. While some studies have documented older age at menarche [1–3], early age at first full-term pregnancy (FFP) [4, 5] and nulliparity [6, 7] to be associated with adverse prognosis in breast cancer patients, others have reported better prognosis in relation to these risk factors [8–12]. Discrepancies in reported associations may be explained by differences in study populations, risk factor distributions, and potential confounders, but could also be due to heterogeneity inherent in breast cancer.

Findings from expression profiling studies have been used to classify breast cancers into intrinsic subtypes (i.e. luminal A, luminal B, human epidermal growth factor receptor 2 (HER2)-enriched, basal-like, and normal-like subtypes), which were associated with different prognoses [13] and can be corroborated by immunohistochemical (IHC) markers for hormone receptors (i.e. estrogen receptor (ER), progesterone receptor [PR]) and HER2. Recently, proxies of the extent of tumor proliferation have been endorsed to refine subgroups that recapitulate the intrinsic subtypes more accurately than using hormone receptors and HER2 alone [14, 15]. Epidemiological studies have shown that associations between breast cancer risk factors vary by tumor subtypes. For example, parity and early age at FFP are associated with decreased risk of luminal breast tumors, but they do not protect and may even increase the risk for ER-negative or triple-negative breast cancers [16–19].

Three previous studies have evaluated the relationship between breast cancer risk factors and survival according to molecular subtype, one among women in Seoul, South Korea [20] and the other two involving analyses of US-based prospective breast cancer cohorts [21, 22]. Results from these studies suggest that the associations between late age at menarche [20], breastfeeding [21], high body mass index (BMI) [22] and survival after breast cancer might differ according to molecular subtype. However, findings from these studies are yet to be validated in independent populations and, to our knowledge, no study has specifically examined risk factors in relation to survival according to subtypes defined by the recent IHC classification scheme accounting for proliferation in an Asian population.

Despite racial and geographic variations in the incidence, presentation, and outcome of breast cancer; so far, most investigations on risk factors in relation to tumor subtypes and survival have been conducted in European populations. This analysis, therefore, aims to evaluate the association between breast cancer risk factors and tumor molecular subtypes, defined by hormone receptors and HER2 in conjunction with histologic grade; and to examine the relationship between risk factors and survival by molecular subtype among women in Sarawak, Malaysia.

Methods

Study population

Sarawak is a Malaysian state on Borneo with a multiethnic composition, comprising of native Borneo populations (51%), Chinese (25%) and Malays (24%) [23]. Overall, 3355 women with invasive breast cancer diagnosed and treated between 2003 and 2016 in the Department of Radiotherapy, Oncology, and Palliative Care, Sarawak General Hospital where ~ 93% of all breast cancer cases diagnosed in Sarawak are treated, were recruited for this study. Of these, 106 (~ 3%) did not participate by not filling the questionnaire leading to a participating rate of ~ 97%. Of the 3249 who participated, 168 (~ 5%) were lost to follow-up and 69 did not have complete information on ER, PR, HER2, and grade that is needed to generate breast cancer subtypes hence were excluded from further analysis. Ultimately, 3012 women representing ~ 90% of the original population were included in the current analysis. Information on lifestyle and environmental risk factors were obtained from questionnaires that were administered to participants at enrollment, which was approximately 4 weeks after diagnosis, while information on tumor characteristics was obtained from clinical records. Weight and height measurements were obtained in the clinic as part of the clinical workup for the calculation of chemotherapy doses. Recordings were performed by a trained member of staff using a weighing scale. Patients were given follow-up appointments to the clinic during which recurrence was evaluated and clinically confirmed. For those living in the outskirts of the city, if recurrence was suspected, the patients were referred to our clinic for further evaluation. Furthermore, a research assistant made regular calls to check the patient's status, whether alive or dead. The current analysis included a follow-up period of 153 months (median follow-up = 24 months). Ethical approval for this project was provided by the Ethics Committee of the National Institutes of Health, Malaysia. This study did not involve the use of personal identifying information; hence, it was exempted from review by the National Institutes of Health (NIH) Office of Human Subject Research Protections [23].

Breast cancer subtype definition

IHC staining for ER, PR, and HER2 was performed on formalin-fixed, paraffin-embedded tissue sections as has been previously described [24]. Molecular subtypes were defined using the St Gallen classification, proposed for the recapitulation of the intrinsic subtypes using IHC and proliferation markers [14, 15]. According to the St Gallen classification scheme, luminal breast cancers can be further distinguished into subgroups based on their level of proliferation (using KI67 or histologic grade) and hormone receptor expression patterns. Accordingly, luminal tumors that homogeneously express hormone receptors (i.e. ER+ and PR+) and low proliferation are classified as luminal A-like while those that heterogeneously express hormone receptors (i.e. ER^+/PR^- or ER^-/PR^+) and/or those that homogeneously or heterogeneously express hormone receptors (i.e. ER+ and/or PR +) but are also high proliferating (high KI67 or grade 3) and/or HER2+ are classified as luminal B. In keeping with this definition, we utilized ER, PR, and HER2 in addition to histologic grade [25], to define subtypes as follows: Luminal A-like: ER^+ and PR^+, $HER2^-$ and low grade (histologic grade 1 or 2); Luminal B-like: ER^+ and/or PR^+, $HER2^-$ and high-grade (histologic grade 3) or ER^+ and/or PR^+, $HER2^+$ (regardless of levels of histologic grade); HER2-enriched: ER^- and PR^- and $HER2^+$; and triple-negative: ER^- and PR^- and $HER2^-$.

Statistical analysis

Frequency tables were used to assess the distribution of risk factors and clinicopathological characteristics among the different subtypes. The chi-square test was used to assess differences for categorical variables and the Kruskal-Wallis test was used for continuous variables.

We categorized risk factors based on what is the convention for each variable and in accordance with what has been published in large-scale studies of breast cancer [18, 26]. We categorized age at menarche [≤12 years (early menarche), 13, 14 and ≥ 15 years (late menarche)]; family history of breast cancer in a first-degree relative [yes and no]; age at FFP [< 21, 21–24.9, 25–30, > 30 years] and age at menopause [≤ 50 and > 50 years] similarly as in previously published articles [18, 26]. For BMI, we adopted the World Health Organization classification [< 18.5 kg/m² (underweight); 18.5–24.9 kg/m² (normal weight); 25–29.9 kg/m² (overweight) and ≥ 30 kg/m² (obese)]. To test for associations between risk factors and molecular subtypes, we constructed a polytomous logistic regression model with tumor subtype as the outcome (luminal A-like subtype as the reference category) and risk factors (age at menarche [≤ 12 years (early menarche, reference category), 13, 14, and ≥ 15 years (late menarche)], parity and breastfeeding [nulliparity (reference category), parity but no breastfeeding, parity and breastfeeding], age at FFP [< 21 (reference category), 21–24.9, 25–30, > 30 years], family history [yes and no (reference category)], and BMI [< 18.5 kg/m² (underweight); 18.5–24.9 kg/m² (normal weight, reference category); 25–29.9 kg/m² (overweight) and ≥ 30 kg/m² (obese)] as explanatory variables, with adjustment for age at

diagnosis (< 35, 35–45, 45–55, 55–65, 65–75, > 75 years) and ethnicity (Chinese, Malay, Native).

The association between breast cancer subtypes and all-cause mortality/recurrence was determined using Kaplan-Meier survival curves and Cox-proportional hazards regression models, which included adjustments for standard prognostic parameters including age at diagnosis, ethnicity, BMI, histologic grade, TNM stage I–IV [i.e. size (T), nodal status (N) and metastasis (M)], systemic therapy (endocrine (tamoxifen or aromatase inhibitor (AI)) and chemotherapy), radiotherapy and surgery. Follow-up started at diagnosis of breast cancer and ended at time of event (recurrence/death) or censoring (end of follow-up or, for the recurrence analysis, also death). For all-cause mortality, we censored at 10 years because this is the threshold at which most breast cancers are, by convention, considered cured in the absence of recurrence or death. We adopted a two-step approach in our survival analyses. In the first step, each of the above risk factors was modeled separately in basic models adjusted for standard prognostic factors separately for each tumor subtype. To test for heterogeneity in risk factor and survival relationships by subtype, we included an interaction term between each risk factor and tumor subtype. Violation of the proportionality assumption of the hazard model was tested by modeling each risk factor as a time-varying covariate. In the second step, it was decided, a priori, that factors that were associated with survival with $P < 0.1$ in the basic model were to be mutually adjusted for in a multivariable model that included the standard prognostic factors mentioned above. Using likelihood ratio (LR) test, we compared this model with one containing only the clinicopathological factors. For sensitivity analysis, we conducted survival analysis for women stratified into two age groups (< 50 yrs and ≥ 50 yrs). Also, we performed additional sensitivity analysis by excluding women with stage IV disease from our multivariate analyses for both all-cause mortality and recurrence. Results were very similar from these sensitivity analyses as compared to analyses including all women and we therefore presented results from all patients. All analyses were two-sided and performed using Stata statistical software version 14.0 (StataCorp, College Station, TX, USA).

Results

In total, our analysis included 3012 invasive breast cancer cases, with a total of 579 deaths in 10 years and 314 recurrence events in 5 years. The mean age at diagnosis was 52 years and mean BMI was 25 kg/m². The majority of the patients were Chinese (48%) and had early-stage (I and II, 56%) and HR-positive (66%) tumors (Table 1). Of the 3012 patients, 1016 (34%) were luminal A-like, 989 (33%) were luminal B-like, 387 (13%) were

Table 1 Distribution of risk factors and clinicopathological characteristics by tumor subtype

Characteristic	Overall (%)	A-like (N = 1016/34%)	%	B-like (N = 989/33%)	%	HER2-enriched (N = 387/13%)	%	Triple-neg. (N = 620/20%)	%	P value[a]
Age, yrs										
Mean (range)	51.6 (19, 91)	52.6 (24–90)		51.1 (19, 90)		51.6 (23, 91)		51.5 (21, 87)		
< 35	180 (5)	47	4.6	49	5.0	26	6.7	40	6.5	**0.01**
35–45	711 (21)	192	18.9	219	22.1	76	19.7	144	23.2	
45–55	1204 (36)	368	36.2	366	37.0	136	35.1	203	32.7	
55–65	806 (24)	241	23.7	246	24.9	105	27.1	143	23.1	
65–75	364 (11)	135	13.3	90	9.1	35	9.1	65	10.5	
> 75	90 (3)	33	3.3	19	1.9	9	2.3	25	4.0	
Ethnicity										
Chinese	1626 (48)	567	55.8	435	44	180	46.5	275	44.4	**< 0.0001**
Malay	801 (24)	204	20.1	263	26.6	104	26.9	155	25	
Native	928 (28)	245	24.1	291	29.4	103	26.6	190	30.6	
Menarche										
≤ 12 yrs	1105 (33)	344	34.1	326	33.2	118	30.8	190	30.9	0.20
13 yrs	1117 (34)	318	31.5	340	34.7	148	38.6	201	32.7	
14 yrs	548 (16)	163	16.2	167	17	60	15.7	111	18	
≥ 15 yrs	559 (17)	184	18.2	148	15.1	57	14.9	113	18.4	
Menopause										
≤ 50 yrs	428 (29)	146	32.7	128	29.7	38	23.2	87	31.6	0.14
> 50 yrs	1031 (71)	301	67.3	303	70.3	126	76.8	188	68.4	
Parity										
Nulliparous	745 (22)	242	23.8	224	22.6	77	19.9	128	20.6	0.29
Parous	2601 (78)	774	76.2	765	77.4	310	80.1	492	79.4	
Age at FFP[b], yrs										
< 21	466 (18)	116	15	158	20.7	54	17.4	95	19.3	**0.02**
21–24.9	1011 (39)	284	36.7	287	37.5	129	41.6	199	40.5	
25–30	864 (33)	275	35.5	248	32.4	103	33.2	154	31.4	
> 30	259 (10)	99	12.8	72	9.4	24	7.7	43	8.7	
Breastfeeding										
No	377 (14)	133	17.2	103	13.5	31	10	64	13	**0.01**
Yes	2224 (86)	641	82.9	662	86.5	279	90	428	87	
Breastfeeding duration										
< 6 months	927 (52)	285	54.2	280	51.8	111	49.6	175	51.3	0.40
6–10 months	374 (21)	112	21.3	122	22.6	48	21.4	62	18.2	
> 10 months	489 (27)	129	24.5	138	25.6	65	29.0	104	30.5	
BMI, kg/m²										
< 18.5	1253 (39)	373	37.8	336	35.1	163	43.7	240	40.2	**0.03**
18.5–24.9	565 (17)	160	16.2	172	18	68	18.2	114	19.1	
25–29.9	998 (31)	317	32.2	301	31.4	104	27.9	177	29.6	
≥ 30	433 (13)	136	13.8	148	15.5	38	10.2	66	11.1	
Family history										
No	2835 (86)	840	84	854	87.8	338	88	516	84.9	**0.05**
Yes	468 (14)	160	16	119	12.2	46	12	92	15.1	

Table 1 Distribution of risk factors and clinicopathological characteristics by tumor subtype *(Continued)*

Characteristic	Overall (%)	A-like (N = 1016/ 34%)	%	B-like (N = 989/ 33%)	%	HER2-enriched (N = 387/13%)	%	Triple-neg. (N = 620/ 20%)	%	P value[a]
Histological grade										
Well diff.	365 (11)	212	20.9	67	6.8	10	2.6	27	4.4	**< 0.0001**
Moderately diff.	1790 (55)	781	76.9	442	44.7	180	46.5	238	38.4	
Poorly diff.	1123 (34)	–	–	473	47.8	192	49.6	344	55.5	
Stage										
I	454 (14)	222	22.1	100	10.3	34	8.9	61	10	**< 0.0001**
II	1353 (42)	444	44.2	395	40.6	136	35.6	249	40.9	
III	1005 (31)	241	24	330	33.9	150	39.3	203	33.3	
IV	421 (13)	78	7.8	139	14.3	57	14.9	91	14.9	
Tumor size										
< 2 cm	2137 (64)	761	75.6	620	63.3	210	54.7	353	57.8	**< 0.0001**
2–5 cm	522 (16)	121	12	150	15.3	83	21.6	104	17	
> 5 cm	660 (20)	125	12.4	209	21.4	91	23.7	154	25.2	
Node status										
0	1517 (46)	566	55.7	368	37.2	146	37.7	272	43.9	**< 0.0001**
1	922 (28)	249	24.5	310	31.3	95	24.5	163	26.3	
2	480 (15)	120	11.8	156	15.8	70	18.1	94	15.2	
≥ 3	375 (11)	72	7.1	139	14.1	68	17.6	75	12.1	
Endocrine										
None	1248 (40)	48	5.1	126	14.2	357	97.5	584	97.2	**< 0.0001**
Tamoxifen	1456 (47)	687	72.9	591	66.7	7	1.9	15	2.5	
Aromatase Inhibitor	395 (13)	207	22.0	169	19.1	2	0.6	2	0.3	
Chemotherapy										
No	799 (24)	371	37.3	177	18.3	62	16.4	95	15.5	**< 0.0001**
Yes	2483 (76)	625	62.7	789	81.7	317	83.6	519	84.5	
Surgery										
No	389 (12)	80	10.2	106	15.8	53	19.4	87	16.3	**< 0.0001**
Yes	2841 (88)	913	89.8	833	84.2	312	80.6	519	83.7	
Radiotherapy										
No	800 (26)	261	27.7	218	24.6	79	23.9	149	26.4	**0.01**
Yes	2235 (74)	683	72.3	669	75.4	252	76.1	416	73.6	

Breast cancer subtypes were defined based on 2013 St Gallen criteria by using hormone receptor (ER and PR) and HER2 in conjunction with histologic grade. In bold are statistically significant P values (< 0.05)
[a]P values are for chi-square tests
[b]FFP first full-term pregnancy

HER2-enriched, and 620 (20%) were triple-negative, respectively.

Distribution of risk factors and clinicopathological characteristics by tumor subtype

As shown in Table 1, women with the luminal A-like subtype were slightly older than those with other subtypes. The distributions of ethnicity (P value < 0.001), age at FFP (P value = 0.019), breastfeeding practices (P value = 0.01), family history (P value = 0.05) and BMI (P value = 0.03) differed by subtype. No differences were observed in the distributions of age at menarche, age at menopause and parity according to subtype. The frequencies of all clinicopathological parameters differed by subtype, with low-grade, small, early-stage and node-negative tumors being more frequent for the luminal A-like subtype (Table 1).

Table 2 shows the associations between examined risk factors and molecular subtype in the multivariable polytomous regression model. Compared with women with

Table 2 OR and 95% CI from a polytomous logistic regression model testing the associations between breast cancer risk factors and tumor molecular subtype

Risk factor	Subtype						
	A-like (comparison group)	B-like		HER2-enriched		Triple-negative	
	N	N	OR[a] (95% CI)	N	OR (95% CI)	N	OR (95% CI)
Ethnicity							
Chinese	567	435	1.00 (reference)	180	1.00 (reference)	275	1.00 (reference)
Malay	204	263	**1.50 (1.18, 1.90)**	104	**1.54 (1.13, 2.11)**	155	**1.51 (1.14, 1.98)**
Native	245	291	**1.39 (1.10, 1.76)**	103	1.21 (0.88, 1.66)	190	**1.50 (1.15, 1.95)**
P value			**0.001**		0.10		**< 0.001**
Menarche							
≤ 12 yrs	344	326	1.00 (reference)	118	1.00 (reference)	190	1.00 (reference)
13 yrs	318	340	1.14 (0.91, 1.43)	148	1.31 (0.98, 1.77)	201	1.15 (0.88, 1.49)
14 yrs	163	167	1.04 (0.79, 1.38)	60	1.02 (0.70, 1.48)	111	1.18 (0.86, 1.61)
≥ 15 yrs	184	148	0.83 (0.63, 1.10)	57	0.87 (0.59, 1.28)	113	1.10 (0.80, 1.50)
P value			0.43		0.51		0.31
Parity and BF[b]							
Nulliparous	242	224	1.00 (reference)	77	1.00 (reference)	128	1.00 (reference)
Parous and No BF	133	103	1.26 (0.84, 1.90)	31	1.07 (0.76, 1.52)	64	1.25 (0.77, 2.00)
Parous and BF	641	662	**1.44 (1.05, 1.98)**	279	**1.64 (1.06, 2.55)**	428	**1.54 (1.07, 2.22)**
P value			0.17		**0.005**		0.12
Age at FFP[c]							
< 21 yrs	116	158	1.00 (reference)	54	1.00 (reference)	95	1.00 (reference)
21–24.9 yrs	284	287	0.78 (0.57, 1.05)	129	1.01 (0.67, 1.51)	199	0.90 (0.64, 1.26)
25–30 yrs	275	248	0.77 (0.57, 1.06)	103	0.91 (0.60, 1.38)	154	0.77 (0.54, 1.09)
> 30 yrs	99	72	**0.63 (0.42, 0.94)**	24	0.57 (0.32, 1.02)	43	**0.58 (0.36, 0.93)**
P value			0.35		0.06		0.38
Family history							
No	840	854	1.00 (reference)	338	1.00 (reference)	516	1.00 (reference)
Yes	160	119	**0.72 (0.55, 0.94)**	46	0.71 (0.49, 1.02)	92	0.92 (0.69, 1.23)
P value			**0.02**		**0.05**		0.62
BMI, kg/m²							
18.5–24.9	160	172	1.00 (reference)	68	1.00 (reference)	114	1.00 (reference)
< 18.5	373	336	0.89 (0.69, 1.17)	163	1.07 (0.76, 1.51)	240	0.96 (0.72, 1.29)
P value			0.38		0.65		0.76
25–29.9	317	301	0.86 (0.65, 1.12)	104	0.74 (0.51, 1.06)	177	0.75 (0.55, 1.02)
P value			0.27		0.13		0.08
≥ 30	136	148	0.90 (0.65, 1.24)	38	**0.55 (0.34, 0.89)**	66	**0.59 (0.40, 0.88)**
P value			0.62		**0.02**		**0.01**

Statistically significant (P value < 0.05) estimates are indicated in bold
[a]OR and corresponding estimates are from a single polytomous logistic regression model that was mutually adjusted for ethnicity, menarche, parity and breastfeeding, age at FFP, family history, BMI and age
[b]BF breastfeeding
[c]FFP first full-term pregnancy

the luminal A-like subtype, women with the luminal B-like, HER2-enriched and triple-negative tumors were significantly more likely to be Malay and Native than Chinese. Furthermore, women with other tumor subtypes were more likely to be parous and have breast-fed [odds ratio (OR) (95% CI) parity and breastfeeding vs nulliparity = 1.44 (1.05, 1.98); 1.64 (1.06, 2.25); and 1.54 (1.07, 2.22) for luminal B, HER2-enriched and triple-negative subtypes, respectively] and less likely to experience their FFP after the age of 30 years [OR (95% CI) > 30 years vs < 21 years = 0.63 (0.42, 0.94); 0.57 (0.32, 1.02); and 0.58 (0.36, 0.93) for luminal B, HER2-enriched and triple-negative subtypes, respectively] than those with the luminal A-like subtype. Women with HER2-enriched [OR (95% CI) BMI > 30 kg/m^2 vs 18.5–24.9 kg/m^2 = 0.55 (0.34, 0.89); P value = 0.02] and triple-negative [OR (95% CI) BMI > 30 kg/m^2 vs 18.5–24.9 kg/m^2 = 0.59 (0.40, 0.88); P value = 0.01] tumors were significantly less likely to be obese than those with the luminal A-like subtype.

Breast cancer risk factors in relation to all-cause mortality and recurrence by subtype

Overall, all-cause mortality and recurrence differed significantly by tumor subtype. In general, women with luminal A-like tumors had better survival outcomes than those with the other subtypes (Fig. 1). As shown in Table 3, in basic models for each risk factor (with adjustment for standard prognostic factors in addition to age, ethnicity and BMI), later age at menarche, parity/breastfeeding, and being underweight were significantly associated with 10-year all-cause mortality in the luminal A-like but not any of the other subtypes. Also, later age at FFP showed a suggestive association with mortality in luminal A-like patients (P trend = 0.08) but not the other subtypes. Results were similar in basic models for recurrence (Table 4).

In the multivariable model with the mutual adjustment for ethnicity, menarche, parity/breastfeeding, age at FFP, family history, and BMI in addition to standard clinicopathological factors and treatment variables, increasing age at menarche [hazard ratio (HR) (95% confidence interval (CI) ≥15 years vs ≤ 12 years = 2.28 (1.05, 4.95);

P value for trend (P trend) = 0.06]; parity/breastfeeding [HR (95% CI) vs nulliparity = 0.48 (0.27, 0.85); P trend = 0.01]; older age at FFP [HR (95% CI) > 30 vs < 21 years = 0.20 (0.04, 0.90); P trend = 0.06]; and being underweight [HR (95% CI) vs normal weight = 3.46 (1.21, 9.89); P value = 0.02] or overweight [HR (95% CI) vs normal weight = 3.14 (1.04, 9.50); P value = 0.04] remained significantly associated with 10-year all-cause mortality in women with the luminal A-like subtype (Table 5 and Fig. 2). For these women, the addition of age at menarche, parity/breastfeeding, and BMI, provided significantly better fit to a model containing clinicopathological factors alone [LRχ^2 (8df) = 21.78; P value = 0.005]. In general, the results were consistent in relation to recurrence (Table 5).

When we examined the association between duration of breastfeeding and all-cause-mortality/recurrence for luminal A-like cases with complete information on breastfeeding duration (N = 719), we observed an inverse association between each breastfeeding duration category and all-cause mortality [HR (95% CI) vs nulliparity = 0.37 (0.18, 0.85), 0.86 (0.35, 2.11), 0.53 (0.24, 1.17) for < 6, 6–10, and > 10 months, respectively (P trend = 0.38)] and recurrence [HR (95% CI) vs nulliparity = 0.47 (0.19, 1.16), 0.73 (0.23, 2.37), 0.05 (0.01, 0.42) for < 6, 6–10, and > 10 months, respectively (P trend = 0.002)]. Among women who breastfed, all-cause mortality did not significantly vary by breastfeeding durations (comparing > 10 months to < 6 months, P value = 0.38) but women who breastfed for > 10 months tended to have better recurrence outcomes [HR (95% CI) vs < 6 months = 0.11 (0.01, 0.93); P value = 0.04].

Discussion

In this study involving over 3000 invasive breast cancer cases from a population-based case series in Sarawak,

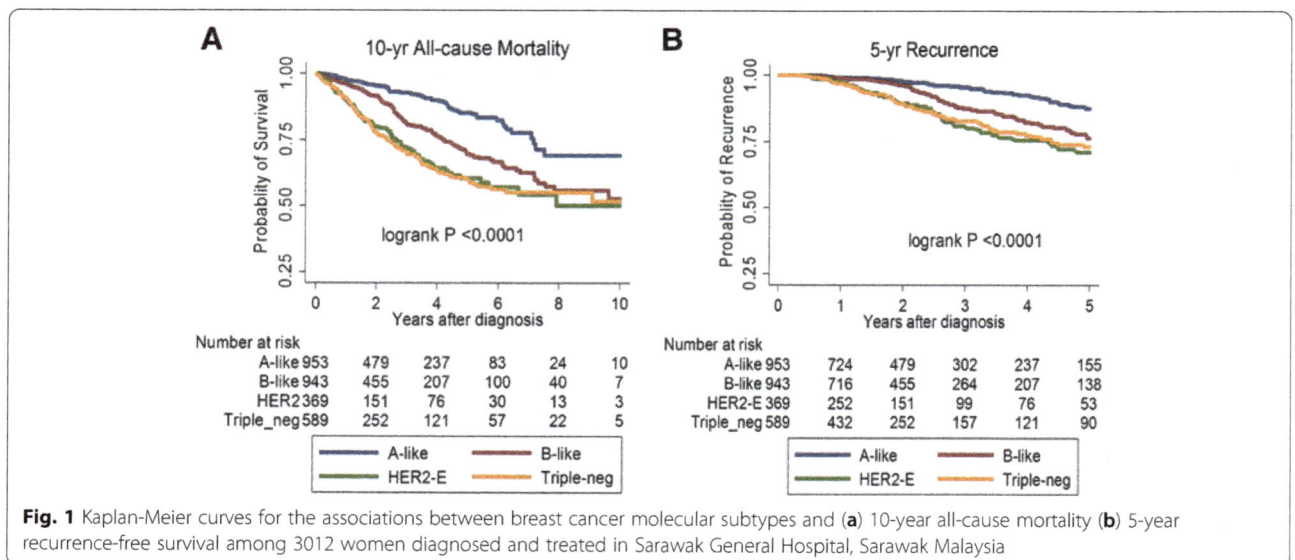

Fig. 1 Kaplan-Meier curves for the associations between breast cancer molecular subtypes and (**a**) 10-year all-cause mortality (**b**) 5-year recurrence-free survival among 3012 women diagnosed and treated in Sarawak General Hospital, Sarawak Malaysia

Table 3 HR and 95% CI for the associations between risk factors and 10-year all-cause mortality by tumor molecular subtype

Risk factor[1a]	10-year all-cause mortality								P het[d]
	A-like		B-like		HER2-enriched		Triple-negative		
	N/events	HR (95% CI)	N/events	HR (95% CI)	N/events	HR (95% CI)	N/events	HR (95% CI)	
Ethnicity									
Chinese	567/39	1.00 (reference)	435/41	1.00 (reference)	180/38	1.00 (reference)	275/57	1.00 (reference)	0.81
Malay	204/17	1.23 (0.65, 2.34)	263/70	**2.32 (1.49, 3.60)**	104/29	1.11 (0.63, 1.96)	155/54	1.22 (0.79, 1.89)	
Native	245/19	1.04 (0.52, 2.05)	291/39	1.68 (1.02, 2.77)	103/20	0.93 (0.48, 1.79)	190/41	1.06 (0.67, 1.67)	
P value		0.80		**0.03**		0.87		0.77	
Menarche									
≤ 12 yrs	344/14	1.00 (reference)	326/52	1.00 (reference)	118/23	1.00 (reference)	190/46	1.00 (reference)	0.06
13 yrs	318/26	1.53 (0.76, 3.11)	340/44	0.88 (0.55, 1.40)	148/29	0.84 (0.45, 1.57)	201/46	1.21 (0.76, 1.92)	
14 yrs	163/11	1.25 (0.54, 2.91)	167/27	0.86 (0.50, 1.48)	60/22	0.92 (0.47, 1.80)	111/26	1.05 (0.61, 1.80)	
≥ 15 yrs	184/23	**2.25 (1.06, 4.78)**	148/27	0.84 (0.49, 1.42)	57/11	0.49 (0.21, 1.11)	113/31	0.89 (0.52, 1.55)	
P value		**0.06**		0.49		0.15		0.66	
Parity and BF[b]									
Nulliparous	242/24	1.00 (reference)	224/36	1.00 (reference)	77/18	1.00 (reference)	128/40	1.00 (reference)	0.28
Parous and No BF	133/10	0.59 (0.27, 1.32)	103/12	0.81 (0.37, 1.75)	31/8	0.87 (0.34, 2.25)	64/20	1.02 (0.52, 1.96)	
Parous and BF	641/41	**0.46 (0.26, 0.81)**	662/102	0.99 (0.64, 1.56)	279/61	0.61 (0.33, 1.14)	428/92	0.86 (0.55, 1.34)	
P value		**0.009**		0.91		0.11		0.48	
Age at FFP[c]									
< 21 yrs	116/10	1.00 (reference)	158/32	1.00 (reference)	54/13	1.00 (reference)	95/19	1.00 (reference)	0.22
21–24.9 yrs	284/14	0.99 (0.38, 2.55)	287/33	1.30 (0.75, 2.25)	129/28	0.83 (0.37, 1.84)	199/42	0.71 (0.39, 1.29)	
25–30 yrs	275/23	0.85 (0.41, 1.73)	248/39	1.14 (0.69, 1.90)	103/22	0.77 (0.40, 1.49)	154/41	0.98 (0.60, 1.60)	
> 30 yrs	99/4	0.36 (0.10, 1.29)	72/10	1.34 (0.64, 2.81)	24/6	0.78 (0.25, 2.46)	43/9	0.53 (0.23, 1.24)	
P value		**0.08**		0.92		0.15		0.58	
Family history									
No	840/56	1.00 (reference)	854/131	1.00 (reference)	338/73	1.00 (reference)	516/122	1.00 (reference)	0.25
Yes	160/17	1.70 (0.93, 3.08)	119/17	1.05 (0.59, 1.88)	46/13	1.47 (0.76, 2.82)	92/22	0.77 (0.46, 1.27)	
P value		**0.08**		0.86					
BMI, kg/m²									
18.5–24.9	160/6	1.00 (reference)	172/25	1.00 (reference)	68/15	1.00 (reference)	114/25	1.00 (reference)	0.80
< 18.5	373/38	**3.42 (1.20, 9.71)**	336/43	1.06 (0.62, 1.82)	163/37	0.83 (0.44, 1.57)	240/63	1.15 (0.70, 1.91)	
P value		**0.02**		0.83		0.58		0.56	
25–30	317/21	2.88 (0.97, 8.59)	301/49	1.30 (0.77, 2.20)	104/19	0.80 (0.39, 1.64)	177/40	0.92 (0.54, 1.57)	
P value		**0.06**		0.32		0.54		0.77	
> 30	136/7	1.30 (0.37, 4.52)	148/23	1.12 (0.61, 2.05)	38/10	1.23 (0.52, 2.90)	66/18	1.21 (0.63, 2.32)	
P value		0.68		0.71		0.63		0.57	

In bold are variables which met our criteria (P value < 0.1) for inclusion in multivariate models

[a]Each risk factor was adjusted for age, ethnicity, BMI, tumor stage, histologic grade, surgery, systemic therapy (endocrine (tamoxifen or AI versus none), chemotherapy (any regimen versus none)) and radiotherapy (received versus none)

[b]BF breastfeeding

[c]FFP first full-term pregnancy

[d]P value for heterogeneity (P-het) of HR estimates according to molecular subtypes

Malaysia, with detailed demographic, risk factor, pathology, and follow-up data, we investigated several established breast cancer risk factors in relation to tumor subtypes and patient outcomes. We found differences in the prevalence of parity and breastfeeding, age at FFP, family history of breast cancer and obesity across different breast tumor subtypes. In general, traditional breast cancer risk factors (older age at FFP, higher BMI, lower

Table 4 HR and 95% CI for the associations between risk factors and 5-year recurrence by tumor molecular subtype

Risk factor[a]	Recurrence after 5 years								P-het[d]
	A-like		B-like		HER2-enriched		Triple-negative		
	N/events	HR (95% CI)	N/events	HR (95% CI)	N/events	HR (95% CI)	N/events	HR (95% CI)	
Ethnicity									
Chinese	567/34	1.00 (reference)	435/49	1.00 (reference)	180/30	1.00 (reference)	275/38	1.00 (reference)	0.96
Malay	204/8	1.01 (0.39, 2.60)	263/30	0.81 (0.45, 1.45)	104/17	0.69 (0.31, 1.51)	155/24	1.11 (0.61, 2.02)	
Native	245/16	1.17 (0.49, 2.79)	291/22	0.84 (0.46, 1.55)	103/10	0.47 (0.18, 1.23)	190/22	0.67 (0.34, 1.34)	
P value		0.75		0.55		0.11		0.32	
Menarche									
≤ 12 yrs	344/13	1.00 (reference)	326/38	1.00 (reference)	118/14	1.00 (reference)	190/34	1.00 (reference)	0.07
13 yrs	318/17	1.55 (0.57, 4.23)	340/31	1.03 (0.58, 1.82)	148/21	1.52 (0.69, 3.33)	201/24	0.72 (0.38, 1.37)	
14 yrs	163/14	2.51 (0.86, 7.33)	167/21	0.81 (0.40, 1.64)	60/9	0.56 (0.16, 1.92)	111/13	0.65 (0.30, 1.43)	
≥ 15 yrs	184/13	**3.26 (1.08, 9.92)**	148/11	0.77 (0.35, 1.68)	57/12	1.11 (0.38, 3.28)	113/12	0.61 (0.27, 1.36)	
P value		**0.02**		0.41		0.81		0.18	
Parity and BF[c]									
Nulliparous	242/19	1.00 (reference)	224/16	1.00 (reference)	77/12	1.00 (reference)	128/19	1.00 (reference)	0.56
Parous and No BF	133/7	0.55 (0.20, 1.50)	103/14	1.86 (0.76, 4.56)	31/7	1.35 (0.39, 4.64)	64/17	1.57 (0.67, 3.66)	
Parous and BF	641/32	**0.27 (0.12, 0.58)**	662/71	1.63 (0.81, 3.28)	279/38	0.58 (0.25, 1.34)	428/48	0.77 (0.39, 1.52)	
P value		**0.001**		0.23		0.15		0.28	
Age at FFP[d]									
< 25	400/13	1.00 (reference)	445/44	1.00 (reference)	183/30	1.00 (reference)	294/41	1.00 (reference)	0.52
≥ 25	374/26	1.69 (0.66, 4.34)	320/41	1.32 (0.78, 2.22)	127/15	0.50 (0.21, 1.16)	197/23	0.75 (0.41, 1.39)	
P value		0.27		0.28		0.10		0.36	
Family history									
No	840/42	1.00 (reference)	854/85	1.00 (reference)	338/49	1.00 (reference)	516/66	1.00 (reference)	0.94
Yes	160/13	0.77 (0.29, 2.03)	119/14	1.17 (0.60, 2.28)	46/7	1.24 (0.45, 3.35)	92/12	0.85 (0.43, 1.70)	
P value		0.60		0.64		0.67			
BMI, kg/m^2									
18.5–24.9	160/6	1.00 (referent)	172/14	1.00 (referent)	68/11	1.00 (referent)	114/16	1.00 (referent)	0.98
< 18.5	373/30	3.97 (0.91, 17.34)	336/29	1.37 (0.62, 3.03)	163/21	0.50 (0.20, 1.27)	240/30	1.01 (0.51, 2.01)	
P value		**0.06**		0.43		0.15		0.97	
25–30	317/16	3.40 (0.75, 15.42)	301/37	2.02 (0.95, 4.29)	104/15	0.70 (0.27, 1.81)	177/24	0.83 (0.39, 1.73)	
P value		0.11		**0.06**		0.46		0.62	
> 30	136/5	1.65 (0.27, 10.15)	148/15	1.28 (0.53, 3.12)	38/7	1.41 (0.46, 4.27)	66/13	0.89 (0.35, 2.25)	
P value		0.59		0.58		0.55		0.81	

In bold are variables which met our criteria (P-value < 0.1) for inclusion in multivariate models
[a]Each risk factor was adjusted for age, ethnicity, BMI, tumor stage, histologic grade, surgery, systemic therapy (endocrine (tamoxifen or AI versus none), chemotherapy (any regimen versus none)) and radiotherapy (received versus none)
[b]BF breastfeeding
[c]FFP first full-term pregnancy. Due to sample size considerations age at FFP was dichotomized
[d]P value for heterogeneity (P-het) of HR estimates according to molecular subtypes

parity, lack of breastfeeding) seem to show higher frequencies among women with the luminal A-like subtype compared with women with other subtypes. Further, we found that age at menarche, breastfeeding, and BMI were independent prognostic factors for both overall mortality and breast cancer recurrence but only for women with the luminal A-like subtype, which had better survival and recurrence outcomes than the other subtypes.

Our findings that nulliparity and older age at FFP were more prevalent in luminal A-like patients are consistent with those reported in studies in Western countries [16, 27]. However, unlike the observation of higher BMI and shorter breastfeeding duration in triple-negative

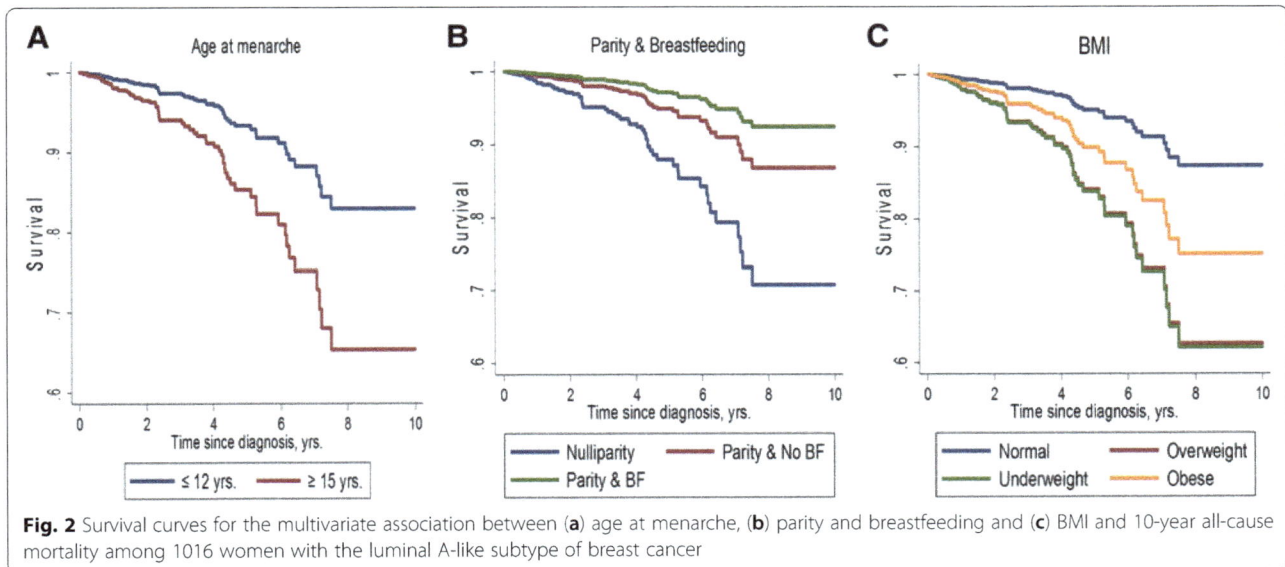

Fig. 2 Survival curves for the multivariate association between (**a**) age at menarche, (**b**) parity and breastfeeding and (**c**) BMI and 10-year all-cause mortality among 1016 women with the luminal A-like subtype of breast cancer

patients among Western, especially African American, women [18, 19, 28, 29], we found lower frequencies of obesity and breastfeeding among HR⁻ (HER2-enriched and triple-negative) than luminal A-like tumors, which may be reflective of population/ethnic differences. In line with this hypothesis, a previous study conducted in South Korea [30] also showed a higher frequency of breastfeeding among women with luminal B or HER2-enriched than those with luminal A disease. In another study involving 730 Mexican women with breast cancer, Martinez and colleagues [31] reported the prevalence of breastfeeding to be higher among women with triple-negative than luminal A tumors. Similarly, results from a multiethnic study showed an inverse association between triple-negative tumors and breastfeeding in White, Hispanic and African American but, notably, not in Asian women, for whom breastfeeding for > 2 months was associated with an 86% increased likelihood of triple-negative tumors [32].

The prevalence of obesity is still much lower in most Asian populations compared with other race/ethnicity groups. In contrast to the reduced breast cancer risk associated with higher BMI among premenopausal Western women, obesity is associated with increased risk for both premenopausal and postmenopausal Asian women [33–35]. The heterogeneity of obesity by tumor subtype among Asian cases remains unclear. Results from both our study and the South Korean study [30] suggest that obesity was less frequent among patients with HER2-enriched tumors. In combination with our finding that women with the HER2-enriched subtype were more likely to be parous and to have breastfed than women with the luminal A-like subtype, our data suggest that these factors (parity, breastfeeding, and low BMI) may

not protect against HER2-enriched breast cancers. The decreasing prevalence of these factors associated with the adoption of westernized lifestyles may, therefore, not affect the incidence of this subtype, which is known to be more prevalent among Asian women [36, 37]. More research to understand the risk factors associated with the HER2-enriched subtype is warranted.

Most epidemiological studies considering the prognostic significance of age at menarche in breast cancer have treated the disease as a homogeneous entity, and results from these studies are largely conflicting [1–3, 8, 38]. We found that older age at menarche was associated with worse prognosis but only among women with the luminal A-like subtype. This finding is consistent with results from a previous study of women in East Asia [20] that also evaluated relationships between risk factors and survival according to subtypes. It is unclear why late menarche and younger age at FFP lead to worse survival outcomes in women with the luminal A-like subtype since they are well known protective factors in terms of breast cancer risk. One possibility is that because early menarche and late age at FFP increase breast cancer risk through prolonged and sustained exposure of the mammary epithelium to the mitogenic effects of reproductive hormones [39, 40], these factors predispose more strongly to HR⁺ tumors which have better prognosis than HR⁻ tumors [18, 41]. Although this association was confined to the luminal A-like subtype, which, by definition, is HR⁺, expression of hormone receptors in tumors occurs in a spectrum. Whereas some tumors have very high expression levels, others have lower levels despite crossing the threshold for consideration as HR⁺. Due to differences in cumulative lifetime exposure to endogenous estrogens, luminal A-like tumors occurring

Table 5 Multivariate HR and 95% CI for the association between breast cancer risk factors and 10-year all-cause mortality and 5-year recurrence among women with luminal A-like subtype breast cancer

Risk factor	10-year all-cause mortality		5-year recurrence	
	N/events	HR[1] (95% CI)	N/events	HR[a] (95% CI)
Ethnicity				
Chinese	539/38	1.00 (reference)	399/21	1.00 (reference)
Malay	194/16	1.14 (0.59, 2.20)	154/7	0.81 (0.29, 2.27)
Native	235/17	0.87 (0.41, 1.85)	190/11	0.90 (0.35, 2.29)
P value		0.95		0.74
Menarche				
≤ 12 yrs	338/13	1.00 (reference)	260/8	1.00 (reference)
13 yrs	302/25	1.45 (0.70, 3.01)	235/13	1.69 (0.59, 4.81)
14 yrs	156/10	1.23 (0.52, 2.92)	119/8	2.64 (0.87, 7.99)
≥ 15 yrs	172/23	**2.28 (1.05, 4.95)**	129/10	**3.52 (1.10, 11.23)**
P value		0.06		**0.02**
Parity and BF[b]				
Nulliparous	229/23	1.00 (reference)	180/15	1.00 (reference)
Parous and No BF	127/9	0.61 (0.26, 1.42)	87/5	0.53 (0.17. 1.59)
Parous and BF	612/39	**0.48 (0.27, 0.85)**	476/19	**0.28 (0.13, 0.64)**
P value		**0.01**		**0.002**
Age at FFP[c]				
< 21 yrs	111/9	1.00 (reference)	85/4	1.00 (reference)
21–24.9 yrs	276/14	0.85 (0.31, 2.31)	220/4	0.40 (0.06, 2.28)
25–30 yrs	262/22	0.71 (0.27, 1.82)	201/17	1.26 (0.30, 5.22)
> 30 yrs	95/4	**0.20 (0.04, 0.90)**	73/1	0.26 (0.02, 3.09)
P value		0.06		0.95
Family history				
No	804/53	1.00 (reference)	629/31	1.00 (referent)
Yes	155/17	1.68 (0.91, 3.10)	122/7	0.75 (0.28, 2.02)
P value		0.10		0.57
BMI				
18.5–24.9 kg/m²	160/6	1.00 (reference)	117/2	1.00 (reference)
< 18.5 kg/m²	365/37	**3.46 (1.21, 9.89)**	285/22	4.31 (0.94, 19.83)
P value		**0.02**		0.06
25–29.9 kg/m²	310/21	**3.14 (1.04, 9.50)**	235/12	**4.74 (1.00, 22.64)**
P value		**0.04**		**0.05**
≥ 30 kg/m²	133/7	1.38 (0.39, 4.86)	106/3	2.16 (0.34, 13.78)
P value		0.61		0.41

In bold are statistically significant estimates (P value < 0.05)

[a]HR was mutually adjusted for ethnicity, menarche, parity and breastfeeding, age at FFP, family history, BMI, age, TNM stage, histologic grade, surgery, systemic therapy (endocrine (tamoxifen or AI versus none), chemotherapy (any regimen vs and radiotherapy (received versus none)

[b]BF breastfeeding

[c]FFP first full-term pregnancy

among women with late menarche may have lower levels of hormone receptor expression, hence worse survival/recurrence outcomes, than those occurring among women with early menarche. Indeed, this is consistent with the finding by Song et al. that longer duration of endogenous estrogen exposure was associated with better survival [30]. On the other hand, late menarche and early age at FFP may be indicative of lower socioeconomic status (SES) which, in turn, may be reflective of less exposure to "westernized" environments/lifestyles.

Nonetheless, adjustment of known surrogates for SES did not change the associations between these factors and survival. That late age at menarche and early age at FFP were not associated with survival/recurrence in the other subtypes may be due to the masking effect of other more aggressive tumor features, which are inherent in these subtypes.

Our findings of breastfeeding being associated with better outcomes are generally consistent with previous reports [2, 12, 42]. A distinctive feature of luminal A-like tumors defined in our analysis is the low levels of proliferation, indicated by low histologic grade. Findings from one previous study showed that the protective effect of breastfeeding on breast cancer mortality was stronger for tumors with low expression of proliferation genes [21]. In our study, breastfeeding was associated with a preponderance of lobular carcinoma and small size tumors, both of which are highly correlated with low levels of proliferation [43–45].

Results from several studies, summarized in two comprehensive reviews and meta-analyses [46, 47], are supportive of the prognostic value of BMI in breast cancer. The association between BMI and survival after breast cancer is thought to be U-shaped [47–49], with underweight and overweight/obese women more likely to suffer worse survival outcomes than their normal weight counterparts. In our study, being underweight and overweight, but not obese, were suggestively associated with worse prognosis, but this might be due to the low frequency of obesity in this population (13%). Compared with overweight/obesity, the effect of underweight in breast cancer survival is less well-studied. Overall, our finding of an association between underweight and worse survival outcomes in breast cancer is in line with those of several other studies involving Asian populations [49–52]. Whilst insulin resistance, chronic inflammation, and altered adipokine and cytokine production have been proposed to underlie the obesity-cancer link [53], the precise mechanisms underpinning the relationship between underweight BMI and disease progression are not well understood. Chronic, pre-diagnostic, malnutrition may contribute to weight loss in cancer patients and may independently influence outcomes in the disease. However, when we examined the impact of indicators of socioeconomic deprivation, as surrogates for chronic malnutrition, our estimates remained unchanged.

Strengths of this study include: a population-based breast cancer case series in an understudied Asian population and the collection of detailed questionnaire information, which allowed us to account for various confounding variables including sociodemographic factors. Several limitations of this study should be noted. First, we did not include controls in our study and

therefore our case-case comparisons could not be translated into relative risk estimates. Second, relatively small sample sizes for some of the subtypes may have affected our power to detect significant associations. Third, data on the specific cause of death were not available and, therefore, we only evaluated risk factors in relation to all-cause, but not breast cancer-specific, mortality even though some of the risk factors, such as BMI, are important predictors of death from other causes [54]. Nonetheless, the consistency of our results for all-cause mortality and for breast cancer recurrence indicate that these factors may contribute to breast cancer-specific mortality in a similar manner.

Conclusions

In conclusion, our data indicate that risk factors for breast cancer are differentially associated with tumor subtypes and exert subtype-specific influence on survival/recurrence from the disease. Specifically, we observed that menarche after the age of 15 years, FFP after 30 years, underweight or overweight BMI, and breastfeeding practices were associated with survival/recurrence only among women with luminal A-like tumors. These findings are supportive of the prognostic value of reproductive and lifestyle-related factors in tumors with biologically favorable profiles, and could have implications for clinical counseling and for the development of subtype-specific prognostic tools. Future prospective studies are needed to delineate the role of lifestyle modification, especially changes in BMI, in improving clinical outcomes for women with luminal A-like breast cancer.

Abbreviations
ACM: All-cause mortality; BMI: Body mass index; CI: Confidence interval; ER: Estrogen receptor; FFP: First full-term pregnancy; HER2: Human epidermal growth factor receptor 2; HR: Hazard ratio; IHC: Immunohistochemical; KM: Kaplan-Meier; LR: Likelihood ratio; OR: Odds ratio; PR: Progesterone receptor

Acknowledgements
The authors acknowledge Julie Buckland and Jane Demuth at Information Management Systems for data management support.

Funding
This research was supported by the Intramural Research Program of the National Institutes of Health, National Cancer Institute, Division of Cancer Epidemiology and Genetics.

Competing interests
The authors declare that they have no competing interests.

Author details
[1]Integrative Tumor Epidemiology Branch, Division of Cancer Epidemiology and Genetics, National Cancer Institute (NCI), National Institutes of Health, 9609 Medical Center Drive, Rockville, MD 20850, USA. [2]Surveillance and Health Services Research, American Cancer Society, 250 Williams Street NW, Atlanta, GA 30303, USA. [3]Department of Radiotherapy, Oncology and Palliative Care, Sarawak General Hospital, Kuching, Sarawak, Malaysia. [4]Division of Cancer Control & Population Sciences, National Cancer Institute, National Institutes of Health, Rockville, MD, USA.

References
1. Caleffi M, Fentiman IS, Birkhead BG. Factors at presentation influencing the prognosis in breast cancer. Eur J Cancer Clin Oncol. 1989;25(1):51–6.
2. Trivers KF, Gammon MD, Abrahamson PE, Lund MJ, Flagg EW, Kaufman JS, et al. Association between reproductive factors and breast cancer survival in younger women. Breast Cancer Res Treat. 2007;103(1):93–102.
3. Orgéas CC, Hall P, Rosenberg LU, Czene K. The influence of menstrual risk factors on tumor characteristics and survival in postmenopausal breast cancer. Breast Cancer Res. 2008;10(6):R107.
4. Schouten LJ, Hupperets PS, Jager JJ, Volovics L, Wils JA, Verbeek AL, et al. Prognostic significance of etiological risk factors in early breast cancer. Breast Cancer Res Treat. 1997;43(3):217–23.
5. Kroman N, Wohlfahrt J, West Andersen K, Mouridsen HT, Westergaard T, Melbye M. Parity, age at first childbirth and the prognosis of primary breast cancer. Br J Cancer. 1998;78(11):1529–33.
6. Papatestas AE, Mulvihill M, Josi C, Ioannovich J, Lesnick G, Aufses AH. Parity and prognosis in breast cancer. Cancer. 1980;45(1):191–4.
7. Green A, Beral V, Moser K. Mortality in women in relation to their childbearing history. Br Med J. 1988;297(6645):391–5.
8. Korzeniowski S, Dyba T. Reproductive history and prognosis in patients with operable breast cancer. Cancer. 1994;74(5):1591–4.
9. Black MM, Hankey BF, Barclay THC. Parity as a prognostic factor in young breast Cancer Patients2. J Natl Cancer Inst. 1983;70(1):27–30.
10. Mohle-Boetani JC, Grosser S, Whittemore AS, Malec M, Kampert JB, Paffenbarger RS. Body size, reproductive factors, and breast cancer survival. Prev Med. 1988;17(5):634–42.
11. Olson SH, Zauber AG, Tang J, Harlap S. Relation of time since last birth and parity to survival of young women with breast Cancer. Epidemiology. 1998; 9(6):669–71.
12. Phillips K-A, Milne RL, Friedlander ML, Jenkins MA, McCredie MRE, Giles GG, et al. Prognosis of premenopausal breast Cancer and childbirth prior to diagnosis. J Clin Oncol. 2004;22(4):699–705.
13. Parker JS, Mullins M, Cheang MC, Leung S, Voduc D, Vickery T, et al. Supervised risk predictor of breast cancer based on intrinsic subtypes. J Clin Oncol. 2009;27(8):1160–7.
14. Goldhirsch A, Winer EP, Coates AS, Gelber RD, Piccart-Gebhart M, Thürlimann B, et al. Personalizing the treatment of women with early breast cancer: highlights of the St Gallen International Expert Consensus on the Primary Therapy of Early Breast Cancer 2013. Ann Oncol. 2013;24(9):2206–23.
15. Senkus E, Kyriakides S, Penault-Llorca F, Poortmans P, Thompson A, Zackrisson S, et al. Primary breast cancer: ESMO clinical practice guidelines for diagnosis, treatment and follow-up. Ann Oncol. 2013; 24(6):vi7–vi23.
16. Millikan RC, Newman B, Tse C-K, Moorman PG, Conway K, Smith LV, et al. Epidemiology of basal-like breast cancer. Breast Cancer Res Treat. 2008; 109(1):123–39.
17. Jatoi I, Anderson WF. Qualitative age interactions in breast cancer studies: a mini-review. Future Oncol. 2010;6(11):1781–8.
18. Yang XR, Chang-Claude J, Goode EL, Couch FJ, Nevanlinna H, Milne RL, et al. Associations of breast cancer risk factors with tumor subtypes: a pooled analysis from the breast Cancer association consortium studies. J Natl Cancer Inst. 2011;103(3):250–63.
19. Anderson WF, Pfeiffer RM, Wohlfahrt J, Ejlertsen B, Jensen M-B, Kroman N. Associations of parity-related reproductive histories with ER± and HER2± receptor-specific breast cancer aetiology. Int J Epidemiol. 2017;46(1):373.
20. Song N, Choi J-Y, Sung H, Jeon S, Chung S, Song M, et al. Tumor subtype-specific associations of hormone-related reproductive factors on breast Cancer survival. PLoS One. 2015;10(4):e0123994.
21. Kwan ML, Bernard PS, Kroenke CH, Factor RE, Habel LA, Weltzien EK, et al. Breastfeeding, PAM50 Tumor Subtype, and Breast Cancer Prognosis and Survival. J Natl Cancer Inst. 2015;107(7):djv087–djv.
22. Cespedes Feliciano EM, Kwan ML, Kushi LH, Chen WY, Weltzien EK, Castillo AL, et al. Body mass index, PAM50 subtype, recurrence, and survival among patients with nonmetastatic breast cancer. Cancer. 2017;123(13):2535–42.
23. Yang XR, Devi BCR, Sung H, Guida J, Mucaki EJ, Xiao Y, et al. Prevalence and spectrum of germline rare variants in BRCA1/2 and PALB2 among breast cancer cases in Sarawak, Malaysia. Breast Cancer Res Treat. 2017;165(3):687–97.
24. Devi CRB, Tang TS, Corbex M. Incidence and risk factors for breast cancer subtypes in three distinct south-east Asian ethnic groups: Chinese, Malay and natives of Sarawak, Malaysia. Int J Cancer. 2012;131(12):2869–77.
25. Tamimi RM, Colditz GA, Hazra A, Baer HJ, Hankinson SE, Rosner B, et al. Traditional breast cancer risk factors in relation to molecular subtypes of breast cancer. Breast Cancer Res Treat. 2012;131(1):159–67.
26. Mustapha A, Jenny C-C, Raza AH, Nilanjan C, Penny C, Frances D, et al. Etiology of hormone receptor positive breast cancer differs by levels of histologic grade and proliferation. Int J Cancer. 2018;143(4):746–57.
27. Anderson KN, Schwab RB, Martinez ME. Reproductive risk factors and breast cancer subtypes: a review of the literature. Breast Cancer Res Treat. 2014; 144(1):1–10.
28. Chen L, Li CI, Tang M-TC, Porter P, Hill DA, Wiggins CL, et al. Reproductive factors and risk of luminal, HER2-overexpressing, and triple-negative breast Cancer among multiethnic women. Cancer epidemiology biomarkers & Prevention. 2016;25(9):1297–304.
29. Kwan ML, Kushi LH, Weltzien E, Maring B, Kutner SE, Fulton RS, et al. Epidemiology of breast cancer subtypes in two prospective cohort studies of breast cancer survivors. Breast Cancer Res. 2009;11(3):1–13.
30. Song N, Choi J-Y, Sung H, Chung S, Song M, Park SK, et al. Heterogeneity of epidemiological factors by breast tumor subtypes in Korean women: a case-case study. Int J Cancer. 2014;135(3):669–81.
31. Martinez ME, Wertheim BC, Natarajan L, Schwab R, Bondy ML, Daneri-Navarro A, et al. Reproductive factors, heterogeneity, and breast tumor subtypes in women of Mexican descent. Cancer Epidemiol Biomarkers Prev. 2013;22(10):1853–61.
32. Shinde SS, Forman MR, Kuerer HM, Yan K, Peintinger F, Hunt KK, et al. Higher parity and shorter breastfeeding duration. Cancer. 2010;116(21): 4933–43.
33. Wada K, Nagata C, Tamakoshi A, Matsuo K, Oze I, Wakai K, et al. Body mass index and breast cancer risk in Japan: a pooled analysis of eight population-based cohort studies. Ann Oncol. 2014;25(2):519–24.
34. Bandera EV, Maskarinec G, Romieu I, John EM. Racial and ethnic disparities in the impact of obesity on breast Cancer risk and survival: a global perspective. Adv Nutr. 2015;6(6):803–19.
35. Amadou A, Ferrari P, Muwonge R, Moskal A, Biessy C, Romieu I, et al. Overweight, obesity and risk of premenopausal breast cancer according to ethnicity: a systematic review and dose-response meta-analysis. Obes Rev. 2013;14(8):665–78.
36. Clarke CA, Keegan THM, Yang J, Press DJ, Kurian AW, Patel AH, et al. Age-specific incidence of breast Cancer subtypes: understanding the black–white crossover. J Natl Cancer Inst. 2012;104(14):1094–101.
37. Horne HN, Beena Devi CR, Sung H, Tang TS, Rosenberg PS, Hewitt SM, et al. Greater absolute risk for all subtypes of breast cancer in the US than Malaysia. Breast Cancer Res Treat. 2015;149(1):285–91.
38. Juret P, Couette JE, Mandard AM, Carre A, Delozier T, Brune D, et al. Age at menarche as a prognostic factor in human breast cancer. Eur J Cancer. 1976;12(9):701–4.

39. Pike MC, Krailo MD, Henderson BE, Casagrande JT, Hoel DG. Hormonal risk factors, breast tissue age and the age-incidence of breast cancer. Nature. 1983;303(5920):767–70.

40. Colditz GA. Relationship between estrogen levels, use of hormone replacement therapy, and breast Cancer. J Natl Cancer Inst. 1998;90(11):814–23.

41. Althuis MD, Fergenbaum JH, Garcia-Closas M, Brinton LA, Madigan MP, Sherman ME. Etiology of hormone receptor–defined breast Cancer: a systematic review of the literature. Cancer Epidemiol Biomarkers Prev. 2004; 13(10):1558–68.

42. Alsaker MDK, Opdahl S, Asvold BO, Romundstad PR, Vatten LJ. The association of reproductive factors and breastfeeding with long term survival from breast cancer. Breast Cancer Res Treat. 2011;130(1):175–82.

43. Urruticoechea A, Smith IE, Dowsett M. Proliferation marker Ki-67 in early breast cancer. J Clin Oncol. 2005;23(28):7212–20.

44. Reed A, Kutasovic J, Lakhani S, Simpson P. Invasive lobular carcinoma of the breast: morphology, biomarkers and 'omics. Breast Cancer Res. 2015;17(1):12.

45. Arpino G, Bardou V, Clark G, Elledge R. Infiltrating lobular carcinoma of the breast: tumor characteristics and clinical outcome. Breast Cancer Res. 2004; 6(3):R149–R56.

46. Chlebowski RT, Aiello E, McTiernan A. Weight loss in breast Cancer patient management. J Clin Oncol. 2002;20(4):1128–43.

47. Chan DSM, Vieira AR, Aune D, Bandera EV, Greenwood DC, McTiernan A, et al. Body mass index and survival in women with breast cancer—systematic literature review and meta-analysis of 82 follow-up studies. Ann Oncol. 2014;25(10):1901–14.

48. Nechuta S, Chen WY, Cai H, Poole EM, Kwan ML, Flatt SW, et al. A pooled analysis of post-diagnosis lifestyle factors in association with late estrogen-receptor–positive breast cancer prognosis. Int J Cancer. 2016;138(9):2088–97.

49. Zhang M, Cai H, Bao P, Xu W, Qin G, Shu XO, et al. Body mass index, waist-to-hip ratio and late outcomes: a report from the shanghai breast Cancer survival study. Sci Rep. 2017;7(1):6996.

50. Moon H-G, Han W, Noh D-Y. Underweight and breast Cancer recurrence and death: a report from the Korean breast Cancer society. J Clin Oncol. 2009;27(35):5899–905.

51. Kawai M, Minami Y, Nishino Y, Fukamachi K, Ohuchi N, Kakugawa Y. Body mass index and survival after breast cancer diagnosis in Japanese women. BMC Cancer. 2012;12(1):149.

52. Kawai M, Tomotaki A, Miyata H, Iwamoto T, Niikura N, Anan K, et al. Body mass index and survival after diagnosis of invasive breast cancer: a study based on the Japanese National Clinical Database—Breast Cancer Registry. Cancer Med. 2016;5(6):1328–40.

53. Iyengar NM, Hudis CA, Dannenberg AJ. Obesity and inflammation: new insights into breast Cancer development and progression. Am Soc Clin Oncol Educ Book. 2013;33:46–51.

54. Thomas F, Bean K, Pannier B, Oppert J-M, Guize L, Benetos A. Cardiovascular mortality in overweight subjects. The Key Role of Associated Risk Factors. 2005;46(4):654–9.

8

Thyroid hormones and breast cancer association according to menopausal status and body mass index

Carolina Ortega-Olvera[1], Alfredo Ulloa-Aguirre[2], Angélica Ángeles-Llerenas[3], Fernando Enrique Mainero-Ratchelous[4], Claudia Elena González-Acevedo[1], Ma. de Lourdes Hernández-Blanco[1], Elad Ziv[5,6], Larissa Avilés-Santa[7], Edelmiro Pérez-Rodríguez[8] and Gabriela Torres-Mejía[3,9]* ⓘ

Abstract

Background: Thyroxine (T4) has been positively associated with tumor cell proliferation, while the effect of triiodothyronine (T3) on cell proliferation has not been well-established because it differs according to the type of cell line used. In Mexico, it has been reported that 14.5% of adult women have some type of thyroid dysfunction and abnormalities in thyroid function tests have been observed in a variety of non-thyroidal illnesses, including breast cancer (BC). These abnormalities might change with body mass index (BMI) because thyroid hormones are involved in the regulation of various metabolic pathways and probably by menopausal status because obesity has been negatively associated with BC in premenopausal women and has been positively associated with BC in postmenopausal women.

Methods: To assess the association between serum thyroid hormone concentration (T4 and T3) and BC and the influence of obesity as an effect modifier of this relationship in premenopausal and postmenopausal women, we measured serum thyroid hormone and thyroid antibody levels in 682 patients with incident breast cancer (cases) and 731 controls, who participated in a population-based case-control study performed from 2004 to 2007 in three states of Mexico. We tested the association of total T4 (TT4) and total T3 (TT3) stratifying by menopausal status and body mass index (BMI), and adjusted for other health and demographic risk factors using logistic regressions models.

Results: Higher serum total T4 (TT4) concentrations were associated with BC in both premenopausal (odds ratio (OR) $_{per\ standard\ deviation}$ = 5.98, 95% CI 3.01–11.90) and postmenopausal women (OR $_{per\ standard\ deviation}$ = 2.81, 95% CI 2.17–3.65). In premenopausal women, the effect of TT4 decreased as BMI increased while the opposite was observed in postmenopausal women. The significance of the effect modification was marginal ($p = 0.059$) in postmenopausal women and was not significant in premenopausal women ($p = 0.22$). Lower TT3 concentrations were associated with BC in both premenopausal and postmenopausal women and no effect modification was observed.

Conclusions: There is a strong association between BC and serum concentrations of TT3 and TT4; this needs to be further investigated to understand why it happens and how important it is to consider these alterations in treatment.

Keywords: Thyroid hormones, Triiodothyronine, Thyroxine, Obesity, Breast cancer

* Correspondence: gtorres@insp.mx
[3]Centro de Investigación en Salud Poblacional, Instituto Nacional de Salud Pública, Av. Universidad No. 655, Col. Santa María Ahuacatitlán, Cuernavaca C.P. 62100, Morelos, México
[9]Instituto Nacional de Salud Pública, Centro de Investigación en Salud Poblacional, Avenida Universidad 655, Col. Santa María Ahuacatitlán, C.P. 62100 Cuernavaca, Morelos, México
Full list of author information is available at the end of the article

Background

The association between thyroid hormones and the risk of breast cancer (BC) has been reported in epidemiological studies [1, 2]. A positive association has been reported between thyroxine (T4) and risk of BC, which is more pronounced in overweight and obese women [1]. Negative associations have been reported between triiodothyronine (T3) and BC among premenopausal women; in contrast, positive associations have been observed among postmenopausal women [2]. It has been shown that in in vitro studies, thyroid hormones affect the growth of BC-derived cell lines [3], lung cancer [4], and glioblastoma [5]. T4 has been shown to increase cell proliferation through the $\alpha v \beta 3$ integrin receptor found on the plasma membrane of cells [3]. In contrast, the effect of T3 on cell proliferation has not been well-established because it differs by the type of cell line used [6–8]. These effects are important, since abnormalities in thyroid function tests have been observed in a variety of non-thyroidal illnesses, without preexisting thyroid or hypothalamic-pituitary disease [9]. Furthermore, these abnormalities might change with body mass index (BMI) because thyroid hormones are involved in the regulation of various metabolic pathways (e.g., adaptive thermogenesis and glucose metabolism) that are relevant for resting energy expenditure and changes in body weight [10, 11].

Worldwide, obesity has increased to epidemic proportions in recent years. According to the World Health Organization (WHO) in 2014, 40% of women over age 18 years were obese and 15% were overweight [12]. By 2016, in Mexico, 37% of women older than 20 years were overweight, and the prevalence of obesity was 38.6% [13]. Obesity has been linked to various chronic diseases and to the development of different types of cancer, including BC [14]. One study indicated that if the BMI had remained at 1982 levels, nearly a quarter (118,000 cases) of all obesity-related cancers in 2012 could have been avoided worldwide [15].

Obesity, as measured by BMI, has been associated with BC risk, but conflicting effects have been reported in premenopausal and postmenopausal women [16–19]. In premenopausal women, BMI is associated with decreased BC risk [20–27], whereas in postmenopausal women, it has been associated with an increased BC risk [28–30]. Recently, genetically predicted BMI was inversely associated with BC risk in both, premenopausal and postmenopausal women [31]. The mechanisms behind these associations have not been fully explained [27]. Several metabolic conditions associated with body fat can influence the BC risk differently in premenopausal and postmenopausal women [27, 32].

In a cohort study conducted in Swedish women, Tosovic et al. (2012) reported a positive association between serum concentrations of free T4 (FT4) and BC prior to diagnosis, particularly in women with a BMI ≥ 25, while for free T3 (FT3), the protective effect was higher in women with BMI < 25; however, most of the associations were not statistically significant [1]. White adipose tissue actively produces various hormones and cytokines (e.g., leptin and growth factors, among others) [33], which are important in the homeostasis and regulation of thyroid hormones [34]. Several studies in euthyroid women have reported that serum free thyroxine (FT4) concentration is inversely correlated with BMI [35–37], while FT3 has been positively associated with visceral fat [38, 39] and BMI ≥ 40 [40], negatively with body fat measured using bioimpedance [41], and not correlated with BMI [36].

In the present case-control study, we examined the association between serum concentrations of thyroid hormones and BC in 2074 Mexican women who participated in the *Cáncer de Mama* (CAMA) study. We also examined obesity as an effect modifier of this relationship in premenopausal and postmenopausal women.

Methods

Study population

The present study is derived from the population-based case-control study "Risk factors for BC in Mexico: mammographic patterns, C-peptide, and growth factors, a multicenter study" (CAMA), which was conducted in three cities of Mexico (Monterrey, Veracruz, and Mexico City) from January 2004 to December 2007 [42]. In summary, the CAMA study included consecutive women with incident BC (cases ($n = 1000$)), aged 35–69 years, who were required to have had a minimum of 5 years of residency in the study cities and who were recruited from 12 public hospitals (5 from the Mexican Social Security Institute (*Instituto Mexicano de Seguro Social – IMSS*), 2 from the Institute of Security and Social Services of State Workers (*Instituto de Seguridad y Servicios Sociales de los Trabajadores de Estado – ISSSTE*), and 5 from the Ministry of Health (*Secretaría de Salud – SS*)). Nurses from the field staff were based at each hospital Monday to Friday from January 2004 to December 2007. The inclusion criteria for the cases were (a) histopathological confirmation of BC (median of 3 days between diagnosis and inclusion in the study); (b) no previous treatment (radiotherapy, chemotherapy, or antiestrogens) in the last 6 months; and (c) absence of pregnancy. The response rate of patients with BC was 94%. Controls ($n = 1074$) were selected based on a probabilistic multistage design and were randomly selected considering the catchment area of each of the participating hospitals. Mammography was performed and women with Breast Imaging Reporting and Data System (BI-RADS) categories I and II were included in the study. The response rate of controls was 87%. The control group was matched to the patients according to quinquennial age, health institution affiliation, and state of residence. In-person interviews were conducted at the hospital with the patients and at the homes of the controls to obtain information on their sociodemographics, reproductive health, breast pathology, lifestyle, and co-morbidities. Information on the perception of body image in different stages of life (six stages) was also included. The perception was measured with the use of six pictograms that represent silhouettes from very thin to very obese. In both the patients and the controls, blood samples and anthropometric measurements were obtained at participating hospitals by personnel following standardized procedures and who were blinded to the study hypotheses. For the analyses of the present study, out of 1000 cases and 1070 controls we excluded 50 and 45 women, respectively, because they answered "yes" to the question "Has a doctor diagnosed you with thyroid disease?" In the remaining 950 cases and 1029 controls, we determined serum thyroid hormone concentrations in a random subsample of 645 cases, among whom 3 % had in situ BC, and 697 controls (Fig. 1). Characteristics (e.g., age, residence, breastfeeding,

first-degree BC family history, BMI, and parity) of the sub-sample and the total population from the CAMA study were not statistically different (data not shown).

Blood measurements
Blood samples were obtained from the participants after they had fasted for at least 8 h. The samples were centrifuged at 3200 rpm at room temperature for 15 min, and the serum was separated and maintained at – 20 °C for 3 weeks and then at – 80 °C until use. Total concentrations of total T3 (TT3), total T4 (TT4), thyroid stimulating hormone (TSH), thyroglobulin (Tg), and thyroid peroxidase (TPO) and thyroglobulin (Tg) antibodies (TgAb) were determined in triplicate using a chemiluminescence assay in a Beckman Coulter UniCel DxI 800 system (Brea, CA, USA) according to the manufacturer's instructions. The coefficients of intra-assay and inter-assay variation were less than 6% for the hormones TT3, TT4, TSH, and Tg. In addition, at the Children's Hospital Oakland Research Institute, 106 ancestry information markers were genotyped using multiplex polymerase chain reaction (PCR) and Sequenom's

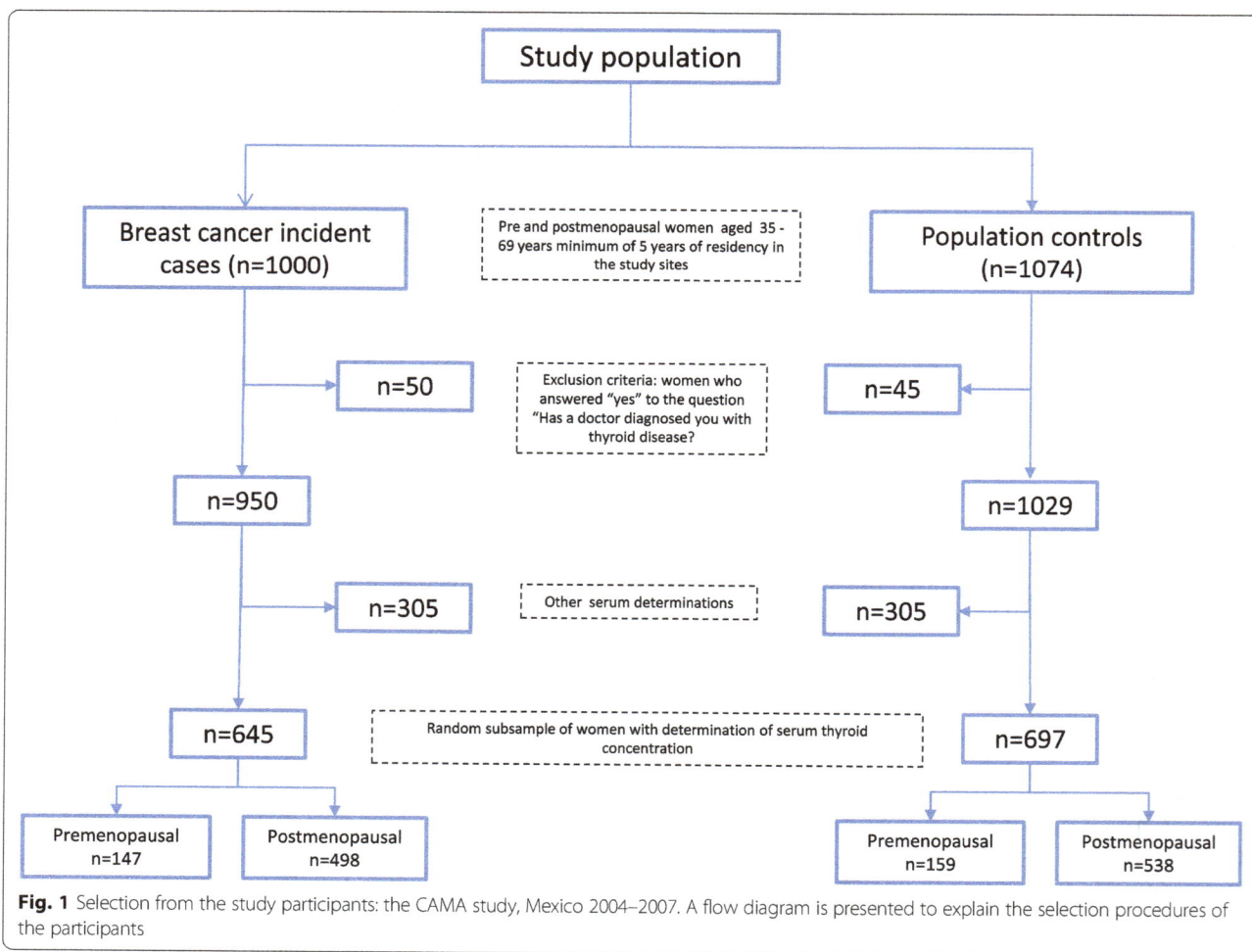

Fig. 1 Selection from the study participants: the CAMA study, Mexico 2004–2007. A flow diagram is presented to explain the selection procedures of the participants

unique baseline extension methodology (Sequenom Inc., San Diego, CA, USA). The details of these markers have been published elsewhere [43, 44]. The laboratory personnel who performed the measurements were blinded to the condition (case or control) of each participant.

Anthropometric measurements

In order to obtain high-quality body measurements, trained nurses were assessed for intra-observer and inter-observer reliability until consistent and accurate anthropometric measurements were obtained. We used validated and standardized protocols and calibrated instruments according to Lohaman's recommendations [45]. Weight was measured using a digital scale (Tanita Corporation of America, Inc., Arlington Heights, IL, USA) and recorded to the nearest 0.1 kg. Height was measured using a stadiometer (SECA, Hamburg, Germany) to the nearest millimeter. Waist circumference was measured at the level of the navel with the patient in standing position, and the hip circumference was measured at the most prominent level of the buttocks with the woman in a standing position. The BMI was calculated as the weight (in kilograms) divided by the height (in meters) squared. The waist-to-hip ratio (WHR) was calculated by dividing the waist circumference (in centimeters) by the hip circumference (in centimeters). The cutoff points used to estimate the association for BMI, waist circumference, hip circumference, and WHR were established according to the distribution of control patients into tertiles, while the cases were assigned according to the controls' cutoff points. Tertiles were used for the anthropometric variables because Mexican women are mostly in the overweight and obesity categories. In addition, the participating women were asked to select the silhouette that best represented their body shape (using six pictograms that represent body shape from very thin to extremely obese) at different stages of their lives (before and immediately after menarche, between 18 and 20 years of age, before their first pregnancy, between 25 and 35 years, and their current body shape at the time of the interview). The correlation between BMI and silhouette has been reported as 0.67 in adult women [46], and in the study population, the correlation was $p = 0.69$ ($p \leq 0.001$). A trajectory analysis based on a group approach was performed as proposed by Nagin [47]; this approach is based on the identification of groups with different individual trajectories in the study population over time and looks for the most homogeneous clusters. To identify the optimal model (number of groups and trajectories), we used the Bayesian information criterion (BIC) [47, 48]. To place enough subjects in each category for the statistical analysis, the body shape silhouettes were combined into

categories. At childhood, at adolescence, at age 18–20 years, and at age before first pregnancy, the thin category included the women who selected silhouette 1. Silhouette 2 was included for the median category, and for obesity, the women who selected silhouettes 3, 4, 5, and 6 were included. For body silhouettes of women aged 25–35 years and for their current body silhouette, the thin category included the women who selected silhouette 1 and 2. Silhouette 3 was included for the median category, and for obesity, the women who selected silhouettes 4, 5, and 6 were included [48].

Diet

A semi-quantitative Food Frequency Questionnaire (FFQ) adapted from Willett [49] to the Mexican population and validated in Mexico City [49, 50] was used for the present study. To measure caloric consumption, participants were asked to report frequency of consumption of a typical serving of 104 items in the past year, and responses were converted to average daily consumption. To calculate intakes, we used the nutrient database developed by the National Institute of Nutrition in Mexico [51] and, when necessary, the US Department of Agriculture food composition tables [52].

Physical activity

To measure physical activity, a semi-structured interview to estimate an individual's time spent performing different physical activities (sleep and light-, moderate-, and vigorous-intensity physical activity) was applied. The interview was based on the 7-day recall questionnaire proposed by Sallis et al. (1985) [53]. For the present study, weekly hours of moderate-intensity physical activity (activities that are tiresome but that do not result in breathlessness) were used. The patients were asked to report physical activity in a typical week 1 year before the appearance of signs and symptoms, to reduce the possibility of reverse causation bias, whereas the controls were asked to report physical activity for the year prior to the survey [42].

Statistical analysis

Descriptive statistics (medians, interquartile ranges, means, SD and proportions) were calculated for both the premenopausal and postmenopausal women who were categorized as either cases or controls. We described sociodemographic, reproductive health, anthropometry, breast pathology, lifestyle, comorbidities, thyroid function parameters and clinical characteristics of the patients (cases) in terms of clinical stage (early $\leq$ IIA; advanced $\geq$ IIB) and histological grade (1, 2, or 3).

To assess the association between BC and TT3 or TT4 serum concentrations, two logistic regression models were used, one for premenopausal and one for postmenopausal women. To build each model, bivariate models were constructed for each variable of interest and potential confounders, then variables with a p value ≤0.20 in the bivariate models were included in each final model. In order to build the most parsimonious models that still explain the data, we left the variables with a p value <0.05 [54, 55]. The dependent variable was BC (yes/no), and the independent variables of interest were TT3 and TT4, which were incorporated into the models as standardized continuous variables $(Z = (x-\mu)/\sigma)$. For each model, odds ratios (OR) and 95% confidence intervals (95% CI) were obtained. For continuous variables such as thyroid function parameters and calorie consumption, we estimated the odds of BC for each increase in SD.

The following are the variables that were considered as potential confounders: (a) sociodemographic variables: age (years), entitlement to a health institution (IMSS, ISSSTE, and Ministry of Health), city of residence (Mexico City, Monterrey, or Veracruz), economic index (low, medium, or high), and educational level (last complete school grade); (b) reproductive health: age at menarche (years), age at menopause (years), time of exposure to endogenous hormones (age at menopause in years to age of menarche in years), parity (number of children born alive), ever use of hormonal contraception (yes/no), age at first full-term pregnancy (years), use of hormones for menopause for more than 1 month (yes/no), and breastfeeding (months); (c) anthropometric measurements: height (cm); (d) breast pathology: personal history of benign breast disease (yes/no) and family history of BC (mother, grandmother, or sisters) (yes/no); (e) lifestyles: hours of moderate-intensity physical activity per week [42, 53], alcohol consumption (consumed on average one or more alcoholic drinks a month for a year (yes/no)), tobacco consumption (smoked at least 100 cigarettes in her lifetime (yes/no)), and daily calorie intake (Kcal) [49–52, 56]; (f) percentage of indigenous ancestry informative markers [44, 57]; (g) comorbidities: diabetes mellitus diagnosed by a physician (yes/no); and (h) the other thyroid function parameters: TSH, Tg, and Tg and thyroperoxidase TPO antibodies (TPO Ab) $(Z = (x-\mu)/\sigma)$. The percentage of ancestry informative markers was considered as a potential confounder due to its potential association with the thyroid hormone profile [57] and because it has been associated with BC [44].

The effect modification of obesity (BMI, waist circumference, hip circumference, WHR, and trajectories according to the silhouettes) was assessed for the association between TT3 or TT4 and BC in premenopausal and postmenopausal women. Multiplicative interactions were evaluated, which considered the thyroid hormones as continuous variables, the anthropometric variables in tertiles (waist circumference (tertiles), hip circumference (tertiles), BMI (tertiles), WHR (tertiles)), and the different trajectories of weight change (constantly low, constantly mid-range,

moderate increase, strong increase, or constantly high). We focus our results on the potential effect modification by BMI since this variable has been associated more consistently as a protector against BC in premenopausal women and as a risk factor in postmenopausal women [23, 58–79]. The results for the rest of the anthropometric variables are presented in additional tables. Given that missing values were lower than 5%, we did not include them in the analysis of multiple models. All models were then analyzed with goodness of fit, model specification, collinearity, and influential values tests according to the procedure proposed by Hosmer and Lemeshow [55]. The analysis was performed using the STATA v13 software (StataCorp, College Station, TX, USA).

Results

The characteristics of the study population are presented separately for premenopausal and postmenopausal women in Table 1. Compared to controls, premenopausal patients (cases), were more likely to have completed professional and postgraduate studies (data not shown). Among postmenopausal women, a higher percentage of patients completed secondary, high school, and postgraduate studies compared with the controls (data not shown). Parity, history of benign breast disease, physical activity, alcohol consumption, and history of diabetes mellitus are associated with BC according to the literature. In both premenopausal and postmenopausal women, waist circumference and hip circumference were smaller in the patients than in the controls. BMI was lower in the patients than in the controls. Table 2, shows that in both the premenopausal and postmenopausal women, the serum TT3 concentration was lower in the patients than in the controls, whereas the serum TT4 concentration was higher in the patients than in the controls. Table 3, shows that more than 40% of the study participants were diagnosed at an advanced clinical stage.

In the premenopausal women who were stratified by tertiles of the anthropometric variables (BMI, waist and hip measurements, and WHR), the median serum TT3 concentration was lower in the patients than in the controls, whereas TT4 concentrations were higher in the patients than in the controls, and serum TSH concentrations were similar in both groups. The same relationship was observed in postmenopausal women (data not shown).

Multiple models, minimally adjusted for age, health institution, and city of residence, showed that when all the women were analyzed, the serum concentration of the TT3 hormone was negatively associated with BC (OR $_{per\ standard\ deviation}$ = 0.16, 95% CI 0.13–0.20), and this association was maintained when the patients were stratified into the premenopausal (OR $_{per\ standard\ deviation}$ = 0.07, 95% CI 0.04–0.12) and postmenopausal groups (OR $_{per\ standard\ deviation}$ = 0.20, 95% CI 0.16–0.25) (data not shown). However, the

Table 1 Characteristics of study participants by menopausal status in the CAMA study, Mexico, 2004–2007

| | Premenopausal women, n = 306 | | | | Postmenopausal women, n = 1036 | | | |
| | Cases, n = 147 | | Controls, n = 159 | | Cases, n = 498 | | Controls, n = 538 | |
	Number	(%)[a]	Number	(%)[a]	Number	(%)[a]	Number	(%)[a]
Sociodemographic								
Age (years)[b]	44.1	38.6–47.3	44.1	40.6–47.8	58.0	52.9–64.3	57.4	52.3–62.1
Wealth index								
Low	52	(35.4)	45	(28.3)	155	(31.1)	199	(37.0)
Medium	38	(25.9)	49	(30.8)	125	(25.1)	187	(34.8)
High	57	(38.8)	65	(40.9)	218	(43.8)	152	(28.3)
Indigenous ancestry percent								
0–25%	3	(2.0)	4	(2.5)	21	(4.2)	10	(1.9)
26–50%	38	(25.9)	41	(25.8)	130	(26.1)	125	(23.2)
51–75%	49	(33.3)	77	(48.4)	188	(37.8)	245	(45.5)
76–100%	18	(12.2)	33	(20.8)	79	(15.9)	139	(25.8)
Reproductive health								
Time of exposure to endogenous hormones (years)[b]					34	30–37	34	29–37
Parity								
None	21	(14.3)	13	(8.2)	62	(12.4)	23	(4.3)
1–3	93	(63.3)	98	(61.6)	227	(45.6)	209	(38.8)
≥4	32	(21.8)	47	(29.6)	205	(41.2)	306	(56.9)
Use of contraception at any point at life								
No	85	(57.8)	86	(54.1)	294	(59.0)	299	(55.6)
Yes	62	(42.2)	73	(45.9)	202	(40.6)	239	(44.4)
Use of hormones for menopause for more than 1 month								
No	–	–	–	–	380	(76.3)	456	(84.8)
Yes	–	–	–	–	114	(22.9)	81	(15.1)
Breastfeeding in months[b]	9	2–25	12	4–34	12	1–42	24	6–57
Anthropometry								
Waist circumference (cm)[b,c]	93.3	84.8–101.5	97.7	92–107.0	97.0	90.3–104.8	99.5	91.65–108.0
Hip circumference (cm)[b,c]	103.1	97.2–111.0	107.9	102–115.7	106.25	100.3–114.6	108.0	101–117.0
Height (cm)[b,c]	154.5	150.5–158.5	153.8	149.7–158.0	151.8	147.3–156.0	150.5	146.7–154.4
Weight (kg)[b,c]	65.8	59.5–74.2	70.2	64.0–79.6	67.2	60.2–76.6	67.8	60.4–77.4
Body mass index (weight in kg/height squared)[b,c]	27.4	24.9–31.5	29.8	27.1–33.4	29.2	26.4–33.2	30.2	27.1–33.8
Waist-hip ratio[b,c]	0.90	0.86–0.94	0.91	0.87–0.95	0.91	0.87–0.96	0.91	0.87–0.97

Table 1 Characteristics of study participants in the CAMA study, Mexico, 2004–2007 (Continued)

	Premenopausal women, n = 306				Postmenopausal women, n = 1036			
	Cases, n = 147		Controls, n = 159		Cases, n = 498		Controls, n = 538	
	Number	(%)[a]	Number	(%)[a]	Number	(%)[a]	Number	(%)[a]
Silhouette trajectory								
Group 1, constantly low	19	(12.9)	28	(17.6)	76	(15.3)	94	(17.5)
Group 2, constantly mid-range	57	(38.8)	56	(35.2)	199	(40.0)	200	(37.2)
Group 3, moderate increase	27	(18.4)	32	(20.1)	101	(20.3)	117	(21.7)
Group 4, Strong increase	41	(27.9)	37	(23.3)	104	(20.9)	113	(21.0)
Group 5, constantly high	3	(2.0)	6	(3.8)	18	(3.6)	14	(2.6)
Breast pathology								
Personal history of benign breast disease								
No	126	(85.7)	140	(88.1)	425	(85.3)	506	(94.1)
Yes	20	(13.6)	16	(10.1)	65	(13.1)	27	(5.0)
Family history of breast cancer (mother, grandmother, and sisters)								
No	137	(93.2)	148	(93.1)	466	(93.6)	525	(97.6)
Yes	10	(6.8)	11	(6.9)	32	(6.4)	13	(2.4)
Lifestyle								
Hours of moderate-intensity physical activity per week[b,d]	9.0	3.5–18.0	12.0	2.0–25.5	5.5	1.0–10.5	12.0	2.0–22.0
Consumed on average one or more alcoholic drinks a month for a year								
No	108	(73.5)	139	(87.4)	403	(80.9)	472	(87.7)
Yes	39	(26.5)	18	(11.3)	70	(14.1)	47	(8.7)
Smoked at least 100 cigarettes in her lifetime								
No	119	(81.0)	113	(71.1)	370	(74.3)	442	(82.2)
Yes	28	(19.0)	46	(28.9)	128	(25.7)	96	(17.8)
Daily total consumption of calories (Kcal)[b,d]	2262.6	1776.1 – 2704.1	1853.0	1514.8–2302.6	2014.9	1631.1–2557.1	1748.5	1396.0–2160.4
Comorbidities								
Diagnosed with diabetes mellitus by a physician								
No	123	(84.4)	130	(82.4)	330	(66.3)	399	(74.2)
Yes	15	(10.2)	18	(11.3)	126	(25.3)	107	(19.9)

CAMA study Risk factors for breast cancer in Mexico: mammographic patterns, C peptide, and growth factors, a multicenter study

[a]Percentages do not necessarily add up to 100% due to missing values

[b]Values correspond to the median and interquartile range

[c]Missing values in percentage: waist: premenopausal women: cases 0%, controls 3.1%; postmenopausal women: cases 2%, controls 0%; height: premenopausal women: cases 2%, controls 0%; postmenopausal women: cases 0%, controls 0%; body mass index: premenopausal women: cases 2%, controls 0%; postmenopausal women: cases 0%, controls 0%; waist-to-hip ratio: premenopausal women: cases 2.0%, controls 3.1%; postmenopausal women: cases 3.8%, controls 2.0%

[d]Missing values: hours of moderate-intensity physical activity per week: premenopausal women: cases 0%, controls 0%; postmenopausal women: cases 0.2%, controls 0%; daily total consumption of calories (Kcal): premenopausal women: cases 10.9%, controls 10.1%; postmenopausal women cases 5.6%, controls 7,6%

Table 2 Thyroid function parameters of study participants by menopausal status in the CAMA study, Mexico, 2004–2007

| | Premenopausal women, n = 306 | | | | Postmenopausal women, n = 1036 | | | |
| | Cases, n = 147 | | Controls, n = 159 | | Cases, n = 498 | | Controls, n = 538 | |
	Median	Interquartile range	Median	Interquartile range	Median	Interquartile range	Median	Interquartile range
Thyroid function parameters								
Total triiodotyronine (TT3) nmol/L[a]	1.6	1.3–1.9	2.4	1.9–2.8	1.7	1.4–2.1	2.6	2.1–3.0
Mean (SD)	1.7	0.5	2.4	0.6	1.8	0.7	2.6	0.6
Total thyroxin (TT4) nmol/L[a]	103.4	87.4–123.1	93.1	83.7–109.7	104.6	89.8–122.3	96.7	84.4–112.2
Mean (SD)	107.3	27.3	97.2	22	108.6	29.5	100.5	25.7
TSH µUI/mL[a]	1.6	1.1–2.1	1.7	1.1–2.3	1.8	1.1–2.8	1.8	1.1–2.9
Mean (SD)	1.8	1.4	2.3	3.3	2.9	9.6	2.9	6.8
Thyroglobulin ng/mL[a]	6.4	4.0–10.2	7.1	4.5–12.2	7.4	3.9–14.5	7.4	4.0–14.5
Mean (SD)	8.9	9.3	9.9	10.9	17.8	70.1	15.9	47.1
Anti-peroxidase antibodies UI/mL[b]	0.1	0.5–2.5	1.10	0.6–3.1	1.1	0.6–3.9	1.1	0.6–3.5
Mean (SD)	46.4	266.2	222.3	1373.8	111.1	444.6	95.0	346.3
Anti-thyroglobulin antibodies[b,c]								
Negative	73	(49.7)	59	(37.1)	135	(27.1)	133	(24.7)
Positive	71	(48.3)	100	(62.9)	221	(44.4)	240	(44.6)
Median UI/mL (interquartile range)[d]	0.9	0.3–3.1	1.0	0.04–3.0	1.0	0.3–4.6	0.8	0.4–2.8
Mean (SD)[d]	17.7	106.4	4.7	9.8	23.1	165.1	14.4	102.4

CAMA study Risk factors for breast cancer in Mexico: mammographic patterns, C peptide, and growth factors, a multicenter study, *TSH* thyroid stimulating hormone
[a]There are no missing values for TT3, TT4, TSH and thyroglobulin
[b]Results correspond to 147 cases and 159 controls (premenopausal women), respectively; and to 356 cases and 373 controls (postmenopausal)
[c]Number and (percentage) of women with negative/positive anti-thyroglobulin antibodies
[d]The values correspond to women with positive results for anti-thyroglobulin antibodies

protective effect was much higher in premenopausal than in postmenopausal women. The association between serum TT4 concentration and BC was positive when all the women were analyzed (OR $_{per\ standard\ deviation}$ = 1.71, 95% CI 1.48–1.98), and this association was maintained when the patients were stratified by menopausal status; however, stronger association was seen in premenopausal women (OR $_{per\ standard\ deviation}$ = 1.97, 95% CI 1.38–2.82) compared with postmenopausal women (OR $_{per\ standard\ deviation}$ = 1.71, 95% CI 1.48–1.98) (data not shown). No significant associations were found with any other thyroid function parameters (TSH, Tg, Tg Ab, or TPO Ab).

Table 4 presents the multiple model stratified by menopausal status, adjusted by BMI and Table 5 presents the models stratified by both menopausal status and BMI. In Table 4, a negative association was

Table 3 Clinical characteristics of patients with breast cancer (cases) by menopausal status in the CAMA study, Mexico, 2004–2007

| | Premenopausal cases, n = 147 | | Premenopausal cases, n = 498 | |
	Number	Percentage[a]	Number	Percentage[a]
Clinical characteristics				
Clinical stage				
Early (≤ IIA)	43	(29.3)	175	(35.1)
Advanced (≥ IIB)	73	(49.7)	206	(41.4)
Histological grade				
1	4	(2.7)	8	(1.6)
2	29	(19.7)	108	(21.7)
3	9	(6.1)	49	(9.8)

CAMA study Risk factors for breast cancer in Mexico: mammographic patterns, C peptide, and growth factors, a multicenter study
[a]Percentages do not add up to 100% due to missing values

Table 4 Associations between thyroid function tests and breast cancer adjusted by BMI in the CAMA study, Mexico, 2004–2007

	Premenopausal women[a]			Postmenopausal women[b]		
	case/control	OR	95% CI	case/control	OR	95% CI
TT3[c]	128/142	0.03	0.01–0.07	382/498	0.17	0.13–0.22
TT4[c]		5.98	3.01–11.90		2.81	2.17–3.65
BMI						
Tertile 1 (BMI < 27.88)	67/47	1.00		145/166	1.00	
Tertile 2 (BMI 27.88–32.05)	35/48	0.56	0.23–1.37	106/168	0.98	0.63–1.52
Tertile 3 (BMI ≥ 32.06)	26/47	0.28	0.11–0.75	131/164	1.16	0.75–1.80

CAMA study Risk factors for breast cancer in Mexico: mammographic patterns, C peptide, and growth factors, a multicenter study. *TT3* total triiodothyroxine, *TT4* total thyroxine, *BMI* body mass index

[a]Logistic regression model in premenopausal women: dependent variable, breast cancer (yes/no); independent variables, TT3 (nmol/L) and TT4 (nmol/L); potential confounders, age (years), city of residence (Mexico City (reference category), Veracruz and Monterrey), health institution (IMSS: Mexican Social Security Institute (reference category); ISSSTE: Institute of Security and Social Services of State Workers; SS: Ministry of Health), daily total consumption of calories (Kcal) and BMI (tertiles). Hormone concentrations and calorie consumption were standardized to allow interpretation of the odds of breast cancer development per increment of standard deviation, $Z = (x-\mu)/\sigma$

[b]Logistic model in postmenopausal women: dependent variable, breast cancer (yes/no); independent variables, TT3 (nmol/L) and TT4 (nmol/L); potential confounders: age (years), city of residence (Mexico City (reference category), Veracruz and Monterrey), health institution (IMSS: Mexican Social Security Institute (reference category); ISSSTE: Institute of Security and Social Services of State Workers; SS: Ministry of Health), thyroid stimulating hormone (continuous), parity (continuous), consumed on average one or more alcoholic drinks a month for a year (yes/no) and smoked at least 100 cigarettes in her lifetime (yes/no), indigenous ancestry (continuous) and BMI (tertiles). Hormone concentrations and calorie consumption were standardized to allow interpretation of the odds of breast cancer development per increment of standard deviation, $Z = (x-\mu)/\sigma$

[c]TT3 (mean 1.7 SD 0.5); TT4 (mean 103.4 SD 27.3)

observed between the serum TT3 concentration and BC in both premenopausal and postmenopausal women, and a positive association was observed between the serum TT4 concentration and BC. The association was stronger in premenopausal women than in postmenopausal women for both hormones. These associations were similar when each of the remaining anthropometric variables and the trajectory of the silhouettes were independently adjusted (Additional file 1: Table S1).

Table 5 Association between thyroid function tests and breast cancer modified by obesity in the CAMA study, Mexico, 2004–2007

	Premenopausal women[a]			Postmenopausal women[b]		
	Case/control	OR	95% CI	Case/control	OR	95% CI
Multiple model stratified by BMI tertiles						
Tertile 1 (BMI < 27.88)	67/47			145/166		
TT3[c]		0.02	0.003–0.09		0.18	0.11–0.28
TT4[c]		11.97	3.43–41.80		2.62	1.67–4.09
Tertile 2 (BMI 27.88–32.05)	35/48			106/168		
TT3[c]		0.04	0.0–0.16		0.15	0.09–0.25
TT4[c]		8.34	2.03–34.24		3.03	1.83–5.02
Tertile 3 (BMI ≥ 32.06)	26/47			131/164		
TT3[c]		0.01	0.0004–0.08		0.10	0.06–0.18
TT4[c]		2.23	0.39–12.66		3.52	2.15–5.75
p value for interaction between TT4 and BMI tertiles		0.22			0.059	
p value for interaction between TT3 and BMI tertiles		0.12			0.34	

CAMA study Risk factors for breast cancer in Mexico: mammographic patterns, peptide C, and growth factors, a multicenter study, *BMI* body mass index, *TT3* total triiodothyroxine, *TT4* total thyroxine

[a]Logistic regression model in premenopausal women: dependent variable, breast cancer (yes/no); independent variables, TT3 (nmol/L) and TT4 (nmol/L); potential confounders, age (years), city of residence (Mexico City (reference category) Veracruz and Monterrey), health institution (IMSS: Mexican Social Security Institute (reference category); ISSSTE: Institute of Security and Social Services of State Workers; SS: Ministry of Health), daily total consumption of calories (Kcal). Models are presented by each tertile of BMI. Hormone concentrations and calorie consumption were standardized to allow interpretation of the odds of breast cancer development per increment of standard deviation, $Z = (x-\mu)/\sigma$

[b]Logistic regression model in postmenopausal women: dependent variable, breast cancer (yes/no); independent variables, TT3 (nmol/L) and TT4 (nmol/L); potential confounders: age (years), city of residence (Mexico City (reference category) Veracruz and Monterrey), health institution (IMSS: Mexican Social Security Institute (reference category); ISSSTE: Institute of Security and Social Services of State Workers; SS: Ministry of Health), thyroid stimulating hormone (continuous), parity (continuous), consumed on average one or more alcoholic drinks a month for a year (yes/no) and smoked at least 100 cigarettes in her lifetime (yes/no) and indigenous ancestry (continuous). Models are presented by each tertile of BMI. Hormone concentrations and calorie consumption were standardized to allow interpretation of the odds of breast cancer development per increment of standard deviation, $Z = (x-\mu)/\sigma$

[c]TT3 (mean 1.7 SD 0.5); TT4 (mean 103.4 SD 27.3)

When premenopausal women were stratified by BMI (Table 5), it was observed that the association between the serum concentration of TT4 and BC decreased as BMI tertiles increased, until they were no longer significant in the upper tertile (p of interaction = 0.22), while the protective effect of the serum TT3 concentration was maintained in the three tertiles (p of interaction = 0.12). Similarly, the effects of the serum concentrations of TT3 and TT4 were evaluated based on the remainder of the anthropometric variables, and waist circumference ($p = 0.887$), hip circumference ($p = 0.291$), WHR ($p = 0.381$), and the silhouettes trajectory variable ($p = 0.52$) were not statistically significant (Additional file 1: Table S2). In postmenopausal women, stratification by BMI showed that the association between the serum TT4 concentration and BC increased as the BMI tertiles increased (p of interaction = 0.059) (Table 5). For the other anthropometric variables, potential effect modification was observed with hip circumference (tertile 1, OR = 2.17, CI 1.34–3.50; tertile 2, OR = 3.58. CI 2.16–5.95; tertile 3, OR = 3.47, CI 2.12–5.68, p of interaction = 0.02), with WHR (tertile 1, OR = 2.97, CI 1.84–4.80; tertile 2, OR = 4.43. CI 2.38–8.27; tertile 3, OR = 2.46, CI 1.60–3.80, p of interaction = 0.02), and with the silhouettes trajectory (constantly low, OR = 3.87, CI 1.72–8.73; constantly mid-range, OR = 2.12, CI 1.44–3.13; moderately increased, OR = 2.53, CI 1.37–4.66; strong increase, OR = 4.57, CI 2.38–8.86, p of interaction = 0.02), but an effect modification was not observed with waist circumference (p of interaction = 0.51). The interactions between the serum TT3 concentration and the anthropometric variables were also evaluated, but these were not statistically significant for BMI ($p = 0.34$), hip circumference ($p = 0.49$), waist circumference ($p = 0.74$), WHR ($p = 0.38$), or the silhouettes trajectory ($p = 0.36$) (Additional file 1: Table S2).

Discussion

The addition of T4 to BC-derived cell lines has been shown to increase cell proliferation [3], while in the presence of estrogen receptor (ER)-positive BC cell lines the addition of T3 inhibits cell proliferation [7]. These effects are important, as abnormalities in thyroid function tests have been observed in a variety of nonthyroidal illness, without preexisting thyroid or hypothalamic-pituitary disease, including BC [80]. These abnormalities might change by BMI because thyroid hormones are involved in the regulation of various metabolic pathways that are relevant for resting energy expenditure [10, 11]. They could also change by menopausal status because obesity has been negatively associated with BC in premenopausal women [20–27] and has been positively associated with BC in postmenopausal women [30]. It is important to assess the modifying effect of obesity in this association because of the implications for treatment in

populations in where the prevalence of obesity and thyroid dysfunction is high.

We analyzed the association between thyroid hormones and BC and the modification effects of general obesity (BMI), central or intra-abdominal obesity (waist circumference, hip circumference, and waist-hip ratio), and trajectories of change in body shape. Initially, we observed that in both the premenopausal and postmenopausal women, the serum TT4 concentration was positively associated with BC, whereas the serum TT3 concentration was inversely associated with BC. These associations were stronger in the premenopausal women. When the premenopausal women were stratified by BMI tertiles, the positive association between the serum TT4 concentration and BC decreased as the BMI tertiles increased; this association was no longer statistically significant in the highest tertile, probably due to the smaller sample size. In contrast, for the postmenopausal women in the highest tertile of BMI, the strength of the association between the serum TT4 concentration and BC was increased.

A possible explanation for our findings could be related to the difference between premenopausal and postmenopausal women with respect to the possibility or risk of the development of ER-negative (ER-) BC due to BMI [81] and due to the finding that the maintenance of increased cell proliferation caused by T4 requires ER function [82]. Studies that have investigated the association between BMI and different molecular subtypes have suggested that in premenopausal women with a BMI ≥ 25, the prevalence of luminal tumors (ER positive (ER+) or progesterone receptor-positive (PR+)), human epidermal growth factor receptor 2 positive or negative (HER2+ or HER2-) and triple-negative tumors (ER-, PR-, HER2-) is higher than in those with a BMI < 25 [83]. Harris et al. (2011) consistently showed that in this same group of women, the risk of development of ER- BC was higher in those in the upper quintiles of waist and hip circumference and of WHR than in those in the lower quintile [27]. In contrast, in postmenopausal women, compared with women with a BMI < 25, the possibility of the development of luminal BC was greater in those with a BMI ≥ 25 [83]. Additionally, a pooled analysis of 35,568 women with invasive BC who participated in 34 studies showed that in those ≤ 50 years of age, the likelihood of observing ER- tumors was higher in obese women (BMI ≥ 30 kg/m^2) than in women who were not obese (BMI < 25 kg/m^2), and this association was statistically significant [81]. This same association was not statistically significant in women > 50 years of age [81].

Tang et al. observed that both the T4 hormone and 17β-estradiol (E2) promoted cell proliferation through the stimulation of the mitogen-activated protein kinase (MAPK) pathway by ER and demonstrated that such proliferation requires ER function to be sustained [82].

In several cell models, it has been observed that at physiological concentrations, T4 is more active than T3 at stimulating the MAPK pathway [84–87]. In premenopausal women, the decrease in the association between TT4 and BC with increasing BMI could be explained by the lower prevalence of ER+ tumors in overweight and obese women [88, 89]. In contrast, in postmenopausal women, the increase in the association between T4 and BC with increasing BMI may be explained by the finding that overweight and obese women are at a greater risk of the development of ER+ breast tumors. However, more studies need to be performed stratifying by menopausal status and BMI. Two cohort studies reported a positive association between the serum T4 concentration and BC. However, in the aforementioned studies no effect modification was assessed for BMI and menopausal status [1, 90].

In our study we observed a negative association between serum TT3 and BC in both premenopausal and postmenopausal women. On the other hand, we did not observe an effect modification of this association by BMI. In addition, our results are consistent with previously published studies. For example, in studies of ER- cell lines that were transfected with ER, T3 inhibited cell proliferation [7]. Also, Tosovic et al., reported a non-statistically significant negative association between serum T3 and BC, independently of menopausal status [1]. That group also observed a negative association when women were stratified by menopausal status and BMI; however, it was not statistically significant [1].

The findings that we report need to be interpreted within the context of certain limitations. The number of premenopausal women was not sufficient for the identification of a statistically significant effect modification by BMI or other obesity measurements; moreover, the confidence intervals after stratification were broad, particularly for other anthropometric measurements that are presented in additional tables. Given the characteristics of Mexican women, among whom more than 70% were overweight and obese, it was not possible to use the cut-off points proposed by the WHO for anthropometric measurements; hence, we stratified the controls by tertiles for each measurement. Our study personnel were trained to measure weight and height and the other anthropometric variables using a standardized approach in both cases and controls, and in the cases, the measurements were performed at the time of the diagnosis. As BMI can be modified by the presence of cancer, this study is not free of reverse causality. However, the median number of days from the diagnosis until the women entered the study and the anthropometric variables were determined was 3 days. Additionally, we measured TT4. Free T4 (FT4) is unbound and is the active component of TT4, therefore further studies should be performed using FT4. Approximately 75% of the T4 in serum is bound to thyroid-binding globulin (TBG), and a smaller fraction is bound to transthyretin or albumin; so less than 0.1% remains free or unbound [91]. Given that postmenopausal hormone therapy and the use of hormonal contraceptives at any point in life lead to increased thyroid binding globulin (TBG) binding capacity [92], we considered adjusting for these variables in our models. However, we did not include them in the final models because they did not confound our main results. We did not include the ER status because when recruiting the patients (cases), ER status was not determined in all women. Tosovic et al., (2014) found statistically significant positive associations between higher pre-diagnostic T3 concentration and negative ER status [93]. However, further analysis needs to be performed because the sample size was very small and they did not adjust or stratify by BMI.

Our findings are congruent with previously observed altered T3 and T4 measurements in diseases such as BC [9]. In those circumstances, there is dysregulation of thyrotrophic feedback control [9], in which T3 and/or T4 are at unusual levels, but the thyroid gland does not appear to be dysfunctional. Thus, the lower levels of T3 and higher levels of T4 in BC cases may be due to the effect of BC on thyroid function rather than T3 and T4 acting as risk factors for BC. If so, these findings may still be of interest to understand whether the levels of T3 and T4 could be related to tumor stage or have other implications for prognosis.

Our findings need to be replicated in other studies, including those with larger sample sizes and to investigate other possible mechanisms by which the association between T4 and BC is potentially modified by BMI in premenopausal and postmenopausal women. In particular, prospective cohort studies in which T3 and T4 are collected prior to cancer diagnosis may be helpful in understanding the causal relationship between BC and thyroid hormones. In addition, a prospective study may also help to improve understanding of the relationship among thyroid hormones, BC, and obesity.

To the best of our knowledge, this is the first study that has evaluated the effect modification by BMI of the relationship between thyroid hormones and BC, both in premenopausal and postmenopausal women. The results of the present study open a new line of research with which to evaluate the effect modification by obesity of the association between thyroid hormones and BC.

Conclusions

There is a strong association between BC and serum concentrations of TT3 and TT4; the latter differed by BMI and menopausal status. This needs to be further investigated to understand why it happens and how important it is to consider these alterations in treatment.

Thyroid hormones and breast cancer association according to menopausal status and body...

107

Abbreviations

BC: Breast cancer; bFGF: Fibroblast growth factor; BIC: Bayesian information criterion; BMI: Body mass index; CAMA: Risk factors for breast cancer in Mexico: mammographic patterns, C peptide, and growth factors, a multicenter study; E2: 17β-estradiol; ER: Estrogen receptor; FT3: Free triiodothyronine; FT4: Free thyroxine; HER2: Human epidermal growth factor receptor 2; IMSS: Instituto Mexicano de Seguro Social; ISSSTE: Instituto de Seguridad y Servicios Sociales de los Trabajadores del Estado; MAPK: Mitogen-activated protein kinase; OR: Odds ratio; PR: Progesterone receptor; RIC: Interquartile range; SS: Secretaría de Salud; T3: Triiodothyronine; T4: Thyroxine; TBG: Thyroid binding globulin; Tg: Thyroglobulin; Tg Ab: Thyroglobulin antibodies; TPO Ab: Thyroperoxidase antibodies; TSH: Thyroid stimulating hormone; TT3: Total triiodothyronine; TT4: Total thyroxine; VEGF: Vascular endothelial growth factor; WHO: World Health Organization; WHR: Waist-to-hip ratio

Acknowledgments

We would like to acknowledge CONACyT (CONACyT-SALUD-2002 C01-7462) y DGPOP 2011 (Dirección General de Programación Organización y Presupuesto, Ejercicio fiscal 2011, Ramo 12 Salud) for the financial support provided for this work and all physicians responsible for the project in the different participating hospitals: Dr Germán Castelazo (IMSS, Ciudad de México, DF), Dr Sinhué Barroso Bravo (IMSS, Ciudad de México, DF), Dr Joaquín Zarco Méndez (ISSSTE, Ciudad de México, DF), Dr Jesús Pablo Esparza Cano (IMSS, Monterrey, Nuevo León), Dr Heriberto Fabela (IMSS, Monterrey, Nuevo León), Dr Fausto Hernández Morales (ISSSTE, Veracruz, Veracruz), Dr Pedro Coronel Brizio (CECAN SS, Xalapa, Veracruz) and Dr Vicente A Saldaña Quiroz (IMSS, Veracruz, Veracruz).

Funding

This work was funded by the National Council of Science and Technology (grant CONACyT-SALUD-2002 C01-7462) and DGPOP 2011, Dirección General de Programación Organización y Presupuesto, Ejercicio fiscal 2011, Ramo 12 Salud.

Authors' contributions

COO and GTM conceived the study, interpreted the data, and wrote the manuscript. COO, GTM, and AALL were involved with collection of data. COO carried out all data analysis. FMR and EPR facilitated the contact with patients. COO, AUA, AALL, FMR, CEGA, MLHB, EZ, LAS, EPR, and GTM were all involved in data interpretation, critical revisions of the manuscript, and approval of the final version.

Competing interests

The authors declare that they have no competing interests.
The views expressed in this manuscript are those of the authors and do not necessarily represent the views of the National Heart, Lung, and Blood Institute; the National Institutes of Health; or the U.S. Department of Health and Human Services.

Author details

[1]Universidad Autónoma de San Luis Potosí, Facultad de Enfermería y Nutrición, Niño Artillero #130, Zona Universitaria, C.P. 78240 San Luis Potosí, S.L.P., México. [2]Red de Apoyo a la Investigación, Universidad Nacional Autónoma de México-Instituto Nacional de Ciencias Médicas y Nutrición Salvador Zubirán, calle Vasco de Quiroga No. 15, Col. Belisario Domínguez Sección XVI, Del. Tlalpan, C.P. 14080 Ciudad de México, México. [3]Centro de Investigación en Salud Poblacional, Instituto Nacional de Salud Pública, Av. Universidad No. 655, Col. Santa María Ahuacatitlán, Cuernavaca C.P. 62100, Morelos, México. [4]Hospital de Ginecología y Obstetricia No. 4 Luis Castelazo Ayala, Instituto Mexicano del Seguro Social, Avenida Río Magdalena No. 289, Col. Tizapán, San Angel, Ciudad de México C.P. 01090, México. [5]Department of Medicine, Division of General Internal Medicine, Institute for Human Genetics, Helen Diller Family Comprehensive Cancer Center, University of California, San Francisco, 1450 3rd St, San Francisco, CA 94143, USA. [6]Department of Epidemiology and Biostatistics, Helen Diller Family Comprehensive Cancer Center, University of California, San Francisco, 1450 3rd St, San Francisco, CA 94143, USA. [7]National Heart, Lung, and Blood Institute at the National Institutes of Health, 6701 Rockledge, Room 10188, Bethesda, MD 20892, USA. [8]Hospital Universitario "Dr José Eleuterio González". Madero y Dr. Aguirre Pequeño, Col. Mitras, C.P. 64460 Monterrey, N.L., México. [9]Instituto Nacional de Salud Pública, Centro de Investigación en Salud Poblacional, Avenida Universidad 655, Col. Santa María Ahuacatitlán, C.P. 62100 Cuernavaca, Morelos, México.

References

1. Tosovic A, Becker C, Bondeson AG, Bondeson L, Ericsson UB, Malm J, et al. Prospectively measured thyroid hormones and thyroid peroxidase antibodies in relation to breast cancer risk. Int J Cancer. 2012;131:2126–33.
2. Tosovic A, Bondeson AG, Bondeson L, Ericsson UB, Malm J, Manjer J. Prospectively measured triiodothyronine levels are positively associated with breast cancer risk in postmenopausal women. Breast Cancer Res. 2010;12:R33.
3. Davis PJ, Goglia F, Leonard JL. Nongenomic actions of thyroid hormone. Nat Rev Endocrinol. 2016;12:111–21.
4. Meng R, Tang HY, Westfall J, London D, Cao JH, Mousa SA, et al. Crosstalk between integrin alphavbeta3 and estrogen receptor-alpha is involved in thyroid hormone-induced proliferation in human lung carcinoma cells. PLoS One. 2011;6:e27547.
5. Lin HY, Sun M, Tang HY, Lin C, Luidens MK, Mousa SA, et al. L-thyroxine vs. 3,5,3'-triiodo-L-thyronine and cell proliferation: activation of mitogen-activated protein kinase and phosphatidylinositol 3-kinase. Am J Physiol Cell Physiol. 2009;296:C980–91.
6. Nogueira CR, Brentani MM. Triiodothyronine mimics the effects of estrogen in breast cancer cell lines. J Steroid Biochem Mol Biol. 1996;59:271–9.
7. Cestari SH, Figueiredo NB, Conde SJ, Clara S, Katayama ML, Padovani CR, et al. Influence of estradiol and triiodothyronine on breast cancer cell lines proliferation and expression of estrogen and thyroid hormone receptors. Arq Bras Endocrinol Metabol. 2009;53:859–64.
8. Hall LC, Salazar EP, Kane SR, Liu N. Effects of thyroid hormones on human breast cancer cell proliferation. J Steroid Biochem Mol Biol. 2008;109:57–66.
9. McIver B, Gorman CA. Euthyroid sick syndrome: an overview. Thyroid. 1997; 7:125–32.
10. Reinehr T. Obesity and thyroid function. Mol Cell Endocrinol. 2010;316:165–71.
11. Longhi S, Radetti G. Thyroid function and obesity. J Clin Res Pediatr Endocrinol. 2013;5(Suppl 1):40–4.
12. Obesity and overweight. 2018. [http://www.who.int/mediacentre/factsheets/fs311/en/]. Accessed 19 July 2018.
13. Hernández Ávila M, Rivera Dommarco J, Shamah Levy T, Cuevas Nasu L, Gómez Acosta L, Gaona Pineda E, Romero Martínez M, Méndez Gómez-Humarán I, Saturno Hernández P, Villalpando Hernández S, et al. Encuesta Nacional de Salud y Nutrición de Medio Camino 2016 (ENSANUT 2016). Instituto Nacional de Salud Pública; 2016. http://promocion.salud.gob.mx/dgps/descargas1/doctos_2016/ensanut_mc_2016-310oct.pdf. Accessed 19 July 2018.
14. Renehan AG, Tyson M, Egger M, Heller RF, Zwahlen M. Body-mass index and incidence of cancer: a systematic review and meta-analysis of prospective observational studies. Lancet. 2008;371:569–78.
15. Arnold M, Pandeya N, Byrnes G, Renehan AG, Stevens GA, Ezzati M, et al. Global burden of cancer attributable to high body-mass index in 2012: a population-based study. Lancet Oncol. 2015;16:36–46.

16. Cheraghi Z, Poorolajal J, Hashem T, Esmailnasab N, Doosti IA. Effect of body mass index on breast cancer during premenopausal and postmenopausal periods: a meta-analysis. PLoS One. 2012;7:e51446.

17. Feng YH. The association between obesity and gynecological cancer. Gynecology and Minimally Invasive Therapy. 2015;4:102–5.

18. Picon-Ruiz M, Morata-Tarifa C, Valle-Goffin JJ, Friedman ER, Slingerland JM. Obesity and adverse breast cancer risk and outcome: Mechanistic insights and strategies for intervention. CA Cancer J Clin. 2017;67:378–97.

19. Kyrgiou M, Kalliala I, Markozannes G, Gunter MJ, Paraskevaidis E, Gabra H, et al. Adiposity and cancer at major anatomical sites: umbrella review of the literature. BMJ. 2017;356:j477.

20. Harvie M, Hooper L, Howell A. Central obesity and breast cancer risk: a systematic review. Obes Rev. 2003;4:157–73.

21. Palmer JR, Adams-Campbell LL, Boggs DA, Wise LA, Rosenberg L. A prospective study of body size and breast cancer in black women. Cancer Epidemiol Biomarkers Prev. 2007;16:1795–802.

22. Slattery ML, Sweeney C, Edwards S, Herrick J, Baumgartner K, Wolff R, et al. Body size, weight change, fat distribution and breast cancer risk in Hispanic and non-Hispanic white women. Breast Cancer Res Treat. 2007;102:85–101.

23. Van Den Brandt PA, Spiegelman D, Yaun S-S, Adami H-O, Beeson L, Folsom AR, et al. Pooled analysis of prospective cohort studies on height, weight, and breast cancer risk. Am J Epidemiol. 2000;152:514–27.

24. Berstad P, Coates RJ, Bernstein L, Folger SG, Malone KE, Marchbanks PA, et al. A case-control study of body mass index and breast cancer risk in white and African-American women. Cancer epidemiology, biomarkers & prevention: a publication of the American Association for Cancer Research, cosponsored by the American Society of Preventive Oncology. 2010;19:1532–44.

25. Ng EH, Gao F, Ji CY, Ho GH, Soo KC. Risk factors for breast carcinoma in Singaporean Chinese women: the role of central obesity. Cancer. 1997;80:725–31.

26. Ogundiran TO, Huo D, Adenipekun A, Campbell O, Oyesegun R, Akang E, et al. Case-control study of body size and breast cancer risk in Nigerian women. Am J Epidemiol. 2010;172:682–90.

27. Harris H, Willett W, Terry K, Michels K. Body fat distribution and risk of premenopausal breast cancer in the Nurses' Health Study II. J Natl Cancer Inst. 2011;103:273–8.

28. La Vecchia C, Giordano SH, Hortobagyi GN, Chabner B. Overweight, obesity, diabetes, and risk of breast cancer: interlocking pieces of the puzzle. Oncologist. 2011;16:726–9.

29. World Cancer Research Fund/American Institute for Cancer Research: Continuous update project report: diet, nutrition, physical activity and breast cancer; 2017.

30. Chow LWC, Lui KL, Chan JCY, Chan TC, Ho PK, Lee WY, et al. Association between body mass index and risk of formation of breast cancer in Chinese women. Asian J Surg. 2005;28:179–84.

31. Guo Y, Warren Andersen S, Shu XO, Michailidou K, Bolla MK, Wang Q, et al. Genetically predicted body mass index and breast cancer risk: Mendelian randomization analyses of data from 145,000 women of European descent. PLoS Med. 2016;13:e1002105.

32. Amadou A, Hainaut P, Romieu I. Role of obesity in the risk of breast cancer: lessons from anthropometry. J Oncol. 2013;2013:906495.

33. Trayhurn P. Endocrine and signalling role of adipose tissue: new perspectives on fat. Acta Physiol Scand. 2005;184:285–93.

34. Ahima RS, Flier JS. Adipose tissue as an endocrine organ. Trends Endocrinol Metab. 2000;11:327–32.

35. Shon HS, Jung ED, Kim SH, Lee JH. Free T4 is negatively correlated with body mass index in euthyroid women. Korean J Intern Med. 2008;23:53–7.

36. Knudsen N, Laurberg P, Rasmussen LB, Bulow I, Perrild H, Ovesen L, et al. Small differences in thyroid function may be important for body mass index and the occurrence of obesity in the population. J Clin Endocrinol Metab. 2005;90:4019–24.

37. Makepeace AE, Bremner AP, O'Leary P, Leedman PJ, Feddema P, Michelangeli V, et al. Significant inverse relationship between serum free T4 concentration and body mass index in euthyroid subjects: differences between smokers and nonsmokers. Clin Endocrinol. 2008;69:648–52.

38. Guan B, Chen Y, Yang J, Yang W, Wang C. Effect of bariatric surgery on thyroid function in obese patients: a systematic review and meta-analysis. Obes Surg. 2017;27:3292–305.

39. Nam JS, Cho M, Park JS, Ahn CW, Cha BS, Lee EJ, et al. Triiodothyronine level predicts visceral obesity and atherosclerosis in euthyroid, overweight and obese subjects: T3 and visceral obesity. Obes Res Clin Pract. 2010;4: e247–342.

40. Montoya-Morales DS, de los Angeles Tapia-Gonzalez M, Alamilla-Lugo L, Sosa-Caballero A, Munoz-Solis A, Jimenez-Sanchez M. Alterations of the thyroid function in patients with morbid obesity. Rev Med Inst Mex Seguro Soc. 2015;53(Suppl 1):S18–22.

41. Kumar HK, Yadav RK, Prajapati J, Reddy CV, Raghunath M, Modi KD. Association between thyroid hormones, insulin resistance, and metabolic syndrome. Saudi Med J. 2009;30:907–11.

42. Angeles-Llerenas A, Ortega-Olvera C, Perez-Rodriguez E, Esparza-Cano JP, Lazcano-Ponce E, Romieu I, et al. Moderate physical activity and breast cancer risk: the effect of menopausal status. Cancer Causes Control. 2010;21:577–86.

43. Fejerman L, Romieu I, John EM, Lazcano-Ponce E, Huntsman S, Beckman KB, et al. European ancestry is positively associated with breast cancer risk in Mexican women. Cancer Epidemiol Biomark Prev. 2010;19:1074–82.

44. Fejerman L, John EM, Huntsman S, Beckman K, Choudhry S, Perez-Stable E, et al. Genetic ancestry and risk of breast cancer among U.S. Latinas. Cancer Res. 2008;68:9723–8.

45. Lohmann TG, Roche AF, Martorell R. Anthropometric standardization reference manual. Champaign: Human Kinetics Books; 1988.

46. Osuna-Ramírez I, Hernández-Prado B, Campuzano JC, Salmerón J. Indice de masa corporal y percepción de la imagen corporal en una población adulta mexicana: la precisión del autorreporte. Salud Publica Mex. 2006;48:94–103.

47. Nagin DS. Analyzing developmental trajectories: a semiparametric, group-based approach. Psychol Methods. 1999;4:139–57.

48. Amadou A, Torres Mejia G, Fagherazzi G, Ortega C, Angeles-Llerenas A, Chajes V, et al. Anthropometry, silhouette trajectory, and risk of breast cancer in Mexican women. Am J Prev Med. 2014;46:S52–64.

49. Hernandez-Avila M, Romieu I, Parra S, Hernandez-Avila J, Madrigal H, Willett W. Validity and reproducibility of a food frequency questionnaire to assess dietary intake of women living in Mexico City. Salud Publica Mex. 1998;40: 133–40.

50. Romieu I, Parra S, Hernandez JF, Madrigal H, Willett W, Hernandez M. Questionnaire assessment of antioxidants and retinol intakes in Mexican women. Arch Med Res. 1999;30:224–39.

51. Morales de León J, Bourges Rodríguez H, Camacho Parra M. Tables of composition of Mexican foods and food products (Condensed version 2015). Instituto Nacional de Ciencias Médicas y Nutrición Salvador Zubirán. 2016. http://www.innsz.mx/2017/Tablas/index.html#page/1. Accessed 19 July 2018.

52. Food Composition Databases. United States Department of Agriculture, Maryland. 2008. https://www.ars.usda.gov/northeast-area/beltsville-md-bhnrc/beltsville-human-nutrition-researchcenter/nutrient-data-laboratory/docs/usda-national-nutrient-database-for-standard-reference/. Accessed 19 July 2018.

53. Sallis JF, Haskell WL, Wood PD, Fortmann SP, Rogers T, Blair SN, et al. Physical activity assessment methodology in the Five-City project. Am J Epidemiol. 1985;121:91–106.

54. Martinez-González M, Sánchez-Villegas A, Faulin-Fajardo J. Bioestadistica Amigable. 2da ed. España: Diaz de Santos; 2006.

55. Hosmer D, Lemeshow S. Applied logistic regression. 2nd ed: John Wiley & Sons; 2000.

56. Willett W. Nutritional epidemiology. 2nd ed. New York: Oxford University Press; 1998.

57. Qu HQ, Li Q, Lu Y, Fisher-Hoch SP, McCormick JB. Translational genomic medicine: common metabolic traits and ancestral components of Mexican Americans. J Med Genet. 2012;49:544–5.

58. Bruning PF, Bonfrer JM, Hart AA, van Noord PA, van der Hoeven H, Collette HJ, et al. Body measurements, estrogen availability and the risk of human breast cancer: a case-control study. Int J Cancer. 1992;51:14–9.

59. Franceschi S, Favero A, La Vecchia C, Baron AE, Negri E, Dal Maso L, et al. Body size indices and breast cancer risk before and after menopause. Int J Cancer. 1996;67:181–6.

60. Harris RE, Namboodiri KK, Wynder EL. Breast cancer risk: effects of estrogen replacement therapy and body mass. J Natl Cancer Inst. 1992;84:1575–82.

61. Huang Z, Hankinson SE, Colditz GA, Stampfer MJ, Hunter DJ, Manson JE, et al. Dual effects of weight and weight gain on breast cancer risk. JAMA. 1997;278:1407–11.

62. Kaaks R, Van Noord PA, Den Tonkelaar I, Peeters PH, Riboli E, Grobbee DE. Breast-cancer incidence in relation to height, weight and body-fat distribution in the Dutch "DOM" cohort. Int J Cancer. 1998;76:647–51.

63. Lahmann PH, Lissner L, Gullberg B, Olsson H, Berglund G. A prospective study of adiposity and postmenopausal breast cancer risk: the Malmo diet and cancer study. Int J Cancer. 2003;103:246–52.

64. Michels KB, Terry KL, Willett WC. Longitudinal study on the role of body size in premenopausal breast cancer. Arch Intern Med. 2006;166:2395–402.

65. Morimoto LM, White E, Chen Z, Chlebowski RT, Hays J, Kuller L, et al. Obesity, body size, and risk of postmenopausal breast cancer: the Women's Health Initiative (United States). Cancer Causes Control. 2002;13:741–51.

66. Sonnenschein E, Toniolo P, Terry MB, Bruning PF, Kato I, Koenig KL, et al. Body fat distribution and obesity in pre- and postmenopausal breast cancer. Int J Epidemiol. 1999;28:1026–31.

67. Tehard B, Lahmann PH, Riboli E, Clavel-Chapelon F. Anthropometry, breast cancer and menopausal status: use of repeated measurements over 10 years of follow-up-results of the French E3N women's cohort study. Int J Cancer. 2004;111:264–9.

68. Vatten LJ, Kvinnsland S. Prospective study of height, body mass index and risk of breast cancer. Acta Oncol. 1992;31:195–200.

69. Weiderpass E, Braaten T, Magnusson C, Kumle M, Vainio H, Lund E, et al. A prospective study of body size in different periods of life and risk of premenopausal breast cancer. Cancer Epidemiol Biomark Prev. 2004;13:1121–7.

70. Friedenreich CM. Review of anthropometric factors and breast cancer risk. Eur J Cancer Prev. 2001;10:15–32.

71. Tehard B, Clavel-Chapelon F. Several anthropometric measurements and breast cancer risk: results of the E3N cohort study. Int J Obes. 2006;30:156–63.

72. Bouchardy C, Le MG, Hill C. Risk factors for breast cancer according to age at diagnosis in a French case-control study. J Clin Epidemiol. 1990;43:267–75.

73. Hu YH, Nagata C, Shimizu H, Kaneda N, Kashiki Y. Association of body mass index, physical activity, and reproductive histories with breast cancer: a case-control study in Gifu, Japan. Breast Cancer Res Treat. 1997;43:65–72.

74. London SJ, Colditz GA, Stampfer MJ, Willett WC, Rosner B, Speizer FE. Prospective study of relative weight, height, and risk of breast cancer. JAMA. 1989;262:2853–8.

75. Swanson CA, Brinton LA, Taylor PR, Licitra LM, Ziegler RG, Schairer C. Body size and breast cancer risk assessed in women participating in the breast cancer detection demonstration project. Am J Epidemiol. 1989;130:1133–41.

76. Tornberg SA, Holm LE, Carstensen JM. Breast cancer risk in relation to serum cholesterol, serum beta-lipoprotein, height, weight, and blood pressure. Acta Oncol. 1988;27:31–7.

77. Tretli S. Height and weight in relation to breast cancer morbidity and mortality. A prospective study of 570,000 women in Norway. Int J Cancer. 1989;44:23–30.

78. Vatten LJ, Kvinnsland S. Body mass index and risk of breast cancer. A prospective study of 23,826 Norwegian women. Int J Cancer. 1990;45:440–4.

79. Willett WC, Browne ML, Bain C, Lipnick RJ, Stampfer MJ, Rosner B, et al. Relative weight and risk of breast cancer among premenopausal women. Am J Epidemiol. 1985;122:731–40.

80. Huang J, Jin L, Ji G, Xing L, Xu C, Xiong X, et al. Implication from thyroid function decreasing during chemotherapy in breast cancer patients: chemosensitization role of triiodothyronine. BMC Cancer. 2013;13:334.

81. Yang XR, Chang-Claude J, Goode EL, Couch FJ, Nevanlinna H, Milne RL, et al. Associations of breast cancer risk factors with tumor subtypes: a pooled analysis from the Breast Cancer Association consortium studies. J Natl Cancer Inst. 2011;103:250–63.

82. Tang HY, Lin HY, Zhang S, Davis FB, Davis PJ. Thyroid hormone causes mitogen-activated protein kinase-dependent phosphorylation of the nuclear estrogen receptor. Endocrinology. 2004;145:3265–72.

83. Li H, Sun X, Miller E, Wang Q, Tao P, Liu L, et al. BMI, reproductive factors, and breast cancer molecular subtypes: a case-control study and meta-analysis. J Epidemiol. 2017;27:143–51.

84. Lin HY, Davis FB, Gordinier JK, Martino LJ, Davis PJ. Thyroid hormone induces activation of mitogen-activated protein kinase in cultured cells. Am J Phys. 1999;276:C1014–24.

85. Davis PJ, Shih A, Lin HY, Martino LJ, Davis FB. Thyroxine promotes association of mitogen-activated protein kinase and nuclear thyroid hormone receptor (TR) and causes serine phosphorylation of TR. J Biol Chem. 2000;275:38032–9.

86. Shih A, Lin HY, Davis FB, Davis PJ. Thyroid hormone promotes serine phosphorylation of p53 by mitogen-activated protein kinase. Biochemistry. 2001;40:2870–8.

87. Lin HY, Shih A, Davis FB, Davis PJ. Thyroid hormone promotes the phosphorylation of STAT3 and potentiates the action of epidermal growth factor in cultured cells. Biochem J. 1999;338(Pt 2):427–32.

88. Kawai M, Malone KE, Tang MT, Li CI. Height, body mass index (BMI), BMI change, and the risk of estrogen receptor-positive, HER2-positive, and triple-negative breast cancer among women ages 20 to 44 years. Cancer. 2014;120:1548–56.

89. Quigley DA, Tahiri A, Luders T, Riis MH, Balmain A, Borresen-Dale AL, et al. Age, estrogen, and immune response in breast adenocarcinoma and adjacent normal tissue. Oncoimmunology. 2017;6:e1356142.

90. Angelousi A, Diamanti-Kandarakis E, Zapanti E, Nonni A, Ktenas E, Mantzou A, et al. Is there an association between thyroid function abnormalities and breast cancer? Arch Endocrinol Metab. 2017;61:54–61.

91. Mendel CM, Weisiger RA, Jones AL, Cavalieri RR. Thyroid hormone-binding proteins in plasma facilitate uniform distribution of thyroxine within tissues: a perfused rat liver study. Endocrinology. 1987;120:1742–9.

92. Utiger RD. Estrogen, thyroxine binding in serum, and thyroxine therapy. N Engl J Med. 2001;344:1784–5.

93. Tosovic A, Bondeson AG, Bondeson L, Ericsson UB, Manjer J. T3 levels in relation to prognostic factors in breast cancer: a population-based prospective cohort study. BMC Cancer. 2014;14:536.

9

Novel 18-gene signature for predicting relapse in ER-positive, HER2-negative breast cancer

Richard Buus[1,2]* [iD], Belinda Yeo[3,4], Adam R. Brentnall[5], Marie Klintman[6], Maggie Chon U. Cheang[7], Komel Khabra[8], Ivana Sestak[5], Qiong Gao[1], Jack Cuzick[5] and Mitch Dowsett[1,2]

Abstract

Background: Several prognostic signatures for early oestrogen receptor-positive (ER+) breast cancer have been established with a 10-year follow-up. We tested the hypothesis that signatures optimised for 0–5-year and 5–10-year follow-up separately are more prognostic than a single signature optimised for 10 years.

Methods: Genes previously identified as prognostic or associated with endocrine resistance were tested in publicly available microarray data set using Cox regression of 747 ER+/HER2− samples from post-menopausal patients treated with 5 years of endocrine therapy. RNA expression of the selected genes was assayed in primary ER+/HER2 − tumours from 948 post-menopausal patients treated with 5 years of anastrozole or tamoxifen in the TransATAC cohort. Prognostic signatures for 0–10, 0–5 and 5–10 years were derived using a penalised Cox regression (elastic net). Signature comparison was performed with likelihood ratio statistics. Validation was done by a case-control (POLAR) study in 422 samples derived from a cohort of 1449.

Results: Ninety-three genes were selected by the modelling of microarray data; 63 of these were significantly prognostic in TransATAC, most similarly across each time period. Contrary to our hypothesis, the derived early and late signatures were not significantly more prognostic than the 18-gene 10-year signature. The 18-gene 10-year signature was internally validated in the TransATAC validation set, showing prognostic information similar to that of Oncotype DX Recurrence Score, PAM50 risk of recurrence score, Breast Cancer Index and IHC4 (score based on four IHC markers), as well as in the external POLAR case-control set.

Conclusions: The derived 10-year signature predicts risk of metastasis in patients with ER+/HER2− breast cancer similar to commercial signatures. The hypothesis that early and late prognostic signatures are significantly more informative than a single signature was rejected.

Keywords: Breast cancer, Oestrogen receptor, Prognostic tests, Biomarkers, Late recurrence

Background

Five years of adjuvant endocrine therapy is standard treatment for patients with primary oestrogen receptor-positive (ER+) breast cancer, and it clearly improves prognosis [1]. Multiparametric molecular assays are increasingly used to estimate prognosis and guide treatment decisions of patients with primary ER+ breast cancer. These include the

Oncotype DX (OncotypeIQ/Genomic Health, Inc., Redwood City, CA, USA) Recurrence Score (RS) [2], Prosigna PAM50 (NanoString Technologies, Seattle, WA, USA) [3], Breast Cancer Index (BCI) [4], EndoPredict (Myriad Genetics, Zurich, Switzerland) [5] and IHC4 [6]. All of them have been evaluated in the TransATAC series of samples that were established from patients with ER+ primary breast cancer randomised to treatment with 5 years of anastrozole or tamoxifen in the ATAC (Arimidex, Tamoxifen, Alone or in Combination) trial [7]. It has become clear that, following surgery, the risk of recurrence in ER+ primary breast cancer is not constant, which is underlined by molecular

* Correspondence: richard.buus@icr.ac.uk; richard.buus@icr.ac.uk
[1]The Breast Cancer Now Toby Robins Research Centre at the Institute of Cancer Research, 237 Fulham Road, London SW3 6JB, UK
[2]Ralph Lauren Centre for Breast Cancer Research, Royal Marsden Hospital, London, UK
Full list of author information is available at the end of the article

differences. In TransATAC we have previously shown that the oestrogen module of RS was prognostic within 5 years of surgery (during endocrine therapy), however it became non-informative for recurrences beyond 5 years, thus weakening the overall prognostic value of RS [8]. In the same data set, patients with high ER expression by RT-PCR were twice as likely to have a relapse 5–10 years after surgery than within the first 5 years. Bianchini et al. reported risk stratification by integrating the mitotic kinase score (MKS) and an oestrogen receptor-related score (ERS), both based on genes constituting the proliferation and oestrogen modules of RS. Women with high MKS and ERS tumours were at greater risk of late recurrence [9]. More recently, improved risk estimation beyond 5 years by RS was reported when integrated with dichotomised ER expression assessed by RT-PCR [10].

Extending endocrine therapy beyond 5 years has been shown to reduce late-recurrence rate [11, 12], however those most likely to benefit from such therapy need to be identified. Although some of the widely used prognostic assays for ER+ patients have been shown to be prognostic for risk beyond 5 years [13–16], none of them have been optimised to quantify residual risk after 5 years free from recurrence, and their ability to predict late relapse varies substantially [17]. The different time-dependent performance of multiparametric molecular signatures indicates that molecular features of ER+ breast cancers may be identified to improve prediction of residual risk in order to spare those patients with significantly low risk of late recurrence from extended endocrine therapy.

We therefore hypothesised that prognostic signatures optimised specifically for the early (0–5 years) and late (5–10 years) follow-up periods, respectively, would be more prognostic than a single signature optimised for the whole 10-year follow-up period. To test this hypothesis, we developed time-dependent prognostic signatures in patient samples from the TransATAC series for early, late and 10-year follow-up periods. The prognostic performance was tested in an independent sample set and against commercial signatures already assessed in TransATAC. Our primary aim was to compare the prognostic value of the newly developed signature(s) added to Clinical Treatment Score (CTS) [6] with that of PAM50 risk of recurrence (ROR) based on subtype and proliferation added to CTS.

Methods

Patient cohorts

Our initial analysis drew from four published breast cancer cohorts (GSE6532, GSE9195, GSE17705, GSE26971) analysed on either of the Affymetrix Human Genome HG-U133A (GPL96) and HG-U133 Plus 2.0 (GPL570) microarray platforms (Affymetrix, Santa Clara, CA, USA). The two platforms shared 22,277 probes to which we restricted our analyses. This cohort had 747 unique patient samples that matched our selection criteria: ER+, HER2−, treated with 5 years of endocrine therapy, chemotherapy-naive, with information on either distant metastasis-free survival (DMFS) or relapse-free survival (RFS) available with a long follow-up. Details of the inclusion criteria are listed in Additional file 1: Methods, and a full list of samples included in the analysis is shown in Additional file 2: Table S1.

In the TransATAC cohort, RNA was available from 948 formalin-fixed, paraffin-embedded (FFPE) tumours from the ATAC trial, previously extracted by Genomic Health Inc. (GHI) [18]. Eligibility required hormone receptor-positive/HER2− disease, without chemotherapy treatment and at least 500 ng of RNA available. One hundred eighty-three recurrence events were recorded for this cohort. This study was approved by the South-East London Research Ethics Committee, and all patients gave informed consent.

The POLAR (Predictors Of early versus LAte Recurrence in ER+ breast cancer) samples were identified from archives of Royal Marsden Hospital (RMH), London, UK, and Lund University Hospital Biobank, Lund, Sweden. Eligibility criteria were patients with ER+/HER2− early breast cancer diagnosed between January 2000 and December 2004, treated with curative intent and with a follow-up data cut-off at May 2014. Patients must have received 5 years of adjuvant endocrine therapy (unless relapse occurred within this time); (neo)-adjuvant chemotherapy was permitted. A 422-sample case-control design was used; control subjects were randomly selected according to matching criteria from among the remaining cohort of patients who did not relapse during follow-up. The total number of patients drawn upon was 1449. The following four matching criteria were used in this study: (1) age at diagnosis (< 50 or > 50 years), (2) Nottingham Prognostic Index (NPI) category (< 3.4, 3.4–5.4, > 5.4), (3) type of adjuvant endocrine therapy (tamoxifen only vs. any aromatase inhibitor [AI]) and (4) chemotherapy use (yes or no). Two-hundred forty-seven recurrence events were recorded. The POLAR study was approved by the RMH Research Ethics Committee (CCR 4122) and the ethics committee of Lund University Hospital (LU 240-01).

Study endpoints

The primary endpoint was time to any recurrence, which was defined as locoregional (ipsilateral breast, contralateral breast and regional lymph nodes) and/or distant recurrence. Secondary endpoint was time to distant recurrence, which was the time from diagnosis until metastasis from the primary tumour at distant organs, excluding contralateral disease and locoregional and ipsilateral recurrences. Death before recurrence was treated as a censoring event for both endpoints.

Analytic procedures

In the microarray data set, 454 probes representing 454 genes (Additional file 2: Table S3) were analysed at univariate level; those significant in univariate analyses in a particular setting were entered into multivariable analyses. Further details are provided in Additional file 1: Methods.

For TransATAC, RNA was extracted by GHI for the RS study [18]. RNA (100 ng) was used with the nCounter platform (NanoString Technologies) to assay the 93 endogenous and 7 reference genes selected in the process of the microarray expression analysis in 948 TransATAC samples.

For POLAR, RNA was extracted from three 3×10-µm unstained sections with more than 40% tumour cellularity using the RNeasy FFPE kit (Qiagen, Hilden, Germany) according to the manufacturer's instructions. RNA was quantified by using a NanoDrop instrument (Thermo Fisher Scientific, Wilmington, DE, USA). Between 50 and 200 ng of RNA was used to profile the expression of 27 endogenous and 5 reference genes with the NanoString nCounter.

NanoString expression data were background-corrected by subtracting the mean of the eight negative control probes, normalised with the geometric mean of five reference genes that had a correlation of Pearson's $r > 0.8$ with all endogenous genes. The data set was then logarithmically (base 2) transformed and z-score-transformed. The *KIF20A* gene was detected in $< 10\%$ of samples in the TransATAC cohort and was removed from the data set. CTS, which carries information on tumour size, nodal status, grade, age and type of endocrine therapy, was calculated as published previously [6].

We trained separate early, late and 10-year signatures by performing elastic net analysis in the TransATAC training cohort. Our objective was to test if the early and late signatures had statistically significantly more prognostic power than the 10-year signature. If so, we would test the validity of the early and late signatures in the non-chemotherapy-treated subpopulation of POLAR and also test their performance in the chemotherapy-treated POLAR cohort. If the early and late signatures were not statistically significantly more prognostic than the overall signature, we would test the validity of the overall signature in the chemotherapy-naive POLAR group and explore its performance in the chemotherapy-treated POLAR group.

Statistical analyses of the cohort with microarray data were carried out at the Institute of Cancer Research (ICR) using R version 3.03 software (R Foundation for Statistical Computing, Vienna, Austria). Statistical analyses using the TransATAC cohort were performed at Queen Mary University of London with STATA version 13.1 (StataCorp, College Station, TX, USA) and R version 3.0.3 software. Statistical work on POLAR was carried out at RMH using the Statistical Analysis Plan version 2.0 and Prism

6.0c (GraphPad Software, La Jolla, CA, USA) software. Before data analysis took place, the statistical analysis plan for the TransATAC study was approved by the Long-term Anastrozole vs Tamoxifen Treatment Effects committee and that for the POLAR study was approved by the RMH Committee for Clinical Research, and these plans are described in Additional file 1: Methods. All statistical tests were two-sided.

Results

We performed the following steps in our study. We used publicly available microarray data to generate lists of prognostic genes to be analysed in the TransATAC cohort. We developed early, late and 10-year prognostic signatures in a training data set (two-thirds of TransATAC) while setting aside a test set (one-third of TransATAC) so that the performance of the newly trained signatures could be evaluated. This internal validation included comparison with commercial signatures of BCI, Oncotype DX RS, PAM50 ROR and IHC4. Finally, we conducted an external validation in the POLAR case-control sample set.

Candidate gene selection and microarray expression data analysis

In order to derive time-dependent prognostic signatures, we shortlisted 585 candidate genes representing proliferation, oestrogen signalling, immune infiltration and immune signalling. These genes were tested for prognostic significance in publicly available gene expression sets of ER+ endocrine therapy-treated breast cancer. A flowchart illustrating the approach is shown in Fig. 1. Sixty-seven genes of interest that are part of the PAM50, Oncotype DX RS, EndoPredict and BCI profilers were also included. Additional genes likely to be related to benefit from endocrine therapy were identified from 81 patients by re-analysing our previously published neoadjuvant endocrine therapy-treated set of samples [19] (https://www.synapse.org/#!Synapse:syn16243). From this dataset, we identified 164 candidate genes by examining correlation of individual gene expression from untreated biopsies with change in the following after 2 weeks of AI treatment: (1) Ki-67, (2) proliferation-associated gene cluster, (3) oestrogen-associated gene cluster, and (4) expression of the modified version of the Global Index of Dependence on Estrogen [20] genes. An additional 354 genes were selected on the basis of literature searches. Genes from published gene modules of the proliferation-associated gene cluster, oestrogen-associated gene cluster and inflammatory response signature [19], the tumour invasion/metastasis module (*PLAU*) [21] and IGG-14 module (immunoglobulin-gamma) [22] were also included. The complete list of candidate genes and the reason for their inclusion are detailed in Additional file 2: Table S1.

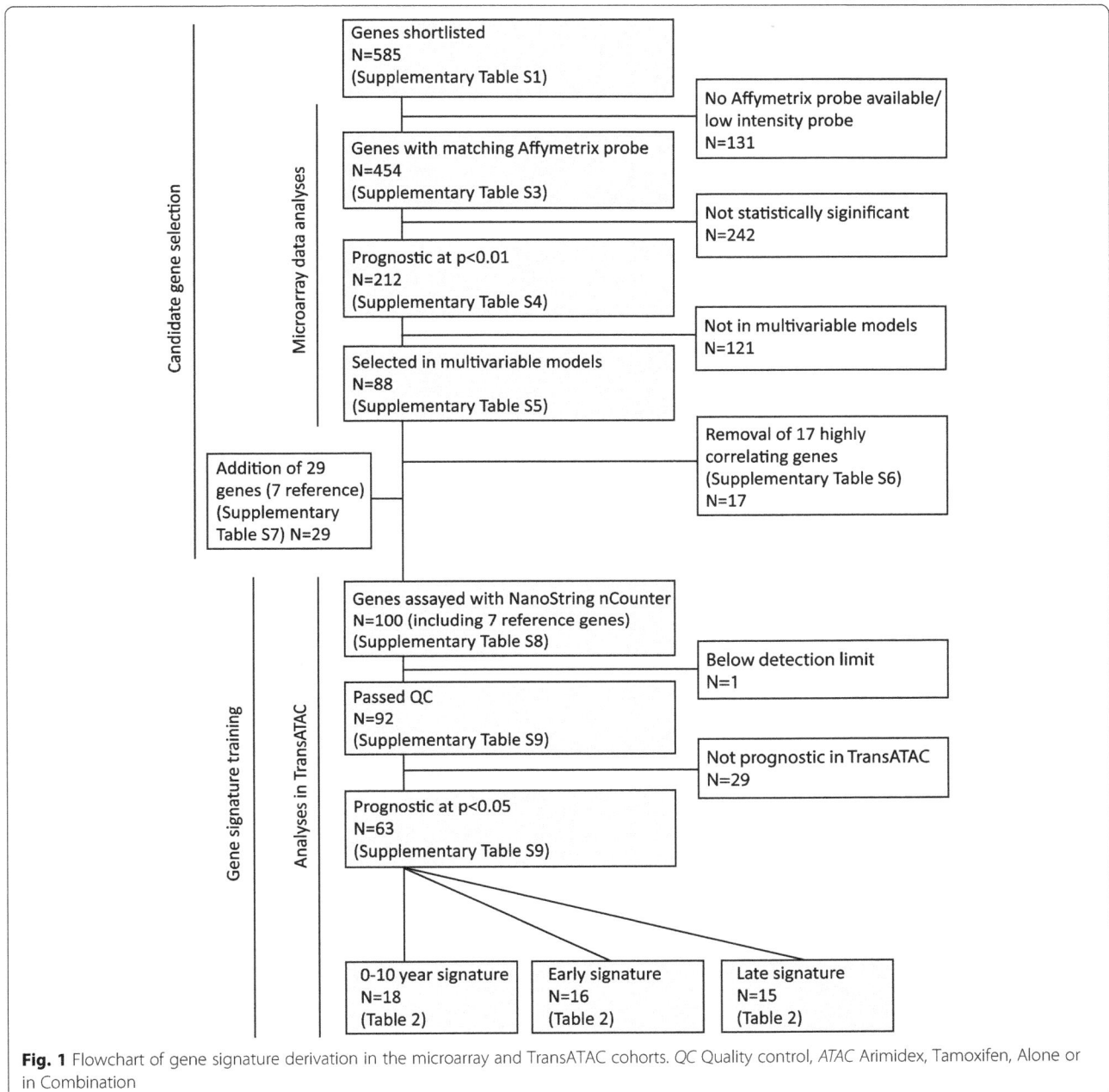

Fig. 1 Flowchart of gene signature derivation in the microarray and TransATAC cohorts. *QC* Quality control, *ATAC* Arimidex, Tamoxifen, Alone or in Combination

Seven hundred forty-seven samples from the microarray expression dataset were compiled from four publicly available breast cancer cohorts to investigate the relationship between genes and outcome (Additional file 2: Table S2) [5, 23–25]. Expression data were available for 454 genes (Additional file 2: Table S3). We performed univariate Cox proportional hazards regression analyses for early, late and 10-year follow-up periods using RFS and DMFS as endpoints, respectively (six analyses), that identified 212 genes that were significant at $p < 0.01$ in any of the analyses (Additional file 2: Table S4). Genes significantly prognostic in a particular time period were taken forward for

multivariable analyses performed by Cox proportional hazards regression with DMFS and RFS as endpoints, respectively, in the early, late and 10-year follow-up settings (six analyses). This resulted in 88 genes being selected in the models (Additional file 2: Table S5), of which 17 genes were removed owing to high correlation of expression with other candidates already selected (Additional file 2: Table S6). An additional 29 genes were added that included candidates without probes available in the microarray expression data analyses, some recently emerging candidates and also seven reference genes (Additional file 2: Table S7).

Expression profiling and signature building in TransATAC
Sample availability in TransATAC is shown in Fig. 2a. Expression data for the 100 selected genes (including housekeeping genes) (Additional file 2: Table S9) were obtained for 948 patient samples in TransATAC using the NanoString nCounter. We assessed the prognostic value of these molecular variables in TransATAC for early, late and 10-year time periods for RFS. Sixty-three genes were statistically significant in at least one of the time windows assessed (Additional file 2: Table S7, Additional file 3: Figure S1). We found different prognostic properties between early and late periods for 20 genes. Six genes were prognostic early but not in the late period (*CD79, IL6ST, LRRC48, MPZL1, PGR* and *PIGV*), and 14 genes were not significantly prognostic early but gained prognostic significance in the late setting (*ANP32E, ANXA1, CTSL2, EPB41L2, ESR1, FOXA1, ICOS, IL17RB, MMP9, MYCBP2, NR2F1, PDZK1, SLAMF8* and *TCF7L2*).

The TransATAC cohort was then randomly split into two-thirds (n = 634) training and one-third (n = 314) validation sets while ensuring that the recurrence rate

was similar in the two subgroups. Demographics for the training, validation and overall cohorts are presented in Table 1. We aimed to select prognostic variables independent of clinicopathological features that are commonly used for prognosis. To achieve this, on top of the 63 statistically significant genes in univariate analyses, CTS was also entered into multivariable selections for early, late and 10-year time-periods, respectively. Elastic net penalised Cox regression with leave-one-out cross-validation was used for feature selection in the TransATAC training set. CTS was selected in all three signatures in addition to 18 genes in the 10-year, 16 genes in the early, and 15 genes in the late follow-up analyses. The variables and their coefficients derived from the elastic net models are listed in Table 2. CTS had the highest coefficient in each of the time periods.

Comparison of time period-optimised prognostic signatures in TransATAC validation set
TransATAC was used to validate and compare the prognostic information of the three time period-dependent

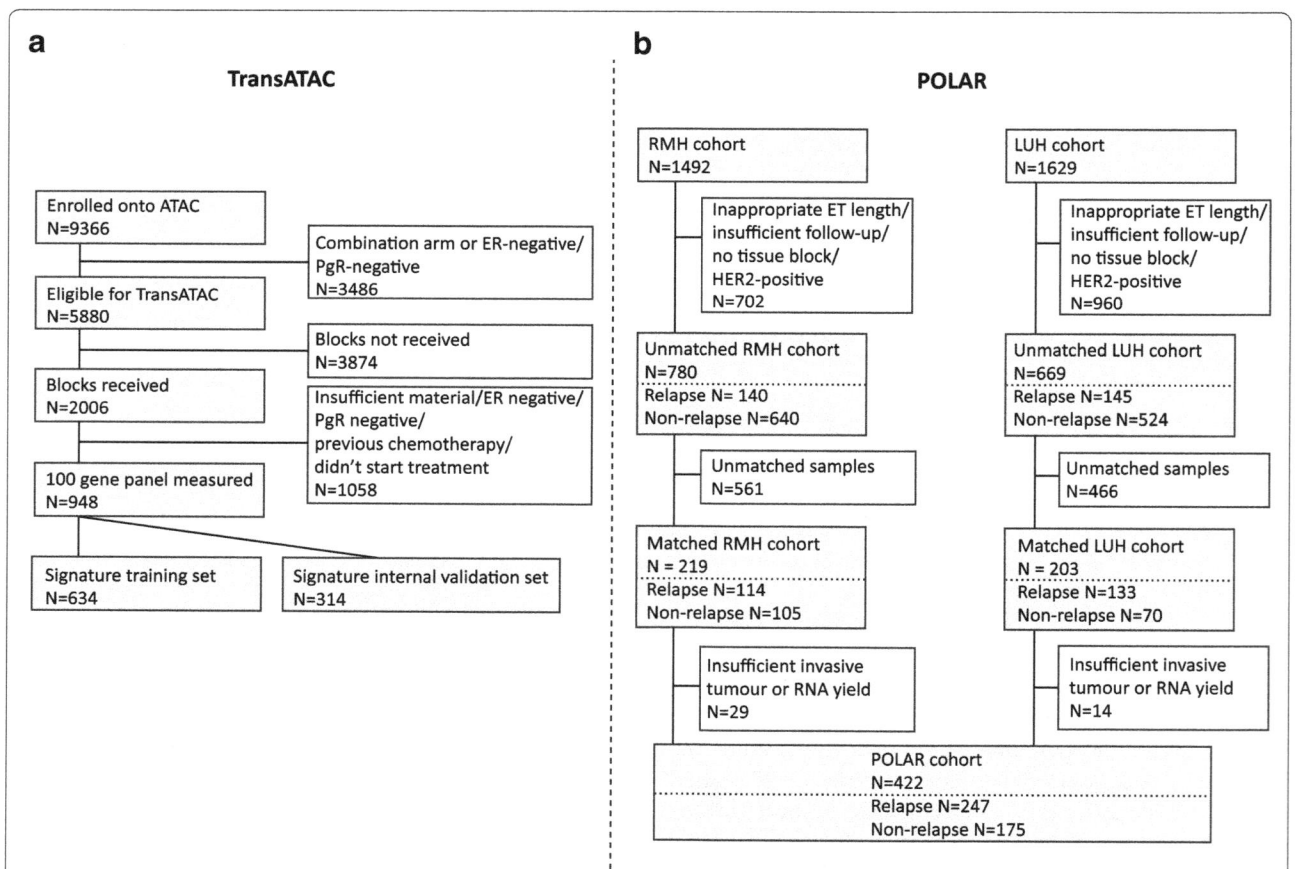

Fig. 2 Consolidated Standards of Reporting Trials (CONSORT) diagram of the availability of samples for analysis from (**a**) the ATAC trial and (**b**) the POLAR collection of samples. *POLAR* Molecular Predictors Of early versus LAte Recurrence in ER-positive breast cancer, *ATAC* Arimidex, Tamoxifen, Alone or in Combination, *ER* Oestrogen receptor, *PgR* Progesterone receptor, *RMH* Royal Marsden Hospital, *LUH* Lund University Hospital, *ET* Endocrine therapy, *HER2* Human epidermal growth factor receptor 2

Table 1 Demographics of TransATAC and POLAR cohorts

Patient group	TransATAC			POLAR								
				POLAR RMH			POLAR LUH			Total POLAR (RMH + LUH)		
	Training	Validation	Total	Cases	Controls	Total	Cases	Controls	Total	Cases	Controls	Total
Number of patients	634	314	948	114	105	219	133	70	203	247	175	422
Age at diagnosis, years[a]												
Mean, years	64	65	65	56	58	57	62	60	61	59	58	59
Median, years	64	64	64	54	58	56	61	58	61	58	58	58
Range, years	48–89	47–86	47–89	29–93	28–88	28–93	35–100	35–87	35–100	29–100	28–88	28–100
Tumour size												
< 2 cm	427 (67%)	207 (66%)	634 (67%)	40 (35%)	43 (41%)	83 (38%)	40 (30%)	27 (39%)	67 (33%)	80 (32%)	70 (40%)	150 (36%)
2–5 cm	194 (31%)	101 (32%)	295 (31%)	63 (55%)	54 (51%)	117 (53%)	89 (67%)	40 (57%)	129 (64%)	152 (62%)	94 (54%)	246 (58%)
> 5 cm	13 (2%)	6 (2%)	19 (2%)	11 (10%)	8 (8%)	19 (9%)	4 (3%)	3 (4%)	7 (3%)	15 (6%)	11 (6%)	26 (6%)
Grade												
1	177 (28%)	88 (28%)	265 (28%)	12 (11%)	14 (13%)	26 (12%)	9 (7%)	11 (16%)	20 (10%)	21 (9%)	25 (14%)	46 (11%)
2	368 (58%)	169 (54%)	537 (57%)	48 (42%)	52 (50%)	100 (46%)	72 (54%)	35 (50%)	107 (53%)	120 (49%)	87 (50%)	207 (49%)
3	89 (14%)	57 (18%)	146 (15%)	54 (47%)	39 (37%)	93 (42%)	52 (39%)	24 (34%)	76 (37%)	106 (43%)	63 (36%)	169 (40%)
Histological subtype												
IDC	492 (78%)	230 (73%)	722 (76%)	80 (70%)	75 (71%)	155 (71%)	104 (78%)	55 (79%)	159 (78%)	184 (74%)	130 (74%)	314 (74%)
ILC	86 (14%)	60 (19%)	146 (15%)	22 (19%)	18 (17%)	40 (18%)	27 (20%)	15 (21%)	42 (21%)	49 (20%)	33 (19%)	82 (19%)
Other	56 (9%)	24 (8%)	80 (8%)	12 (11%)	12 (11%)	24 (11%)	2 (2%)	0 (0%)	2 (1%)	14 (6%)	12 (7%)	26 (6%)
Nodal status												
Node negative	441 (70%)	224 (71%)	665 (70%)	60 (53%)	56 (53%)	116 (53%)	42 (32%)	29 (41%)	71 (35%)	102 (41%)	85 (49%)	187 (44%)
1–3 positive nodes	136 (22%)	63 (20%)	199 (21%)	25 (22%)	34 (32%)	59 (27%)	54 (41%)	31 (44%)	85 (42%)	79 (32%)	65 (37%)	144 (34%)
4 or more nodes	57 (9%)	27 (9%)	84 (9%)	29 (25%)	15 (14%)	44 (20%)	37 (28%)	10 (14%)	47 (23%)	66 (27%)	25 (14%)	91 (22%)
PgR												
Negative	114 (18%)	46 (15%)	160 (17%)	5 (4%)	7 (7%)	12 (5%)	25 (19%)	9 (13%)	34 (17%)	30 (%)	16 (%)	46 (11%)
Positive	513 (81%)	268 (85%)	781 (82%)	20 (18%)	23 (22%)	43 (20%)	102 (77%)	56 (80%)	158 (78%)	122 (%)	79 (%)	201 (48%)
Unknown	7 (1%)	–	7 (1%)	89 (78%)	75 (71%)	164 (75%)	6 (5%)	5 (7%)	11 (5%)	95 (%)	80 (%)	175 (41%)
NPI category[a]												
≤ 3.4	298 (47%)	140 (45%)	438 (46%)	25 (22%)	26 (25%)	51 (23%)	15 (11%)	13 (19%)	28 (14%)	40 (16%)	39 (22%)	79 (19%)
3.4–5.4	281 (44%)	147 (47%)	428 (45%)	49 (43%)	50 (48%)	99 (45%)	77 (58%)	42 (60%)	119 (59%)	126 (51%)	92 (53%)	218 (52%)
> 5.4	55 (9%)	27 (9%)	82 (9%)	40 (35%)	29 (28%)	69 (32%)	41 (31%)	15 (21%)	56 (28%)	81 (33%)	44 (25%)	125 (30%)
Endocrine therapy[a]												
Tamoxifen only	301 (47%)	163 (52%)	464 (49%)	80 (70%)	72 (69%)	152 (69%)	96 (72%)	50 (71%)	146 (72%)	176 (71%)	122 (70%)	298 (71%)
AI	333 (53%)	151 (48%)	484 (51%)	34 (30%)	33 (31%)	67 (31%)	37 (28%)	20 (29%)	57 (28%)	71 (29%)	53 (30%)	124 (29%)
Chemotherapy[a]												
No	634 (100%)	314 (100%)	948 (100%)	54 (47%)	49 (47%)	103 (47%)	94 (71%)	55 (79%)	149 (73%)	148 (60%)	104 (59%)	252 (60%)
Yes	0	0	0	60 (53%)	56 (53%)	116 (53%)	39 (29%)	15 (21%)	54 (27%)	99 (40%)	71 (41%)	170 (40%)

Abbreviations: AI Aromatase inhibitor, *IDC* Invasive ductal carcinoma, *ILC* Invasive lobular carcinoma, *PgR* Progesterone receptor, *NPI* Nottingham Prognostic Index, *RMH* Royal Marsden Hospital, *LUH* Lund University Hospital, *POLAR* Molecular Predictors Of early versus LAte Recurrence in ER+ breast cancer

[a] Denotes matching criteria in POLAR

Table 2 Variables and corresponding beta-coefficients of the time-dependent 10-year, early and late signatures

Variable	10-Year signature	Early signature	Late signature
ALDH1A1			−0.194
ANP32E	0.143	0.010	0.083
CRABP2	0.084	0.207	
CXCL12		−0.183	
CXCR4	0.142		0.056
EGFR			−0.030
ELF5	−0.046	−0.001	
FGF2	−0.178		−0.232
IGF1	−0.029	−0.017	
IGJ	−0.086	−0.037	−0.030
IL6ST		−0.044	
LINC00341	−0.463	−0.362	−0.392
LRRC48		−0.104	
MMP9	0.043		0.064
MPZL1	0.276	0.066	0.043
NUSAP1	0.088	0.065	
PBX1	0.159		0.375
PDZK1	−0.011		−0.063
PGR		−0.073	
PRC1		0.019	
RGL1	−0.429	−0.166	−0.161
RRM2	0.077	0.124	
SFRP1	−0.017		−0.278
STC2	−0.087	−0.068	
TNF	−0.029		−0.026
ZEB2			−0.138
CTS	0.514	0.409	0.516

Positive coefficients are associated with higher recurrence risk; negative coefficients are associated with lower recurrence risk. Beta-coefficients were normalised by dividing them by the SD of the respective variables in the training population

signatures (Table 3). In the 0–10-year follow-up period, all three newly derived signatures were significantly prognostic, with the late signature being significantly less informative than the 10-year signature (10-year signature likelihood ratio chi-square test $[LR\chi^2] = 28.0$; early signature $LR\chi^2 = 33.4$; late signature $LR\chi^2 = 18.1$). In the 0–5-year period, the 10-year signature and early signature were equally prognostic and significantly more than the late signature ($LR\chi^2$ for 10-year signature = 14.1; $LR\chi^2$ for early signature = 14.9; $LR\chi^2$ for late signature = 8.9). In the late setting, the early signature was the most prognostic, followed by the 10-year and late signatures ($LR\chi^2$ for 10-year signature = 13.9; $LR\chi^2$ for early signature = 18.6; $LR\chi^2$ for late signature = 9.3). CTS was

strongly prognostic in all three time periods (CTS 0–10-year $LR\chi^2 = 48.7$; CTS 0–5-year $LR\chi^2 = 29$; CTS 5–10-year $LR\chi^2 = 19.8$).

For the 0–10-year period, all three signatures added statistically significant prognostic information beyond that of the CTS ($\Delta LR\chi^2$ for 10-year signature = 7.9; $\Delta LR\chi^2$ for early signature = 10.3; $\Delta LR\chi^2$ for late signature = 4.3). In the 0–5-year period none of the signatures added significant prognostic information to CTS. However, in the 5–10-year period, the 10-year and early signatures added statistically significant prognostic information to CTS (10-year signature $\Delta LR\chi^2 = 4.8$; early signature $\Delta LR\chi^2 = 8.0$; late signature $\Delta LR\chi^2 = 2.7$).

Given that the early and the late signatures were not statistically significantly more prognostic than the 10-year signature in the respective periods they were optimised for, we rejected our primary hypothesis that signatures optimised separately for the early and the late follow-up periods, respectively, are more prognostic than a 10-year signature, but we proceeded to assess the validity of the 18-gene, 10-year signature in an independent cohort and to compare its performance with that of commercial signatures.

Signature test of 10-year validity in POLAR cohort

A matched case-control set of samples was compiled from RMH and Lund University Hospital archives (POLAR) to validate the 10-year signature (Fig. 2b, Table 1). Our aims were to test the validity the 10-year signature in an endocrine therapy-only cohort similar to the training set and also to explore if the prognostic property (if any) extends to a higher-risk, chemotherapy-treated population. The latter cohort was of interest in the 5–10-year period because of the potential for its use in selecting patients for extended adjuvant endocrine therapy.

Despite having matched cases and controls on NPI category, the CTS was still higher in cases than in control subjects: 201.9 ± 98 (SD) vs. 170.8 ± 87.6 ($p = 0.0009$), respectively. In a univariate analysis, CTS had an OR of 1.004 (95% CI, 1.001–1.006) for a one-unit increase. We assessed a multivariable model with CTS with and the 10-year signature, and both were found to be statistically significant: 10-year signature OR = 1.851 (95% CI, 1.194–2.868), $p = 0.006$; CTS OR = 1.003 (1.001–1.005), $p = 0.012$.

We also assessed whether the 10-year signature added significant prognostic information above CTS alone using LR tests (Table 4, Additional file 4: Table S10). In the overall POLAR cohort ($n = 422$), CTS was prognostic across 10 years and in the early follow-up period (CTS 0–10-year period $LR\chi^2 = 11.23$; 0–5-year period $LR\chi^2 = 22.09$), but not in the 5–10-year period. The 10-year signature was prognostic in all three follow-up periods and contributed to CTS with significant prognostic information in the 10-year and early periods (0–10-year period $\Delta LR\chi^2$, CTS

Table 3 Statistical analysis of TransATAC validation cohort

Score	No. of patients (relapses)	Univariate comparisons					Multivariable comparisons				
							CTS + signature vs CTS				CTS + signature
		$LR\chi^2$	p Value	HR (95% CI)	P diff	C-index (SE)	$\Delta LR\chi^2$	p Value	HR (95% CI)	P diff	C-index (SE)
0–10 years											
CTS	314 (59)	48.7	< 0.001	2.16 (1.79–2.62)	–	0.674 (0.018)	–	–	–	–	–
10-Year signature		28	< 0.001	1.98 (1.54–2.55)	Reference	0.671 (0.026)	7.9	0.005	1.49 (1.13–1.96)	Reference	0.709 (0.021)
Early signature		33.4	< 0.001	2.06 (1.62–2.61)	0.334	0.678 (0.024)	10.3	0.001	1.55 (1.19–2.02)	0.48	0.711 (0.020)
Late signature		18.1	< 0.001	1.72 (1.34–2.20)	0.000	0.642 0(.029)	4.3	0.037	1.33 (1.02–1.74)	0.004	0.700 (0.022)
0–5 years											
CTS	314 (26)	29	< 0.001	2.04 (1.53–2.74)	–	0.679 (0.023)	–	–	–	–	–
10-Year signature		14.1	< 0.001	2.05 (1.41–2.98)	0.833	0.678 (0.037)	3.2	0.073	1.46 (0.97–2.19)	0.77	0.712 (0.029)
Early signature		14.9	< 0.001	2.00 (1.42–2.81)	Reference	0.672 (0.035)	2.8	0.096	1.40 (0.95–2.06)	Reference	0.705 (0.028)
Late signature		8.9	0.003	1.77 (1.22–2.57)	0.138	0.648 (0.042)	1.7	0.19	1.31 (0.87–1.97)	0.65	0.705 (0.031)
5–10 years											
CTS	270 (33)	19.8	< 0.001	1.84 (1.33–2.54)	–	0.657 (0.026)	–	–	–	–	–
10-Year signature		13.9	< 0.001	1.93 (1.37–2.72)	0.027	0.663 (0.036)	4.8	0.028	1.53 (1.05–2.22)	0.14	0.696 (0.030)
Early signature		18.6	< 0.001	2.11 (1.52–2.94)	0.091	0.681 (0.032)	8	0.005	1.70 (1.19–2.43)	0.14	0.708 (0.028)
Late signature		9.3	0.002	1.68 (1.21–2.34)	Reference	0.636 (0.038)	2.7	0.099	1.36 (0.95–1.94)	Reference	0.686 (0.031)

CTS Clinical Treatment Score, *LR* Likelihood ratio
Both univariate and multivariable analyses are presented for years 0–10, years 0–5, and years 5–10 separately. Likelihood ratio test based on Cox proportional hazards models for univariate and multivariable analyses. Differences in likelihood ratio values ($\Delta LR\chi^2$) were used. CTS was used as a covariate in the multivariable regressions. For each score, HRs per SD change are presented

+ 10-year signature vs. CTS = 7.74; 0–5-year period $\Delta LR\chi^2$, CTS + 10-year signature vs. CTS = 7.59), but not in the 5–10-year period. Both CTS and the 10-year signature were marginally more informative across the 10 years in the chemotherapy-treated POLAR cohort than in the endocrine therapy-only population, despite the latter having more patients and events (patients, $n = 170$ vs. $n = 252$; events, 99 vs. 148). Additionally, the 10-year signature added significantly more prognostic information to CTS in the chemotherapy-treated group ($\Delta LR\chi^2$: CTS + 10-year signature vs. CTS = 6.71) than among those receiving endocrine therapy only ($\Delta LR\chi^2$, CTS + 10-year signature vs. CTS = 2.47).

Prognostic properties of the 18 individual genes constituting the 10-year signature were assessed in POLAR and compared with data obtained in TransATAC. In POLAR, only 8 of the 18 genes were significantly prognostic at the univariate level (Fig. 3), but all genes except tumour

Table 4 Statistical analysis of three groups of POLAR validation set for 0–10 years of follow-up

			All POLAR patients	Chemotherapy-treated	Chemotherapy-naive
0–10 Years					
No. of patients (relapses)			$n = 422$ (247)	$n = 170$ (99)	$n = 252$ (148)
Univariate	CTS	$LR\chi^2$	11.23	7.75	6.1
		P	< 0.001	0.005	0.014
		C-index (SE)	0.594 (0.028)	0.623 (0.044)	0.590 (0.036)
	10-Year signature	$LR\chi^2$	12.44	7.73	5.39
		P	< 0.004	0.005	0.020
		C-index (SE)	0.593 (0.028)	0.619 (0.044)	0.578 (0.037)
Multivariable comparisons	CTS + 10-year signature vs CTS	$\Delta LR\chi^2$	7.74	6.71	2.47
		P	0.005	0.001	0.116
	CTS + 10-year signature	C-index (SE)	0.617 (0.028)	0.669 (0.042)	0.598 (0.036)

Abbreviations: POLAR Molecular Predictors Of early versus LAte Recurrence in ER-positive breast cancer, *CTS* Clinical Treatment Score, *LR* Likelihood ratio, *SE* standard error
Both univariate and multivariable analyses are presented for years 0–10, years 0–5, and years 5–10 separately. Likelihood ratio test based on Cox proportional hazards models for univariate and multivariable analyses. Differences in likelihood ratio values ($\Delta LR\chi^2$) were used. CTS was used as a covariate in the multivariable regressions

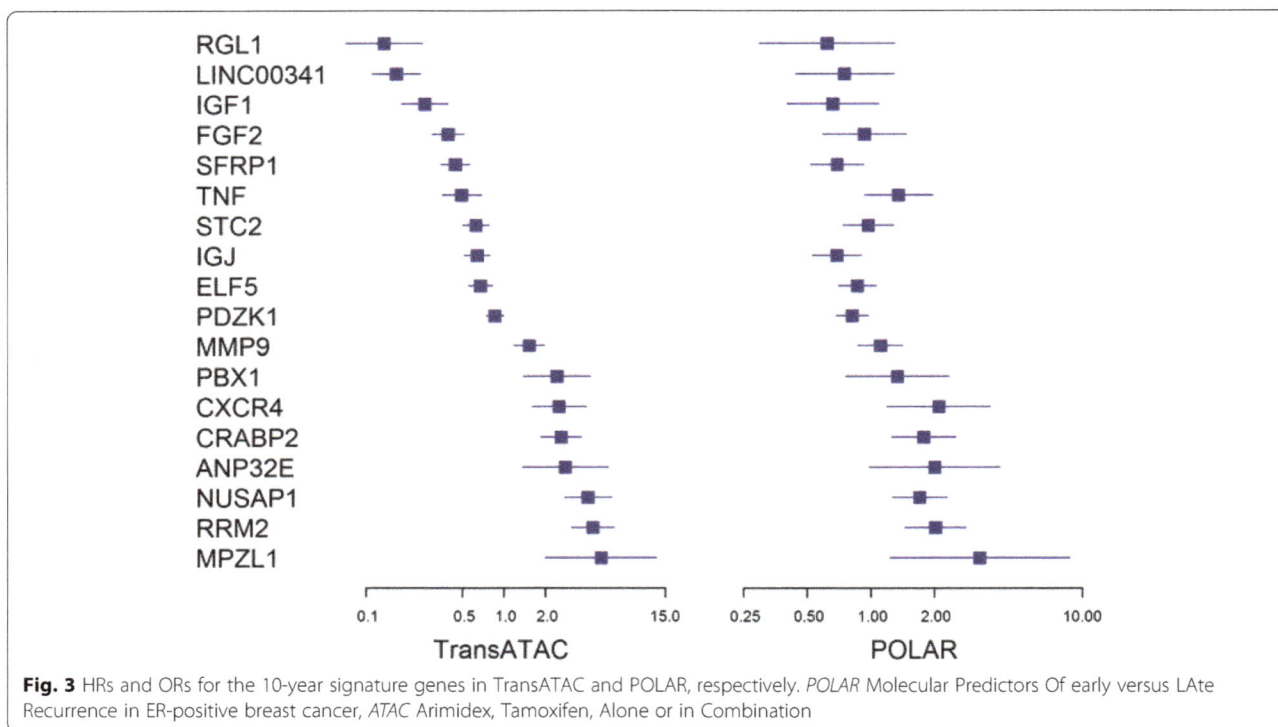

Fig. 3 HRs and ORs for the 10-year signature genes in TransATAC and POLAR, respectively. *POLAR* Molecular Predictors Of early versus LAte Recurrence in ER-positive breast cancer, *ATAC* Arimidex, Tamoxifen, Alone or in Combination

necrosis factor-alpha (TNF) showed the same prognostic direction both in TransATAC and in POLAR.

Comparison of the 10-year signature with CTS, RS, PAM50 ROR, BCI and IHC4 in TransATAC

We have previously published data on the prognostic performance of CTS, RS, PAM50 ROR, BCI and IHC4 in TransATAC [6, 15, 18, 26]; data for all scores were available for 271 patients in the validation cohort. We assessed their prognostic information for 10 years after surgery using any recurrence and distant recurrence as endpoints, respectively, and compared them with the newly developed 10-year signature (Table 5). For both any and distant recurrence, the BCI provided the most added information beyond the CTS in this set (any recurrence, CTS $LR\chi^2 = 37.4$; BCI $\Delta LR\chi^2 = 9.5$; distant recurrence, CTS $LR\chi^2 = 46.7$; BCI $\Delta LR\chi^2 = 14.5$, respectively). The novel 10-year signature performed similarly to the other three scores in this respect.

Discussion

We developed novel time-specific prognostic signatures for early, late and 10-year follow-up periods for ER+/HER2– patients treated with endocrine therapy alone to allow us to test the hypothesis that sequentially applying early and late signatures could be more prognostic for risk of relapse than a single newly developed 10-year signature. This hypothesis was based largely on our observation that the performance of some components in many of the commercially available

signatures varied between these time periods. For example, we found that ESR1 and the oestrogen module overall in the RS was less prognostic in years 5–10 than in years 0–5 [8]. Analogous findings were reported by Bianchini et al. [9]. Very recently, the Early Breast Cancer Trialists' Collaborative Group (EBCTCG) published data on clinicopathological and limited immunohistochemical data on over 60,000 women who were treated with 5 years of endocrine therapy [27]. Although progesterone receptor showed strong prognostic performance in years 0–5, it showed no significant relationship with prognosis thereafter. These data on markers associated with hormone responsiveness support the contention, but by no means prove, that cessation of endocrine treatment at 5 years may lead to increased recurrence risk in more hormonally responsive tumours. We therefore included in our assessment genes that we and others have found to be associated with the anti-proliferative response of primary ER+ breast cancer to oestrogen deprivation. Our work involved a discovery set of 747 samples; training and test sets of 634 and 314 TransATAC samples, respectively; and independent case-control series from 1449 eligible samples. As such, this was one of the largest original gene expression analyses undertaken for evaluating prognosis in ER+ breast cancer.

Of the 92 genes selected from microarray data and assessed in univariate analyses in TransATAC, we found 63 to be significantly prognostic ($p < 0.05$) in any of the three time periods, which is considerably more than expected by chance after allowing for multiple testing

Table 5 Statistical analysis for all and distant recurrences in the TransATAC validation cohort

Score	Univariate				Multivariable comparisons			
					CTS + signature vs CTS			CTS + signature
	$LR\chi^2$	p Value	HR (95% CI)	C-index (SE)	$\Delta LR\chi^2$	p Value	HR (95% CI)	C-index (SE)
All recurrences ($n = 271$, AR = 55)								
CTS	37.4	< 0.001	1.94 (1.57–2.40)	0.664 (0.020)	–	–	–	–
10-Year signature	20.7	< 0.001	1.85 (1.42–2.41)	0.657 (0.029)	5.7	0.017	1.42 (1.07–1.89)	0.695 (0.023)
BCI	25.0	< 0.001	2.07 (1.54–2.77)	0.679 (0.029)	9.5	0.002	1.62 (1.19–2.21)	0.711 (0.024)
RS	11.1	< 0.001	1.52 (1.21–1.91)	0.607 (0.027)	5.8	0.016	1.35 (1.07–1.71)	0.683 (0.021)
ROR	18.3	< 0.001	1.77 (1.36–2.31)	0.650 (0.030)	6.0	0.014	1.42 (1.07–1.87)	0.700 (0.024)
IHC4	14.4	< 0.001	1.63 (1.28–2.10)	0.629 (0.029)	7.5	0.006	1.46 (1.12–1.91)	0.696 (0.023)
Distant recurrences ($n = 271$, DR = 41)								
CTS	46.7	< 0.001	2.25 (1.79–2.82)	0.689 (0.019)	–	–	–	–
10-Year signature	26.4	< 0.001	2.24 (1.64–3.06)	0.694 (0.029)	8.5	0.004	1.65 (1.18–2.30)	0.733 (0.023)
BCI	34.0	< 0.001	2.71 (1.91–3.84)	0.726 (0.028)	14.5	< 0.001	2.03 (1.40–2.95)	0.754 (0.023)
RS	10.7	< 0.001	1.58 (1.23–2.03)	0.616 (0.029)	5.1	0.024	1.38 (1.06–1.79)	0.707 (0.020)
ROR	21.3	< 0.001	2.05 (1.50–2.79)	0.680 (0.031)	7.5	0.006	1.58 (1.14–2.21)	0.736 (0.024)
IHC4	17.9	< 0.001	1.87 (1.41–2.49)	0.658 (0.031)	9.8	0.002	1.68 (1.22–2.31)	0.731 (0.023)

Abbreviations: AR All recurrences, *DR* Distant recurrences, *CTS* Clinical Treatment Score, *BCI* Breast Cancer Index, *RS* Recurrence score, *ROR* Risk of recurrence, *LR* Likelihood ratio

Both univariate and multivariable analyses are presented. For each score, HRs per SD change are presented. Likelihood ratio test based on Cox proportional hazards models for univariate and multivariable analyses. Differences in likelihood ratio values ($\Delta LR\chi^2$) were used. CTS was used as a covariate in the multivariable regressions

errors. For most genes, the same prognostic pattern was observed for early and late periods, however we observed some possibly different prognostic properties for 20 genes. Notably, consistent with the above arguments, higher levels of ESR1 and its pioneer factor FOXA1 showed a shift at 5 years to be associated with worse prognosis beyond 5 years, but surprisingly over the 10-year period, the two genes were associated with poor prognosis. The complementary role whereby upon stimulus ER binding to chromatin is dependent on the presence of FOXA1 is well established [28]. In our dataset, FOXA1 and ESR1 correlated highly (Pearson's $R = 0.65$); the possibility that increased expression of one or both may put patients at increased risk of late relapse merits further investigation, particularly with regard to whether the genes also identify patients who benefit from extended adjuvant therapy.

The optimised time-dependent signatures derived in the TransATAC training set were rather similar to one another in makeup. All genes in the 10-year signature featured in either (or both) of the early and late signatures with their coefficients being in the same direction. The early and late signatures had five and three variables, respectively, not present in the 10-year signature, suggesting that the early and late signatures may not have captured time-specific features or that such time-specific features that exist exert a minor modulatory influence on the overall prognosis over 10 years. It is notable that CTS was consistently the most prognostic variable in the three time-dependent models

and that its contribution was similar in both early and late recurrence. This is consistent with the data of the EBCTCG that classical clinicopathological features retain their strong prognostic influence beyond 5 years [27].

Given that the 10-year signature captured prognostic features of both early and late events, it is perhaps not surprising that no improvement was seen in the use of early and late signatures compared with the overall 10-year signature that led to the rejection of our hypothesis. Also, it should be noted that splitting of the 0–10-year time period into 0–5- and 5–10-year periods markedly reduces the power to detect prognostic contributions. At least a contributory factor for the lack of improvement may be the dominance of proliferation-related genes in our and other signatures. As shown in our earlier analysis of the RS, each of the individual proliferation genes and the integrated module are equally prognostic before and after 5 years [8]. Notably, this is also supported by the observation by the EBCTCG that Ki-67 was equally prognostic before and after 5 years in their overview analysis of late recurrence [27].

The 10-year signature was nonetheless validated in the POLAR sample set and provided significant prognostic information in both chemotherapy-naive and chemotherapy-treated cohorts. Moreover, it added independent prognostic information beyond that of CTS in the POLAR cohort. Comparison of the information provided by each gene showed that 8 of the 18 genes were significantly prognostic at univariate level in POLAR (4 genes at $P < 0.05$, 2 genes at $P < 0.01$ and 3 genes at $P < 0.001$). TNF showed an opposite prognostic direction in training and validation sets, thus weakening the performance of the signature in POLAR. TNF is a versatile pro-inflammatory cytokine that has both pro- and anti-tumour activities promoting lymphocytic infiltration and activating the nuclear factor-κB, c-Jun N-terminal kinase and mitogen-activated protein kinase pathways, and it is capable of inducing apoptosis through TNF receptors 1 and 2 [29]. It may be that the inclusion of higher-risk, chemotherapy-treated patients in POLAR contributed to the difference in TNF's prognostic pattern; further investigation is needed to explain the relationship of TNF and risk of relapse in these cohorts.

The 10-year signature was compared with established prognostic signatures in the TransATAC validation set. Importantly, the 10-year signature was developed for the endpoint of any recurrence contrary to the endpoint of distant recurrence used in the development of RS, PAM50, ROR, BCI and IHC4. In univariate assessments, BCI and the 10-year signatures were the most informative for both all and distant recurrence. When added to CTS, all signatures assessed provided similar amounts of information, with CTS + BCI being the most informative for distant recurrence. This new signature did not outperform the established signatures, even though it was based on a large and wide-ranging analysis of both established prognostic genes and novel genes with a clear rationale for inclusion. Larger studies may be needed to fully optimise novel prognostic signatures with improved prognostic information, however the data from our studies indicate that the gain is unlikely to be large. Other approaches that assess response to treatment or integrate mutational and DNA copy number profiles or by the use of circulating tumour DNA are likely to be more fruitful.

The results presented here support the mounting evidence that better risk estimation can be achieved by combining molecular profilers with clinicopathological factors. For the three time-dependent signatures derived in TransATAC, CTS was the most prognostic in all three time-dependent signatures and provided more prognostic information than RS, ROR, BCI and IHC4, respectively. Additionally, all profilers added significant prognostic information to CTS, leading to combined signatures being significantly more informative. There is emerging evidence for genetic differences affecting outcome amongst various racial groups [30]. Although this is an important question with practical consequences, the cohort presented here was > 99% Caucasian and did not provide us with the opportunity to examine within TransATAC.

Our study has strengths and limitations. An advantage was that a large discovery cohort of 634 samples was used for signature training. All tumours were ER+/HER2− from post-menopausal patients who had received 5 years of endocrine therapy without chemotherapy. This was a homogeneous group of breast cancers, which reduced confounding factors such as tumour subtype and differing treatment lengths and types. Data for the clinical prognostic tests were obtained by the same methods as set out by the tests' developers. The same batch of RNA was used for the newly developed signatures presented here and for the clinical prognostic tests used in the comparisons, reducing intra-sample variation. The clinical data were derived from a registration standard trial with comprehensive follow-up over 10 years. Limitations include that the candidate gene selection based on microarray data and associated clinical information from multiple studies did not allow the assessment of candidates by taking multiple clinical variables into account; this may have limited the performance of derived signatures that ultimately included CTS as a variable. Also, CTS, IHC4 and the 10-year signature were derived in TransATAC; therefore, their performance in the comparisons was slightly overestimated compared with what we would see in independent cohorts. Finally, although this study was relatively large compared with others, the splitting of the data into early and late signatures decreased the statistical power for comparisons within those time periods. The approach we have taken is likely to have somewhat overfitted the 10-year signature to the TransATAC population. An alternative approach for the derivation and validation of the 10-year signature would have been to fit the signature to the whole of the TransATAC cohort and validate it in the POLAR cohort. However, the approach we took allowed the comparison of the 10-year signature with commercially available signatures in the TransATAC test set. Had the 10-year signature not at least matched these, it would not have been worth proceeding further.

Conclusions

In summary, we found that early and late signatures are unlikely to be more informative for predicting relapse than a single signature optimised for 10 years. Larger studies may be needed to fully optimise novel gene expression signatures for prognosis in endocrine-treated ER+ patients with breast cancer, however a substantial improvement in performance is unlikely.

Additional files

Additional file 1: Methods. Additional methods. (DOCX 21 kb)

Additional file 2: Table S1. List of 585 candidate genes. **Table S2.** List and identifiers for the 747-patient microarray expression data cohort. **Table S3.** List of 454 Affymetrix probes studied. **Table S4.** List of 212 genes significantly prognostic ($p < 0.01$) in any of the three time periods in the microarray data. **Table S5.** List of 88 genes by multivariable selections in any of the three time periods in the microarray data. Nodal status was used as a covariate in the regressions. **Table S6.** List of 17 genes manually removed from the multivariable list. **Table S7.** List of 29 genes added to the candidate list. **Table S8.** Details of the 100-probe NanoString code set used in TransATAC. **Table S9.** HRs, CIs and p values for the 92 genes assessed in TransATAC in univariate analyses. (XLSX 130 kb)

Additional file 3: Figure S1. Forest plot of HRs and CIs for the 92 genes assessed in TransATAC in univariate analyses. Asterisk denotes significance. (PDF 1497 kb)

Additional file 4: Table S10. Likelihood ratio (LR) χ^2 and p values for CTS and 10-year signature in three groups of POLAR validation set for 0–5 and 5–10 years of follow-up. Both univariate and multivariable analyses are presented for years 0–10, years 0–5, and years 5–10 separately. LR test based on Cox proportional hazards models for univariate and multivariable analyses. Differences in LR values ($\Delta LR\chi^2$) were used. CTS was used as a covariate in the multivariable regressions. *POLAR* Molecular Predictors Of early versus LAte Recurrence in ER-positive breast cancer, *CTS* Clinical Treatment Score. (DOCX 15 kb)

Abbreviations

AI: Aromatase inhibitor; ATAC: Arimidex, Tamoxifen, Alone or in Combination; BCI: Breast Cancer Index; CTS: Clinical Treatment Score; DMFS: Distant metastasis-free survival; EBCTCG: Early Breast Cancer Trialists' Collaborative Group; ER: Oestrogen receptor; ERS: Oestrogen receptor-related score; FFPE: Formalin-fixed, paraffin-embedded; GHI: Genomic Health Inc.; HR: Hormone receptor; IHC4: Score based on four IHC markers; LR: Likelihood ratio; LUH: Lund University Hospital; MKS: Mitotic kinase score; NPI: Nottingham Prognostic Index; POLAR: Predictors Of early versus LAte Recurrence in ER+ breast cancer; RFS: Relapse-free survival; RMH: Royal Marsden Hospital; ROR: Risk of recurrence; RS: Oncotype DX Recurrence Score; TNF: Tumour necrosis factor

Acknowledgements

We acknowledge Professor Mårten Fernö and Professor Per Malmström for their work in providing data and samples for the Lund cohort. We thank Genomic Health Inc., NanoString Technologies and BioTheranostics for the data of their respective gene signatures. The authors acknowledge Kabir Mohammed's work on calculating C-indices in the POLAR cohort.

Funding

This work was supported by Breast Cancer Now working in partnership with Walk the Walk, as well as by the National Institute for Health Research Royal Marsden/ICR Biomedical Research Centre. ARB was funded by Cancer Research UK (grant number C569/A16891). The study was supported by funds from Skåne County Council's Research and Development Foundation, Governmental Funding of Clinical Research within the National Health Service (grant number ALFSKANE-350191 [to MK]), the Swedish Breast Cancer Association (BRO), the Mrs Berta Kamprad Foundation and The Inger Persson Research Foundation. IS and JC were supported by Cancer Research UK (programme grant C569/A10404).

Authors' contributions

MD, JC and RB conceived of and designed study. BY and MK identified and acquired clinical samples. RB and BY performed experiments. RB, ARB, MCUC, KK, IS, BY and QG performed statistical analyses. RB and MD wrote and edited the manuscript. All authors read and approved the final version of the manuscript.

Competing interests

MCUC reports patents, royalties, other intellectual property: PAM50 patent. The other authors declare that they have no competing interests.

Author details

[1]The Breast Cancer Now Toby Robins Research Centre at the Institute of Cancer Research, 237 Fulham Road, London SW3 6JB, UK. [2]Ralph Lauren Centre for Breast Cancer Research, Royal Marsden Hospital, London, UK. [3]Olivia Newton-John Cancer Research Institute, Melbourne, Australia. [4]Austin Health, Melbourne, Australia. [5]Centre for Cancer Prevention, Wolfson Institute of Preventive Medicine, Queen Mary University of London, London, UK. [6]Lund University, Skane University Hospital, Faculty of Medicine, Department of Clinical Sciences Lund, Oncology and Pathology, Lund, Sweden. [7]Clinical Trials and Statistic Unit, The Institute of Cancer Research, London, UK. [8]Research Data Management and Statistics Unit, Royal Marsden Hospital, London, UK.

References

1. Early Breast Cancer Trialists' Collaborative Group (EBCTCG). Aromatase inhibitors versus tamoxifen in early breast cancer: patient-level meta-analysis of the randomised trials. Lancet. 2015;386(10001):1341–52.
2. Paik S, Shak S, Tang G, Kim C, Baker J, Cronin M, Baehner FL, Walker MG, Watson D, Park T, et al. A multigene assay to predict recurrence of tamoxifen-treated, node-negative breast cancer. N Engl J Med. 2004;351(27):2817–26.
3. Parker JS, Mullins M, Cheang MC, Leung S, Voduc D, Vickery T, Davies S, Fauron C, He X, Hu Z, et al. Supervised risk predictor of breast cancer based on intrinsic subtypes. J Clin Oncol. 2009;27(8):1160–7.
4. Ma XJ, Salunga R, Dahiya S, Wang W, Carney E, Durbecq V, Harris A, Goss P, Sotiriou C, Erlander M, et al. A five-gene molecular grade index and HOXB13:IL17BR are complementary prognostic factors in early stage breast cancer. Clin Cancer Res. 2008;14(9):2601–8.
5. Filipits M, Rudas M, Jakesz R, Dubsky P, Fitzal F, Singer CF, Dietze O, Greil R, Jelen A, Sevelda P, et al. A new molecular predictor of distant recurrence in ER-positive, HER2-negative breast cancer adds independent information to conventional clinical risk factors. Clin Cancer Res. 2011;17(18):6012–20.
6. Cuzick J, Dowsett M, Pineda S, Wale C, Salter J, Quinn E, Zabaglo L, Mallon E, Green AR, Ellis IO, et al. Prognostic value of a combined estrogen receptor, progesterone receptor, Ki-67, and human epidermal growth factor receptor 2 immunohistochemical score and comparison with the Genomic Health recurrence score in early breast cancer. J Clin Oncol. 2011;29(32):4273–8.
7. Forbes JF, Cuzick J, Buzdar A, Howell A, Tobias JS, Baum M. Effect of anastrozole and tamoxifen as adjuvant treatment for early-stage breast cancer: 100-month analysis of the ATAC trial. Lancet Oncol. 2008;9(1):45–53.
8. Dowsett M, Sestak I, Buus R, Lopez-Knowles E, Mallon E, Howell A, Forbes JF, Buzdar A, Cuzick J. Estrogen receptor expression in 21-gene recurrence score predicts increased late recurrence for estrogen-positive/HER2-negative breast Cancer. Clin Cancer Res. 2015;21(12):2763–70.
9. Bianchini G, Pusztai L, Karn T, Iwamoto T, Rody A, Kelly C, Muller V, Schmidt S, Qi Y, Holtrich U, et al. Proliferation and estrogen signaling can distinguish patients at risk for early versus late relapse among estrogen receptor positive breast cancers. Breast Cancer Res. 2013;15:R86.
10. Wolmark N, Mamounas EP, Baehner FL, Butler SM, Tang G, Jamshidian F, Sing AP, Shak S, Paik S. Prognostic impact of the combination of recurrence score and quantitative estrogen receptor expression (ESR1) on predicting late distant recurrence risk in estrogen receptor-positive breast cancer after 5 years of tamoxifen: results from NRG Oncology/National Surgical Adjuvant Breast and Bowel Project B-28 and B-14. J Clin Oncol. 2016;34(20):2350–8.
11. Goss PE, Ingle JN, Martino S, Robert NJ, Muss HB, Piccart MJ, Castiglione M, Tu D, Shepherd LE, Pritchard KI, et al. A randomized trial of letrozole in postmenopausal women after five years of tamoxifen therapy for early-stage breast cancer. N Engl J Med. 2003;349(19):1793–802.
12. Davies C, Pan H, Godwin J, Gray R, Arriagada R, Raina V, Abraham M, Medeiros Alencar VH, Badran A, Bonfill X, et al. Long-term effects of continuing adjuvant tamoxifen to 10 years versus stopping at 5 years after

diagnosis of oestrogen receptor-positive breast cancer: ATLAS, a randomised trial. Lancet. 2013;381(9869):805–16.

13. Dubsky P, Brase JC, Jakesz R, Rudas M, Singer CF, Greil R, Dietze O, Luisser I, Klug E, Sedivy R, et al. The EndoPredict score provides prognostic information on late distant metastases in ER+/HER2– breast cancer patients. Br J Cancer. 2013;109(12):2959–64.

14. Sestak I, Dowsett M, Zabaglo L, Lopez-Knowles E, Ferree S, Cowens JW, Cuzick J. Factors predicting late recurrence for estrogen receptor-positive breast cancer. J Natl Cancer Inst. 2013;105(19):1504–11.

15. Sgroi DC, Sestak I, Cuzick J, Zhang Y, Schnabel CA, Schroeder B, Erlander MG, Dunbier A, Sidhu K, Lopez-Knowles E, et al. Prediction of late distant recurrence in patients with oestrogen-receptor-positive breast cancer: a prospective comparison of the breast-cancer index (BCI) assay, 21-gene recurrence score, and IHC4 in the TransATAC study population. Lancet Oncol. 2013;14(11):1067–76.

16. Sestak I, Cuzick J, Dowsett M, Lopez-Knowles E, Filipits M, Dubsky P, Cowens JW, Ferree S, Schaper C, Fesl C, et al. Prediction of late distant recurrence after 5 years of endocrine treatment: a combined analysis of patients from the Austrian Breast and Colorectal Cancer Study Group 8 and Arimidex, Tamoxifen Alone or in Combination randomized trials using the PAM50 risk of recurrence score. J Clin Oncol. 2015;33(8):916–22.

17. Zhao X, Rodland EA, Sorlie T, Vollan HK, Russnes HG, Kristensen VN, Lingjaerde OC, Borresen-Dale AL. Systematic assessment of prognostic gene signatures for breast cancer shows distinct influence of time and ER status. BMC Cancer. 2014;14:211.

18. Dowsett M, Cuzick J, Wale C, Forbes J, Mallon EA, Salter J, Quinn E, Dunbier A, Baum M, Buzdar A, et al. Prediction of risk of distant recurrence using the 21-gene recurrence score in node-negative and node-positive postmenopausal patients with breast cancer treated with anastrozole or tamoxifen: a TransATAC study. J Clin Oncol. 2010;28(11):1829–34.

19. Dunbier AK, Ghazoui Z, Anderson H, Salter J, Nerurkar A, Osin P, A'Hern R, Miller WR, Smith IE, Dowsett M. Molecular profiling of aromatase inhibitor-treated postmenopausal breast tumors identifies immune-related correlates of resistance. Clin Cancer Res. 2013;19(10):2775–86.

20. Mackay A, Urruticoechea A, Dixon JM, Dexter T, Fenwick K, Ashworth A, Drury S, Larionov A, Young O, White S, et al. Molecular response to aromatase inhibitor treatment in primary breast cancer. Breast Cancer Res. 2007;9(3):R37.

21. Desmedt C, Haibe-Kains B, Wirapati P, Buyse M, Larsimont D, Bontempi G, Delorenzi M, Piccart M, Sotiriou C. Biological processes associated with breast cancer clinical outcome depend on the molecular subtypes. Clin Cancer Res. 2008;14(16):5158–65.

22. Fan C, Prat A, Parker JS, Liu Y, Carey LA, Troester MA, Perou CM. Building prognostic models for breast cancer patients using clinical variables and hundreds of gene expression signatures. BMC Med Genet. 2011;4:3.

23. Loi S, Haibe-Kains B, Desmedt C, Lallemand F, Tutt AM, Gillet C, Ellis P, Harris A, Bergh J, Foekens JA, et al. Definition of clinically distinct molecular subtypes in estrogen receptor-positive breast carcinomas through genomic grade. J Clin Oncol. 2007;25(10):1239–46.

24. Loi S, Haibe-Kains B, Desmedt C, Wirapati P, Lallemand F, Tutt AM, Gillet C, Ellis P, Ryder K, Reid JF, et al. Predicting prognosis using molecular profiling in estrogen receptor-positive breast cancer treated with tamoxifen. BMC Genomics. 2008;9:239.

25. Symmans WF, Hatzis C, Sotiriou C, Andre F, Peintinger F, Regitnig P, Daxenbichler G, Desmedt C, Domont J, Marth C, et al. Genomic index of sensitivity to endocrine therapy for breast cancer. J Clin Oncol. 2010;28(27):4111–9.

26. Dowsett M, Sestak I, Lopez-Knowles E, Sidhu K, Dunbier AK, Cowens JW, Ferree S, Storhoff J, Schaper C, Cuzick J. Comparison of PAM50 risk of recurrence score with oncotype DX and IHC4 for predicting risk of distant recurrence after endocrine therapy. J Clin Oncol. 2013;31(22):2783–90.

27. Pan H, Gray R, Braybrooke J, Davies C, Taylor C, McGale P, Peto R, Pritchard KI, Bergh J, Dowsett M, Hayes DF, EBCTCG. 20-Year risks of breast-cancer recurrence after stopping endocrine therapy at 5 years. N Engl J Med. 2017;377(19):1836–46.

28. Hurtado A, Holmes KA, Ross-Innes CS, Schmidt D, Carroll JS. FOXA1 is a key determinant of estrogen receptor function and endocrine response. Nat Genet. 2011;43(1):27–33.

29. Wang X, Lin Y. Tumor necrosis factor and cancer, buddies or foes? Acta Pharmacol Sin. 2008;29(11):1275–88.

30. Troester MA, Sun X, Allott EH, Geradts J, Cohen SM, Tse CK, Kirk EL, Thorne LB, Mathews M, Li Y, et al. Racial differences in PAM50 subtypes in the Carolina Breast Cancer Study. J Natl Cancer Inst. 2018;110(2):176–82.

10

Circulating microRNAs in the early prediction of disease recurrence in primary breast cancer

Chara Papadaki[1†], Michalis Stratigos[2†], Georgios Markakis[3], Maria Spiliotaki[1], Georgios Mastrostamatis[1], Christoforos Nikolaou[4,5], Dimitrios Mavroudis[1,2] and Sofia Agelaki[1,2*]

Abstract

Background: In primary breast cancer metastases frequently arise from a state of dormancy that may persist for extended periods of time. We investigated the efficacy of plasma micro-RNA (miR)-21, miR-23b, miR-190, miR-200b and miR-200c, related to dormancy and metastasis, to predict the outcome of patients with early breast cancer.

Methods: miRNAs were evaluated by RT-qPCR in plasma obtained before adjuvant chemotherapy. miRNA expression, classified as high or low according to median values, correlated with relapse and survival. Receiver operating characteristic (ROC) curves were constructed to determine miRNA sensitivity and specificity.

Results: miR-21 ($p < 0.001$), miR-23b ($p = 0.028$) and miR-200c ($p < 0.001$) expression were higher and miR-190 was lower ($p = 0.013$) in relapsed ($n = 49$), compared to non-relapsed patients ($n = 84$). Interestingly, miR-190 was lower ($p = 0.0032$) in patients with early relapse (at < 3 years; $n = 23$) compared to those without early relapse ($n = 110$). On the other hand, miR-21 and miR-200c were higher ($p = 0.015$ and $p < 0.001$, respectively) in patients with late relapse (relapse at ≥ 5 years; $n = 20$) as compared to non-relapsed patients. High miR-200c was associated with shorter disease-free survival (DFS) ($p = 0.005$) and high miR-21 with both shorter DFS and overall survival (OS) ($p < 0.001$ and $p = 0.033$, respectively) compared to low expression. ROC curve analysis revealed that miR-21, miR-23b, miR-190 and miR-200c discriminated relapsed from non-relapsed patients. A combination of of miR-21, miR-23b and miR-190 showed higher sensitivity and specificity in ROC analyses compared to each miRNA alone; accuracy was further improved by adding lymph node infiltration and tumor grade to the panel of three miRs (AUC 0.873). Furthermore, the combination of miR-200c, lymph node infiltration, tumor grade and estrogen receptor predicted late relapse (AUC 0.890).

Conclusions: Circulating miRNAs are differentially expressed among relapsed and non-relapsed patients with early breast cancer and predict recurrence many years before its clinical detection. Our results suggest that miRNAs represent potential circulating biomarkers in early breast cancer.

Keywords: Circulating miRNAs, Breast cancer, Relapse, Metastasis, Dormancy

* Correspondence: agelaki@uoc.gr; oncsec@med.uoc.gr
†Chara Papadaki and Michalis Stratigos contributed equally to this work.
[1]Laboratory of Translational Oncology, School of Medicine, University of Crete, Heraklion, 71003 Heraklion, Crete, Greece
[2]Department of Medical Oncology, University General Hospital of Heraklion, 1352 PO BOX, 711 10 Heraklion, Crete, Greece
Full list of author information is available at the end of the article

Background

Despite significant advances in diagnosis and treatment of early breast cancer, almost 30% of patients will eventually have local or distant recurrence [1–3]. Recurrence is considered to result from cancer cells that persist after surgery and systemic therapy and remain in a dormant state for many years before they start proliferating and form local or distant metastases [4, 5]. Strategies to improve the management of patients with early disease should include the development of novel biomarkers for the early recognition of patients at high risk of relapse.

Clinicopathological parameters are commonly used for the prediction of patients' prognosis; however, they often lack individualized validity for the identification of patients at high risk, due to significant inter-patient heterogeneity [6]. In addition, molecular profiling tests have been developed for prognostication but their routine clinical implementation is problematic [7]. Furthermore, the genetic profiling of solid tumors is currently performed on biopsies that might fail to reflect intra-tumoral heterogeneity and limit the opportunity to track genetic alterations occurring during cancer evolution [8]. Therefore, there is an unmet need to identify novel non-invasive biomarkers for the better prediction of the risk of recurrence in breast cancer.

MicroRNAs (miRNAs), a large family of small (20–22 nucleotides) non-coding RNAs, regulate approximately 30% of the genes in the human genome at the post-transcriptional level, by binding to the complementary sequences of the $3'$- untranslated region (3'-UTR) of their target messenger RNAs (mRNAs), leading to either mRNA degradation or inhibition of protein translation [9]. miRNAs are deregulated in cancer, acting as both oncogenes and tumor suppressor genes [10]. The altered expression of miRNAs has been associated with poor clinical outcome in patients diagnosed with a variety of tumors [11]. In the past decade miRNAs have emerged as promising biomarkers in breast cancer and have been increasingly identified in biological fluids such as serum or plasma as circulating miRNAs [12]. Circulating miRNAs are significantly stable in biological fluids [13, 14] and could potentially serve as a "liquid biopsy" for the real-time evaluation of tumor status.

The assessment of dormancy and metastasis-related miRNAs could be of importance for the identification of patients at high risk of relapse. The mechanisms that lead to dormancy or enable the formation of metastases remain poorly understood. Data from in vitro models or expression analysis in patients with breast cancer suggest that miR-21, miR-23b, miR-190 and the miR-200 family members, such as miR-200b and miR-200c, are important in cancer dormancy and metastasis. An epithelial to mesenchymal transition (EMT)-related gene signature in the primary tumor has been associated with both stromal activation and escape from dormancy in breast cancer [15], suggesting that intrinsic EMT features may regulate the transition of disseminated tumor cells into a dormant phenotype with the ability to outgrow as recurrent disease. In another report, the activation of the EMT program, as orchestrated by the key regulator of EMT, Zeb1, was sufficient to promote escape from latency and stimulate the development of metastases [16]. The miR-200 family regulates EMT by targeting the ZEB1/2-E-cadherin axis [17], whereas in other studies, elevated levels of miR-200 family have induced EMT and promoted metastasis in breast cancer [18]. Several lines of evidence suggest that miR-21 is oncogenic in various types of cancer by suppressing several apoptotic and tumor suppressor genes [19] and by inducing cell proliferation, migration, invasion and metastasis. miR-23b has been shown to promote tumor dormancy in the metastatic niche [20], whereas miR-190 upregulation has been associated with prolonged tumor dormancy in fast-growing tumors such as osteosarcomas and glioblastomas [21].

Based on the above, the aim of the present study was to investigate the expression of miR-21, miR-23b, miR-190, miR-200b and miR-200c in the plasma of patients with early breast cancer and evaluate their role in the prediction of patients' outcomes.

Methods

Patients' characteristics and sample collection

A total of 209 consecutive patients with early breast cancer who underwent surgery followed by adjuvant chemotherapy administered at the Department of Medical Oncology of the University Hospital of Heraklion (Crete, Greece) between years 2003 and 2010 and had available plasma samples, were included in the present study. Plasma samples were obtained after the surgical resection of the primary tumor and before the initiation of adjuvant chemotherapy. Plasma samples were also collected from 23 normal blood donors to serve as controls. All patients and normal donors had provided signed informed consent to participate in the study, which was approved by the Ethics and Scientific Committee of Department of Medical Oncology of the University Hospital of Heraklion (ID 13998/8–10-2104; Crete, Greece). Clinical characteristics and follow-up information for each patient were prospectively collected. Peripheral blood from healthy donors and patients was drawn early in the morning and was collected in EDTA tubes. Plasma was subsequently isolated within 2 h by centrifugation at 2500 rpm for 15 min at 4 °C, followed by a second centrifugation at 2000 g for 15 min at 4 °C to remove cellular debris. Samples were kept in aliquots at 80 °C until further use. Plasma samples presenting a change in color to pink, suggesting the presence of hemolysis, were not processed for further analysis (Fig. 1).

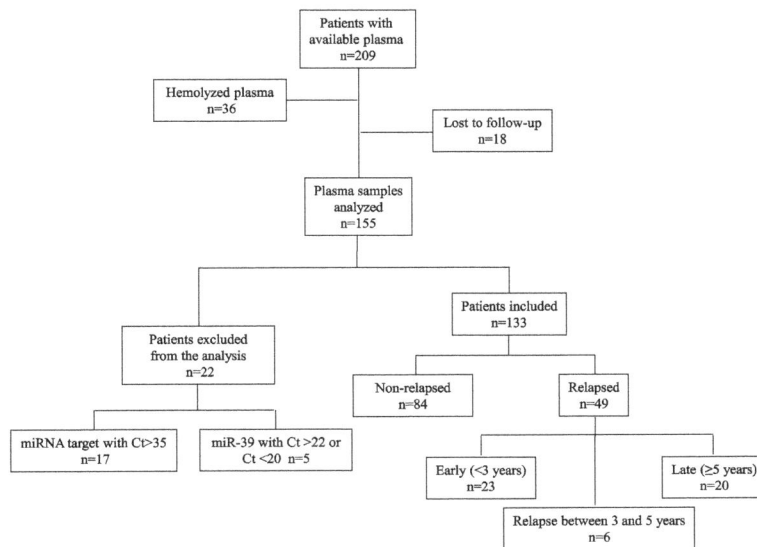

Fig. 1 Flow chart of the study. Ct, cycle threshold

RNA isolation

Plasma samples were thawed on ice and centrifuged at 10000 rpm for 10 min in order to remove cellular debris. Total RNA was extracted from 400 µl of plasma using Trizol LS (Ambion, Life Technologies). After denaturation, 5 µl containing 25 fmoles of a synthetic *Caenorhabditis elegans* miRNA cel-miR-39 (Qiagen Inc., USA) was added to each sample as an endogenous control to allow for normalization of sample-to-sample variation. Aqueous phase was separated from organic phase by adding 250 µl chloroform followed by incubation on ice for 10 min. After centrifugation, an equal volume of 700 µl of supernatant, from each sample, was transferred to an Eppendorf tube. Then, RNA was precipitated by adding 0.7 volumes of isopropanol and 1 µl glycogen followed by incubation at 80 °C, overnight. On the next day, and after centrifugation, RNA pellet was washed three times with 75% ethanol, air dried and finally resuspended in 50 µl RNAse-free water. RNA from all samples was kept in aliquots at 80 °C until further use in the subsequent real-time qPCR.

Quantitative real-time PCR analysis and miRNA expression

Reverse transcription and RT-qPCR was performed according to manufacturer's instructions and as previously described [13]. Total RNA input of 1.67 µl was reverse transcribed using the TaqMan miRNA Reverse Transcription kit and miRNA specific stem-loop primers (Applied Biosystmes, Foster City, CA, USA) in a 5-µl reaction comprising 1 mM dNTPs, 1 × PCR Reverse Transcription Buffer, 0.787 µl H_2O, 3.3 units Multiscribe Reverse Transcriptase, 0.252 units RNase inhibitors and 0.2 × RT-specific stem-loop primers.

The reaction was performed in a Peltier Thermal Cycler PTC-200 at 16 °C for 30 min, 42 °C for 30 min and 85 °C for 5 min. Complementary DNA (cDNA) was diluted at 30 µl and each miRNA was assessed by RT-qPCR in a 5-µl reaction comprising 1 × of TaqMan 2× Universal PCR Mater Mix, No AmpErase UNG, 0.25 µl of TaqMan miRNA Assay and 2.25 µl of diluted cDNA. The quantitative real- time PCR reaction was carried out at 95 °C for 10 min, followed by 40 cycles of 95 °C for 15 min and 60 °C for 1 min on a ViiA 7 Real-Time PCR System (Applied Biosystems, Foster City, CA, USA). All the assays were performed in triplicates. Appropriate negative controls were used in both cDNA synthesis and RT-qPCR reactions where RNA input was replaced by H_2O and no template control was used, respectively. The average expression levels for each miRNA were calculated by the $2^{-\Delta Ct}$ method relative to the average of miR-23a.

Due to the lack of consensus concerning the normalization of circulating miRNAs we used miR-23a as a reference gene that was stably and reproducibly expressed among patients' groups (Mann-Whitney test, $p = 0.458$) and among patients and normal donors (Mann-Whitney test, $p = 0.12$) [22]. Finally, the fold change in target miRNAs relative to miRNAs expressed in normal controls was calculated by the $2^{-\Delta\Delta Ct}$ method [23]. Samples with mean cycle threshold (Ct) > 35 for target miRNAs ($n = 17$) were excluded from the analysis. In addition, samples with mean Ct > 22 or Ct < 20 of cel-miR-39 ($n = 5$), suggesting RNA extraction was not efficient, were also excluded. Moreover, plasma samples were tested for contamination with red blood cells by measuring miR-451 and miR-23a expression levels [24].

Samples contaminated with red blood cells were not processed for further analysis.

Statistical analysis

The statistical analysis was performed using the SPSS software package, version 22.0 (SPSS Inc. Chicago IL, USA). Cutoff points were set at the median value for expression of each miRNA. Patients with miRNA expression above or equal to the median values were characterized as having high expression, whereas patients with miRNA expression below the median were characterized as having low expression. Spearman's test was used to test correlation between expression of the different miRNAs. The Mann-Whitney U-test and Kruskal Wallis test were used to estimate associations between miRNA expression and clinicopathological characteristics. Differences in clinicopathological characteristics between relapsed and non-relapsed patients were evaluated by Pearson's chi-square test. The associations between circulating miRNA expression levels and disease-free survival (DFS) or overall survival (OS) were assessed by the Kaplan-Meier method, log rank test (Mantel-Cox) and Cox proportional hazard regression models. DFS was calculated from the date of surgery until the date of relapse or death from any cause, whereas OS was calculated from the date of surgery until the date of death from any cause or last follow up. The Mann-Whitney test was used to examine the differential expression between the different groups of patients. To evaluate the value of circulating miRNAs in predicting relapse, receiver operating characteristics (ROC) curves were constructed and area under the curve (AUC) calculated. The Youden index (sensitivity + specificity − 1) was used to set the optimal cutoff point. Logistic regression analyses were performed to identify the best discriminating combinations of miRNAs with clinicopathological features. Cross-validation analysis was implemented in R using a generalized linear model for logistic regression, with recurrence/non-relapse as binary target variables (http://www.r-project.org/). Statistical significance was set at $p < 0.05$ (two-sided test). This report is written according to the reporting recommendations for tumor marker prognostic studies (REMARK criteria) [25].

Results

Study design and patients' characteristics

The flow diagram of the study and patients' characteristics are summarized in Fig. 1 and Table 1, respectively. Plasma samples from 155 patients with early breast cancer and from 23 healthy women were processed for RNA extraction. There were 22 patients excluded from the analysis as described above. After a median follow-up period of 94.3 months (range 14.33–159.30),

84 out of the 133 patients with breast cancer who were included in the analysis remained disease-free and 49 had relapsed. Demographics and clinical characteristics were similar between patients who remained disease-free and those who developed recurrence, except for the proportions of patients with tumor size of > 5 cm (T3) and four or more infiltrated axillary lymph nodes, which were higher in patients who had recurrence ($p = 0.015$ and $p = 0.003$, respectively; Table 1). Patients were divided into three groups according to the clinical outcome: (i) patients who remained disease-free during the whole follow-up period ($n = 84$), (ii) patients with early relapse, defined as relapse within 3 years post-surgery (< 3 years; $n = 23$) and (iii) patients with late relapse, defined as relapse presenting at 5 years or more post-surgery (≥ 5 years; $n = 20$). Consequently, 6 out of 49 relapses were observed in between 3 and 5 years. Patients' characteristics for the groups (ii) and (iii) are shown in Table 2. The median age was 52, 55 and 53 years in each group, respectively.

miRNA expression and statistical correlations

No significant associations were observed between miRNA expression (high expression, low expression) and age, menopausal status, tumor size, histological grade, number of infiltrated lymph nodes, estrogen receptor (ER), progesterone receptor (PR) or human epidermal growth factor receptor 2 (HER2) status (chi-square test, $p > 0.05$). However, miR-21 expression was higher in PR-negative as compared to PR-positive patients (63.4% vs 36.6%; chi-square test, $p = 0.038$). As expected, there was strong correlation between expression of miR-200b and miR-200c (Spearman's Rho 0.628; $p < 0.001$) that belong to the same miR-200 family. Moreover, there was strong correlation between miR-21 and miR-200b (Spearman's Rho 0.447; $p < 0.001$) and miR-200c (Spearman's Rho 0.540; $p < 0.001$) expression, as well. Weaker but still significant association was observed between the dormancy-related miR-23b and miR-190 (Spearman's Rho 0.236; $p < 0.001$) (Table 3).

miRNA expression and clinical outcome

Median expression levels of miR-21, miR-23b and miR-200c were significantly higher ($p < 0.001$, $p = 0.028$ and $p < 0.001$, respectively) and median miR-190 expression was significantly lower ($p = 0.013$) in relapsed compared to non-relapsed patients (Fig. 2). No significant difference was observed in the median expression of miR-200b ($p = 0.063$) between the two groups. Subsequently, we evaluated the DFS (Fig. 3) and OS (Fig. 4) in patients classified into high and low expression groups, according to the median value of each miRNA. We found that patients with high miR-21 expression had significantly shorter DFS compared to patients with low

Table 1 Characteristics of patients with early breast cancer

Characteristic	All patients		No relapse		Relapse		P
	Number	Percentage	Number	Percentage	Number	Percentage	
Number of patients	133		84	63	49	37	
Age (years)							ns[a]
Median	54		52		56		
Range	27–79		35–79		27–75		
Menopausal status							ns[a]
Premenopausal	57	42,9	40	47.6	17	34.7	
Postmenopausal	76	57.1	44	52.4	32	65.3	
Tumor size (cm)							0.015[a]
T1	60	45.1	42	50	18	36.7	
T2	66	49.6	41	48.8	25	51	
T3	7	5,3	1	1.2	6	12.3	
Histological grade							ns[a]
I	6	4.5	6	7.1			
II	59	44.5	41	48.8	18	36.7	
III	58	43.6	31	36.9	27	55.1	
Lobular	5	3.7	3	3.6	2	4.1	
Unknown	5	3.7	3	3.6	2	4.1	
Infiltrated lymph nodes							0.001[a]
0	49	36.8	37	44.0	12	24.5	
1–3	44	33.1	28	33.3	16	32.7	
≥ 4	34	25.6	13	15.5	21	42.8	
Unknown	6	4.5	6	7.2			
ER status							
Positive	88	66.2	56	66.7	32	65.3	
Negative	43	32.3	26	31	17	34.7	ns[a]
Unknown	2	1.5	2	2.3			
PR status							ns[a]
Positive	90	67.7	61	72.6	29	59.2	
Negative	41	30.8	21	25	20	40.8	
Unknown	2	1.5	2	2.4			
HER2 status							ns[a]
Positive	15	11.3	7	8.3	8	16.3	
Negative	112	84.2	72	85.7	40	81.6	
Unknown	6	4.5	5	6	1	2.1	
Adjuvant chemotherapy							ns[a]
Anthracycline-based	13	9.8	9	10.7	4	8.2	
Taxanes+anthracyclines	90	67.7	51	60.7	39	79.6	
Taxane-based	21	15.8	15	17.9	6	12.2	
Others	9	6.7	9	10.7			
Hormone therapy							ns[a]
Yes	103	77.5	68	80.9	35	71.4	
No	28	21.0	14	16.7	14	28.6	
Unknown	2	1.5	2	2.4			

ER estrogen receptor, *PR* progesterone receptor, *HER2* human epidermal growth factor receptor 2, *ns* not significant

[a]Pearson's chi-squared test for comparison between patients with relapse and without relapse

Table 2 Characteristics of patients with early (< 3 years) and late (≥ 5 years) relapse

Characteristic	Early (< 3 years)		Late (≥ 5 years)		P
	Number	Percentage	Number	Percentage	
Number of patients	23	17	20	15	
Age (years)					ns[a]
Median	55		53		
Range	27–75		38–74		
Menopausal status					ns[a]
Premenopausal	8	34.8	7	35	
Postmenopausal	15	65.2	13	65	
Tumor size (cm)					ns[a]
T1	7	30.4	8	40	
T2	12	52.2	10	50	
T3	4	17.4	2	10	
Histological grade					ns[a]
I	0		0		
II	10	43.5	6	30	
III	12	52.2	14	70	
Lobular	1	4.3			
Infiltrated lymph nodes					ns[a]
0	7	30.4	3	15	
1–3	9	39.2	6	30	
≥ 4	7	30.4	11	55	
ER					< 0.001[a]
Positive	9	39.2	19	95	
Negative	14	60.8	1	5	
PR					0.006[a]
Positive	10	43.5	17	85	
Negative	13	56.5	3	15	
Unknown					
HER2					ns[a]
Positive	4	17.4	4	20	
Negative	18	78.3	16	80	
Unknown	1	4.3			
Adjuvant chemotherapy					ns[a]
Anthracyclines-based	2	8.7	2	10	
Taxanes+anthracyclines	16	69.6	17	85	
Taxane-based	5	21.7	1	5	
Hormone therapy					0.002[a]
Yes	12	52.2	19	95	
No	11	47.8	1	5	

ER estrogen receptor, PR progesterone receptor, HER2 human epidermal growth factor receptor 2, ns not significant
Pearson's chi-squared test for comparison between patients with relapse and without relapse

expression (105.03 months versus not reached; $p < 0.001$) (Fig. 3a). Similarly, patients with high miR-200c expression had significantly shorter DFS compared to those with low miR-200c (105.03 vs not reached; $p = 0.005$) (Fig. 3e).

Finally, patients with high expression of both miR-21 and miR-200c had shorter DFS compared to patients with only one miRNA high or with both low (81.37 vs 132.9 and not reached, respectively; $p < 0.001$) (Fig. 3f). No significant

Table 3 Coefficients of correlation among five miRNAs

	miR-21	miR-23b	miR-190	miR-200b	miR-200c
miR-21	1.000				
miR-23b	0.109	1.000			
miR-190	0.160	0.236*	1.000		
miR-200b	0.447**	−0.144	0.005	1.000	
miR-200c	0.540**	0.145	0.081	0.628**	1.000

**p < 0.01; *p < 0.05

differences in DFS were found among patients with high or low expression of miR-23b, miR-190 or miR-200b (Fig. 3b-d). Median survival was not reached by patients with either high or low expression of any of the miRNAs evaluated (Fig. 4b-e). Nevertheless, only patients with high miR-21 had significantly shorter OS compared to those with low miR-21 ($p = 0.033$) (Fig. 4a).

To evaluate further the prognostic value of the circulating miRNAs, univariate and multivariate analyses were performed that included demographic and clinical variables and the expression levels of the five miRNAs (classified into high or low). Cox univariate analysis revealed that patients with infiltrated axillary lymph nodes

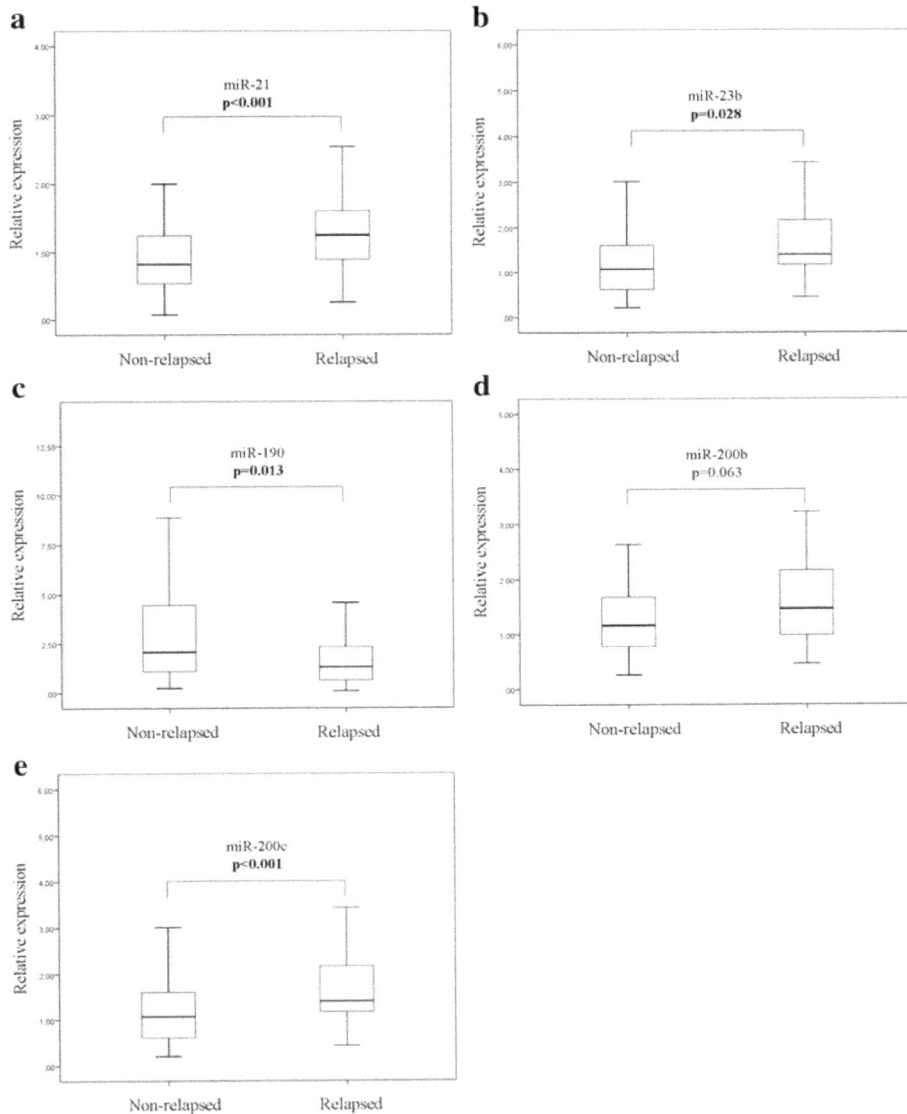

Fig. 2 Relative expression levels of circulating miRNAs in relapsed and non-relapsed patients. Plasma levels of miR-21 (**a**), miR-23 (**b**), miR-190 (**c**), miR-200b (**d**) and miR-200c (**e**) were evaluated by RT-qPCR. Statistically significant differences were determined using the Mann-Whitney test. P values are shown

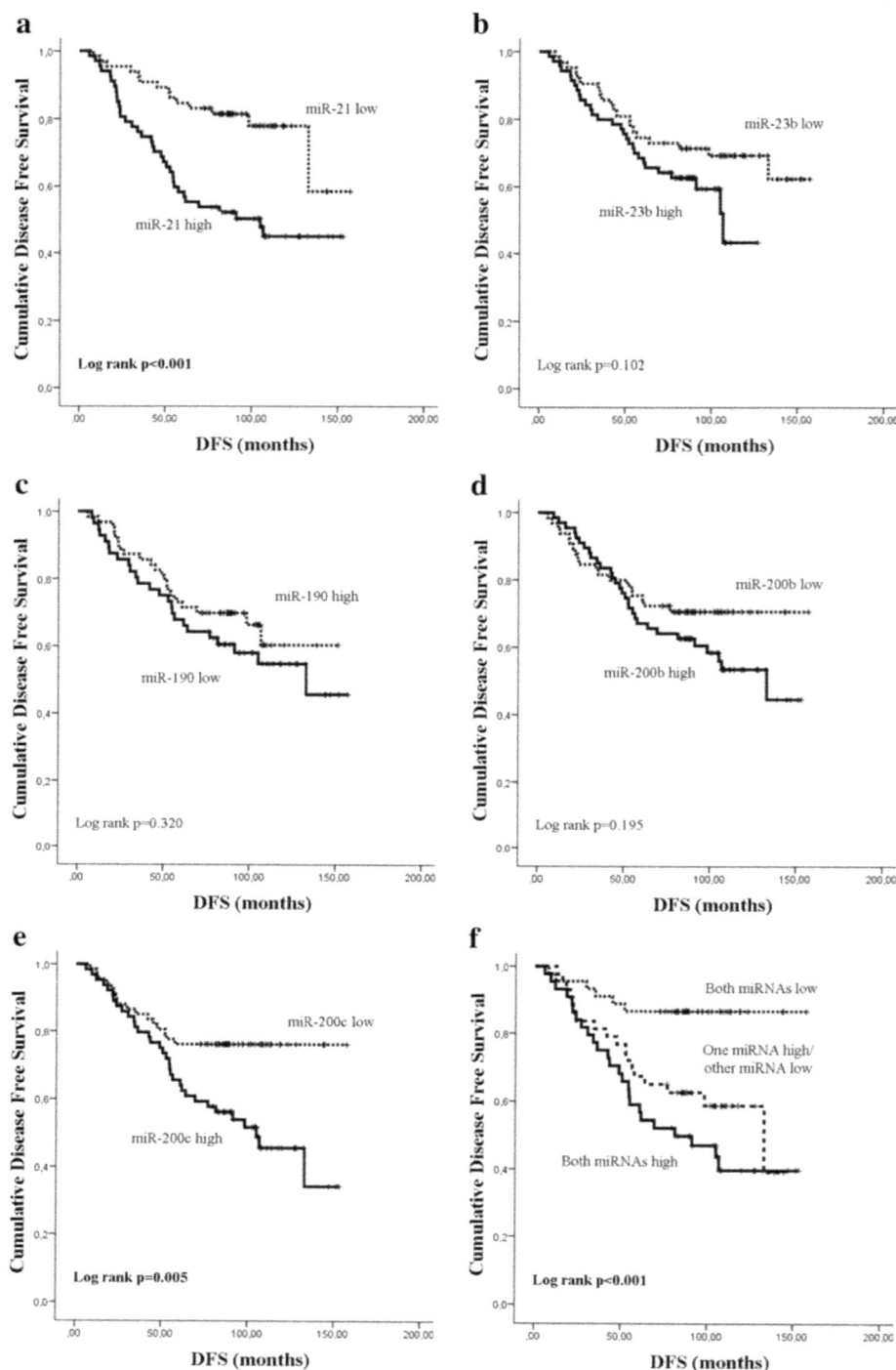

Fig. 3 Kaplan-Meier analysis of disease-free survival (DFS) according to the expression of circulating miRNAs and their combination. DFS in patients with high or low expression of miR-21 (**a**), miR-23b (**b**), miR-190 (**c**), miR-200b (**d**), miR-200c (**e**) and the combination of miR-21 and miR-200c (**f**). Curves were compared using the log rank test. *P* values are shown

and those with negative hormone receptor expression had significantly shorter DFS ($p = 0.013$ and $p = 0.028$, respectively) and OS ($p = 0.044$ and p = 0.01, respectively) (Table 4). High miR-21 and miR-200c expression levels were significantly associated with shorter DFS ($p < 0.001$ and $p = 0.007$, respectively) and only miR-21 high expression was associated with shorter OS ($p = 0.042$) (Table 4). Cox multivariate analysis

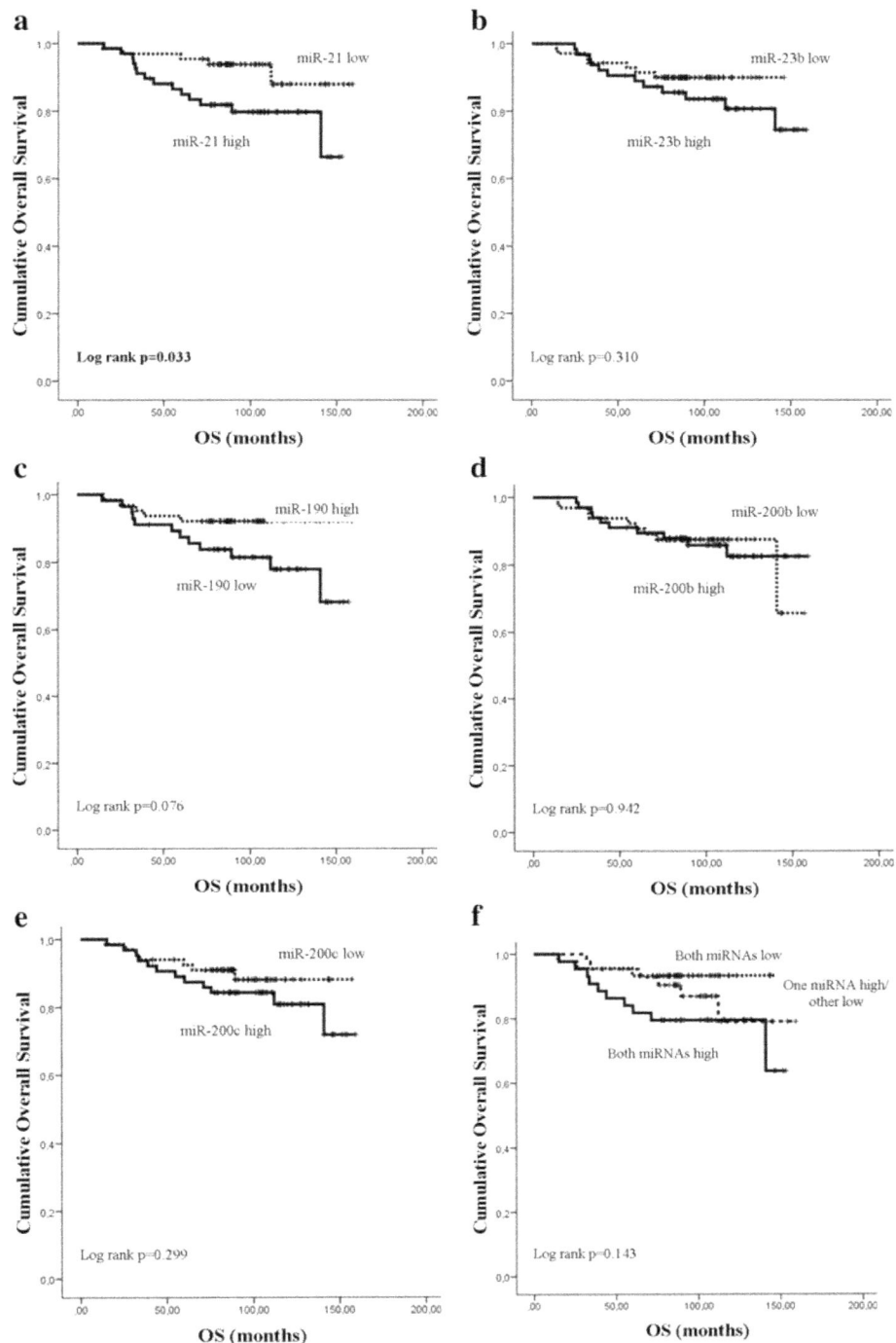

Fig. 4 Kaplan-Meier analysis of overall survival (OS) according to the expression of circulating miRNAs and their combination. OS in patients with high or low expression of miR-21 (**a**), miR-23b (**b**), miR-190 (**c**), miR-200b (**d**), miR-200c (**e**) and the combination of miR-21 and miR-200c (**f**). Curves were compared using the log rank test. *P* values are shown

revealed that the involvement of axillary lymph nodes and hormone receptor negativity were independent prognostic factors for shorter DFS ($p = 0.019$ and $p = 0.012$, respectively) and OS ($p = 0.029$ and $p = 0.006$, respectively)

(Table 4). Furthermore, only high miR-21 and high miR-200c expression emerged as independent prognostic factors associated with shorter DFS ($p = 0.003$ and $p = 0.037$) (Table 4).

Table 4 Univariate and multivariate analysis for DFS and OS in patients with early breast cancer

| | Univariate analysis | | | |
| | DFS | | OS | |
	HR (95% CI)	p value	HR (95% CI)	p value
Tumor size, T2–3 vs T1	1.48 (0.832–2.633)	0.177	1.584 (0.623–4.026)	0.334
Lymph nodes, pos vs neg	2.288 (1.192–4.391)	0.013	3.553 (1.034–12.206)	0.044
Histology grade, III vs I/II	1.650 (0.910–3.003)	0.099	1.276 (0.501–3.251)	0.609
ER, neg vs pos	1.318 (0.731–2.375)	0.359	2.120 (0.857–5.244)	0.104
PR, neg vs pos	2.003 (1.131–3.549)	0.017	2.323 (0.940–5.743)	0.068
ER/PR, neg vs at least one pos	2.010 (1.080–3.741)	0.028	3.324 (1.329–8.314)	0.01
Her2 pos vs neg	1.649 (0.771–3.525)	0.197	1.474 (0.429–5.065)	0.538
miR-21 high vs low	2.896 (1.556–5.390)	<0.001	2.884 (1.038–8.013)	0.042
miR-23b high vs low	1.624 (0.903–2.919)	0.105	1.630 (0.629–4.227)	0.315
miR-190 low vs high	1.342 (0.749–2.405)	0.322	2.511 (0.877–7.186)	0.086
miR-200b high vs low	1.460 (0.821–2.599)	0.198	1.034 (0.417–2.565)	0.942
miR-200c high vs low	2.287 (1.258–4.156)	0.007	1.637 (0.640–4.184)	0.304
Both miR-21/mir-200c high vs others	2.360 (1.346–4.135)	0.003	2.225 (0.902–5.489)	0.082
	Multivariate analysis			
	DFS		OS	
	HR (95% CI)	p value	HR (95% CI)	p value
Lymph nodes, pos vs neg	2.202 (1.138–4.260)	0.019	4.006 (1.151–13.935)	0.029
ER/PR, neg vs at least one pos	2.275 (1.202–4.305)	0.012	3.668 (1.457–9.233)	0.006
miR-21 high vs low	4.557 (1.685–12.869)	0.003	–	–
miR-200c high vs low	3.158 (1.074–9.288)	0.037		

DFS disease-free survival, *OS* overall survival, *pos* positive, *neg* negative, *ER* estrogen receptor, *PR* progesterone receptor, *HER2* human epidermal growth factor receptor 2

miRNA expression according to the timing of recurrence

We examined further whether the five circulating miR-NAs are differentially expressed among patients classified into groups according to the timing of recurrence. For this purpose we compared miRNA expression levels in (i) patients who relapsed early compared to those who did not experience early relapse i.e. in patients who had recurrence within 3 years (n = 23) and those who either relapsed 3 or more years post-surgery or remained disease-free for the whole follow-up period (n = 110) and (ii) in patients with late relapse (at ≥ 5 years; n = 20) compared to those who remained disease-free during the whole follow-up period (n = 84). The Mann-Whitney test revealed that miR-190 expression levels were lower in patients with early relapse (p = 0.0032), whereas no differences were recorded for the remaining miRNAs (Fig. 5). Moreover, miR-21 and miR-200c expression was higher in patients with late relapse as compared to non-relapsed patients (p = 0.015 and p < 0.001, respectively; Fig. 6a and e).

Combination of miRNA expression and clinicopathological characteristics in a relapse-predictive model

Expression levels of various miRNAs were combined with clinicopathological characteristics in relapse-predicting models. We used binary logistic regression incorporating various combinations of miRNAs and used the corresponding ROC curves to determine the sensitivity and the specificity of plasma miRNA expression, to discriminate patients who subsequently had disease recurrence from non-relapsed patients (Fig. 7 and Table 5). When assessing single miRNAs, the ROC curves showed that the expression of miR-21 and miR-200c had the highest performance with an area under the ROC curve (AUC) of 0.685 (sensitivity 71.4%, specificity 63.9% (p < 0.001; 95% CI 0.592–0.777)) and AUC of 0.678 (sensitivity 75.5%, specificity 61% (p < 0.001; 95% CI 0.586–0.769)), respectively (Fig. 7a and e, respectively and Table 5). When assessing combinations of miRNAs, binary logistic regression analysis resulted in a pattern of three miRNAs (miR-21, miR-23b and miR-190) bearing the highest predictive accuracy. The AUC from ROC analysis of this combined model 0.765, with sensitivity 80% and specificity 65.3% (p < 0.001; 95% CI 0.673–0.850) (Fig. 8a and Table 5). Eventually, the combination of the three miR-NAs with the currently used clinical prognostic parameters, axillary lymph node infiltration and tumor grade, resulted in superior discriminatory capability (AUC 0.873, sensitivity 89% and specificity 76.2% (p < 0.001;

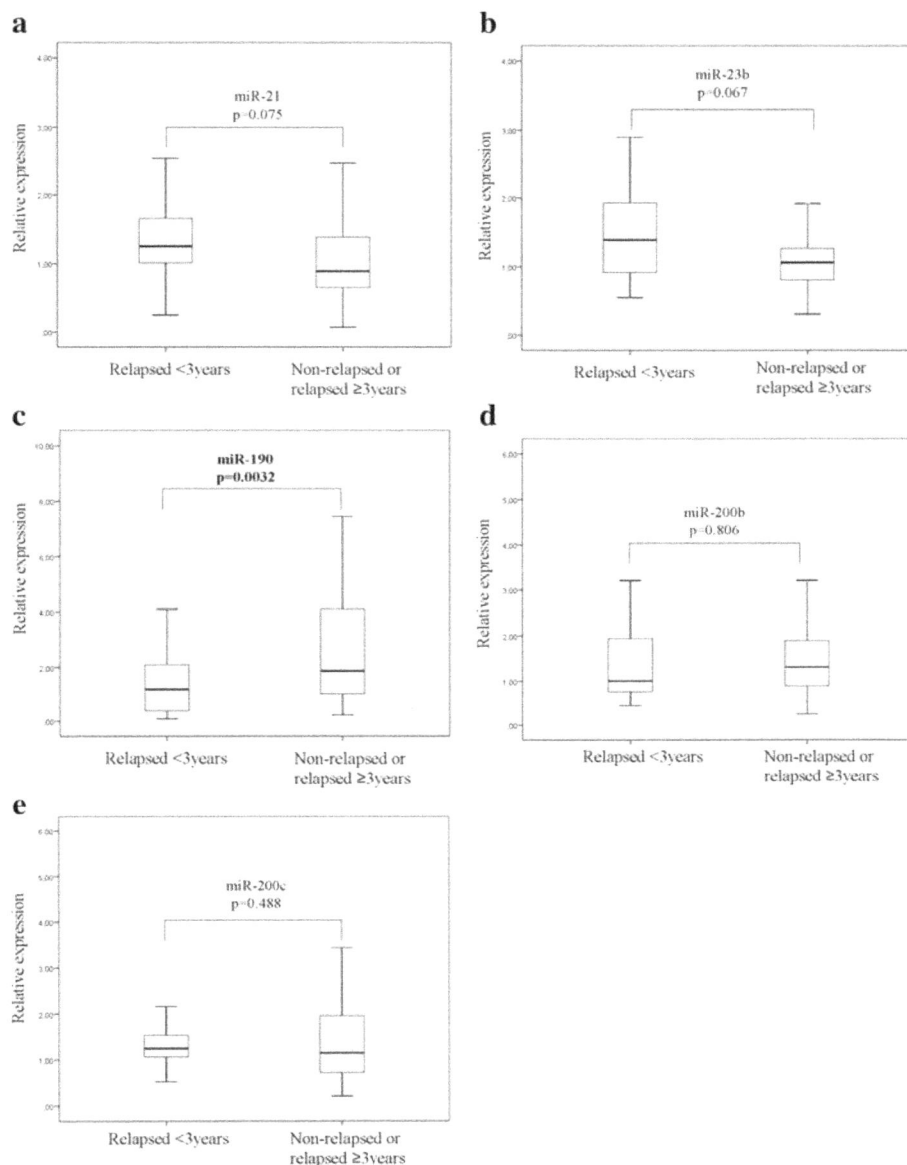

Fig. 5 Differential expression of the five circulating miRNAs in patients with early relapse. Relative expression levels of miR-21 (**a**), miR-23 (**b**), miR-190 (**c**), miR-200b (**d**) and miR-200c (**e**) in plasma from patients that experienced early relapse (< 3 years) compared to those without early relapse. Statistically significant differences were determined using the Mann-Whitney test

95% CI 0.802–0.940)) compared to the expression of the three miRNAs alone or to the clinicopathological features alone (Fig. 8b, c and Table 5). Using the same procedure the combination of miR-200c expression, axillary lymph node infiltration, tumor grade and ER status resulted in an increased AUC of 0.890 with a sensitivity 75% and specificity 89% ($p < 0.001$; 95% CI 0.818–0.972) for the prediction of late disease relapse (Fig. 8d and Table 5). When the same model was fitted to predict early relapse, there were no differences in the discriminatory power when combining miRNAs with clinicopathological parameters.

The robustness of the predictive performance of our models was assessed through a cross-validation strategy. A 10-fold cross-validation with a 70–30 split (70% training data, 30% testing data) was implemented in R and applied on nine different feature combinations of miRNAs and clinicopathological features. Mean AUC values were calculated for each 10-fold cross-validation. The mean AUC was then compared to the AUC calculated from our initial regression analysis. There were no significant differences in the values of AUC in any variable combinations, indicating that the performance of

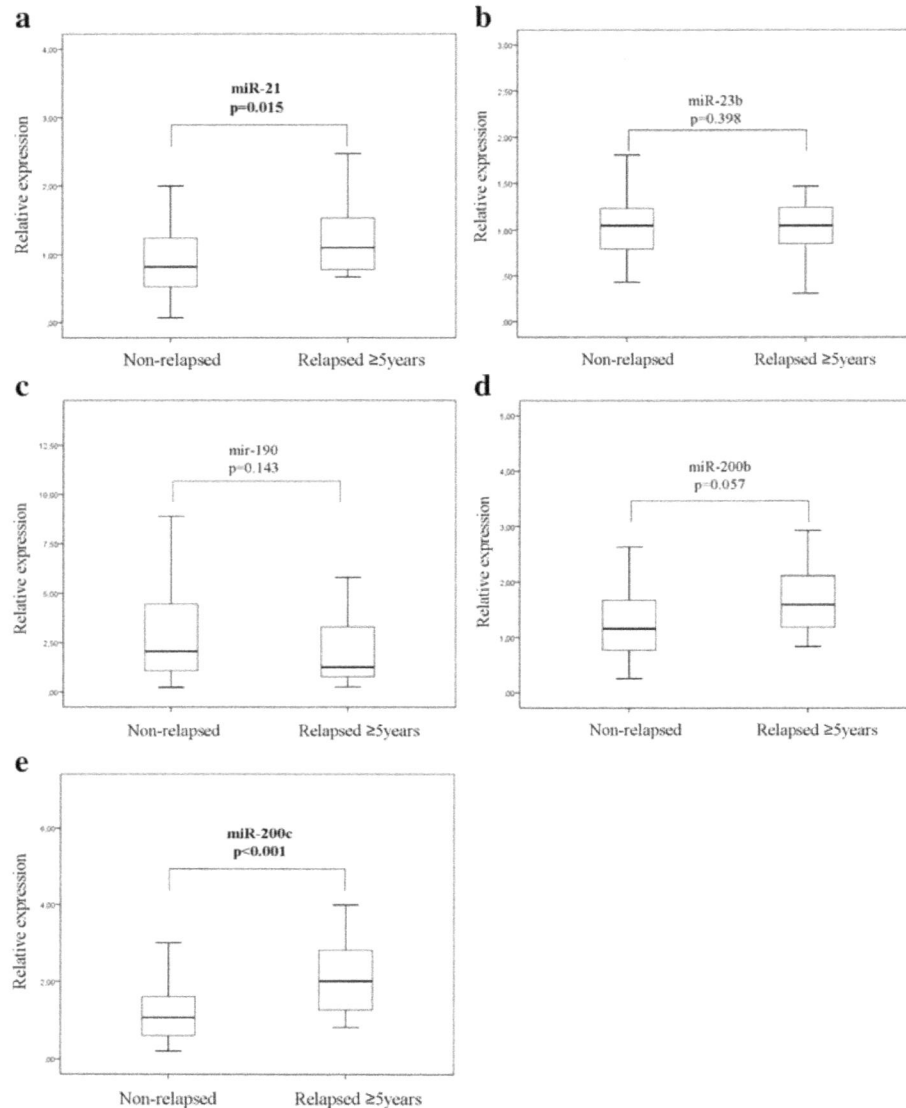

Fig. 6 Differential expression of the five circulating miRNAs in patients with late relapse. Relative expression levels of miR-21 (**a**), miR-23 (**b**), miR-190 (**c**), miR-200b (**d**) and miR-200c (**e**) in plasma from patients who relapsed late (≥ 5 years) compared to patients without relapse during the follow-up. Statistically significant differences were determined using the Mann-Whitney test

these models is robust and can be generalized to independent datasets (Additional file 1: Table S1).

Discussion

An important area in current breast cancer research is the identification of novel biomarkers for the prediction of outcome in patients with early disease. In the present study we investigated the predictive capacity of the dormancy and metastasis-related miR-21, miR-23b, miR-190, miR-200b and miR-200c when determined in the plasma of patients with early breast cancer. We found that miR-21, miR-23b, miR-190 and miR-200c, evaluated before the initiation of adjuvant therapy, were

differentially expressed among patients who subsequently experienced disease recurrence, compared to patients who did not relapse. High expression of miR-21 and miR-200c was associated with shorter DFS compared to patients with low expression, whereas high miR-21 was also associated with shorter OS. Interestingly, miR-21, miR-23b, miR-190 and miR-200c discriminated patients who relapsed from non-relapsed patients. The combination of miR-21, miR-23b and miR-190 in ROC curve analyses had higher sensitivity and specificity compared to each miRNA alone; accuracy was further improved by adding lymph node infiltration and tumor grade to the panel of three miRNAs. Furthermore, the

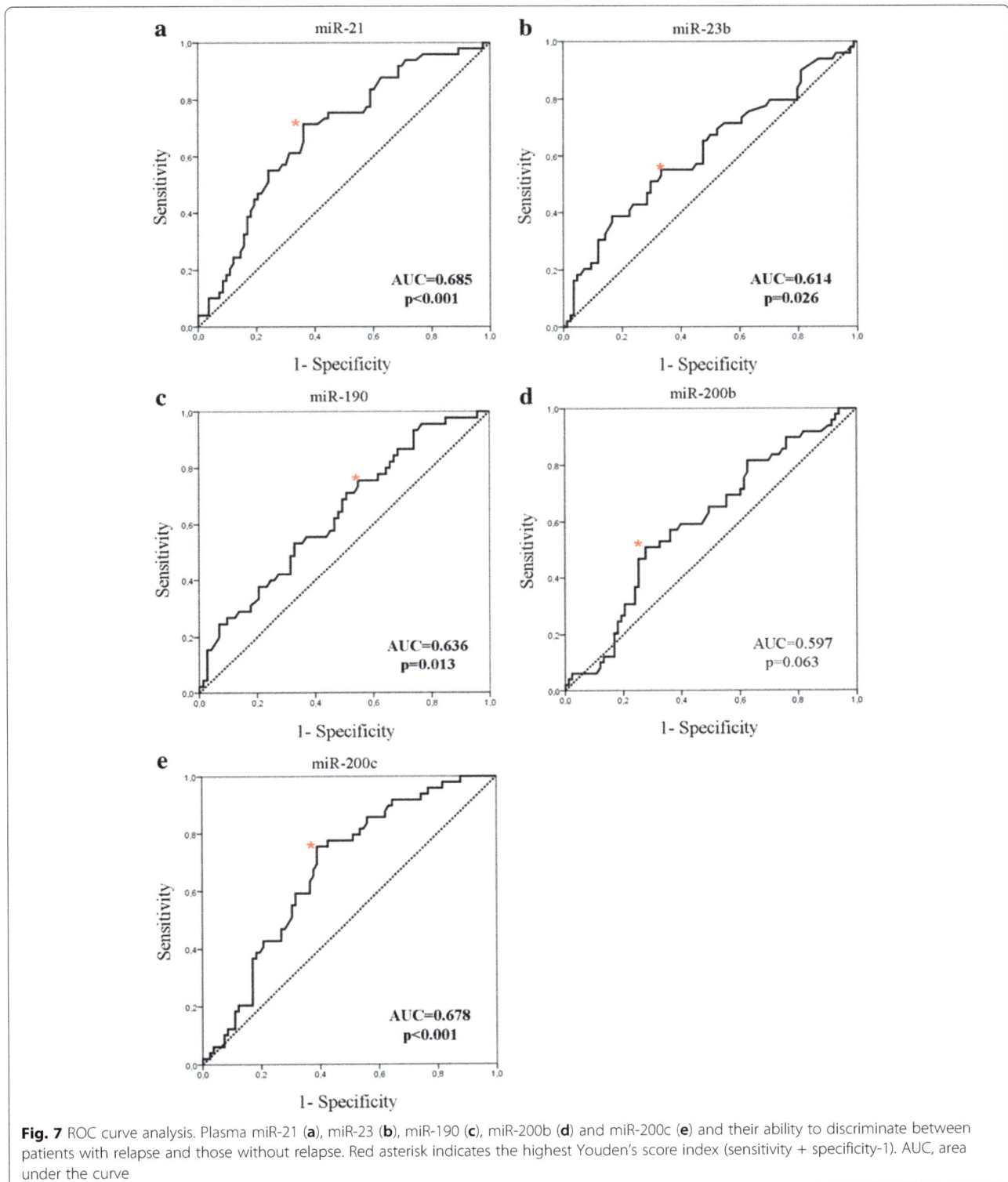

Fig. 7 ROC curve analysis. Plasma miR-21 (**a**), miR-23 (**b**), miR-190 (**c**), miR-200b (**d**) and miR-200c (**e**) and their ability to discriminate between patients with relapse and those without relapse. Red asterisk indicates the highest Youden's score index (sensitivity + specificity-1). AUC, area under the curve

combination of miR-200c, lymph node infiltration, tumor grade and ER status predicted late relapse.

In breast cancer, clinically detectable metastases emerge after a period of dormancy and can last for varying and frequently prolonged periods of time. As miRNAs regulate tumor progression and metastasis we hypothesized that dormant tumors could be distinguished from faster-growing tumors by the differential

Table 5 Performance of miRNAs and their combinations to predict relapse in patients with early breast cancer

Potential predictors	Cutoff value	Sensitivity (%)	Specificity (%)	AUC (95% CI)	p
Early breast cancer					
miR-21	0.98	71.4	63.9	0.685 (0.592–0.777)	< 0.001
miR-23b	1.35	38.8	83.3	0.614 (0.512–0.716)	0.029
miR-190	2.36	75.6	45.2	0.636 (0.534–0.738)	0.013
miR-200b	1.72	51.0	72.3	0.597 (0.498–0.696)	0.063
miR-200c	1.15	75.5	61.0	0.678 (0.586–0.769)	< 0.001
Three miRNAS (miR-21, miR-23b, miR-190)	0.39	80	65.3	0.765 (0.673–0.850)	< 0.001
Lymph nodes and grade	0.29	83	46.7	0.709 (0.614–0.804)	< 0.001
Three miRNAS plus lymph nodes and grade	0.41	89	76.2	0.873 (0.802–0.940)	< 0.001
Late relapse (≥ 5 years)					
miR-200c and lymph nodes, grade and ER status	0.42	75	89	0.89 (0.812–0.972)	< 0.001

AUC area under the receiver operating curve, *ER* estrogen receptor

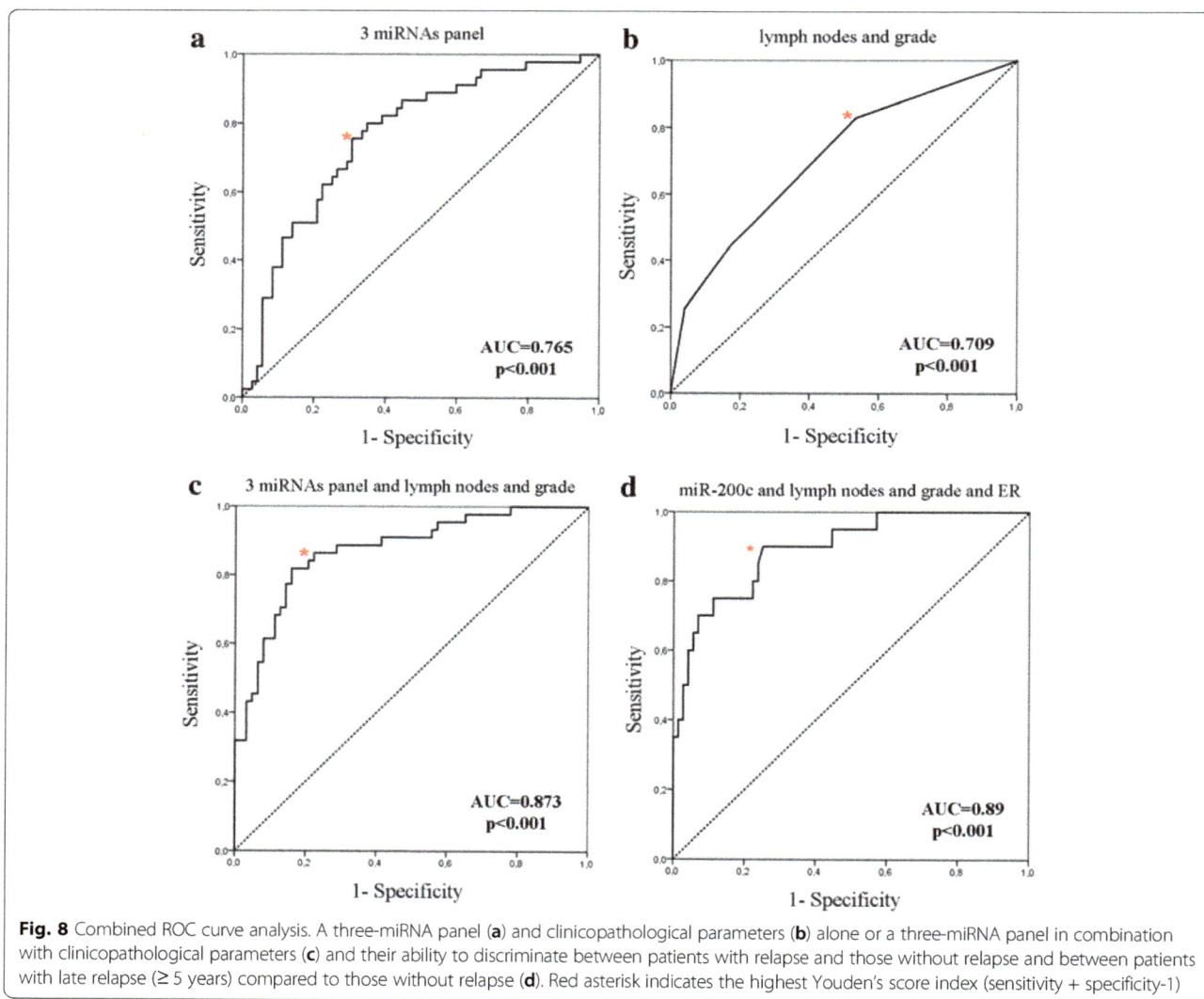

Fig. 8 Combined ROC curve analysis. A three-miRNA panel (**a**) and clinicopathological parameters (**b**) alone or a three-miRNA panel in combination with clinicopathological parameters (**c**) and their ability to discriminate between patients with relapse and those without relapse and between patients with late relapse (≥ 5 years) compared to those without relapse (**d**). Red asterisk indicates the highest Youden's score index (sensitivity + specificity-1)

expression of miRNAs [26]. We show for the first time that miR-190 expression was lower in patients with early relapse, suggesting a potential role for this miRNA in sustaining tumor dormancy in breast cancer. Indeed, miR-190 was among the most upregulated miR-NAs in a dormancy-related miRNA signature [21]. miR-190 is involved in the regulation of the transforming growth factor (TGF)β pathway and in breast cancer TGFβ has been shown to promote bone and lung metastases [27, 28]. Thus, miR-190 could induce tumor dormancy through the modulation of TGFβ signaling [29].

Previous studies showed that miR-23b induced dormant phenotypes in a bone marrow, metastatic, human breast cancer cell line, induced cell cycle arrest in glioma cancer stem cells and suppressed glioma cell migration and invasion [20, 30, 31] . On the contrary, the miR-23b/27b/24 cluster correlated with increased metastatic potential in human breast cancer cell lines and was upregulated in lung metastases from breast cancer [32]. Moreover, high miR-23b/27b/24 expression was associated with poor outcome in breast cancer [33]. Our results demonstrate higher plasma miR-23b expression in patients who relapsed, indicating that it is more likely associated with the development of metastases in breast cancer. Interestingly, the mature sequence of miR-23a differs by just one nucleotide in comparison to its paralog miR-23b, therefore they could share the same putative target genes and similar biological functions. However, there are reports showing distinct function between miR-23a and miR-23b and in contrast to miR-23b, we detected no variations in miR-23a expression levels among the different patient cohorts [34, 35].

Various preclinical studies have established that miR-21 is involved in tumor growth, invasion and migration, extracellular matrix modification and survival [36]. In primary breast cancer, miR-21 expression is associated with tumor progression, advanced clinical stage, lymph node metastasis and poor patient outcome [37, 38]. In support of the tumor-promoting role of miR-21, serum miR-21 distinguishes patients with breast cancer from healthy controls and patients with distant metastasis from those with locoregional disease, and it is associated with poor prognosis in breast cancer [36, 39, 40]. Accordingly, we show that high circulating miR-21 discriminated between patients with early breast cancer who relapsed and those who remained disease-free and specifically, high expression was associated with late relapse. Importantly, patients with high plasma miR-21 expression levels had worse DFS and OS compared to patients with low expression, whereas high miR-21 also emerged as an independent predictive factor for shorter DFS ($p = 0.003$). Iorio et al., demonstrated that the TGFβ gene was a target for miR-21 and Yan et al. showed that TGFβ1 and the receptor TGFβR2 were identified among the putative target

genes of miR-21 [37, 38]. These data suggest that the tumor promoting effects of miR-21 in breast cancer, could be exerted through the regulation of TGFβ signaling.

The miR-200 family (miR-200a, miR-200b, miR-200c, miR-141 and miR-429) has opposing roles in the regulation of EMT and metastasis [41]. On one hand, they negatively regulate the E-cadherin transcriptional repressors ZEB1/2 preventing EMT and on the other, they have been associated with global shifts in gene expression which promote metastatic colonization in breast cancer mouse models [17, 42]. Conflicting results have been also reported on the clinical relevance of miR-200 family members in breast cancer [43, 44]. By adopting a global profiling approach, Madhavan et al. showed that miR-200b and miR-200c were among the panel of six miRNAs with significantly increased expression in patients with early breast cancer who developed metastases [45]. Our results also support the association between the plasma miR-200 family and metastatic progression in breast cancer. Importantly, high miR-200c was associated with late relapse and emerged as an independent prognostic factor for worse DFS ($p = 0.037$).

ROC curve analysis confirmed the value of the plasma miRNAs in the prediction of disease recurrence in breast cancer. The combination of miR-21, miR-23b and miR-190 had higher accuracy compared to each miRNA alone. Moreover, the addition of common clinicopathological prognostic factors further improved the discriminatory capability of the three miRNAs. These results provide novel opportunities for breast cancer therapeutics employing the aforementioned miRNAs in a combinatorial miRNA approach [46]. From a network analysis perspective, further insights might be achieved through the incorporation of information on the expression of the protein-coding mRNA associated to the involved miRNA. The formulation of a model of intervention efficiency based on a combination of miRNA, their gene targets and associated pathways would thus provide complementary information orthogonal to the one obtained from pathological characteristics.

In breast cancer, late relapses are common and impose considerable concern among disease-free patients, and there are no accurate tools to identify patients at risk. Importantly, in our study miR-200c expression combined with the clinical information on axillary lymph node status, tumor grade and ER status yielded an AUC of 0.89 with sensitivity of 75% and specificity of 89% for the prediction of late relapse ($p < 0.001$).

Our study is among the first to demonstrate the potential of metastasis-promoting miRNAs to serve as circulating predictive markers in early breast cancer. Importantly, (a) this patient cohort had long-term follow up, (b) plasma samples and clinical information were obtained prospectively, (c) the prediction of relapse was possible years before metastasis emerged and (d) circulating miRNAs added independent predictive value to common clinicopathological parameters. Furthermore, we considered pre-analytical and analytical parameters very carefully, taking into account the variables that could lead to bias in miRNA quantification [22, 47].

Limitations of our study include that results are derived from the analysis of a relatively small group of patients and lack validation in an independent cohort. However, by performing cross-validation analysis of our data [48], the predictive performance of the aforementioned miRNAs was confirmed, therefore it could probably be verified in an independent dataset. Nevertheless, our results should be viewed as preliminary and warrant prospective validation in a larger cohort of patients with early disease.

Conclusions

Our results suggest that dormancy and metastasis-related miRNAs are differentially expressed in plasma in patients with early breast cancer who experience disease recurrence and in those that will remain disease-free. The identified miRNAs might be of potential use in the development of a multimarker blood-based test to complement and improve prognostication based on clinicopathological characteristics. Furthermore, these results imply that circulating miRNAs could serve as novel surrogate markers for the presence of occult micro metastatic disease and for increased risk of recurrence in early breast cancer. Finally, they provide potential insights into the procedures and pathways involved in the regulation of dormancy and metastasis in breast cancer.

Abbreviations

AUC: Area under the curve; cDNA: Complementary DNA; Ct: Cycle threshold; DFS: Disease-free survival; EMT: Epithelial-mesenchymal transition; ER: Estrogen receptor; HER2: Human epidermal growth factor receptor 2; miR: Micro-RNA; OS: Overall survival; PR: Progesterone receptor; ROC: Receiver operating characteristic; TGF: Transforming growth factor

Acknowledgements

We are grateful to all patients and volunteers who signed the consent form.

Funding

This work was partly supported by Hellenic Society of Medical Oncology (HESMO). Michalis Stratigos is a recipient of a HESMO research fellowship. Work was also partly supported by the Anticancer Research Support Association (ARSA). The funders had no role in study design, data collection and analysis, decision to publish and preparation of the manuscript.

Authors' contributions

CP coordinated the work, performed control experiments and molecular analysis, analyzed the data, interpreted the results and drafted the manuscript. MS collected the patients' clinicopathological data, participated in data acquisition and interpretation and was involved in drafting the manuscript GM provided support in statistical analysis and data interpretation MS was involved in study design and participated in laboratory work. GM participated in laboratory work. CN provided support in statistical analysis and was involved in drafting the revised manuscript. DM was involved in study design and data interpretation, participated in the preparation of the manuscript and provided general support SA designed, coordinated and supervised the study, was involved in data analysis and interpretation and drafted the manuscript. All authors have read and approved the final manuscript.

Competing interests

The authors declare that they have no competing interests.

Author details

[1]Laboratory of Translational Oncology, School of Medicine, University of Crete, Heraklion, 71003 Heraklion, Crete, Greece. [2]Department of Medical Oncology, University General Hospital of Heraklion, 1352 PO BOX, 711 10 Heraklion, Crete, Greece. [3]Department of Agricultural, Technological Education Institute of Heraklion, 72100 Heraklion, Crete, Greece. [4]Computational Genomics Group, Department of Biology, University of Crete, 70013 Heraklion, Greece. [5]Institute of Molecular Biology and Biotechnology, Foundation for Research and Technology, 70013 Heraklion, Crete, Greece.

References

1. Brewster AM, et al. Residual risk of breast cancer recurrence 5 years after adjuvant therapy. J Natl Cancer Inst. 2008;100(16):1179–83.
2. Colleoni M, et al. Annual hazard rates of recurrence for breast cancer during 24 years of follow-up: results from the international breast cancer study group trials I to V. J Clin Oncol. 2016;34(9):927–35.
3. Davies C, et al. Long-term effects of continuing adjuvant tamoxifen to 10 years versus stopping at 5 years after diagnosis of oestrogen receptor-positive breast cancer: ATLAS, a randomised trial. Lancet. 2013;381(9869): 805–16.
4. Aguirre-Ghiso JA. Models, mechanisms and clinical evidence for cancer dormancy. Nat Rev Cancer. 2007;7(11):834–46.
5. Pan H, et al. 20-Year risks of breast-cancer recurrence after stopping endocrine therapy at 5 years. N Engl J Med. 2017;377(19):1836–46.
6. Sestak I, Cuzick J. Markers for the identification of late breast cancer recurrence. Breast Cancer Res. 2015;7:10.
7. Chen N. Incorporate gene signature profiling into routine molecular testing. Appl Transl Genom. 2013;2:28–33.
8. Bedard PL, et al. Tumour heterogeneity in the clinic. Nature. 2013;501(7467): 355–64.
9. Bartel DP. MicroRNAs: target recognition and regulatory functions. Cell. 2009;136(2):215–33.
10. Hayes J, Peruzzi PP, Lawler S. MicroRNAs in cancer: biomarkers, functions and therapy. Trends Mol Med. 2014;20(8):460–9.
11. Peng Y, Croce CM. The role of MicroRNAs in human cancer. Signal Transduction And Targeted Therapy. 2016;1:15004.

12. Schwarzenbach H, et al. Clinical relevance of circulating cell-free microRNAs in cancer. Nat Rev Clin Oncol. 2014;11(3):145–56.

13. Mitchell PS, et al. Circulating microRNAs as stable blood-based markers for cancer detection. Proc Natl Acad Sci U S A. 2008;105(30):10513–8.

14. Turchinovich A, et al. Characterization of extracellular circulating microRNA. Nucleic Acids Res. 2011;39(16):7223–33.

15. Cheng Q, et al. A signature of epithelial-mesenchymal plasticity and stromal activation in primary tumor modulates late recurrence in breast cancer independent of disease subtype. Breast Cancer Res. 2014;16(4):407.

16. De Cock JM, et al. Inflammation triggers Zeb1-dependent escape from tumor latency. Cancer Res. 2016;76(23):6778–84.

17. Gregory PA, et al. The miR-200 family and miR-205 regulate epithelial to mesenchymal transition by targeting ZEB1 and SIP1. Nat Cell Biol. 2008; 10(5):593–601.

18. Dykxhoorn DM, et al. miR-200 enhances mouse breast cancer cell colonization to form distant metastases. PLoS One. 2009;4(9):e7181.

19. Zhu S, et al. MicroRNA-21 targets tumor suppressor genes in invasion and metastasis. Cell Res. 2008;18(3):350–9.

20. Ono M, et al. Exosomes from bone marrow mesenchymal stem cells contain a microRNA that promotes dormancy in metastatic breast cancer cells. Sci Signal. 2014;7(332):ra63.

21. Almog N, et al. Transcriptional changes induced by the tumor dormancy-associated microRNA-190. Transcription. 2013;4(4):177–91.

22. Schwarzenbach H, et al. Data normalization strategies for MicroRNA quantification. Clin Chem. 2015;61(11):1333–42.

23. Schmittgen TD, Livak KJ. Analyzing real-time PCR data by the comparative C(T) method. Nat Protoc. 2008;3(6):1101–8.

24. Blondal T, et al. Assessing sample and miRNA profile quality in serum and plasma or other biofluids. Methods. 2013;59(1):S1–6.

25. McShane LM, et al. Reporting recommendations for tumor marker prognostic studies. J Clin Oncol. 2005;23(36):9067–72.

26. Almog N, et al. Consensus micro RNAs governing the switch of dormant tumors to the fast-growing angiogenic phenotype. PLoS One. 2012;7(8): e44001.

27. Gennarino VA, et al. Identification of microRNA-regulated gene networks by expression analysis of target genes. Genome Res. 2012;22(6):1163–72.

28. Drabsch Y, ten Dijke P. TGF-beta signaling in breast cancer cell invasion and bone metastasis. J Mammary Gland Biol Neoplasia. 2011;16(2):97–108.

29. Bragado P, et al. TGF-beta2 dictates disseminated tumour cell fate in target organs through TGF-beta-RIII and p38alpha/beta signalling. Nat Cell Biol. 2013;15(11):1351–61.

30. Geng J, et al. Methylation mediated silencing of miR-23b expression and its role in glioma stem cells. Neurosci Lett. 2012;528(2):185–9.

31. Loftus JC, et al. miRNA expression profiling in migrating glioblastoma cells: regulation of cell migration and invasion by miR-23b via targeting of Pyk2. PLoS One. 2012;7(6):e39818.

32. Ell B, et al. The microRNA-23b/27b/24 cluster promotes breast cancer lung metastasis by targeting metastasis-suppressive gene prosaposin. J Biol Chem. 2014;289(32):21888–95.

33. Jin L, et al. Prooncogenic factors miR-23b and miR-27b are regulated by Her2/Neu, EGF, and TNF-alpha in breast cancer. Cancer Res. 2013;73(9): 2884–96.

34. Lin R, et al. Targeting miR-23a in CD8+ cytotoxic T lymphocytes prevents tumor-dependent immunosuppression. J Clin Invest. 2014;124(12):5352–67.

35. Li J, et al. The poly-cistronic miR-23-27-24 complexes target endothelial cell junctions: differential functional and molecular effects of miR-23a and miR-23b. Mol Ther Nucleic Acids. 2016;5(8):e354.

36. Aleckovic M, Kang Y. Regulation of cancer metastasis by cell-free miRNAs. Biochim Biophys Acta. 2015;1855(1):24–42.

37. Iorio MV, et al. MicroRNA gene expression deregulation in human breast cancer. Cancer Res. 2005;65(16):7065–70.

38. Yan LX, et al. MicroRNA miR-21 overexpression in human breast cancer is associated with advanced clinical stage, lymph node metastasis and patient poor prognosis. RNA. 2008;14(11):2348–60.

39. Wang G, et al. Quantitative measurement of serum microRNA-21 expression in relation to breast cancer metastasis in Chinese females. Ann Lab Med. 2015;35(2):226–32.

40. Muller V, et al. Changes in serum levels of miR-21, miR-210, and miR-373 in HER2-positive breast cancer patients undergoing neoadjuvant therapy: a translational research project within the Geparquinto trial. Breast Cancer Res Treat. 2014;147(1):61–8.

41. Humphries B, Yang C. The microRNA-200 family: small molecules with novel roles in cancer development, progression and therapy. Oncotarget. 2015; 6(9):6472–98.

42. Korpal M, et al. Direct targeting of Sec23a by miR-200s influences cancer cell secretome and promotes metastatic colonization. Nat Med. 2011;17(9): 1101–8.

43. Song. C, et al. miR-200c inhibits breast cancer proliferation by targeting KRAS. Oncotarget. 2015;6(33):34968–78.

44. Antolin S, et al. Circulating miR-200c and miR-141 and outcomes in patients with breast cancer. BMC Cancer. 2015;15:297.

45. Madhavan D, et al. Circulating miRNAs as surrogate markers for circulating tumor cells and prognostic markers in metastatic breast cancer. Clin Cancer Res. 2012;18(21):5972–82.

46. Kasinski AL, et al. A combinatorial microRNA therapeutics approach to suppressing non-small cell lung cancer. Oncogene. 2015;34(27):3547–55.

47. McDonald JS, et al. Analysis of circulating microRNA: preanalytical and analytical challenges. Clin Chem. 2011;57(6):833–40.

48. Machiela MJ, et al. Evaluation of polygenic risk scores for predicting breast and prostate cancer risk. Genet Epidemiol. 2011;35(6):506–14.

11

Contributions of the RhoA guanine nucleotide exchange factor *Net1* to polyoma middle T antigen-mediated mammary gland tumorigenesis and metastasis

Yan Zuo[1], Arzu Ulu[1], Jeffrey T. Chang[1,2] and Jeffrey A. Frost[1]* (ORCID)

Abstract

Background: The RhoA activating protein Net1 contributes to breast cancer cell proliferation, motility, and invasion in vitro, yet little is known about its roles in mammary gland tumorigenesis and metastasis.

Methods: *Net1* knockout (KO) mice were bred to mice with mammary gland specific expression of the polyoma middle T antigen (PyMT) oncogene. Mammary gland tumorigenesis and lung metastasis were monitored. Individual tumors were assessed for proliferation, apoptosis, angiogenesis, RhoA activation, and activation of PyMT-dependent signaling pathways. Primary tumor cells from wild-type and *Net1* KO mice were transplanted into the mammary glands of wild-type, nontumor-bearing mice, and tumor growth and metastasis were assessed. Gene expression in wild-type and *Net1* KO tumors was analyzed by gene ontology enrichment and for relative activation of gene expression signatures indicative of signaling pathways important for breast cancer initiation and progression. A gene expression signature indicative of Net1 function was identified. Human breast cancer gene expression profiles were screened for the presence of a Net1 gene expression signature.

Results: We show that *Net1* makes fundamental contributions to mammary gland tumorigenesis and metastasis. *Net1* deletion delays tumorigenesis and strongly suppresses metastasis in PyMT-expressing mice. Moreover, we observe that loss of *Net1* reduces cancer cell proliferation, inhibits tumor angiogenesis, and promotes tumor cell apoptosis. *Net1* is required for maximal RhoA activation within tumors and for primary tumor cell motility. Furthermore, the ability of PyMT to initiate oncogenic signaling to ERK1/2 and PI3K/Akt1 is inhibited by *Net1* deletion. Primary tumor cell transplantation indicates that the reduction in tumor angiogenesis and lung metastasis observed upon *Net1* deletion are tumor cell autonomous effects. Using a gene expression signature indicative of Net1 activity, we show that Net1 signaling is activated in 10% of human breast cancers, and that this correlates with elevated proliferation and PI3K pathway activity. We also demonstrate that human breast cancer patients with a high *Net1* gene expression signature experience shorter distant metastasis-free survival.

Conclusions: These data indicate that Net1 is required for tumor progression in the PyMT mouse model and suggest that Net1 may contribute to breast cancer progression in humans.

Keywords: RhoA, Net1, Polyoma middle T antigen, Breast cancer, Metastasis

---

* Correspondence: Jeffrey.a.frost@uth.tmc.edu
[1]Department of Integrative Biology and Pharmacology, University of Texas Health Science Center at Houston, 6431 Fannin St, Houston, TX 77030, USA
Full list of author information is available at the end of the article

Background

Metastasis is the primary cause of death in breast cancer patients, yet there are few therapies directed at this process. As regulators of cell proliferation, cytoskeletal organization, and cell motility, Rho GTPases are essential to dissemination of cancer cells throughout the body. The Rho GTPase family consists of 20 genes in humans, with Cdc42, Rac1, and RhoA being the most thoroughly studied [1, 2]. Rac1, RhoA, and RhoC are commonly overexpressed in human breast cancers and RNAi-mediated knockdown or deletion of these genes inhibits tumorigenesis and metastasis [3–7]. Rac1 and RhoA/C contribute to metastasis by regulating separate types of invasive behavior in cancer cells, with Rac1 driving integrin-dependent, mesenchymal-type movement and RhoA/C driving integrin-independent, amoeboid movement. Importantly, cancer cells switch between these types of movement depending on the extracellular obstacles they are traversing, and inhibition of either of these forms of movement significantly inhibits invasive activity [8–10].

Rho GTPases function as molecular switches, cycling between their active, GTP-bound and inactive, GDP-bound states. When active, Rho proteins interact with downstream proteins, known as effectors, to initiate signaling cascades that control cell motility [11, 12]. Rho GTPase activation is controlled by two families of proteins, known as guanine nucleotide exchange factors (RhoGEFs) and GTPase activating proteins (RhoGAPs). RhoGEFs stimulate GDP release, thereby allowing Rho proteins to bind GTP and become active [13, 14]. Rho-GAPs stimulate the intrinsic GTPase activity of Rho proteins, thereby shutting them off [15]. Because the wild-type forms of Rho proteins are overexpressed in breast cancers, it is commonly assumed that altered function of RhoGAPs and RhoGEFs drives their activation. For example, the RhoGAP DLC-1 is deleted or epigenetically silenced in many breast cancer subtypes, driving aberrant RhoA activation and metastatic spread to the bones [16–18]. Alternatively, the Rac1 GEFs P-Rex1, Vav2/3, and Dock1 have been shown to contribute to metastatic behavior in particular breast cancer subtypes [19–21]. Despite evidence for RhoA and RhoC contributing to breast cancer tumorigenesis and metastasis, RhoA subfamily GEFs that contribute to breast cancer in vivo have not yet been identified.

The neuroepithelial transforming gene 1 (Net1) is a RhoA subfamily GEF that is overexpressed in many human cancers, including breast cancer [22, 23]. We have shown previously that Net1 is required for human breast cancer cell motility and invasive capacity in vitro [24]. In these cells Net1 is dedicated to controlling actomyosin contraction, as inhibition of Net1 expression blocks actomyosin contractility but does not affect other RhoA-regulated events, such as Ezrin phosphorylation. We have also observed that Net1 controls FAK activation, which is necessary for focal adhesion maturation [24]. Furthermore, Net1 has been shown to control cell motility in other cell types, and to regulate actin cytoskeletal rearrangements downstream of ligands such as TGFβ [25–27]. Net1 also controls mitotic progression by regulating Aurora A activation and chromosome alignment during the metaphase [28]. Thus, there is ample evidence to suggest that Net1 may contribute to tumorigenesis and metastasis in vivo; however, the role of Net1 in these processes has not been investigated. Similarly, the role of Net1 in human breast cancer is largely unknown.

In the present work we demonstrate that *Net1* is critical for mammary gland tumorigenesis and metastasis in the mouse mammary tumor virus (MMTV)-PyMT mouse genetic model of breast cancer, and demonstrate obligate signaling pathways that are regulated by *Net1*. Moreover, we identify a gene expression signature indicative of Net1 function and use this signature to demonstrate that Net1 contributes to metastasis in human breast cancer patients. Together these data indicate that Net1 is required for breast cancer progression in the MMTV-PyMT mouse model and may also contribute to human breast tumorigenesis and metastasis.

Methods

Mouse husbandry and care

Mice were housed in the Center for Laboratory Animal Medicine and Care within the Medical School at the University of Texas Health Science Center at Houston, TX, USA. All studies were approved by the Institutional Animal Care and Use Committee (protocol AWC 14-007) and were conducted in accordance with the guidelines of the US Public Health Service Policy for Humane Care and Use of Laboratory Animals.

Mouse strains used, genotyping, and analysis of tumorigenesis

$Net1^{-/-}$ mice in the C57BL/6 strain were as described previously [29]. Male *MMTV-PyMT* mice (Tg(MMTV-PyVT)634Mul) in the FVB/J background were purchased from Jackson Labs. The *MMTV-PyMT* allele was carried by crossing to female FVB/J mice. Mice lacking *Net1* were backcrossed to wild-type FVB/J mice for 10 generations to create a congenic line. Female $Net1^{+/-}$ (FVB/J) mice were mated with male *MMTV-PyMT* (FVB/J) mice to derive $Net1^{+/-}$,*MMTV-PyMT* mice. Female $Net1^{+/-}$ mice were crossed with *male Net1*$^{+/-}$,*MMTV-PyMT* mice to produce a cohort of female littermates with $Net1^{+/+}$,*MMTV-PyMT* and $Net1^{+/-}$,*MMTV-PyMT*, and $Net1^{-/-}$,*MMTV-PyMT* genotypes for tumor studies. Primers for genotyping *Net1*-deficient mice were as follows: forward primer 5GF3, 5′-TGCTATGCTATTGCTGCTT-3′, and reverse primer 3GR1, 5′-AGAACACCACCAAGTAACAA-3′ (amplifies wild-type *Net1*); and forward primer 5GF1, 5'-TTGTTACTTGGTGGTGTTCT-3' and reverse primer TV3-1R, 5'-AAGTGCTAACCTTCCTGC-3' (amplifies *Net$^{-/-}$* allele) [29]. The PyMT transgene was identified using previously published primers: forward, 5'-CGGCGGAGCGAGGAACTGAGGAGAG-3'; and reverse, 5'-TCAGAAGACTCGGCAGTCTTAGGCG-3' [30]. Tumor growth was monitored after weaning. Once palpable tumors had formed, tumor size was measured twice per week using electronic calipers. Tumor volume was calculated using the following equation:

$$V = \left(\text{Length} \times \text{Width}^2\right)/2.$$

Mice were euthanized when the largest tumor reached 2.5 cm^3.

Antibodies
The following antibodies were used: anti-pSer19-MLC2 (3675), anti-Ki67 (12202), anti-cleaved caspase 3 (9661), anti-CD31 (77699), anti-pT696-MYPT1 (5163), anti-MYPT1 (2634), anti-pY461-Src (6943), anti-pT202/Y204ERK1/2 (4370), anti-ERK1/2 (4695), anti-pT308-Akt1 (2965), anti-pS473-Akt1 (4060), anti-Akt (2920), anti-PP2A-C (2038), anti-PP2A-A (2041), anti-Shc (2432), anti-PI3 kinase p85 (4257), and anti-RhoC (3430) (Cell Signaling Technology); anti-β-actin (A5316) (Sigma-Aldrich); anti-PyMT (sc-53,481), anti-GST (sc-138), anti-Src (sc-8056), and normal rat IgG (sc-2026) (SantaCruz Biotechnology); and anti-RhoA (ARH03) (Cytoskeleton, Inc.).

Primary tumor cell isolation and mammary gland transplantation
Individual mammary tumors were isolated from *Net1$^{+/+}$,MMTV-PyMT* and *Net1$^{-/-}$,MMTV-PyMT* mice, manually minced, and incubated in DMEM/F12 (Hyclone) with 2 mg/ml collagenase A (Agilent), and 1× antibiotic–antimycotic (Life Technologies) for 2 h at 37 °C with 150 rpm rotation at a 45° angle. The minced tissues were then shaken vigorously and pipetted up and down to create a cell suspension. The cells were pelleted by centrifugation at $600 \times g$ for 10 min at room temperature, resuspended in DMEM/F12 with 10% fetal bovine serum (FBS) and 1× antibiotic–antimycotic, and passed through a 70-μm cell strainer (ThermoFisher Scientific). The cells were cultured in DMEM/F12 with 10% FBS, 100 U/ml penicillin/streptomycin, 10 μg/ml insulin, and 1× antibiotic–antimycotic. The epithelial marker cytokeratin 8 (CK8) and PyMT were detected in 90–95% of cells by immunofluorescence microscopy.

Confluent primary tumor cells were harvested with 0.25% trypsin and rinsed twice with PBS. 8×10^6 cells were mixed with Matrigel (catalog no. 354,248; Corning) to a final volume of 200 μl, and were injected into the number four fat pad of wild-type female FVB mice, 6–7 weeks old, using a 28.5-G insulin syringe (catalog no. 329,424; BD). Once palpable, tumor sizes were measured twice per week. Mice were euthanized when the tumors reached 2.5 cm in length or diameter. Mammary tumors and lungs were collected for immunohistochemistry (IHC) and IF staining to analyze tumor cell proliferation, apoptosis, and angiogenesis, as described in the following.

Cell motility assays
For migration assays, confluent primary tumor cells were starved in DMEM/F12 plus 0.5% FBS for 16 h prior to trypsinization. 8×10^4 cells were placed in the upper chamber of a Transwell insert with 8-μm pores (BD Biosciences). The medium in the bottom well was supplemented with EGF (100 ng/ml; R&D Systems). Cells were allowed to migrate for 2 h, and then the cells in the upper well were removed using a cotton swab. Cells on the bottom of the membrane were fixed and stained with DAPI (1 μg/ml; Sigma-Aldrich). Cells that had traversed the membrane were counted in 10 random fields using a 20× objective and a Zeiss Axiophot microscope. Images were captured with an Axiocam MRm camera and Axiovision software. Cell numbers were quantified using ImageJ software.

Mammary gland whole mount analysis and tissue immunohistochemistry
After dissection, the fourth inguinal mammary glands were immediately fixed in Carnoy's fixative (60% ethanol, 30% chloroform, 10% glacial acetic acid) for 2–4 h at room temperature. Glands were stained in Carmine alum solution (2 mg/ml carmine, 10.5 mM aluminum potassium sulfate dodecahydrate) overnight with gentle shaking followed by successive dehydration steps in 70%, 95%, and 100% ethanol for 1 h each, at room temperature. Glands were cleared in xylene overnight and mounted on glass slides with Permount (ThermoFisher Scientific). Mammary glands were imaged with an Eclipse 80i digital camera (Nikon) mounted on a SMZ-745 T stereo microscope (Nikon).

For immunohistochemistry (IHC) of hyperplastic regions, number four inguinal mammary glands were immediately fixed in 4% paraformaldehyde overnight at 4 °C and stored in 70% ethanol at 4 °C until paraffin embedding. Tumors were excised and fixed for IHC as already described. Five-micron sections were cut for all tissues, deparaffinized in xylene, and rehydrated. Sections were boiled for 20 min in 10 mM sodium citrate for antigen retrieval, rinsed in PBS, and quenched for 30 min in 3% H_2O_2 at room temperature. Sections were blocked in 5% BSA/0.5% Tween-20, or M.O.M. blocking buffer (BMK2202; Vector Labs), for 1 h at room temperature. Primary antibodies were diluted in blocking solution and sections were incubated with primary antibodies overnight at 4 °C. After washing five times in phosphate buffered saline (PBS), sections were incubated with secondary antibodies for 45 min at room temperature, washed in PBS, and incubated in ABC solution (PK7100; Vector Labs) for 30 min. Sections were then developed in diaminobenzidine (K3468; Dako) and counterstained with hematoxylin (Thermo Fisher Scientific). Images were visualized with Eclipse 80i microscope (Nikon) and Digital Sight DS-VI1 camera (Nikon), and acquired using NIS-Elements Basic Research software (Nikon).

Lung isolation and analysis

Whole lungs were isolated after euthanasia, rinsed with sterile PBS, and immediately fixed in 4% paraformaldehyde overnight at 4 °C. Lungs were stored in 70% ethanol at 4 °C until paraffin embedding. Metastatic foci on the dorsal and ventral surface of lung lobes were counted and imaged with a SMZ-745 T stereo microscope (Nikon) mounted with an Eclipse 80i digital camera (Nikon). Five-micron sections were cut, deparaffinized in xylene, and rehydrated. The lung sections were then stained with hematoxylin and eosin (ThermoFisher Scientific). Sections were visualized with a SMZ-745 T stereo microscope (Nikon), and images were acquired using NIS-Elements Basic Research software (Nikon).

Isolation of tissues and western blotting analysis

Mouse tissues were rinsed quickly in cold PBS, snap frozen in liquid nitrogen, and stored at − 80 °C until use. For extraction of proteins and mRNA, frozen tissues were pulverized with a mortar and pestle under liquid nitrogen and homogenized on ice in SDS lysis buffer for protein extraction (2% SDS, 20 mM Tris–HCl (pH 8.0), 100 mM NaCl, 80 mM β-glycerophosphate, 50 mM NaF, 1 mM sodium orthovanadate, 10 μg/ml pepstatin A, 10 μg/ml leupeptin, 10 μg/ml aprotinin) or TRK lysis buffer (E.Z.N.A.® Total RNA Kit I; Omega Bio-Tek) for RNA extraction, using a rotor-stator homogenizer. For protein analysis, lysed tissue was sonicated and protein concentrations were determined by bicinchoninic acid assay (Pierce). Equal amounts of protein were separated by SDS-PAGE, transferred to polyvinylidene difluoride membrane (PVDF), and analyzed by western blotting.

Immunoprecipitation and GST-RBD assays

For analysis of proteins coprecipitating with PyMT, pulverized mouse tumors were lysed in radioimmunoprecipitation assay (RIPA) buffer with 0.1% SDS (1.0% Triton X-100, 0.1% SDS, 0.5% sodium deoxycholate, 50 mM Tris–HCl (pH 8.0), 150 mM NaCl, 80 mM β-glycerophosphate, 10 μg/ml leupeptin, 10 μg/ml pepstatin A,10 μg/ml aprotinin, 1 mM phenylmethylsulfonyl fluoride), incubated on ice for 10 min, and homogenized using a rotor-stator homogenizer. Insoluble proteins were pelleted by centrifugation (16,000 × g, 10 min, 4 °C). Equal amounts of soluble lysate were precleared by incubation for 30 min at 4 °C with 2 μg of normal rat IgG plus Protein G-Sepharose (Rockland Immunochemicals). Clarified lysates were then incubated with 2 μg of normal rat IgG or rat anti-PyMT plus Protein G-Sepharose for 2 h at 4 °C. Immunoprecipitates were washed three times with wash buffer (20 mM Tris–HCl (pH 8.0), 125 mM NaCl, 5 mM $MgCl_2$, and 0.5% Triton X-100), resuspended in 2 × Laemmli sample buffer, and resolved by SDS-PAGE. Proteins were transferred to a PVDF membrane and analyzed by western blotting analysis as described previously [31].

For GST-RBD assays, pulverized mouse tumors were lysed in 0.5% Triton lysis buffer plus 10 mM $MgCl_2$ (0. 5% Triton X-100, 10 mM $MgCl_2$, 20 mM Tris–HCl (pH 8.0), 100 mM NaCl, 1 mM EDTA, 50 mM NaF, 80 mM β-glycerophosphate, 10 mM $MgCl_2$, 1 mM Na_2VO_3, 10 μg/ml leupeptin, 10 μg/ml pepstatin A,10 μg/ml aprotinin, 1 mM phenylmethylsulfonyl fluoride) and homogenized using a rotor-stator homogenizer. Insoluble proteins were pelleted by centrifugation (16,000 × g, 10 min, 4 °C). Equal amounts of soluble lysate were incubated with 30 μg of GST-Rhotekin-RBD protein beads (Cytoskeleton, Inc.) for 1 h at 4 °C. Precipitates were washed three times with wash buffer (25 mM Tris–HCl (pH 7.5), 30 mM $MgCl_2$, 40 mM NaCl), resuspended in 2 × Laemmli sample buffer, and resolved by SDS-PAGE. Proteins were transferred to a PVDF membrane and analyzed by western blotting.

Gene expression analysis

Gene expression was analyzed by the UTHealth Quantitative Genomics and Microarray Core Facility using an Illumina mouse WG6 Whole-Genome Gene Expression BeadChip. Gene expression values were estimated with the Illumina GenomeStudio software with background subtraction and quantile normalization. Changes in gene expression were initially identified using a Student's t test, and genes were accepted as differentially expressed if they exhibited at least 1.5-fold change with $P < 0.05$ between the wild-type and Net1 knockout samples. Gene Ontology category enrichment analysis was performed using GATHER [32]. We scored the activation of gene expression signatures on gene expression profiles as described previously [33]. Briefly, for a gene expression dataset, we centered and normalized each gene to a mean of 0 and standard deviation of 1, and then averaged the expression of each gene in the signature, after taking the additive inverse of the expression values for genes negatively correlated with the pathway. Finally, we created a Net1 gene expression signature using an empirical Bayes approach [34] to find genes differentially expressed in Net1 knockout mouse tumors with at least

5-fold change and $P < 0.05$. To score this signature on human tumors, we found the human orthologs of the genes in the signature using the Homologene database [35].

Statistical analysis

Unpaired, two-tailed Student t tests were employed for all other statistical tests. $P < 0.05$ was considered significant, as indicated in figure legends. All data are reported as means, and errors are the standard error of the mean. Animal cohort size was chosen based on the work of many other groups using this tumor model and all animals within the cohort were included in the results. No randomization of animals was necessary. No blinding of cohort identity was done.

Results

Net1 is required for tumorigenesis and metastasis in MMTV-PyMT mice

We have shown previously that mice lacking *Net1* are healthy, but experience a short delay in mammary gland development during puberty characterized by reduced estrogen receptor alpha (ERα) expression, reduced proliferation, and less ductal branching. However, these mice are able to nurse their young, indicating that *Net1* is ultimately dispensable for mammary gland function [29]. To determine whether *Net1* is required for mammary gland tumorigenesis or metastasis, we bred mice lacking *Net1* to mice carrying the polyoma middle T antigen under the control of the mouse mammary tumor virus promoter (MMTV-PyMT). The MMTV-PyMT mouse model is an extremely aggressive, well-characterized breast cancer model in which mice develop multifocal mammary tumors at a median age of 6–7 weeks. Moreover, lung metastasis occurs in these mice with 100% penetrance [36]. Importantly, this breast cancer model does not require ERα expression for tumorigenesis or disease progression [37].

To assess the contribution of Net1 to tumorigenesis and metastasis, we bred cohorts of mice lacking one or both *Net1* alleles, and compared the rate of tumor appearance to that of wild-type MMTV-PyMT mice. We observed that loss of one *Net1* allele was sufficient to significantly delay the appearance of palpable tumors, and that loss of both *Net1* alleles caused a more significant effect (Fig. 1a). The effect of deletion of a single *Net1* allele may reflect our prior observation that loss of one allele causes an approximately 70% decrease in *Net1* mRNA expression in the mammary gland [29]. Despite the delay in tumorigenesis, mice lacking *Net1* invariably developed tumors in all mammary glands, with at least one of these tumors reaching maximum allowable size in a time frame similar to wild-type PyMT-expressing mice (Fig. 1b). Moreover, the aggregate tumor weight was similar in all genotypes (Fig. 1c). To determine whether

Net1 deletion affected metastasis, we assessed the lungs of mice within each genotype when mice were euthanized. We observed that loss of *Net1* strongly reduced the number of metastatic nodules observable on the lung surface (Fig. 1d, f). *Net1* deletion also significantly reduced the number of metastases and overall metastatic area in sectioned lungs stained with hematoxylin and eosin (H&E) (Fig. 1e, g, h). These data indicate that *Net1* contributes to mammary gland tumorigenesis and lung metastasis in PyMT-expressing mice.

Net1 is required for cell proliferation in early lesions

Hyperplastic areas begin to appear in the ducts surrounding the nipples in MMTV-PyMT mice as early as 3 weeks of age, and by 5 weeks these hyperplastic regions are large enough to easily observe in mammary gland whole mounts [38]. To determine whether *Net1* deletion affected the incidence of hyperplasia, we analyzed mammary gland whole mounts from MMTV-PyMT mice at 5 weeks of age lacking one or both *Net1* alleles. We observed that loss of just one *Net1* allele was sufficient to reduce the overall area of hyperplasia (Fig. 2a, b). This was not due to a general failure of the mammary duct to develop, as the ductal tree had clearly invaded past the lymph node (Fig. 2a, right panel). Ki67 staining indicated that proliferation in these early-stage legions was clearly reduced in mice lacking *Net1* (Fig. 2c, d). This was not due to altered PyMT expression, as *Net1*$^{-/-}$ mice expressed similar levels of the PyMT transgene (Fig. 2e, f). Proliferation was also significantly reduced in late-stage tumors, indicating that this phenotype was maintained (Fig. 2g, h). These data indicate that *Net1* deletion reduces cell proliferation in early hyperplastic regions and as well as in late-stage tumors.

Net1 deletion results in increased tumor necrosis and reduced tumor angiogenesis

Most tumors in *Net1*$^{-/-}$ mice were less firm than wild-type tumors, suggesting that they contained significant necrotic mass. To determine whether this was the case, we examined the morphology of tumor sections in a range of tumor sizes from less than 0.5 g to greater than 3 g. This analysis indicated that tumors with *Net1* deletion exhibited an increased necrotic area regardless of tumor size (Fig. 3a–c). Necrotic areas were largely confined to the centers of tumors with healthy margins. *Net1* knockout tumors also had an increase in staining for the apoptotic marker cleaved caspase 3 (CC3) (Fig. 3d, e). Because tumor necrosis can be caused by reduced tumor angiogenesis, we examined non-necrotic areas of tumors for expression of the blood vessel endothelial cell marker CD31. This analysis showed that tumors lacking *Net1* had reduced CD31 staining, indicating a reduction in blood vessel content (Fig. 3f, g). These data

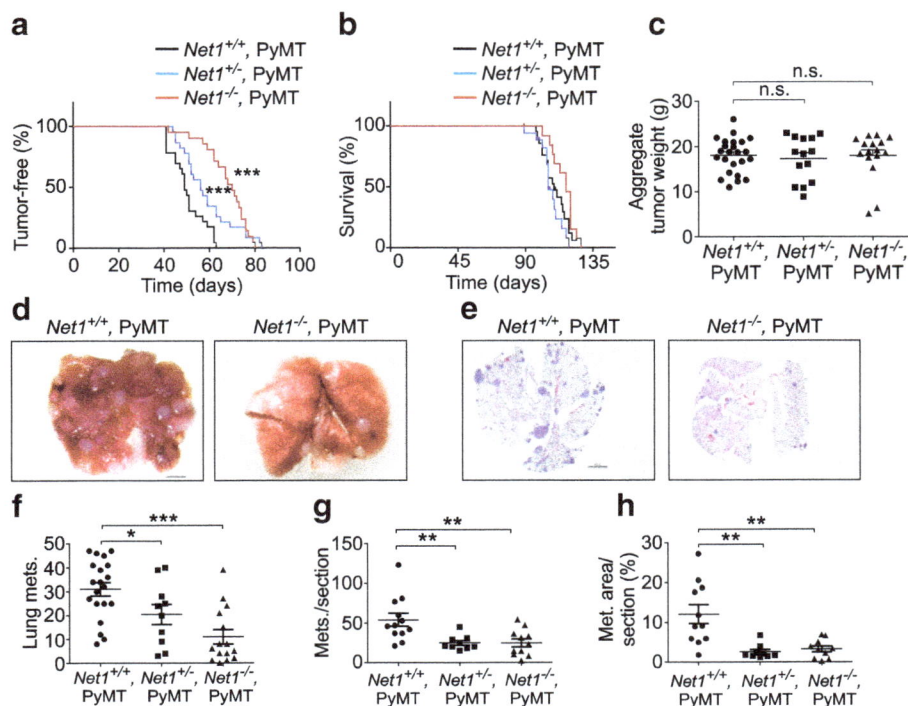

Fig. 1 *Net1* deletion delays tumorigenesis and inhibits metastasis in MMTV-PyMT mice. **a** Kaplan–Meier analysis of tumor onset. *Net1*$^{+/+}$,*PyMT* = 23 mice; *Net1*$^{+/-}$,*PyMT* = 23 mice; *Net1*$^{-/-}$,*PyMT* = 21 mice. **b** Survival analysis. Mice were euthanized when the largest tumor reached 2.5 cm. *Net1*$^{+/+}$,*PyMT* = 18 mice; *Net1*$^{+/-}$,*PyMT* = 14 mice; *Net1*$^{-/-}$,*PyMT* = 14 mice. **c** Aggregate tumor mass in MMTV-PyMT mice. *Net1*$^{+/+}$ = 22 mice; *Net1*$^{+/-}$ = 14 mice; *Net1*$^{-/-}$ = 7 mice. **d** Examples of lungs from *Net1*$^{+/+}$,*MMTV-PyMT* and *Net1*$^{-/-}$,*MMTV-PyMT* mice. Bar = 2 mm. **e** Examples of H&E-stained lung sections from *Net1*$^{+/+}$, *MMTV-PyMT* and *Net1*$^{-/-}$,*MMTV-PyMT* mice. Bar = 2 mm. **f** Quantification of metastatic nodules on lung surface in genotypes shown. *Net1+/+,PyMT* = 20 mice; *Net1+/−,PyMT* = 10 mice; *Net1−/−,PyMT* = 15 mice. **g** Quantification of metastases in lung sections in genotypes shown. *Net1+/+,PyMT* = 12 mice; *Net1+/−,PyMT* = 9 mice; *Net1−/−,PyMT* = 11 mice. **h** Quantification of lung area occupied by metastases in genotypes shown. *Net1+/+,PyMT* = 11 mice; *Net1+/−,PyMT* = 9 mice; *Net1−/−,PyMT* = 10 mice. Bars represent median values. *$P < 0.05$; **$P < 0.01$; ***$P < 0.001$. Met. metastasis, Mets metastases, Net1 neuroepithelial transforming gene 1, n.s. not significant, PyMT polyoma middle T antigen

indicate that loss of *Net1* results in increased tumor necrosis, most likely due to impaired tumor angiogenesis.

Net1 is required for RhoA signaling in tumors

We have observed previously in human breast cancer cells that Net1 controls RhoA activation and actomyosin contractility [24]. Because *Net1*$^{-/-}$ tumors exhibited reduced lung metastasis, we assessed RhoA signaling. RhoA controls actomyosin contraction by promoting the accumulation of phosphorylated myosin light chain (MLC2) [1]. When we examined tumors lacking *Net1* for MLC2 phosphorylation we observed that there was a significant decrease in pMLC2 staining (Fig. 4a, b). Western blotting analysis showed that there was also a decrease in phosphorylation of the regulatory subunit of myosin phosphatase (MYPT1) on its activating site pT696 (Fig. 4c). Moreover, there was a significant decrease in the overall level of RhoA activity in these tumors (Fig. 4d, e). However, RhoC activation was unaffected, indicating that Net1 is specific for RhoA in PyMT tumors (Fig. 4d, f). These data indicate that *Net1*

deletion caused a substantial reduction in RhoA activity and actomyosin contractility in PyMT-expressing tumors. To determine whether this translated into decreased motility of individual tumor cells, we measured the motility of cells isolated from primary tumors in modified Boyden chambers. We observed that *Net1* deletion significantly impaired motility toward EGF (Fig. 4g), suggesting that these cells would have a reduced capacity for motility in vivo.

Net1 is required for PyMT signaling

PyMT is a plasma membrane-associated protein that transforms cells by acting as a scaffold for Shc, the PI3K regulatory subunit p85, and PLCγ (Fig. 5a) [39, 40]. Shc recruitment activates the Ras–Raf–Mek–ERK pathway to promote cell proliferation and tumor growth [41, 42]. p85 recruitment brings the catalytic subunit of PI3K in proximity to the plasma membrane, where it generates phosphatidylinositol (3,4,5)-trisphosphate (PIP$_3$) to promote tumor cell survival [41, 42]. Importantly, both of these pathways must be activated for PyMT to promote

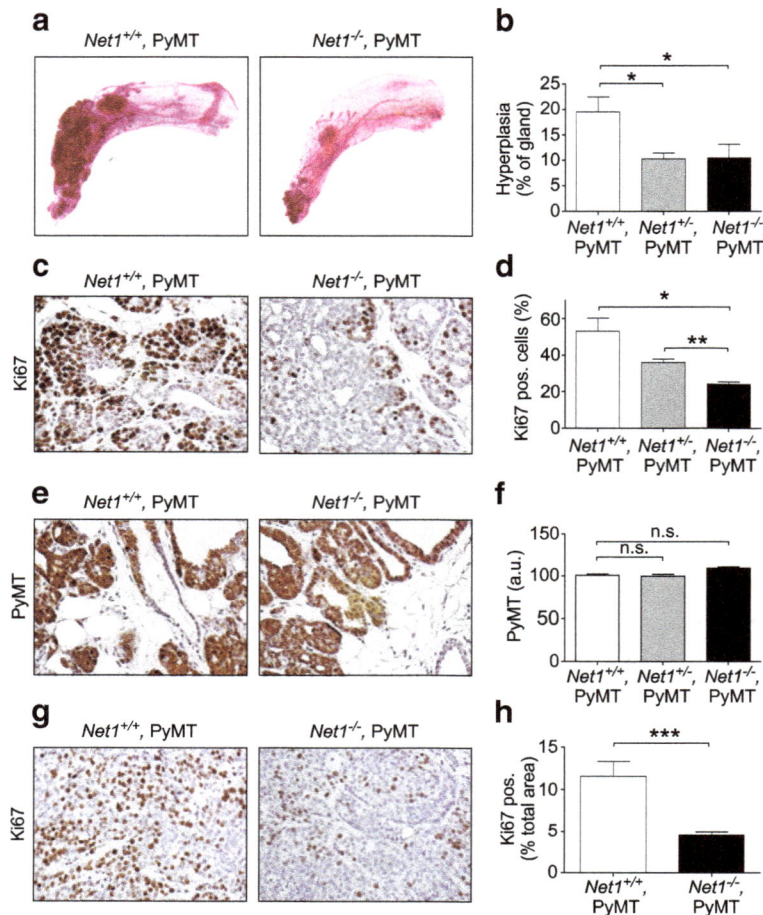

Fig. 2 *Net1* deletion delays mammary gland hyperplasia and inhibits proliferation. **a** Representative examples of inguinal mammary gland whole mounts from *Net1*[+/+],*PyMT* and *Net1*[−/−],*PyMT* mice at 5 weeks of age. **b** Quantification of hyperplastic mammary gland area at 5 weeks in genotypes shown. Six mice per genotype analyzed. **c** Representative examples of Ki67 staining in hyperplastic mammary gland sections from mice at 5 weeks. **d** Quantification of Ki67-positive cells in hyperplastic mammary gland sections at 5 weeks. Five independent regions within each sample quantified, 3–4 animals per genotype. **e** Representative examples of PyMT expression in hyperplastic mammary gland sections at 5 weeks. **f** Quantification of PyMT staining in mammary gland sections. Six independent regions within each sample quantified, 3 animals per genotype. **g** Representative examples of Ki67 staining in tumors at 14 weeks. **h** Quantification of Ki67-positive cells in 14-week tumors. Ki67 staining quantified as percent positive area divided by total area. Five independent regions within each sample quantified, 6 animals per genotype. Errors are standard error of the mean. $*P < 0.05$; $**P < 0.01$; $***P < 0.001$. Net1 neuroepithelial transforming gene 1, n.s. not significant, PyMT polyoma middle T antigen

mammary tumorigenesis [41]. To assess whether *Net1* deletion impaired signaling through these pathways, we examined Src, ERK1/2, and Akt1 activation in wild-type and *Net1* knockout tumors. For these assays we selected healthy, solid sections of tumors from each genotype. We observed a significant decrease in Src activation in *Net1* knockout tumors (Fig. 5b, c). There was also a significant decrease in ERK1/2 activation, as well as phosphorylation of Akt1 on its activating sites T308 and S473 (Fig. 5b, c). These data suggest that the ability of PyMT to stimulate intracellular signaling was impaired by loss of *Net1*.

To initiate cell signaling PyMT must first recruit the A and C subunits of PP2A, which then allows recruitment of Src [43, 44]. Src interaction with PyMT stimulates its

tyrosine kinase activity, promoting phosphorylation of residues within PyMT that serve as docking sites for Shc, p85, and PLCγ [39, 40]. To determine whether the interaction of PyMT with PP2A, Shc, or PI3K was affected by *Net1* deletion, we immunoprecipitated PyMT from wild-type and *Net1* knockout tumors and tested for coprecipitation of each protein. We observed that coprecipitation of the A and C subunits of PP2A was significantly impaired by *Net1* deletion, as was the coprecipitation of total and active Src, Shc, and p85 with PyMT (Fig. 5d). These data indicate that reduced activation of the Shc–ERK1/2 and PI3K–Akt pathways in *Net1* knockout tumors results from impaired recruitment of key signaling molecules to PyMT.

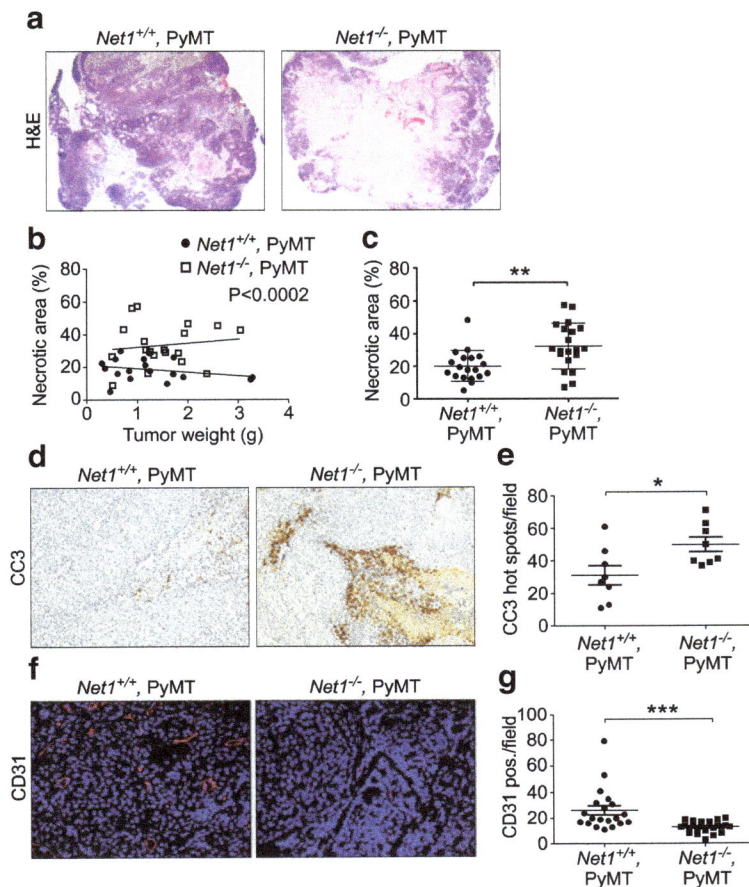

Fig. 3 *Net1* deletion inhibits tumor angiogenesis and causes increased tumor cell death. **a** Representative examples of H&E staining of large tumors in genotypes shown. **b** Quantification of necrotic area in H&E sections over range of tumor sizes for genotypes shown. Five animals per genotype, 4–5 tumors per animal, quantified. **c** Quantification of necrotic area of all tumors per genotype. **d** Representative examples of cleaved caspase 3 (CC3) staining in large tumors from genotypes shown. **e** Quantification of number of CC3 hot spots in large tumors. Entire tumor sections analyzed from 8 mice of each genotype. **f** Examples of cell determinant 31 (CD31) staining (red) in solid tumors from *Net1*^+/+^,*PyMT* and *Net1*^−/−^,*PyMT* mice. DNA shown in blue. **g** Quantification of CD31 staining. Five areas per sample analyzed; tumors from 4 (*Net1*^+/+^,*PyMT*) or 5 (*Net1*^−/−^,*PyMT*) mice assessed. Bars represent median values. *$P < 0.05$; **$P < 0.01$; ***$P < 0.001$. H&E hematoxylin and eosin, Net1 neuroepithelial transforming gene 1, PyMT polyoma middle T antigen

Net1 deletion inhibits tumor angiogenesis and lung metastasis in a tumor cell autonomous manner

To test whether the effects of *Net1* deletion on tumor angiogenesis and metastasis were tumor cell autonomous, primary MMTV-PyMT tumor cells were isolated from wild-type and *Net1* knockout mice and then transplanted into the mammary glands of syngeneic, wild-type FVB mice. Tumors were allowed to grow to the same size, at which time the mice were euthanized. Tumors and lungs were then excised to assess tumor characteristics and lung metastasis. We observed that PyMT tumors lacking *Net1* grew in volume at a similar rate to wild-type tumors (Fig. 6a). However, staining of sectioned tumors for Ki67 indicated that there was a small but significant decrease in the number of cells proliferating in *Net1* knockout tumors (Fig. 6b, c). When

tumors were stained for CD31, we found that there were significantly fewer blood vessels in tumors lacking *Net1*, similar to what was observed in *Net1* knockout mice (Fig. 6d, e). Consistent with this observation, *Net1* knockout tumors generally were less well perfused and lacked blood vessels in the surrounding skin relative to wild-type tumors (Additional file 1: Figure S3). Staining for cleaved caspase 3 indicated that apoptosis was significantly increased in *Net1* knockout tumors (Fig. 6f, g). Moreover, there was a trend toward increased necrotic area in tumors derived from *Net1* knockout cells (Additional file 2: Figure S4). When we analyzed the lungs in mice with wild-type PyMT tumors we observed a significant degree of metastasis. This was generally less than that observed in the MMTV-PyMT genetic mouse model (Fig. 1d–h), but tumors in the cell injection

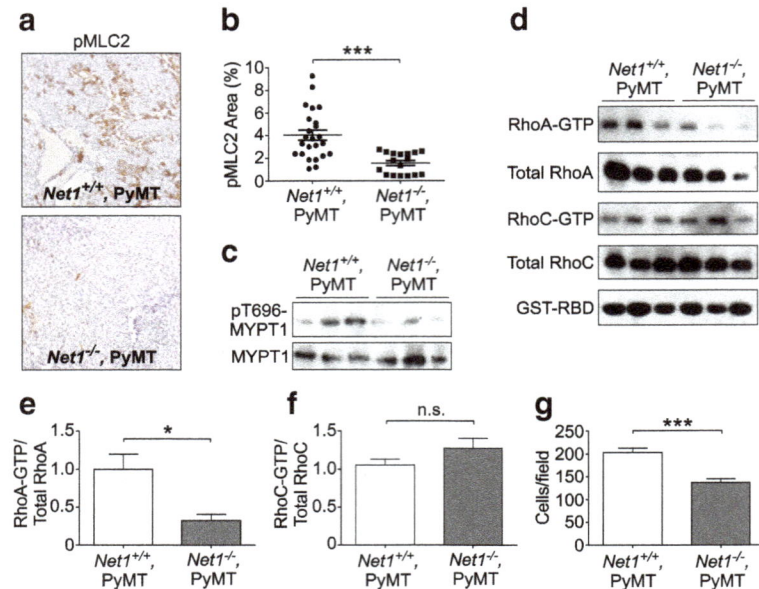

Fig. 4 *Net1* deletion inhibits RhoA activation and myosin light chain phosphorylation in tumors. **a** Representative examples of staining for myosin light chain 2 phosphorylated on serine 19 (pMLC2) in genotypes shown. Only solid tumors analyzed. **b** Quantification of pMLC2 staining as percentage of total area in genotypes shown. Seven areas analyzed, 3 animals per genotype. **c** Analysis of myosin phosphatase 1 (MYPT1) phosphorylation on its activating site T696 in tumor lysates. Each lane represents lysate from a tumor from a separate animal. **d** Analysis of active RhoA and RhoC activation in tumor lysates using GST-Rhotekin binding domain (GST-RBD) pulldowns. Each lane represents lysate from a tumor from a separate animal. **e** Quantification of RhoA-GTP/total RhoA for GST-RBD pulldowns. Six tumors per genotype quantified. **f** Quantification of RhoC-GTP/total RhoC for GST-RBD pulldowns. Six tumors per genotype quantified. **g** Quantification of primary tumor cell motility toward EGF in modified Boyden chambers. Data represent mean number of migrated cells/field from three separate tumors per genotype, isolated from separate mice, performed in duplicate. Errors are standard error of the mean. *$P < 0.05$; ***$P < 0.001$. GST glutathione-S-transferase, MYPT1 myosin phosphatase targeting subunit 1, Net1 neuroepithelial transforming gene 1, n.s. not significant, PyMT polyoma middle T antigen, RBD RhoA binding domain, RhoA Ras homolog family member A, RhoC Ras homolog family member C

model were only allowed to grow for 5 weeks. Importantly, lung metastasis was nearly absent in mice injected with PyMT cells lacking *Net1* (Fig. 6h, i). Taken together these data indicate that *Net1* deletion inhibits tumor angiogenesis and lung metastasis in a tumor cell autonomous nature.

A Net1 gene expression signature predicts PI3K activation, cancer cell proliferation, and distant metastasis-free survival in human breast cancer patients

To perform an unbiased analysis of the mechanism by which Net1 controls PyMT-stimulated tumorigenesis and metastasis, we analyzed global gene expression in wild-type and *Net1*$^{-/-}$ PyMT mammary tumors. RNA was isolated from three tumors of each genotype and analyzed using an Illumina Bead Array for whole genome expression. Based on their expression patterns, we found that 241 genes were upregulated in the *Net1* knockout tumors while 166 genes were downregulated with a 1.5-fold change ($P < 0.05$) (Additional file 3: Table S1). Gene ontology analysis with GATHER [45] indicated that a significant portion of the genes activated in tumors from *Net1*$^{-/-}$ mice corresponded to regulators of metabolism,

mitochondrial function, transcription, and tissue polarity (Fig. 7a). This may reflect adaptation to altered energy demands caused by reduced tumor angiogenesis (Fig. 3f, g). On the other hand, the repressed genes corresponded to cell cycle and mitotic regulators (Fig. 7b), reflecting the reduced proliferation of *Net1*$^{-/-}$ tumor cells (Fig. 2c, d).

To identify cancer pathways that are lost in the *Net1*$^{-/-}$ tumors, we predicted the activity of 52 pathways using previously published gene expression signatures [46] and approaches that we developed previously [32, 33]. A gene expression signature is a characteristic pattern in the transcriptional profile of a tumor that is indicative of the activation of a signaling pathway [47, 48]. Because they reflect the downstream consequences of pathway activity, gene expression signatures provide measures on the functional status of a pathway. Based on these signatures, we observed that three of those pathways, namely p53, PI3K, and proliferation, are consistently decreased in the *Net1* knockout tumors (Fig. 7c). Thus, *Net1*-expressing tumors correlated with the transcriptional profile of p53 mutant tumors, while *Net1*-deleted tumors correlated with transcription in wild-type p53-expressing tumors. Similarly, a PI3K transcriptional signature was

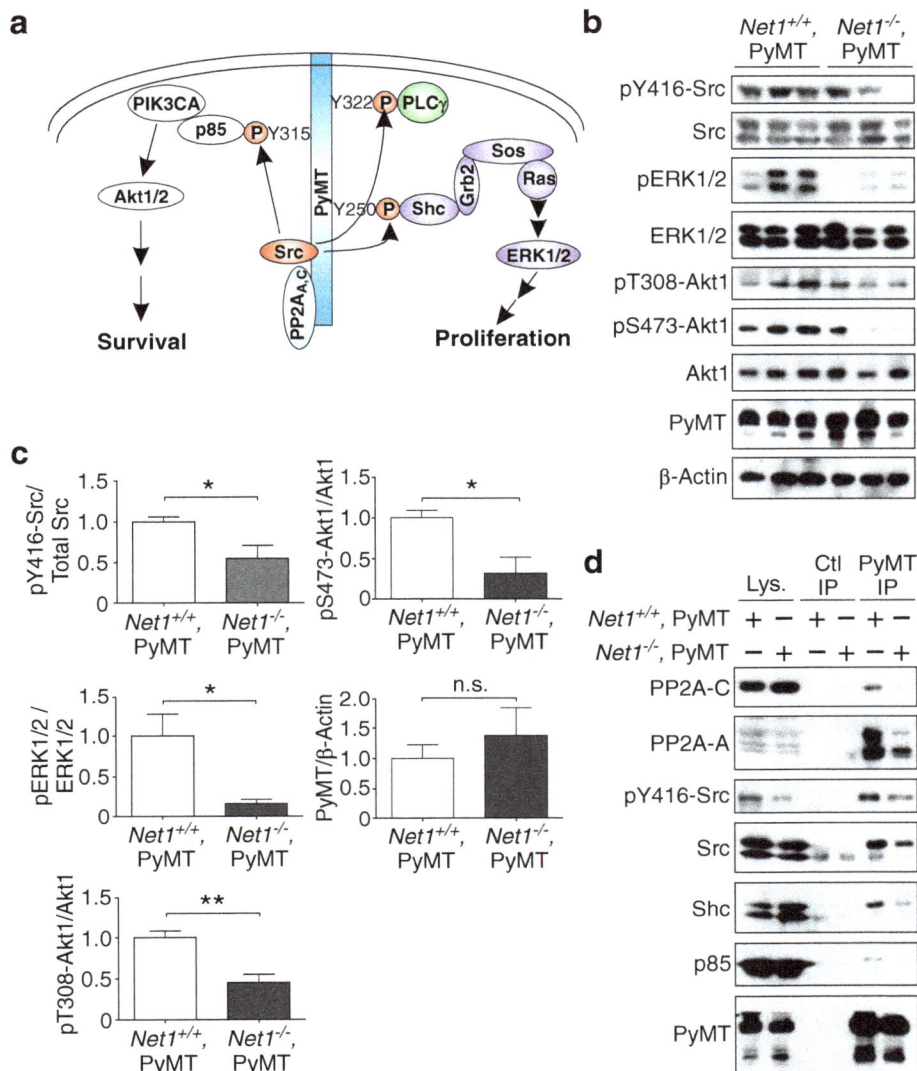

Fig. 5 *Net1* deletion inhibits PyMT-dependent ERK1/2 and Akt1 activation. **a** Schematic depicting PyMT-initiated signaling. **b** Representative analysis of Src, ERK1/2, and Akt1 phosphorylation on their activating sites in whole tumor lysates. Each lane represents a tumor from a distinct animal. **c** Quantification of western blotting in whole tumor lysates. Three to 6 tumors per genotype examined. **d** Western blot analysis of proteins coimmunoprecipitating with PyMT from tumors of genotypes shown. Representative experiment from four independent experiments. Errors are standard error of the mean. *$P < 0.05$; **$P < 0.01$. AKT1 v-akt murine thymoma viral oncogene homolog 1, ERK1 extracellular signal regulated kinase 1, Net1 neuroepithelial transforming gene 1, p85 phosphatidylinositol 3-kinase regulatory subunit p85α, PIK3CA phosphatidylinositol 3-kinase catalytic subunit A, PP2A protein phosphatase 2A, PyMT polyoma middle T antigen, Shc Src homology domain 2 containing, Src SRC proto-oncogene, non-receptor tyrosine kinase

repressed by *Net1* deletion, as was the proliferation-dependent gene expression signature (Fig. 7c). Thus, our observations indicating *Net1* dependence for cell survival, PI3K activity, and proliferation in PyMT-expressing tumors matched the apparent *Net1* dependence for these gene expression pathways.

Because of the importance of PI3K signaling to human breast cancer, we then assessed whether Net1 activation was associated with PI3K activity. To do this, we created a signature for Net1 activity using an empirical Bayes approach to identify the 277 genes (283 probes) that together can predict Net1 activation (Fig. 7d; Additional file 4: Figure S1; Additional file 5: Table S2). We then scored Net1 activity across breast cancer tumors from the TCGA [49] and correlated it with overexpression or mutagenic activation of the PI3K p110α catalytic subunit (PI3KCA) or deletion of the PIP$_3$ phosphatase PTEN. We observed that 10% of all human breast cancers

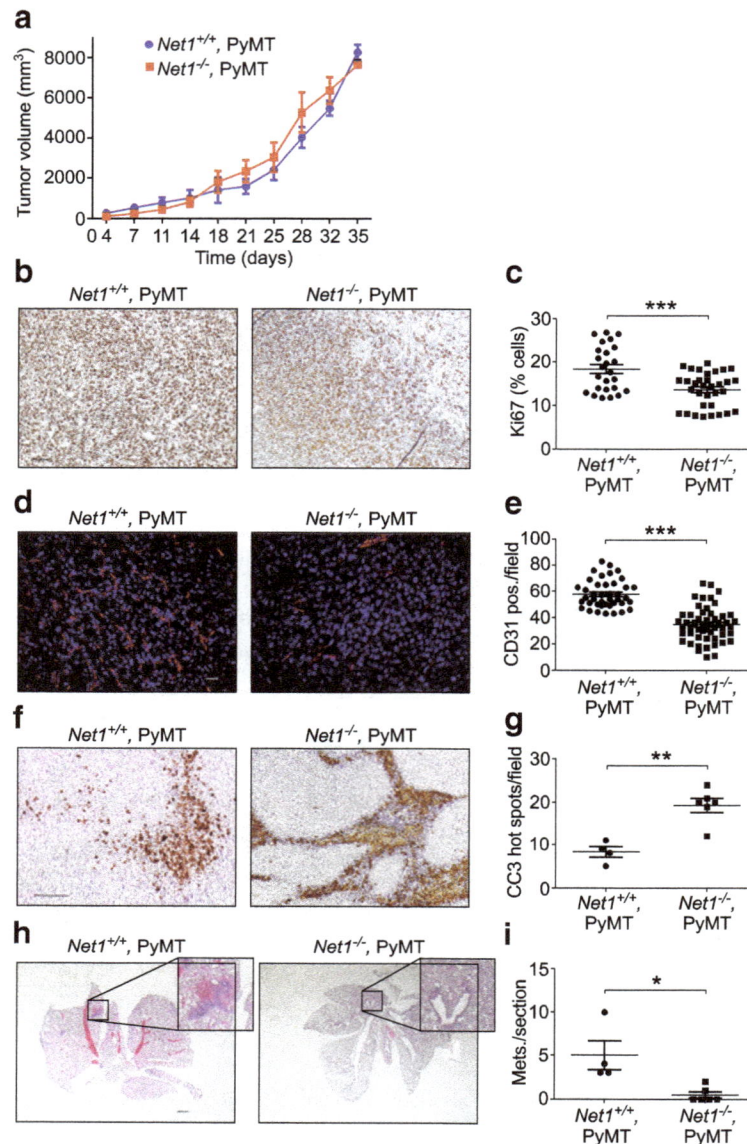

Fig. 6 *Net1* deletion reduces proliferation and angiogenesis, and increases apoptosis in a tumor cell autonomous manner. Wild-type and *Net1* knockout PyMT tumor cells injected into fourth inguinal mammary gland of wild-type FVB mice. **a** Tumor growth. *Net1*$^{+/+}$ = 4 mice; *Net1*$^{-/-}$ = 6 mice. **b** Representative examples of Ki67 staining in *Net1*$^{+/+}$ and *Net1*$^{-/-}$ tumors. Bar = 100 μm. **c** Quantification of Ki67 staining in tumors. Five independent regions within each sample quantified from 4 *Net1*$^{+/+}$ and 6 *Net1*$^{-/-}$ tumors. Bars represent median values. **d** Representative examples of CD31 staining (red) in *Net1*$^{+/+}$ and *Net1*$^{-/-}$ tumors. DNA shown in blue. Bar = 20 μm. **e** Quantification of CD31 staining. Five independent regions from each tumor analyzed in 4 *Net1*$^{+/+}$ and 6 *Net1*$^{-/-}$ tumors. Bars represent median values. **f** Representative examples of CC3 staining in *Net1*$^{+/+}$ and *Net1*$^{-/-}$ tumors. Bar = 100 μm. **g** Quantification of CC3 staining. CC3 hot spots analyzed in 4 *Net1*$^{+/+}$ and 6 *Net1*$^{-/-}$ tumors. Bars represent median values. **h** Representative examples of lung metastasis in mice injected with *Net1*$^{+/+}$ and *Net1*$^{-/-}$ cells. Bar = 1000 μm. **i** Quantification of lung metastasis in 6 *Net1*$^{+/+}$ and 6 *Net1*$^{-/-}$ mice. Bars represent median values. *$P < 0.05$; **$P < 0.01$; ***$P < 0.001$. Mets metastases, Net1 neuroepithelial transforming gene 1, PyMT polyoma middle T antigen

exhibited a high Net1 gene expression signature (Fig. 7e). Similar to previous results, 39% of human breast cancers exhibited PI3KCA activation, while 16% exhibited PTEN loss [49–51]. Importantly, patients with a high Net1 gene expression signature exhibited fewer instances of PI3KCA activation and increased incidence of PTEN loss (Fig. 7f). Coupled with our observation that PI3K signaling is high in wild-type *PyMT* tumors, this suggests that tumors with high Net1 activity did not require PI3KCA overexpression or mutagenic activation, but did tend to cosegregate with PTEN loss, to drive PI3K signaling.

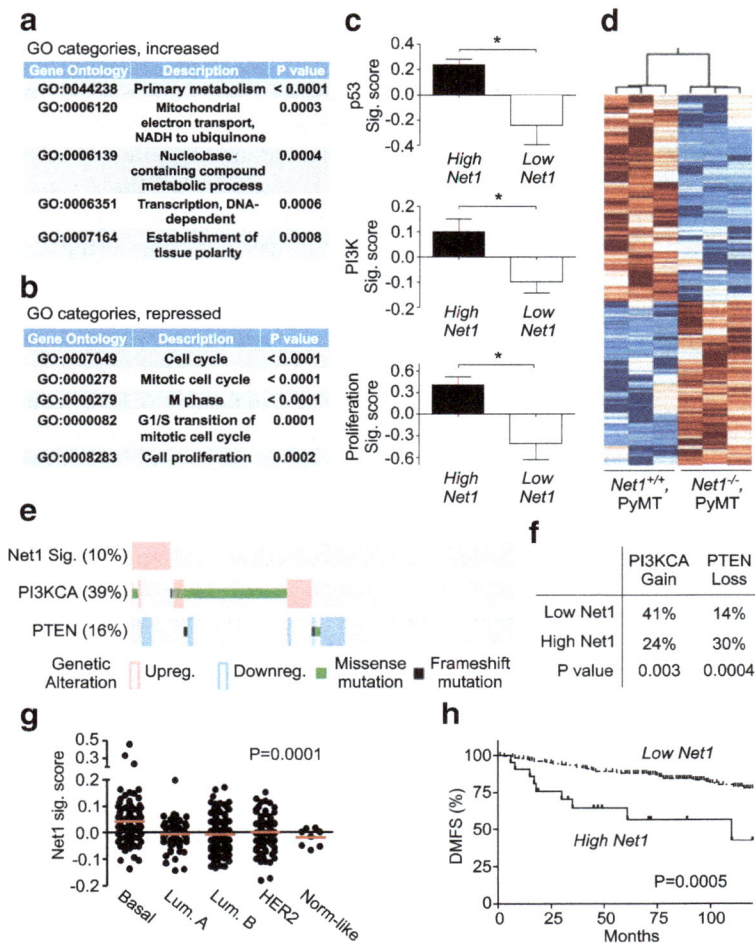

Fig. 7 Identification of Net1-dependent gene signature in mammary gland tumors and analysis of human breast cancer patients. **a** Top 5 GO categories of genes activated in *Net1* knockout, PyMT tumors. **b** Top 5 GO categories of genes repressed in *Net1* knockout, PyMT tumors. **c** Signature scores in p53, PI3K, and proliferation gene expression pathways in wild-type (High Net1) or Net1 knockout (Low Net1) PyMT tumors. **d** Heat map of gene expression comprising Net1 signature in *Net1^{+/+}*,*PyMT* and *Net1^{−/−}*,*PyMT* tumors. **e** Frequency of Net1 gene expression signature, PI3KCA mutation or amplification, and PTEN loss of expression in human breast cancers in TCGA. **f** Correlation of Net1 signature with phosphatidylinositol 3-kinase catalytic subunit A (PIK3CA) overexpression or mutation, or PTEN loss, in human breast cancers. **g** Correlation of Net1 signature with human breast cancer subtypes. Statistical significance assessed by ANOVA. **h** Kaplan–Meier analysis of distant metastasis-free survival (DMFS) in human breast cancer patients with positive and negative Net1 gene expression signatures. GSE11121 analyzed. GO Gene Ontology, Lum. luminal, Net1 neuroepithelial transforming gene 1, PI3K phosphatidylinositol 3-kinase, PTEN phosphatase and tensin homolog, PyMT polyoma middle T antigen

When we assessed whether Net1 is activated in particular subtypes of breast cancer, we observed an increased incidence of a positive Net1 gene expression signature in basal-type breast cancers (Fig. 7g). This is consistent with other studies indicating that basal-type breast cancers tend to have a greater frequency of PI3K pathway activation [49]. We then examined whether a high Net1 gene expression signature correlated with distant metastasis-free survival in human breast cancer patients. We observed that patients with a high Net1 gene expression signature experienced reduced distant metastasis-free survival in a breast cancer dataset [52] (Fig. 7h), consistent with the requirement for *Net1*

expression for metastasis in MMTV-PyMT mice. This result was confirmed in an independent dataset [53] (Additional file 6: Figure S2). Taken together, these data indicate that a Net1 gene expression signature is observed in highly proliferative breast tumors that harbor elevated PI3K signaling and tend to metastasize sooner, consistent with an important role for Net1 in disease progression in human breast cancer patients.

Discussion

Although RhoA signaling is critically important for breast cancer cell motility and invasiveness in vitro, few studies have assessed its role in metastasis in vivo. In the present study we demonstrate that the RhoA subfamily GEF *Net1* contributes to PyMT-driven tumorigenesis and is required for efficient lung metastasis. Moreover, we demonstrate that high Net1 signaling correlates with increased human breast cancer metastasis, indicating that our findings are relevant to human disease progression. To our knowledge, this is the first report of a RhoA GEF promoting breast tumorigenesis or metastasis.

MMTV-PyMT mice model luminal B-type breast tumors [54]. However, the wide incidence of the Net1 gene expression signature in human breast cancers suggests that Net1 function is not limited to this breast cancer subtype. For example, we observed that a high Net1 gene expression signature correlated closely with human basal-type breast cancers (Fig. 7g). Moreover, the reduced distant metastasis-free survival in patients with a high Net1 gene expression signature was observed in a cohort of patients that was not subdivided according to cancer subtype (Fig. 7f). These findings, coupled with our previous results indicating that coexpression of Net1 with the β4 integrin predicted reduced distant metastasis-free survival and reduced overall survival in ERα-positive breast cancer patients [55], indicate that Net1 may promote metastasis in a wide range of breast cancer subtypes. The idea that aberrant RhoA activation drives breast cancer metastasis fits with the findings of others indicating that reduced expression of the RhoA subfamily-specific GAP DLC-1 is predictive of metastatic spread to the bone in all breast cancer subtypes [18]. These findings are distinct from studies focusing on Rac1 activators, which appear to function in a more subtype-specific manner. For example, the Rac1 GEFs P-Rex1 and Vav2/3 contribute to metastasis in luminal subtype breast cancers, while the Rac1 GEF Dock1 controls metastasis in HER2-positive breast cancers [19–21]. The subtype independence of Net1 has important implications for therapeutic approaches, as it suggests that targeting Net1 would be a widely applicable therapeutic strategy for breast cancer. Our data indicating that *Net1* deletion switched tumors to a wild-type p53 gene expression signature (Fig. 6c) may also suggest that targeting Net1 would sensitize breast tumors with wild-type p53 to chemotherapies dependent on p53 function.

A potential caveat of our Net1 gene expression signature is that it may contain components that reflect PyMT signaling, which would also be expected to include PI3K activation. Unfortunately, it is not technically possible to isolate the activity of one pathway from the function of the rest of the signaling network. In our design, we compare the gene expression profile of Net1 within a PyMT background, and, in principle, the contribution of PyMT should not be detected. Nevertheless, the notion that Net1 function is associated with PI3K

signaling and metastasis is logical given the reported roles of Rho GTPase signaling in controlling PI3K activation and extracellular matrix invasion in cell-based studies. Future work will be required to dissect the components of the Net1 gene expression signature that are conserved among different breast cancer models.

It is unclear why there was not a significant increase in the survival of mice with *Net1* deletion, given the observed delay in tumor initiation. On the surface this would suggest that *Net1*-deleted tumors proliferated more rapidly, yet this was clearly not the case as Ki67 staining was reduced in both early and late tumors (Fig. 2), and unbiased gene expression analysis demonstrated significantly reduced expression of proliferation associated genes (Fig. 6b, c). This apparent contradiction most likely reflects the short delay in tumorigenesis (only 20 days), and the fact that *Net1*-deleted tumors tended to be fluid filled and less firm, which may have increased their apparent volume when measuring tumor size with calipers. The observation that they had larger necrotic cores supports this idea (Fig. 3a–c).

The *Net1* mouse model we used is a whole-body deletion of the *Net1* gene, so some of the phenotypes we observed may be due to cancer cell extrinsic as well as intrinsic effects. That being said, our tumor cell transplant experiments indicate that many of the phenotypes we observed are tumor cell autonomous. For example, tumors arising from injection of *Net1* knockout cells exhibited less proliferation, less angiogenesis, and increased apoptosis (Fig. 6b–g). Significantly, there was also less metastasis to the lungs (Fig. 6h, i), indicating that the decrease in metastasis in the genetic $Net1^{-/-}$,PyMT mice was likely not the result of a delay in tumorigenesis. The decrease in proliferation in *Net1* knockout cells is likely attributable to decreased signaling by PyMT (Fig. 5). However, it is less clear how Net1 influences tumor angiogenesis. Presumably, *Net1* deletion inhibits the secretion of one or more angiogenic factors by the tumor cells. Whether this occurs through altered transcription, translation, or secretion is an open question, as RhoA signaling has been shown to impact each of these steps. Future work will be directed at understanding the mechanism by which Net1 controls tumor angiogenesis.

The PyMT oncogene is considered a general model for activated receptor tyrosine kinase (RTK) signaling in oncogenic transformation [39]. Thus, the effects of Net1 on PyMT signaling to PI3K and ERK1/2 may have wider applicability. This idea is supported by our finding that our $Net1^{-/-}$ tumors have reduced gene expression signatures for PI3K and proliferation signaling (Fig. 7c). Signaling by PyMT is initiated through interactions with PP2A and Src, and these interactions are greatly reduced in $Net1^{-/-}$ tumors (Fig. 5d). The mechanism by which Net1 regulates recruitment of PP2A and Src to PyMT is at present unclear, as there is no precedence for regulation of these events by Rho GTPases. *Net1* knockout tumor cells tended to express slightly more PyMT than wild-type cells (Figs. 2 and 5), so reduced recruitment cannot be due to effects on PyMT expression. One possibility is that loss of Net1 inhibits delivery of signaling molecules to the plasma membrane. RhoB has been shown previously to regulate EGF-mediated delivery of Src to the plasma membrane [56]. Moreover, RhoB has been reported to interact with the catalytic subunit of PP2A and to control its ability to recruit the B55 regulatory subunit [57, 58]. Thus, it may be that Net1-dependent recruitment of $PP2A_{A,C}$ to PyMT is also RhoB dependent. In the future it will be important to test whether Net1 is required for recruitment of Src or PI3K to activated RTKs.

Conclusions

These data indicate that *Net1* is important for PyMT-stimulated tumorigenesis and metastasis, and may also contribute to human breast cancer metastasis. Net1 contributes to breast cancer progression through multiple mechanisms, which include promotion of cancer cell proliferation and motility, and tumor angiogenesis.

Additional files

Additional file 1: Figure S3. Representative examples of tumors from FVB mice injected with *Net1$^{+/+}$,PyMT* and *Net1$^{-/-}$,PyMT* cells. (PDF 353 kb)

Additional file 2: Figure S4: (**A**) Representative examples of H&E-stained tumor sections from FVB mice injected with *Net1$^{+/+}$,PyMT* and *Net1$^{-/-}$,PyMT* cells. (**B**) Quantification of necrotic areas from four *Net1$^{+/+}$,PyMT* tumors and six *Net1$^{-/-}$,PyMT* tumors. (PDF 315 kb)

Additional file 3: Table S1. Genes differentially expressed in *Net1 +/+,PyMT* and *Net1-/-,PyMT* tumors, $P < 0.05$. (PDF 114 kb)

Additional file 4: Figure S1. Control analysis of the Net1 signature. (**A**) Signature score for *Net1+/+,PyMT* and *Net1-/-,PyMT* tumors. (**B**) Principal component analysis of gene expression for the Net1 signature. (PDF 17 kb)

Additional file 5: Table S2. Genes comprising the Net1 gene expression signature. Threshold for significance was a 5-fold change between Net1 wild-type and knockout tumors, $P < 0.05$. (PDF 36 kb)

Additional file 6: Figure S2. Correlation of the Net1 gene expression signature with reduced DMSF in breast cancer patients. GSE20685 analyzed. (PDF 13 kb)

Abbreviations

AKT1: v-Akt murine thymoma viral oncogene homolog 1; CC3: Cleaved caspase 3; CD31: Cell determinant 31; CDC42: Cell division cycle 42; DLC-1: Deleted in liver cancer 1; DOCK1: Dedicator of cytokinesis 1; ERα: Estrogen receptor alpha; ERK1: Extracellular signal regulated kinase 1; FAK: Focal adhesion kinase; GST: Glutathione-S-transferase; Ki67: Marker of proliferation Ki-67; MLC2: Myosin regulatory light chain 2; MMTV: Mouse mammary tumor virus; MYPT1: Myosin phosphatase targeting subunit 1; Net1: Neuroepithelial transforming gene 1; p53: Tumor protein p53; p85: Phosphatidylinositol 3-kinase regulatory subunit p85α; PI3K: Phosphatidylinositol 3-kinase; PIP$_3$: Phosphatidylinositol-3,4,5-phosphate; PLCγ: Phospholipase C gamma; PP2A: Protein phosphatase 2A; P-Rex1: Phosphatidylinositol-3,4,5-trisphosphate dependent Rac exchange factor 1; PTEN: Phosphatase and tensin homolog; PyMT: Polyoma middle T antigen;

Rac1: Ras-Related C3 botulinum toxin substrate 1; RBD: RhoA binding domain; RhoA: Ras homolog family member A; RhoB: Ras homolog family member B; RhoC: Ras homolog family member C; RhoGAP: Rho GTPase activating protein; RhoGEF: Rho guanine nucleotide exchange factor; Shc: Src homology domain 2 containing; Src: SRC proto-oncogene, non-receptor tyrosine kinase; TCGA: The Cancer Genome Atlas; TGFβ: Transforming growth factor beta; Vav2: Vav guanine nucleotide exchange factor 2

Acknowledgements

The authors would like to thank Jeffrey Rosen, Jianming Xu, and members of their laboratories for their generous advice.

Funding

This work was funded by NIH grant CA172129 to JAF and CPRIT fellowship RP160015 to AU.

Authors' contributions

YZ and JAF developed the hypotheses, designed the experiments, and drafted the manuscript. YZ performed all experiments associated with the manuscript. AU assisted with animal husbandry, breeding, and genotyping, and contributed to writing of the manuscript. JTC performed all bioinformatics analysis of gene expression in wild-type and *Net1* KO tumors, and assisted with writing of the manuscript. All authors read and approved the final manuscript.

Competing interests

The authors declare that they have no competing interests.

Author details

^{1}Department of Integrative Biology and Pharmacology, University of Texas Health Science Center at Houston, 6431 Fannin St, Houston, TX 77030, USA. ^{2}School of Biomedical Informatics, University of Texas Health Science Center at Houston, 6431 Fannin St, Houston, TX 77030, USA.

References

1. Jaffe AB, Hall A. Rho GTPases: biochemistry and biology. Annu Rev Cell Dev Biol. 2005;21:247–69.
2. Heasman SJ, Ridley AJ. Mammalian Rho GTPases: new insights into their functions from in vivo studies. Nat Rev Mol Cell Biol. 2008;9:690–701.
3. Fritz G, Brachetti C, Bahlmann F, Schmidt M, Kaina B. Rho GTPases in human breast tumours: expression and mutation analyses and correlation with clinical parameters. Br J Cancer. 2002;87:635–44.
4. van Golen KL, Davies S, Wu ZF, Wang Y, Bucana CD, Root H, et al. A novel putative low-affinity insulin-like growth factor-binding protein, LIBC (lost in inflammatory breast cancer), and RhoC GTPase correlate with the inflammatory breast cancer phenotype. Clin Cancer Res. 1999;5:2511–9.
5. Clark EA, Golub TR, Lander ES, Hynes RO. Genomic analysis of metastasis reveals an essential role for RhoC. Nature. 2000;406:532–5.
6. Pille JY, Denoyelle C, Varet J, Bertrand JR, Soria J, Opolon P, et al. Anti-RhoA and anti-RhoC siRNAs inhibit the proliferation and invasiveness of MDA-MB-231 breast cancer cells in vitro and in vivo. Mol Ther. 2005;11:267–74.

7. Hakem A, Sanchez-Sweatman O, You-Ten A, Duncan G, Wakeham A, Khokha R, et al. RhoC is dispensable for embryogenesis and tumor initiation but essential for metastasis. Genes Dev. 2005;19:1974–9.

8. Friedl P, Wolf K. Plasticity of cell migration: a multiscale tuning model. J Cell Biol. 2010;188:11–9.

9. Sanz-Moreno V, Marshall CJ. The plasticity of cytoskeletal dynamics underlying neoplastic cell migration. Curr Opin Cell Biol. 2010;22:690–6.

10. Madsen CD, Sahai E. Cancer dissemination—lessons from leukocytes. Dev Cell. 2010;19:13–26.

11. Bishop AL, Hall A. Rho GTPases and their effector proteins. Biochem J. 2000;348(Pt 2):241–55.

12. Thumkeo D, Watanabe S, Narumiya S. Physiological roles of Rho and Rho effectors in mammals. Eur J Cell Biol. 2013;92:303–15.

13. Rossman KL, Der CJ, Sondek J. GEF means go: turning on RHO GTPases with guanine nucleotide-exchange factors. Nat Rev Mol Cell Biol. 2005;6:167–80.

14. Meller N, Merlot S, Guda C. CZH proteins: a new family of Rho-GEFs. J Cell Sci. 2005;118:4937–46.

15. Tcherkezian J, Lamarche-Vane N. Current knowledge of the large RhoGAP family of proteins. Biol Cell. 2007;99:67–86.

16. Yuan BZ, Miller MJ, Keck CL, Zimonjic DB, Thorgeirsson SS, Popescu NC. Cloning, characterization, and chromosomal localization of a gene frequently deleted in human liver cancer (DLC-1) homologous to rat RhoGAP. Cancer Res. 1998;58:2196–9.

17. Goodison S, Yuan J, Sloan D, Kim R, Li C, Popescu NC, et al. The RhoGAP protein DLC-1 functions as a metastasis suppressor in breast cancer cells. Cancer Res. 2005;65:6042–53.

18. Wang Y, Lei R, Zhuang X, Zhang N, Pan H, Li G, et al. DLC1-dependent parathyroid hormone-like hormone inhibition suppresses breast cancer bone metastasis. J Clin Invest. 2014;124:1646–59.

19. Sosa MS, Lopez-Haber C, Yang C, Wang H, Lemmon MA, Busillo JM, et al. Identification of the Rac-GEF P-Rex1 as an essential mediator of ErbB signaling in breast cancer. Mol Cell. 2010;40:877–92.

20. Citterio C, Menacho-Marquez M, Garcia-Escudero R, Larive RM, Barreiro O, Sanchez-Madrid F, et al. The rho exchange factors vav2 and vav3 control a lung metastasis-specific transcriptional program in breast cancer cells. Sci Signal. 2012;5:ra71.

21. Laurin M, Huber J, Pelletier A, Houalla T, Park M, Fukui Y, et al. Rac-specific guanine nucleotide exchange factor DOCK1 is a critical regulator of HER2-mediated breast cancer metastasis. Proc Natl Acad Sci U S A. 2013;110:7434–9.

22. Shen SQ, Li K, Zhu N, Nakao A. Expression and clinical significance of NET-1 and PCNA in hepatocellular carcinoma. Med Oncol. 2008;25:341–5.

23. Dutertre M, Gratadou L, Dardenne E, Germann S, Samaan S, Lidereau R, et al. Estrogen regulation and physiopathologic significance of alternative promoters in breast cancer. Cancer Res. 2010;70:3760–70.

24. Carr HS, Zuo Y, Oh W, Frost JA. Regulation of FAK activation, breast cancer cell motility and amoeboid invasion by the RhoA GEF Net1. Mol Cell Biol. 2013;33:2773–86.

25. Murray D, Horgan G, MacMathuna P, Doran P. NET1-mediated RhoA activation facilitates lysophosphatidic acid-induced cell migration and invasion in gastric cancer. Br J Cancer. 2008;99:1322–9.

26. Lee J, Moon HJ, Lee JM, Joo CK. Smad3 regulates Rho signaling via NET1 in the transforming growth factor-beta-induced epithelial-mesenchymal transition of human retinal pigment epithelial cells. J Biol Chem. 2010;285:26618–27.

27. Papadimitriou E, Vasilaki E, Vorvis C, Iliopoulos D, Moustakas A, Kardassis D, et al. Differential regulation of the two RhoA-specific GEF isoforms Net1/Net1A by TGF-beta and miR-24: role in epithelial-to-mesenchymal transition. Oncogene. 2011;31(23):2862–75.

28. Menon S, Oh W, Carr HS, Frost JA. Rho GTPase independent regulation of mitotic progression by the RhoGEF Net1. Mol Biol Cell. 2013;24:2655–67.

29. Zuo Y, Berdeaux R, Frost JA. The RhoGEF Net1 is required for normal mammary gland development. Mol Endocrinol. 2014;28:1948–60.

30. Cuevas BD, Winter-Vann AM, Johnson NL, Johnson GL. MEKK1 controls matrix degradation and tumor cell dissemination during metastasis of polyoma middle-T driven mammary cancer. Oncogene. 2006;25:4998–5010.

31. Song EH, Oh W, Ulu A, Carr HS, Zuo Y, Frost JA. Acetylation of the RhoA GEF Net1A controls its subcellular localization and activity. J Cell Sci. 2015;128:913–22.

32. Chang JT, Gatza ML, Lucas JE, Barry WT, Vaughn P, Nevins JR. SIGNATURE: a workbench for gene expression signature analysis. BMC Bioinformatics. 2011;12:443. https://doi.org/10.1186/1471-2105-12-443.

33. Tisza MJ, Zhao W, Fuentes JS, Prijic S, Chen X, Levental I, et al. Motility and stem cell properties induced by the epithelial-mesenchymal transition require destabilization of lipid rafts. Oncotarget. 2016;7:51553–68.

34. Efron B, Tibshirani R, Storey JD, Tusher V. Empirical Bayes analysis of a microarray experiment. Am Stat Assoc. 2001;96:1151–60.

35. NCBI Resource Coordinators. Database resources of the National Center for Biotechnology Information. Nucleic Acids Res. 2016;44:D7–19.

36. Guy CT, Cardiff RD, Muller WJ. Induction of mammary tumors by expression of polyomavirus middle T oncogene: a transgenic mouse model for metastatic disease. Mol Cell Biol. 1992;12:954–61.

37. Toneff MJ, Du Z, Dong J, Huang J, Sinai P, Forman J, et al. Somatic expression of PyMT or activated ErbB2 induces estrogen-independent mammary tumorigenesis. Neoplasia. 2010;12:718–26.

38. Lin EY, Jones JG, Li P, Zhu L, Whitney KD, Muller WJ, et al. Progression to malignancy in the polyoma middle T oncoprotein mouse breast cancer model provides a reliable model for human diseases. Am J Pathol. 2003;163:2113–26.

39. Marcotte R, Muller WJ. Signal transduction in transgenic mouse models of human breast cancer–implications for human breast cancer. J Mammary Gland Biol Neoplasia. 2008;13:323–35.

40. Fluck MM, Schaffhausen BS. Lessons in signaling and tumorigenesis from polyomavirus middle T antigen. Microbiol Mol Biol Rev. 2009;73:542–63.

41. Webster MA, Hutchinson JN, Rauh MJ, Muthuswamy SK, Anton M, Tortorice CG, et al. Requirement for both Shc and phosphatidylinositol 3' kinase signaling pathways in polyomavirus middle T-mediated mammary tumorigenesis. Mol Cell Biol. 1998;18:2344–59.

42. Ong SH, Dilworth S, Hauck-Schmalenberger I, Pawson T, Kiefer F. ShcA and Grb2 mediate polyoma middle T antigen-induced endothelial transformation and Gab1 tyrosine phosphorylation. EMBO J. 2001;20:6327–36.

43. Glover HR, Brewster CE, Dilworth SM. Association between src-kinases and the polyoma virus oncogene middle T-antigen requires PP2A and a specific sequence motif. Oncogene. 1999;18:4364–70.

44. Ogris E, Mudrak I, Mak E, Gibson D, Pallas DC. Catalytically inactive protein phosphatase 2A can bind to polyomavirus middle tumor antigen and support complex formation with pp60(c-src). J Virol. 1999;73:7390–8.

45. Chang JT, Nevins JR. GATHER: a systems approach to interpreting genomic signatures. Bioinformatics. 2006;22:2926–33.

46. Gatza ML, Silva GO, Parker JS, Fan C, Perou CM. An integrated genomics approach identifies drivers of proliferation in luminal-subtype human breast cancer. Nat Genet. 2014;46:1051–9.

47. Bild AH, Yao G, Chang JT, Wang Q, Potti A, Chasse D, et al. Oncogenic pathway signatures in human cancers as a guide to targeted therapies. Nature. 2006;439:353–7.

48. Chang JT, Carvalho C, Mori S, Bild AH, Gatza ML, Wang Q, et al. A genomic strategy to elucidate modules of oncogenic pathway signaling networks. Mol Cell. 2009;34:104–14.

49. The Cancer Genome Atlas Network. Comprehensive molecular portraits of human breast tumours. Nature. 2012;490:61–70.

50. Bachman KE, Argani P, Samuels Y, Silliman N, Ptak J, Szabo S, et al. The PIK3CA gene is mutated with high frequency in human breast cancers. Cancer Biol Ther. 2004;3:772–5.

51. Perren A, Weng LP, Boag AH, Ziebold U, Thakore K, Dahia PL, et al. Immunohistochemical evidence of loss of PTEN expression in primary ductal adenocarcinomas of the breast. Am J Pathol. 1999;155:1253–60.

52. Schmidt M, Bohm D, von TC SE, Puhl A, Pilch H, et al. The humoral immune system has a key prognostic impact in node-negative breast cancer. Cancer Res. 2008;68:5405–13.

53. Kao KJ, Chang KM, Hsu HC, Huang AT. Correlation of microarray-based breast cancer molecular subtypes and clinical outcomes: implications for treatment optimization. BMC Cancer. 2011;11:143. https://doi.org/10.1186/1471-2407-11-143.

54. Pfefferle AD, Herschkowitz JI, Usary J, Harrell JC, Spike BT, Adams JR, et al. Transcriptomic classification of genetically engineered mouse models of breast cancer identifies human subtype counterparts. Genome Biol. 2013;14:R125–14.

55. Gilcrease MZ, Kilpatrick SK, Woodward WA, Zhou X, Nicolas MM, Corley LJ, et al. Coexpression of alpha6beta4 integrin and guanine nucleotide exchange factor Net1 identifies node-positive breast cancer patients at high risk for distant metastasis. Cancer Epidemiol Biomark Prev. 2009;18:80–6.

56. Sandilands E, Cans C, Fincham VJ, Brunton VG, Mellor H, Prendergast GC, et al. RhoB and actin polymerization coordinate Src activation with endosome-mediated delivery to the membrane. Dev Cell. 2004;7:855–69.

57. Lee WJ, Kim DU, Lee MY, Choi KY. Identification of proteins interacting with the catalytic subunit of PP2A by proteomics. Proteomics. 2007;7:206–14.

58. Bousquet E, Calvayrac O, Mazieres J, Lajoie-Mazenc I, Boubekeur N, Favre G, et al. RhoB loss induces Rac1-dependent mesenchymal cell invasion in lung cells through PP2A inhibition. Oncogene. 2016;35:1760–9.

12

Aerobic and resistance exercise improves physical fitness, bone health, and quality of life in overweight and obese breast cancer survivors: a randomized controlled trial

Christina M Dieli-Conwright[1,5]* (iD), Kerry S Courneya[2], Wendy Demark-Wahnefried[3], Nathalie Sami[1], Kyuwan Lee[1], Frank C Sweeney[1], Christina Stewart[1], Thomas A Buchanan[4], Darcy Spicer[5], Debu Tripathy[6], Leslie Bernstein[7] and Joanne E Mortimer[8]

Abstract

Background: Exercise is an effective strategy to improve quality of life and physical fitness in breast cancer survivors; however, few studies have focused on the early survivorship period, minorities, physically inactive and obese women, or tested a combined exercise program and measured bone health. Here, we report the effects of a 16-week aerobic and resistance exercise intervention on patient-reported outcomes, physical fitness, and bone health in ethnically diverse, physically inactive, overweight or obese breast cancer survivors.

Methods: One hundred breast cancer survivors within 6 months of completing adjuvant treatment were assessed at baseline, post-intervention, and 3-month follow-up (exercise group only) for physical fitness, bone mineral density, serum concentrations of bone biomarkers, and quality of life. The exercise intervention consisted of moderate-vigorous (65–85% heart rate maximum) aerobic and resistance exercise thrice weekly for 16 weeks. Differences in mean changes for outcomes were evaluated using mixed-model repeated measure analysis.

Results: At post-intervention, the exercise group was superior to usual care for quality of life (between group difference: 14.7, 95% CI: 18.2, 9.7; $p < 0.001$), fatigue ($p < 0.001$), depression ($p < 0.001$), estimated VO_{2max} ($p < 0.001$), muscular strength ($p < 0.001$), osteocalcin ($p = 0.01$), and BSAP ($p = 0.001$). At 3-month follow-up, all patient-reported outcomes and physical fitness variables remained significantly improved compared to baseline in the exercise group ($p < 0.01$).

Conclusions: A 16-week combined aerobic and resistance exercise program designed to address metabolic syndrome in ethnically-diverse overweight or obese breast cancer survivors also significantly improved quality of life and physical fitness. Our findings further support the inclusion of supervised clinical exercise programs into breast cancer treatment and care.

Keywords: Exercise, quality of life, physical fitness, bone health, breast cancer

* Correspondence: cdieli@usc.edu
[1]Division of Biokinesiology and Physical Therapy, University of Southern California (USC), |1540 E. Alcazar St., CHP 155, Los Angeles, CA 90089, USA
[5]Department of Medicine, Keck School of Medicine, University of Southern California, Los Angeles, CA 90033, USA
Full list of author information is available at the end of the article

Background

Breast cancer survivors are at elevated risk for the development of comorbid conditions such as sarcopenia, osteoporosis, and cardiovascular disease [1] which contribute to declines in quality of life, cardiorespiratory fitness, muscular strength, and bone health. These negative health concerns are partly induced by cancer-related treatments (e.g., chemotherapy, radiation, endocrine therapy) and are exacerbated by obesity and a physically inactive lifestyle. Exercise is an effective non-pharmacologic strategy to mitigate cancer-related treatment side effects and improve quality of life, cardiorespiratory fitness, and muscular strength in breast cancer survivors [2]; however, few studies have focused on the early survivorship period (≤ 6 months post-treatment), minorities, physically inactive and obese women, or tested a combined exercise program and measured bone health.

The overall purpose of this trial was to compare a 16-week supervised moderate-vigorous intensity aerobic and resistance exercise intervention to usual care in physically inactive, overweight and obese breast cancer survivors. We previously reported that the exercise intervention led to significant improvements in metabolic syndrome, sarcopenic obesity, and circulating biomarkers that were maintained at 3-month follow-up [3]. Here, we report the secondary outcomes of physical fitness, bone health, and quality of life. We hypothesized that a combined exercise intervention performed within 6 months of cancer treatment completion would improve patient-reported outcomes, physical fitness, and bone health in ethnically-diverse, physically inactive, overweight/obese breast cancer survivors compared to usual care.

Methods

Participants/Consent

Eligible participants were < 6 months post-treatment for chemo- or radiation-therapy for stage 0-III breast cancer and were non-smokers, physically inactive (< 60 min of structured exercise/week), with BMI ≥ 25.0 kg/m^2 (or body fat > 30%) and waist circumference > 88 cm. Participants were verbally screened for eligibility by phone or in person at time of consent. Treatment history and diagnosis were confirmed by medical record abstraction. Body composition measure were obtained at time of screening per testing methods described below (Covariate Measures).

Recruitment occurred between August 1, 2012 and December 31, 2016 from the USC Norris Comprehensive Cancer Center and Los Angeles County Hospital. The protocol and informed consent were IRB-approved (HS-12-00141) and registered (ClinicalTrials.gov:NCT01140282). A signed informed consent was obtained from each participant.

Participants were randomized to exercise or usual care following the completion of baseline testing using concealed randomization lists.

Experimental Design

This randomized controlled trial compared a progressive combined (aerobic and resistance) exercise intervention versus usual care on baseline to 4-month changes in physical fitness, bone health, and patient-reported outcomes. Detailed methods [4], and primary outcomes related to metabolic syndrome were published previously. Endpoints were assessed at baseline, post-intervention (month 4), and 3-month follow-up (exercise group only). To enhance participation, usual care participants were offered the exercise program following the study period.

Cardiorespiratory Fitness

A single-stage submaximal treadmill test was used to estimate maximal oxygen uptake, VO$_{2max}$ [5]. Participants first performed a 4-min warm up by walking on a treadmill (Desmo Woodway, Waukesha, WI) at a speed (2.0, 3.0, 4.0, or 4.5 mph) that increased their heart rate between 50 and 70% heart rate maximum. This was followed by the 4-min test at the same speed with a 5% grade; heart rate was measured during the final 30 s of the test. Using heart rate, speed, age and gender, estimated maximal oxygen uptake was predicted using the test-specific regression formula [5].

Muscular Strength

Estimated maximal voluntary strength (1-RM) was assessed for the chest press, latissimus pulldown, knee extension, and knee flexion using the 10-repetition maximum (10-RM) method (Tuff Stuff, Pomona, CA). [6] Participants completed a warm-up load of ~ 5–8-RM before attempting 10-RM. A 2-min rest period was given between attempts; 3–5 attempts were performed.

Dual Energy X-Ray Absorptiometry (DXA)

Dual hip and lumbar DXA scans were used to assess bone mineral density (BMD; Lunar GE iDXA, Fairfield, Connecticut).

Blood Collection and Analysis

Fasting (≥ 12 h) blood was obtained by trained phlebotomists. Serum was stored at $- 80°$ until batch analysis at study completion. Biomarkers of bone turnover were analyzed and included bone-specific alkaline phosphatase (BSAP) and osteocalcin as markers of bone formation, C-telopeptide of type 1 collagen (CTX), N-telopeptides of type 1 collagen (NTX) as markers of bone resorption, and receptor activator factor-kappa B (RANK) and receptor activator factor-kappa B ligand (RANKL) as markers of bone remodeling. In addition, we quantified calcium and 25-hydroxyvitamin D.

Osteocalcin (Meso Scale Discovery, Rockville MD, Catalog #K151HHC-1), BSAP (Ostase Assay Catalog #37300, Beckman Coulter, Ontario, Canada), CTX (Immunodiagnostics, Gaithersburg, MD, Catalog #AC-02F1), NTX (MyBioSource, San Diego, CA, Catalog #MBS705111), RANK (MyBioSource, San Diego, CA, Catalog #MBS9308775), and RANKL (MyBio-Source, San Diego, CA, Catalog #MBS2533374) were analyzed by enzyme-linked immunoabsorbent assays. 25-hydroxyvitamin D was detected by high-performance liquid chromatography (Dionex Corporation, Sunnyvale, CA). Calcium was detected using an automated colorimetric technique including an ion-specific assay (abcam, Cambridge, MA Catalog #ab102505) and a colorimetric microplate reader (BioTek, Winooski, VT). Duplicate testing was performed with coefficients of variation for all samples < 10%.

Patient-reported Outcomes

Quality of Life was assessed using the Functional Assessment of Cancer Therapy-Breast (FACT-B) and the Short Form-36 Health Survey (SF-36). The Brief Fatigue Inventory (BFI) was used to assess fatigue, where a lower score indicates less fatigue [7]. Risk for depression and depressive symptoms were assessed using the 20-item Center for Epidemiologic Studies-Depression Scale (CES-D) [8].

Covariate Measures

Weight was measured to the nearest 0.1 kg on an electronic scale with the patient wearing a hospital gown and no shoes and height was measured to the nearest 0.5 cm with a fixed stadiometer in order to calculate BMI. Waist circumference was measured at the midpoint between the lower margin of the last palpable rib and the iliac crest. Physical activity history was assessed at baseline using an interviewer-administered, validated questionnaire to assess historical, past-year, and past-week physical activity [9]. Three-day dietary records (2 weekdays and 1 weekend day) were completed at baseline, post-intervention, and 3-month follow-up (exercise group only) within 1-week of each assessment and analyzed using Nutritionist Pro™ (Woodinville, WA). Participants completed the Charlson Comorbidity questionnaire [10]. Cancer-related information (i.e., time since treatment completion, time since diagnosis, disease stage, hormone-receptor status, endocrine therapy, and surgery) was abstracted from medical records.

Exercise Intervention

The exercise program aligned with ACS/ACSM exercise guidelines for cancer survivors (150 min of aerobic exercise and 2–3 days of resistance exercise training/week) [11]. Participants received 3 supervised one-on-one exercise sessions/week. Days 1 and 3 consisted of aerobic and resistance exercise of ~ 80 min and Day 2 included ~ 50 min of aerobic exercise. All sessions were led by a certified ACS/ACSM Cancer Exercise Trainer. Participants wore a Polar® heart monitor (Lake Success, NY) during each exercise session. Each session began with a 5-min aerobic exercise warm-up at 40–50% estimated VO_2max. Sequenced resistance exercise followed in circuit training fashion with no rest periods between exercises: Leg Press ⇔ Chest Press ⇒ Lunges ⇔ Seated Row ⇒ Leg Extensions ⇔ Triceps Extensions ⇒ Leg Flexion ⇔ Biceps Curl; where ⇔ indicates the two exercises that alternated until all sets were completed, then the following pair of exercises was performed. Initial resistance was set at 80% of the estimated 1-RM for lower body exercises and 60% estimated 1-RM for upper body exercises. When the participant was able to complete three sets of 10 repetitions at the set weight in two consecutive sessions then the weight is increased by 10%. Repetitions increased from 10 (week 4) to 12 (week 8) to 15 (week 12) every 4 weeks to safely build muscular endurance. Compression garments were required during the exercise sessions for all participants who held prescriptions.

Resistance exercises were followed by self-selected aerobic exercise: treadmill walking/running; rowing machine; stationary bicycle. Heart rate (HR) was monitored throughout the aerobic sessions to maintain a HR at 65–80% of maximum HR. Target HR was increased every 4 weeks to safely build cardiorespiratory endurance and to maintain the prescribed intensity as participants improved their cardiorespiratory fitness. Duration of the aerobic sessions was increased from 30 min (week 1) to 50 min (week 16) as cardiorespiratory fitness increased to meet the exercise guidelines for cancer survivors. Participants ended each session with a 5-min cool down at 40–50% estimated VO_2max. The trainers documented attendance and minutes of exercise per session.

Follow-up period (exercise group only)

A 12-week follow-up was instituted in the exercise group to assess intervention durability. During the 12-week period, participants were encouraged to exercise on their own without study team supervision. Participants were asked to maintain weekly physical activity logs and wear an accelerometer on a daily basis during this period; they repeated outcome measure testing upon completion of the 12-week period. Sustainability was assessed at 28-week follow-up in this group by 7-day accelerometer monitoring (Model GT3X Actigraph, Fort Walton Beach, FL). Participants were asked to wear the accelerometer during waking hours for 7 consecutive days, perform their normal or usual activity, and remove the device while bathing, showering, or swimming. Participants received verbal and written instructions and a wear time log to encourage adherence. Devices were returned at time of follow-up testing. Accelerometer data was used to estimate minutes and intensity of physical activity performed according to the manufacturer's directions.

Statistical Analyses

As this is a secondary analysis of the parent trial which focused on metabolic syndrome, the sample size was based on projected changes in insulin [12]. Enrollment of 100 women provided 80% statistical power ($\alpha = 0.05$) to detect a 2.6 μU/ml (SD = 4.0 μU/ml) difference in mean insulin levels assuming 20% drop-out using a two-group t-test.

Within-group differences in mean changes for individual outcomes measured at post-intervention and 3-month follow-up (exercise group only) were evaluated using general linear models repeated-measures ANOVAs. Between-group differences in mean changes for individual outcomes measured at post-intervention were evaluated using mixed-model repeated measure analysis. A priori covariates included type of treatment (chemotherapy, radiation, or both), surgery type, time on hormonal therapy, comorbidities, and BMI were explored in models due to their possible associations with outcomes, but none modified results. Five women using bisphosphonates were excluded when analyzing BMD and other bone biomarkers.

Post-hoc analyses included stratification by menopausal status at time of diagnosis. (women were classified as postmenopausal if amenorrheic over the previous 12 months). Analyses were performed using SAS (Version 9.4, Cary, NC).

Results

The study CONSORT diagram is reported elsewhere. Briefly, we assessed 418 women for eligibility of which 100 were randomized to the exercise or usual care group. Four participants in the exercise group and five participants in the usual care group did not complete the study. Baseline characteristics also are reported elsewhere and were similar across the 2 groups. On average, women were 53.5 ± 10.4 (SD) years old, postmenopausal (60%), Hispanic white (55%) or non-Hispanic white (26%), 6.2 ± 2.1 months from diagnosis, with a BMI = 33.5 ± 5.5 kg/m². Women were diagnosed primarily with stage I (40%) or II (38%) breast cancer and largely treated with both chemo- and radiation- therapy (76%). The weekly average of moderate-to-vigorous physical activity at baseline was 9.6 ± 6.8 min.

Intervention adherence and adverse events are reported elsewhere. High session attendance of 96% (overall average 46 of 48 sessions) was attained by the exercise group. Adherence with aerobic exercise, and with intensity and volume of resistance exercises was 95%. No adverse events were reported over the duration of the study.

Physical Fitness

Physical fitness outcomes are displayed in Table 1. Estimated VO_{2max}, an indicator of cardiorespiratory fitness, significantly increased in the exercise group as compared to baseline and the usual care group (p-value< 0.001). Resting heart rate significantly decreased in the exercise group as compared to baseline and the usual care group (p-value< 0.001). Muscle strength, assessed as estimated 1-RM, significantly increased across all four exercises (leg extension, leg flexion, latissimus pulldown, chest press) in the exercise group as compared to baseline and the usual care group (p-values< 0.001). At follow-up, all physical fitness measures remained significantly improved in the exercise group compared to baseline (p-values< 0.001). The usual care group did not experience changes in any measure of physical fitness (p-values> 0.05).

Bone Health

Table 2 shows baseline, post-intervention, and 3-month follow-up changes in BMD and bone biomarkers by group. Post-intervention, BMD (whole body, lumbar spine, total hip, trochanter, and femoral neck) did not significantly change in the exercise or usual care groups ($p > 0.10$). Calcium and 25-hydroxyvitamin D levels increased ($p = 0.09$) in the exercise group however this did not reach significance. Osteocalcin and BSAP, biomarkers of bone formation, increased in the exercise as compared to baseline ($p = 0.04$, 0.05, respectively) and the usual care group ($p = 0.01$, 0.07, respectively) however, significance was only reached for osteocalcin. Post-intervention, CTX and NTX, biomarkers of bone resorption, and RANK and RANKL, biomarkers of bone remodeling, did not significantly change in the exercise or usual care groups ($p > 0.05$). Stratification by menopausal status did not alter these results.

Patient-Reported Outcomes

Tables 3 and 4 display patient-reported outcomes. Post-intervention, FACT-B scores (Table 3) were significantly improved in exercise vs. usual care (between group difference: 14.7, 95% CI: 18.2, 9.7; $p < 0.001$). FACT-General, trial outcome index, and all subscales were significantly improved in the exercise group when compared to baseline ($p \leq 0.01$) and the usual care group (p < 0.001). All SF-36 subscores (Table 4) significantly

Table 1 Comparison of physical fitness between exercise and usual care groups

	Baseline	Post-intervention		3-month follow-up		Between-group difference post-intervention	
	Mean (SD)	Mean (SD)	P value[a]	Mean (SD)	P value[b]	Mean (95% CI)	P value[c]
Estimated VO$_{2max}$ (mL/kg/min)							
Exercise	23.3 (6.1)	35.1 (8.0)	< 0.001	32.1 (8.2)	< 0.001	11.8 (25.2 to 16.7)	< 0.001
Usual care	22.7 (6.4)	19.3 (8.5)	0.14	–	–		
Resting heart rate (bpm)							
Exercise	87.9 (8.0)	77.5 (8.5)	< 0.001	76.9 (8.9)	< 0.001	−15.4 (−18.1 to −11.7)	< 0.001
Usual care	87.7 (7.7)	88.1 (7.8)	0.67	–	–		
Leg extension (kgs)							
Exercise	45.4 (10.6)	75.7 (10.8)	< 0.001	77.4 (11.5)	< 0.001	30.4 (35.9 to 27.8)	< 0.001
Usual care	44.9 (9.1)	42.9 (9.0)	0.15	–	–		
Leg flexion (kgs)							
Exercise	39.5 (9.6)	63.6 (11.2)	< 0.001	62.4 (12.1)	< 0.001	24.0 (27.2 to 21.6)	< 0.001
Usual care	40.8 (10.1)	39.7 (10.6)	0.23	–	–		
Latissimus pulldown (kgs)							
Exercise	30.6 (4.7)	39.0 (6.1)	< 0.001	38.5 (6.5)	< 0.001	9.6 (11.7 to 6.1)	< 0.001
Usual care	30.3 (4.0)	29.6 (4.4)	0.27	–	–		
Chest press (kgs)							
Exercise	9.1 (2.3)	20.7 (4.5)	< 0.001	19.5 (4.0)	< 0.001	11.6 (15.9 to 7.7)	< 0.001
Usual care	9.2 (2.5)	8.7 (2.4)	0.40	–	–		

Abbreviations: *SD* standard deviation, *CI* confidence interval, *kgs* kilograms
[a]P value for repeated measures ANOVA comparing changes in the exercise group from baseline to post-intervention, and in the usual care group from baseline to post-intervention
[b]P value for repeated measures ANOVA comparing changes in the exercise group from baseline to 3-month follow-up
[c]P value for mixed model analysis comparing changes between the exercise and usual care group from baseline to post-intervention

improved in the exercise group when compared to baseline and the usual care group ($p \leq 0.001$). Fatigue and depression (Table 4) significantly reduced in the exercise group as compared to baseline ($p \leq 0.01$) and the usual care group ($p < 0.001$). At follow-up, all patient-reported outcome measures remained significantly improved in the exercise group compared to baseline ($p < 0.001$).

Discussion

A supervised 16-week aerobic and resistance exercise intervention designed to improve metabolic syndrome also led to significant improvements in quality of life, depression, fatigue, and physical fitness that were maintained at 3-month follow-up among ethnically-diverse, physically inactive, and overweight/obese breast cancer survivors. While the intervention did not alter bone density, osteocalcin and BSAP showed significant improvements. This is the first study to our knowledge to significantly improve these outcomes with a structured combined exercise intervention in an ethnically-diverse sample of overweight or obese breast cancer survivors soon after treatment. These results are impactful given that quality of life, fatigue, and physical deconditioning are some of the most common and persevering symptoms reported by breast cancer survivors [13, 14]. This

work supports the ACS/ACSM exercise guidelines for cancer survivors and demonstrates successful integration of these guidelines for women from different ethnic backgrounds.

Remarkable improvements in patient-reported outcomes were observed for quality of life, fatigue, and depressive symptoms. While our results align with those reported in the literature [15, 16], the exercise-induced reductions in fatigue (effect size $d = 0.91$) and depressive symptomology (effect size $d = 0.97$) are unparalleled with substantially larger effect sizes than the 0.30 and 0.38 reported from recent meta-analyses examining exercise and fatigue [16] and depressive symptoms [17], respectively, in cancer survivors. The marked reduction in these two domains may be due to the inclusion of women within a short period (6 months) of concluding cancer-related treatment, the physically inactive and obese nature of the participants upon enrollment, and the ethnically diverse sample. Further, it is plausible that the combination of aerobic and resistance exercise, in a supervised manner, resulted in greater benefits on patient-reported outcomes than only one mode of exercise. Previous studies have integrated a supervised combined exercise intervention with significant improvements in quality of life [18–23], fatigue [20], and

Table 2 Comparison of bone health between exercise and usual care groups

	Baseline	Post-intervention		3-month follow-up		Between-group difference post-intervention	
	Mean (SD)	Mean (SD)	P value[a]	Mean (SD)	P value[b]	Mean (95% CI)	P value[c]
Calcium (mg/dL)							
Exercise	10.3 (2.6)	13.7 (1.9)	0.09	13.4 (1.7)	0.10	3.4 (5.0 to 1.6)	0.10
Usual care	10.5 (2.5)	9.9 (2.6)	0.67	–	–		
25(OH)D (ng/dL)							
Exercise	21.7 (4.4)	27.8 (6.7)	0.09	27.4 (6.5)	0.09	6.1 (9.8 to 4.3)	0.10
Usual care	21.5 (4.1)	20.9 (4.0)	0.57	–	–		
Osteocalcin (ng/mL)							
Exercise	12.1 (3.1)	15.0 (4.1)	0.01	14.7 (3.5)	0.01	3.1 (5.6 to 1.5)	0.01
Usual care	12.3 (3.4)	12.0 (3.0)	0.61	–	–		
BSAP (ng/mL)							
Exercise	16.1 (4.6)	18.0 (5.0)	0.01	17.7 (4.6)	0.01	1.9 (2.4 to 0.55)	0.001
Usual care	16.2 (4.3)	15.9 (4.2)	0.55	–	–		
CTX (ng/mL)							
Exercise	0.48 (0.1)	0.44 (0.2)	0.07	0.44 (0.2)	0.07	−0.04 (−0.10 to −0.06)	0.10
Usual care	0.47 (0.1)	0.48 (0.2)	0.74	–	–		
NTX (nM BCE/L)							
Exercise	18.6 (3.1)	17.7 (2.8)	0.10	17.8 (2.7)	0.11	−0.90 (−1.1 to − 0.6)	0.12
Usual care	18.4 (2.7)	18.3 (2.5)	0.67	–	–		
RANK (pg/mL)							
Exercise	27.4 (6.8)	26.7 (6.4)	0.14	26.6 (6.1)	0.14	−0.70 (−0.9 to − 0.4)	0.20
Usual care	26.9 (6.6)	26.4 (6.5)	0.34	–	–		
RANKL (pmol/L)							
Exercise	142.5 (18.9)	146.1 (16.1)	0.09	145.7 (16.2)	0.09	3.6 (5.1 to 1.2)	0.14
Usual care	139.8 (18.1)	148.8 (18.9)	0.47	–	–		
Whole body BMD (g/cm^2)							
Exercise	1.22 (0.1)	1.27 (0.1)	0.15	1.26 (0.1)	0.16	0.05 (0.04 to 0.02)	0.15
Usual care	1.20 (0.1)	1.19 (0.1)	0.29	–	–		
Lumbar spine BMD (g/cm^2)							
Exercise	1.16 (0.09)	1.20 (0.09)	0.09	1.20 (0.1)	0.09	0.04 (0.03 to 0.01)	0.10
Usual care	1.15 (0.09)	1.14 (0.09)	0.57	–	–		
Total hip BMD (g/cm^2)							
Exercise	0.91 (0.09)	0.94 (0.09)	0.17	0.94 (0.09)	0.17	0.03 (0.03 to 0.00)	0.18
Usual care	0.90 (0.09)	0.89 (0.08)	0.23	–	–		
Trochanter BMD (g/cm^2)							
Exercise	0.72 (0.07)	0.74 (0.07)	0.18	0.74 (0.07)	0.20	0.02 (0.03 to 0.00)	0.22
Usual care	0.71 (0.06)	0.70 (0.06)	0.43	–	–		
Femoral neck BMD (g/cm^2)							
Exercise	0.88 (0.1)	0.90 (0.1)	0.21	0.88 (0.7)	0.24	0.02 (0.03 to 0.00)	0.21
Usual care	0.87 (0.1)	0.86 (0.1)	0.23	–	–		

Abbreviations: *SD* standard deviation, *CI* confidence interval, *BMD* bone mineral density, *RANK* receptor activator factor-kappa B, *RANKL* receptor activator factor-kappa B ligand

[a]*P* value for repeated measures ANOVA comparing changes in the exercise group from baseline to post-intervention, and in the usual care group from baseline to post-intervention

[b]*P* value for repeated measures ANOVA comparing changes in the exercise group from baseline to 3-month follow-up

[c]*P* value for mixed model analysis comparing changes between the exercise and usual care group from baseline to post-intervention

Table 3 Comparison of breast cancer-specific quality of life between exercise and usual care groups

	Baseline Mean (SD)	Post-intervention Mean (SD)	P value[a]	3-month follow-up Mean (SD)	P value[b]	Between-group difference post-intervention Mean (95% CI)	P value[c]
Physical well-being							
Exercise	19.2 (3.1)	23.2 (3.0)	< 0.001	23.1 (3.2)	< 0.001	3.9 (7.2 to 1.7)	0.003
Usual care	19.1 (3.4)	19.1 (3.5)	0.74	–	–		
Social well-being							
Exercise	19.7 (3.0)	23.0 (3.2)	< 0.001	23.0 (3.0)	< 0.001	3.3 (6.9 to 1.1)	0.005
Usual care	19.6 (3.1)	19.5 (3.0)	0.81	–	–		
Emotional well-being							
Exercise	18.4 (2.6)	20.1 (3.1)	0.01	20.1 (3.5)	0.01	1.7 (3.4 to 0.8)	0.01
Usual care	18.3 (2.5)	18.2 (2.7)	0.75	–	–		
Functional well-being							
Exercise	19.9 (3.4)	22.0 (3.2)	0.01	21.9 (3.1)	0.01	2.0 (4.2 to 0.6)	0.01
Usual care	20.0 (3.6)	19.9 (3.3)	0.83	–	–		
Additional concerns							
Exercise	21.1 (4.7)	24.7 (4.1)	0.002	24.0 (4.5)	0.001	3.6 (7.7 to 2.0)	0.002
Usual care	21.7 (4.4)	19.6 (10.4)	0.43	–	–		
FACT-General							
Exercise	77.2 (9.0)	88.3 (9.9)	< 0.001	88.1 (9.2)	< 0.001	11.1 (16.4 to 7.7)	< 0.001
Usual care	77.0 (9.1)	76.7 (9.0)	0.54	–	–		
FACT-Breast							
Exercise	98.3 (14.1)	113.0 (13.0)	< 0.001	112.1 (13.2)	< 0.001	14.7 (18.2 to 9.7)	< 0.001
Usual care	98.7 (14.4)	96.3 (14.5)	0.44	–	–		
Trial outcome index							
Exercise	60.2 (7.3)	69.9 (7.5)	< 0.001	69.0 (7.7)	< 0.001	8.8 (15.3 to 4.3)	< 0.001
Usual care	60.8 (7.5)	58.6 (7.4)	0.64	–	–		

Abbreviations: *SD* standard deviation, *CI* confidence interval, *FACT* Functional Assessment of Cancer Therapy
[a]P value for repeated measures ANOVA comparing changes in the exercise group from baseline to post-intervention, and in the usual care group from baseline to post-intervention
[b]P value for repeated measures ANOVA comparing changes in the exercise group from baseline to 3-month follow-up
[c]P value for mixed model analysis comparing changes between the exercise and usual care group from baseline to post-intervention

depression [18] yet achieved a magnitude of improvement lower than our results. Differences in exercise duration, intensity, and frequency may underlie the various magnitudes of change across outcomes.

Physical function, described as the ability of an individual to perform common daily activities has been shown to predict survival and mortality in breast cancer survivors [24, 25], and thus is gaining support as a relevant prognostic indicator among cancer survivors. One determinant of physical function is one's level of physical fitness, thereby improving physical fitness as a means to improve physical function is of high importance. We found notable improvements in estimated VO_{2max} (52%) and muscular strength (> 30%) following exercise. For example, estimated 1-RM for chest press increased by 133%. Previous studies utilizing a supervised combined exercise intervention have produced significant improvements in physical fitness [18–23, 26] yet to a lesser

degree than our results. Various exercise fitness testing methodologies (i.e., six-minute walk test, 12-min walk test, Aerobic Power Index cycle test, modified Bruce treadmill test) were used across studies, challenging the interpretation of results and between-study comparisons. Moreover, we used indirect assessment of VO_{2max} that involved the use of a regressions formula which may have influenced our results.

Our large exercise-induced effects on physical fitness may be due to the high rate of physically inactive behavior at baseline, and subsequent low physical fitness levels at baseline, the early survivorship phase, high adherence, a supervised environment, and inclusion of both aerobic and resistance exercise. In particular, most (95%) of our Hispanic white participants had no history of physical activity and therefore may have experienced greater gains in the outcomes from the intervention. The large increase in maximal strength for the chest press may be

Table 4 Comparison of health status, fatigue, and depression between exercise and usual care groups

| | Baseline | Post-intervention | | 3-month follow-up | | Between-group difference post-intervention | |
	Mean (SD)	Mean (SD)	P value[a]	Mean (SD)	P value[b]	Mean (95% CI)	P value[c]
SF-36 SUBSCORES							
Physical functioning							
Exercise	65.3 (9.4)	74.1 (9.5)	0.001	73.9 (8.9)	0.001	9.2 (12.3 to 7.7)	0.001
Usual care	65.0 (9.7)	64.1 (9.8)	0.77	–	–		
Role-physical							
Exercise	68.4 (8.6)	75.7 (9.1)	0.002	74.4 (9.5)	0.003	7.3 (10.9 to 4.8)	0.001
Usual care	67.9 (9.1)	66.9 (8.7)	0.55	–	–		
Bodily pain							
Exercise	50.5 (9.6)	63.3 (11.2)	0.001	62.1 (12.1)	0.001	13.2 (17.2 to 9.6)	0.001
Usual care	50.8 (10.1)	49.7 (10.3)	0.23	–	–		
General health							
Exercise	60.1 (11.7)	67.2 (11.1)	0.002	67.0 (10.5)	0.001	7.1 (11.7 to 4.0)	0.002
Usual care	59.7 (11.0)	57.6 (10.4)	0.43	–	–		
Mental health							
Exercise	69.1 (12.3)	77.7 (12.5)	0.003	75.5 (11.0)	0.001	8.6 (12.9 to 5.7)	0.001
Usual care	69.7 (12.5)	68.7 (13.0)	0.60	–	–		
Role-emotional							
Exercise	70.1 (11.3)	83.7 (12.5)	0.001	82.0 (12.0)	0.001	12.1 (15.6 to 7.3)	0.001
Usual care	70.2 (11.5)	68.7 (10.4)	0.44	–	–		
Social functioning							
Exercise	79.1 (14.3)	87.7 (14.5)	0.001	85.5 (14.0)	0.001	8.6 (14.9 to 5.7)	0.002
Usual care	79.4 (14.5)	78.7 (12.4)	0.67	–	–		
Vitality							
Exercise	49.4 (9.3)	56.8 (9.5)	0.001	55.5 (9.0)	0.001	7.4 (12.9 to 4.3)	0.001
Usual care	49.2 (9.5)	48.7 (9.4)	0.63	–	–		
Physical component summary							
Exercise	66.1 (9.3)	72.7 (10.5)	0.003	72.0 (10.0)	0.001	6.6 (12.3 to 4.1)	0.001
Usual care	65.8 (9.0)	63.7 (9.4)	0.27	–	–		
Mental component summary							
Exercise	67.1 (11.0)	72.7 (12.1)	0.004	72.4 (12.4)	0.001	5.5 (9.6 to 3.3)	0.001
Usual care	69.2 (11.7)	68.7 (11.4)	0.56	–	–		
BFI							
Exercise	7.1 (2.0)	2.9 (1.5)	< 0.001	3.1 (1.9)	0.0001	−4.2 (−6.1 to −2.4)	< 0.001
Usual care	7.2 (2.1)	7.7 (2.4)	0.30	–	–		
CES-D							
Exercise	15.1 (3.3)	9.7 (2.5)	< 0.001	9.5 (3.0)	0.0001	6.6 (11.9 to 3.1)	< 0.001
Usual care	15.2 (3.5)	16.7 (3.4)	0.11	–	–		

Abbreviations: *SD* standard deviation, *CI* confidence interval; Short form-36 Health Status, *SF-36*; Brief Fatigue Index, *BFI*; Center for Epidemiological Studies Depression; *CES-D*

[a]P value for repeated measures ANOVA comparing changes in the exercise group from baseline to post-intervention, and in the usual care group from baseline to post-intervention

[b]P value for repeated measures ANOVA comparing changes in the exercise group from baseline to 3-month follow-up

[c]P value for mixed model analysis comparing changes between the exercise and usual care group from baseline to post-intervention

attributed to the deconditioned status of the participants enrolled within 6 months of the completion of cancer treatment. Our adherence of 96% exceeds the 70–80% noted in other trials [27–29], and could be attributed to flexible session timing (5 am – 8 pm, 7d/wk), one-on-one supervision, and the provision of parking permits or bus passes to overcome transportation barriers. Intentionally, we conducted the intervention in a controlled clinical setting under direct supervision to ensure exercise safety and dose intensity needed to elicit greater benefits in our outcomes.

Bone loss occurs as a consequence of breast cancer treatment [30]. Premenopausal breast cancer survivors may experience chemotherapy-induced amenorrhea or pharmacologic ovarian suppression treatment, predisposing them to further bone loss [30]. While we did not observe improvements in BMD, this may be explained by the short duration of our intervention. Interventions similar to ours that included aerobic and resistance exercise produced conflicting results and involved varying durations of exposure to exercise. Thomas et al. did not observe significant improvements in BMD following a 12-month aerobic and resistance exercise intervention in breast cancer survivors taking aromatase inhibitors (change from baseline: 0.001, 95% CI: -0.009, 0.010) [31]. Almstedt and Tarleton [32] observed improvements in T-scores at the femoral neck and whole body following 13 weeks of aerobic and resistance exercise + whole body vibration in female cancer survivors (breast cancer $n = 5$). It is probable that the incorporation of whole body vibration contributed to the improvements BMD observed by Almstedt and Tarleton. Notably, we did observe a significant increase in osteocalcin and BSAP, a biomarkers of bone formation, so perhaps a longer intervention of a minimum of 6 months would elicit a positive effect on BMD.

Strengths of our study include the focus on high-risk breast cancer survivors with high rates of inactivity and obesity, targeting the early survivorship period, the ethnically-diverse sample, the randomized controlled trial design, the high adherence rate, and the modest loss-to-follow up. Limitations include lack of direct physical function and physical fitness measures (i.e., 1-RM and VO2max), and lack of an attention control group.

Conclusions

In summary, a combined exercise intervention designed to improve metabolic syndrome in ethnically diverse, overweight or obese BCS also demonstrated significant improvements in patient-reported outcomes and physical fitness. Based on our findings, supervised clinical exercise programs that adhere to the ACS/ACSM exercise guidelines should be incorporated into breast cancer treatment and early survivorship care plans.

Abbreviations
ACS: American Cancer Society; ACSM: American College of Sports Medicine; ANOVA: analysis of variance; BFI: Brief Fatigue Inventory; BMD: bone mineral density; BMI: body mass index; BSAP: bone-specific alkaline phosphatase; CES-D: Center for Epidemiologic Studies-Depression Scale; CTX: C-telopeptide of type 1 collagen; DXA: dual energy x-ray absorptiometry; FACT-B: Functional Assessment of Cancer Therapy-Breast; HR: heart rate; IRB: institutional review board; NTX: N-telopeptides of type 1 collagen; RANK: Receptor activator factor-kappa B; RANKL: Receptor activator factor-kappa B ligand; RM: repetition maximum; SD: standard deviation; SF-36: Short Form-36 Health Survey

Acknowledgements
We acknowledge the Clinical Investigations Support Office of the Norris Comprehensive Cancer Center for their support of this investigation, the extraordinary generosity of our study participants- without their participation our study would not have been possible, and the exercise training staff for delivering an engaging and uniform intervention.

Funding
This work was supported by grants K07CA160718 from the National Cancer Institute, UL1TR001855 and UL1TR000130 from the National Center for Advancing Translational Science (NCATS) of the U.S. National Institutes of Health.

Authors' contributions
CMDC was responsible for conceptualization, funding acquisition, project administration, methodology, data curation, writing- original draft, review and editing. KSC was responsible for conceptualization, methodology, writing- original draft, review and editing. WDW was responsible for conceptualization, methodology, writing- original draft, review and editing. NS was responsible for project administration, methodology, data curation, writing- review and editing. KL was responsible for project administration, methodology, data curation, writing- review and editing. FCS was responsible for project administration, methodology, data curation, writing- review and editing. CS was responsible for project administration, methodology, data curation, writing- review and editing. TAB was responsible for conceptualization, methodology, writing- original draft, review and editing. DS was responsible for methodology, writing- original draft, review and editing. DT was responsible for methodology, writing-original draft, review and editing. LB was responsible for funding acquisition, methodology, writing- original draft, review and editing. JEM was responsible for conceptualization, funding acquisition, methodology, writing-original draft, review and editing. All authors read and approved the final manuscript.

Competing interests
The authors declare that they have no competing interests.

Author details
[1]Division of Biokinesiology and Physical Therapy, University of Southern California (USC), |1540 E. Alcazar St., CHP 155, Los Angeles, CA 90089, USA. [2]Faculty of Kinesiology, Sport, and Recreation, University of Alberta, Edmonton, AB T6G 2H9, Canada. [3]Department of Nutrition Sciences, University of Alabama at Birmingham, Birmingham, AL 35294, USA. [4]Division

of Endocrinology and Diabetes, Keck School of Medicine, USC, Los Angeles, CA 90033, USA. [5]Department of Medicine, Keck School of Medicine, University of Southern California, Los Angeles, CA 90033, USA. [6]Department of Breast Medical Oncology, The University of Texas MD Anderson Cancer Center, Houston, TX 77030, USA. [7]Division of Biomarkers of Early Detection and Prevention, Beckman Research Institute, City of Hope (COH), Duarte, CA 91010, USA. [8]Division of Medical Oncology and Experimental Therapeutics, COH, Duarte, CA 91010, USA.

References

1. Ording AG, Garne JP, Nystrom PM, Froslev T, Sorensen HT, Lash TL. Comorbid diseases interact with breast cancer to affect mortality in the first year after diagnosis--a Danish nationwide matched cohort study. PLoS One. 2013;8(10):e76013.
2. Speck RM, Courneya KS, Masse LC, Duval S, Schmitz KH. An update of controlled physical activity trials in cancer survivors: a systematic review and meta-analysis. J Cancer Surviv. 2010;4(2):87–100.
3. Dieli-Conwright CM, Courneya KS, Demark-Wahnefried W, Sami N, Lee K, Buchanan TA, et al. Effects of Aerobic and Resistance Exercise on Metabolic Syndrome, Sarcopenic Obesity, and Circulating Biomarkers in Overweight or Obese Survivors of Breast Cancer: A Randomized Controlled Trial. J Clin Oncol. 2018;36(9):875–83.
4. Dieli-Conwright CM, Mortimer JE, Schroeder ET, Courneya K, Demark-Wahnefried W, Buchanan TA, et al. Randomized controlled trial to evaluate the effects of combined progressive exercise on metabolic syndrome in breast cancer survivors: rationale, design, and methods. BMC Cancer. 2014;14:238.
5. Ebbeling CB, Ward A, Puleo EM, Widrick J, Rippe JM. Development of a single-stage submaximal treadmill walking test. Med Sci Sports Exerc. 1991;23(8):966–73.
6. Brzycki M. Strength testing: Predicting a one-rep max from repetition-to-fatigue. J Physic Educ Recreat Dance. 1993;64:88–90.
7. Mendoza TR, Wang XS, Cleeland CS, Morrissey M, Johnson BA, Wendt JK, et al. The rapid assessment of fatigue severity in cancer patients: use of the Brief Fatigue Inventory. Cancer. 1999;85(5):1186–96.
8. Radloff LS. The CES-D Scale: A Self-Report Depression Scale for Research in the General Population. Appl Psychol Meas. 1977;1(3):385–401.
9. Kriska AM, Knowler WC, LaPorte RE, Drash AL, Wing RR, Blair SN, et al. Development of questionnaire to examine relationship of physical activity and diabetes in Pima Indians. Diabetes Care. 1990;13(4):401–11.
10. Charlson ME, Pompei P, Ales KL, MacKenzie CR. A new method of classifying prognostic comorbidity in longitudinal studies: development and validation. J Chronic Dis. 1987;40(5):373–83.
11. Schmitz KH, Courneya KS, Matthews C, Demark-Wahnefried W, Galvao DA, Pinto BM, et al. American College of Sports Medicine roundtable on exercise guidelines for cancer survivors. Med Sci Sports Exerc. 2010;42(7):1409–26.
12. Ligibel JA, Campbell N, Partridge A, Chen WY, Salinardi T, Chen H, et al. Impact of a mixed strength and endurance exercise intervention on insulin levels in breast cancer survivors. J Clin Oncol. 2008;26(6):907–12.
13. Bower JE, Ganz PA, Desmond KA, Bernaards C, Rowland JH, Meyerowitz BE, et al. Fatigue in long-term breast carcinoma survivors: a longitudinal investigation. Cancer. 2006;106(4):751–8.
14. Crosswell AD, Lockwood KG, Ganz PA, Bower JE. Low heart rate variability and cancer-related fatigue in breast cancer survivors. Psychoneuroendocrinology. 2014;45:58–66.
15. Battaglini CL, Mills RC, Phillips BL, Lee JT, Story CE, Nascimento MG, et al. Twenty-five years of research on the effects of exercise training in breast cancer survivors: A systematic review of the literature. World J Clin Oncol. 2014;5(2):177–90.
16. Mustian KM, Alfano CM, Heckler C, Kleckner AS, Kleckner IR, Leach CR, et al. Comparison of Pharmaceutical, Psychological, and Exercise Treatments for Cancer-Related Fatigue: A Meta-analysis. JAMA Oncol. 2017;3(7):961–8.
17. Patsou ED, Alexias GD, Anagnostopoulos FG, Karamouzis MV. Effects of physical activity on depressive symptoms during breast cancer survivorship: a meta-analysis of randomised control trials. ESMO Open. 2017;2(5):e000271.
18. Dolan LB, Barry D, Petrella T, Davey L, Minnes A, Yantzi A, et al. The Cardiac Rehabilitation Model Improves Fitness, Quality of Life, and Depression in Breast Cancer Survivors. J Cardiopulm Rehabil Prev. 2017;38(4):246-252.
19. Smith TM, Broomhall CN, Crecelius AR. Physical and Psychological Effects of a 12-Session Cancer Rehabilitation Exercise Program. Clin J Oncol Nurs. 2016;20(6):653–9.
20. De Luca V, Minganti C, Borrione P, Grazioli E, Cerulli C, Guerra E, et al. Effects of concurrent aerobic and strength training on breast cancer survivors: a pilot study. Public Health. 2016;136:126–32.
21. Campbell A, Mutrie N, White F, McGuire F, Kearney N. A pilot study of a supervised group exercise programme as a rehabilitation treatment for women with breast cancer receiving adjuvant treatment. Eur J Oncol Nurs. 2005;9(1):56–63.
22. Milne HM, Wallman KE, Gordon S, Courneya KS. Effects of a combined aerobic and resistance exercise program in breast cancer survivors: a randomized controlled trial. Breast Cancer Res Treat. 2008;108(2):279–88.
23. Mutrie N, Campbell AM, Whyte F, McConnachie A, Emslie C, Lee L, et al. Benefits of supervised group exercise programme for women being treated for early stage breast cancer: pragmatic randomised controlled trial. BMJ. 2007;334(7592):517.
24. Brown JC, Harhay MO, Harhay MN. Physical function as a prognostic biomarker among cancer survivors. Br J Cancer. 2015;112(1):194–8.
25. Sehl M, Lu X, Silliman R, Ganz PA. Decline in physical functioning in first 2 years after breast cancer diagnosis predicts 10-year survival in older women. J Cancer Surviv. 2013;7(1):20–31.
26. Knobf MT, Jeon S, Smith B, Harris L, Thompson S, Stacy MR, et al. The Yale Fitness Intervention Trial in female cancer survivors: Cardiovascular and physiological outcomes. Heart Lung. 2017;46(5):375–81.
27. Courneya KS, Segal RJ, Gelmon K, Reid RD, Mackey JR, Friedenreich CM, et al. Predictors of supervised exercise adherence during breast cancer chemotherapy. Med Sci Sports Exerc. 2008;40(6):1180–7.
28. Arem H, Sorkin M, Cartmel B, Fiellin M, Capozza S, Harrigan M, et al. Exercise adherence in a randomized trial of exercise on aromatase inhibitor arthralgias in breast cancer survivors: the Hormones and Physical Exercise (HOPE) study. J Cancer Surviv. 2016;10(4):654–62.
29. Schmitz KH, Ahmed RL, Hannan PJ, Yee D. Safety and efficacy of weight training in recent breast cancer survivors to alter body composition, insulin, and insulin-like growth factor axis proteins. Cancer Epidemiol Biomark Prev. 2005;14(7):1672–80.
30. Santen RJ. Clinical review: Effect of endocrine therapies on bone in breast cancer patients. J Clin Endocrinol Metab. 2011;96(2):308–19.
31. Thomas GA, Cartmel B, Harrigan M, Fiellin M, Capozza S, Zhou Y, et al. The effect of exercise on body composition and bone mineral density in breast cancer survivors taking aromatase inhibitors. Obesity (Silver Spring). 2017;25(2):346–51.
32. Almstedt HC, Tarleton HP. Mind the gaps: missed opportunities to promote bone health among cancer survivors. Support Care Cancer. 2015;23(3):611–4.

13

Targeted next-generation sequencing identifies clinically relevant somatic mutations in a large cohort of inflammatory breast cancer

Xu Liang[1,2], Sophie Vacher[2], Anais Boulai[2], Virginie Bernard[3], Sylvain Baulande[4], Mylene Bohec[4], Ivan Bièche[2,5], Florence Lerebours[6] and Céline Callens[2*]

Abstract

Background: Inflammatory breast cancer (IBC) is the most aggressive form of primary breast cancer. Using a custom-made breast cancer gene sequencing panel, we investigated somatic mutations in IBC to better understand the genomic differences compared with non-IBC and to consider new targeted therapy in IBC patients.

Methods: Targeted next-generation sequencing (NGS) of 91 candidate breast cancer-associated genes was performed on 156 fresh-frozen breast tumor tissues from IBC patients. Mutational profiles from 197 primary breast tumors from The Cancer Genome Atlas (TCGA) were used as non-IBC controls for comparison analysis. The mutational landscape of IBC was correlated with clinicopathological data and outcomes.

Results: After genotype calling and algorithmic annotations, we identified 392 deleterious variants in IBC and 320 variants in non-IBC cohorts, respectively. IBC tumors harbored more mutations than non-IBC (2.5 per sample vs. 1.6 per sample, $p < 0.0001$). Eighteen mutated genes were significantly different between the two cohorts, namely *TP53*, *CDH1*, *NOTCH2*, *MYH9*, *BRCA2*, *ERBB4*, *POLE*, *FGFR3*, *ROS1*, *NOTCH4*, *LAMA2*, *EGFR*, *BRCA1*, *TP53BP1*, *ESR1*, *THBS1*, *CASP8*, and *NOTCH1*. In IBC, the most frequently mutated genes were *TP53* (43.0%), *PIK3CA* (29.5%), *MYH9* (8.3%), *NOTCH2* (8.3%), *BRCA2* (7.7%), *ERBB4* (7.1%), *FGFR3* (6.4%), *POLE* (6.4%), *LAMA2* (5.8%), *ARID1A* (5.1%), *NOTCH4* (5.1%), and *ROS1* (5.1%). After grouping 91 genes on 10 signaling pathways, we found that the DNA repair pathway for the triple-negative breast cancer (TNBC) subgroup, the RTK/RAS/MAPK and cell cycle pathways for the HR⁻/HER2⁺ subgroup, the DNA repair, RTK/RAS/MAPK, and NOTCH pathways for the HR⁺/HER2⁻ subgroup, and the DNA repair, epigenome, and diverse pathways for the HR⁺/HER2⁺ subgroup were all significantly differently altered between IBC and non-IBC. *PIK3CA* mutation was independently associated with worse metastasis-free survival (MFS) in IBC since the median MFS for the *PIK3CA* mutant type was 26.0 months and for the *PIK3CA* wild type was 101.1 months ($p = 0.002$). This association was observed in TNBC ($p = 0.04$) and the HR⁻/HER2⁺ subgroups ($p = 0.0003$), but not in the HR⁺/HER2⁻ subgroup of IBC.

Conclusions: Breast cancer-specific targeted NGS uncovered a high frequency of deleterious somatic mutations in IBC, some of which may be relevant for clinical management.

Keywords: Inflammatory breast cancer, Targeted NGS, Somatic mutation, Prognosis

* Correspondence: celine.callens@curie.fr
[2]Pharmacogenomic Unit, Department of Genetics, Curie Institute, PSL
Research University, 26 rue d'Ulm, 75005 Paris, France
Full list of author information is available at the end of the article

Background

Inflammatory breast cancer (IBC) is a breast adenocarcinoma defined by a rapid onset of inflammatory signs involving at least one-third of the breast, such as erythema and edema (also known as 'peau d'orange') [1]. Although IBC is rare, constituting 1–5% of breast cancer cases, it harbors aggressive behavior with poor a prognosis and accounts for roughly 10% of breast cancer mortality annually [2]. Compared to non-IBC, IBC frequently presents resistance to conventional therapies and early recurrence. Although therapeutic progress in the past two decades in the context of non-IBC has also had a positive impact in women with IBC, with a more than 22-month improvement in median breast cancer-specific survival (BCSS) and a 14% improvement in 2-year BCSS [3], IBC is still a challenge for breast cancer physicians because of poor survival and lack of specific treatment. The clinical presentation and outcome of IBC are obviously different from those of non-IBC but there is no significant difference in treatment between IBC and stage III non-IBC. The poor understanding of the specific biological and molecular characteristics of IBC precludes specific therapeutic interventions. We urgently need to identify how and why IBC is distinct from non-IBC.

The ability to exploit the genetic information of a tumor for any clinical potential has only recently become evident. In this evidence-based precision medicine, genetic data have been exploited to identify therapies appropriate for an individual and has led to changes in drug oversight policy and the way certain drugs have been designated. As a special case of breast cancer mostly defined by clinical symptoms, IBC genome-specific maps are barely understood. Thus far, in previous studies, the IBC gene expression profiles demonstrated high transcriptional heterogeneity and heavy overall mutation burden compared with non-IBC [4, 5]. The largest molecular biology research on IBC mainly focused on the transcriptome and demonstrated the presence of molecular subtypes similar to those of non-IBC tumors, although with over-representation of human epidermal growth factor receptor 2 (HER2)-enriched tumors and a low prevalence of Luminal A tumors, and suggested the deregulation of the expression of few genes in IBC compared with non-IBC, in particular those involved in cell motility, invasion, inflammatory pathways, and transforming growth factor (TGF)Beta signaling [6–8]. Recently, some studies reported a higher frequency of *TP53*, *PIK3CA*, and *ERBB2* mutations in IBC than in non-IBC [9, 10], but these studies were performed in a small series and need further study to draw any conclusions.

Therefore, there is a need to extensively describe the genomic alterations in IBC to identify pathways involved in metastatic processes and drug resistance and to generate new treatment strategies for IBC patients. We have designed a breast cancer and targeted treatment-associated gene panel and performed targeted next-generation sequencing (NGS) in a large cohort of 156 IBC samples. Using the clinicopathological data and long-term survival follow-up, the association of the IBC mutational landscape with clinical outcomes was studied.

Methods

Samples

Tumor samples were collected from 156 women with IBC who underwent core biopsies at the Curie Institute/ Rene Huguenin Hospital (Saint-Cloud, France) between 1988 and 2012. Each patient signed a written informed consent form and the study was approved by the Curie Institute/Rene Huguenin Hospital ethics committee. Tumor samples were immediately stored in liquid nitrogen after biopsy or surgery until DNA extraction. The samples analyzed contained more than 70% tumor cells.

Criteria for the diagnosis of IBC were the simultaneous presence of diffuse erythema and edema (peau d'orange) involving at least one-third of the breast with or without a measurable breast mass (staged T4d according to the AJCC classification) [1]. All patients with IBC tumors prospectively collected between 1988 and 2012 (with only 27 IBC samples collected between 1988 and 2003) received anthracycline-based ± taxane induction chemotherapy associated after 2003 with trastuzumab for HER2-positive tumors. Thirty-two of 43 HER2-positive patients (74.4%) received trastuzumab combined chemotherapy. Mastectomy with axillary node dissection was performed in all nonmetastatic patients following first-line systemic therapy. Radiation therapy was performed in all patients and hormone therapy was administered when indicated.

Public data for 197 invasive breast carcinomas from The Cancer Genome Atlas (TCGA) were used as a non-IBC dataset. This cohort was obtained using http://www.cbioportal.org [11, 12]. We extracted stage III and stage IV patients from 1105 samples in the clinical file downloaded from the TCGA data matrix (Breast invasive carcinoma, TCGA Provisional 2016), and we filtered out male patients, patients without completed cancer status information, and inflammatory breast cancer which was shown to be T4d. Of the 226 patients selected, somatic mutations detected by whole-exome sequencing were available for 197 patients and the clinical characteristics are shown in Additional file 1 (Table S1).

Identification of breast cancer subtypes

Estrogen receptor (ER) and progesterone receptor (PR) status were determined by immunohistochemical (IHC) staining of paraffin-embedded tissue with monoclonal antibodies as part of the routine diagnostic procedure. Nuclear staining of 10% of the invasive cells was considered positive. Hormone receptor (HR) positivity was defined as ER and/or PR positivity. The HER2 status was determined by IHC staining and fluorescence in-situ hybridization (FISH). HER2 positivity was defined as 3+ IHC staining intensity (strong membranous staining in 10% of cells) or gene amplification (a HER2/CEP17 gene copy ratio of 2.0) using FISH. The subtypes were assessed for the primary tumor site.

Somatic mutation data collection

Targeted NGS was applied to a custom-made panel of 91 'breast cancer-specific' genes selected for their involvement in breast cancer. This BreastCurie panel was made up of the most frequently mutated genes (mutation frequency greater than 1%) in breast cancer from TCGA [13] and genes with potential therapeutic-targeted mutation based on the agreement of biologic specialists of the Institut Curie. The BreastCurie panel includes 91 genes (Additional file 2: Table S2) which were grouped into nine different signaling pathways: PIK3CA/AKT/mTOR, RTK/RAS/MAPK, cell cycle and apoptosis, DNA repair, NOTCH, ER, extracellular matrix, transcription, and epigenome. The genes *KEAP1*, *LDLRAP1*, *STMN2*, *MYO3A*, *VHL*, *AGTR2*, *CTNNB1*, *APC*, *SF3B1*, and *MYH9* all have different functionalities and were thus grouped into a pathway called "diverse".

For each sample, coding exons and intron-exon boundaries of all genes were amplified using two ultra-high-multiplex polymerase chain reaction (PCR) primer pools (4834 amplicons) based on Ion AmpliSeq Targeted Sequencing Technology (ThermoFisher Scientific, USA). DNA libraries were prepared using the TruSeq nano DNA kit (Illumina, San Diego, CA, USA). Targeted NGS was performed on an Illumina Hiseq2500 sequencer according to the manufacturer's instructions using the paired-end 120 nucleotide (PE120) sequencing mode. Sequence data were aligned to the human reference genome (hg19) using the Bowtie2 algorithm. The single nucleotide variants (SNVs) and indels were called using the GATK UnifiedGenotyper with default parameters. Known variants found in dbsnp129 and dbsnp137 with a variant allele frequency (VAF) superior to 1% (1000 g or ESP6500) were removed. Filtered retained variants had to have a total coverage depth of greater than or equal to 100 reads and a VAF of at least 5%. The sequencing results were analyzed for base substitutions, short insertions and deletions (INDELs), and copy number alterations (focal amplifications and homozygous deletions) as previously described [14, 15]. Further confirmation of detected variants was performed with a comparison to public databases (cbioportal, tumorportal), and potential pathogenicity was evaluated with four different public algorithms (Polyphen2, Sift, Mutation Assessor, Mutation Taster). We annotated all variants detected with the 'treatment algorithms' as previously

described [14, 16], and which was performed in SHIVA [17], SAFIR01 [18], and SAFIR02 (trial in progress). Briefly, only hotspots missense, splice-site mutation revealing in-frame exon skipping, in-frame micro-deletions, or micro-insertions that were well established to be activating mutations should be considered functionally relevant for oncogenes. Meanwhile, for tumor suppressor gene, nonsense mutations, splice-site mutation, or frameshift insertion/deletions were considered pathogenic; missense mutations were considered relevant if they were established inactivating mutations in silico or in the literature [14]. Eventually, detected mutations were classified as pathogenic variants, unknown pathogenic variants, and nonpathogenic variants. The mutational profile of the 197 non-IBC cohort from TCGA was obtained after exclusion of all genes that were not included in our 91 genes panel. The same algorithms and classification were used to annotate the somatic variants of non-IBC cohort from TCGA.

DNA copy number estimation

We estimated the copy number variations (CNV) using ONCOCNV, a computed method and software tool for high-quality base counting of the sequenced genes, as previously described [15]. Only mapping and base quality more than 20 were considered. The total number of reads covering each gene area was summarized and then normalized twice: first, by the total number of reads covering the analyzed sample, and then by the median coverage of the 155 other samples. We considered marked amplification if 80% of the captured gene areas had a normalized count of 2 or more. We considered homozygous deletion if 80% of the captured gene areas had a normalized count of 0.5 or less.

Statistical analysis

Statistical analyses were performed using GraphPad Prism (version 5.01) software. The results were considered statistically significant at a p value < 0.05. We constructed contingency tables and performed a χ^2 test for the association between clinical features and gene mutation or pathway alteration and to compare the mutation profiles between IBC and non-IBC patients, and Fisher's exact tests were used when a cell contained less than five. Follow-up was measured from the date of diagnosis to the date of last news for patients without any event. Metastasis-free survival (MFS) was determined as the interval between initial diagnosis and detection of the first distant metastasis, with an interval less than 6 months being excluded. Survival distributions were estimated by the Kaplan-Meier method, and survival was compared between groups with the log-rank test. The p values were based on the Wald test, and patients with one or more missing data were excluded. The Cox proportional hazards regression model was used to assess prognostic significance in the multivariate analysis and the results are presented as hazard ratios. All statistical tests were two sided at the 5% level of significance.

Results

Patients characteristics

Pathological and clinical characteristics available for 156 IBC are provided in Table 1. All patients were female. Median age at IBC diagnosis was 53 years (age range

Table 1 Pathological and clinical characteristics of the inflammatory breast cancer (IBC) cohort

	IBC
Total, n (%)	156 (100)
Age (years)	
Median	53
Range	23–84
≤50, n (%)	63 (40.5)
>50, n (%)	93 (59.5)
Sex, n (%)	
Female	156 (100)
Male	0 (0)
Stage, n (%)	
III	120 (76.9)
IV	36 (23.1)
ER status, n (%)	
Negative	89 (57.1)
Positive	67 (42.9)
PR status, n (%)	
Negative	111 (71.2)
positive	45 (28.8)
Her2 status, n (%)	
Negative	113 (72.4)
Positive	43 (27.6)
Subgroups, n (%)	
TNBC	51 (32.7)
HR⁻/Her2⁺	33 (21.2)
HR⁺/Her2⁻	62 (39.7)
HR⁺/Her2⁺	10 (6.4)
Distant metastases, n (%)	
Yes	98 (62.8)
No	58 (37.2)
SBR histological grade, n (%)	
I	2 (1.3)
II	63 (40.4)
III	91 (58.3)

ER estrogen receptor, *Her2* human epidermal growth factor receptor 2, *HR* hormone receptor, *PR* progesterone receptor, *SBR* Scarf Bloom Richardson classification, *TNBC* triple-negative breast cancer

23–84 years). Median follow-up was 50.4 months (range 3.0 to 212.4 months) for IBC patients. Thirty-six of the 156 IBC patients (23.1%) had stage IV disease at diagnosis. Metastases were detected in 62.8% (98/156) of IBC patients and 26.9% (53/197) of non-IBC patients ($p <$ 0.0001). Patients from the IBC and non-IBC cohorts were respectively classified into four subgroups according to hormone receptor (HR) and HER2 status. We also combined HR⁺/HER2⁻ and HR⁺/HER2⁺ to be HR⁺ (72 patients, 46.2%), triple-negative breast cancer (TNBC) and HR⁻/HER2⁺ to be HR⁻ (72 patients, 53.8%), and HR⁻/HER2⁺ and HR⁺/HER2⁺ to be HER2⁺ subtypes (43 patients, 27.6%) during the IBC analysis.

IBC mutation profiling

Among the 91 sequenced genes from 156 IBC samples, we detected 777 somatic mutations comprising 733 point mutations and 44 indels. Point mutations included 666 missense, 59 nonsense, and 8 splice-site mutations, and the 44 indels included 28 frame-shift and 16 in-frame. They corresponded to 516 different mutations in 84 genes, and 152 samples exhibited at least one mutation. After annotation of all these mutations, 392 mutations in 73 genes on 144 samples were predicted to have high probability of being deleterious, and were thus classified as pathogenic variants and unknown pathogenic variants (Fig. 1a). In the non-IBC, a total of 320 deleterious mutations in 56 genes on 146 samples was identified (Fig. 1b). All pathogenic variants and unknown pathogenic variants were considered as mutations for further research.

Comparison of mutation frequency between IBC and non-IBC

The average number of mutations per sample was higher in IBC than in non-IBC (2.5 vs. 1.6, $p = 0.0009$). We observed a significantly different mutation frequency between IBC and non-IBC patients for the following genes: *TP53, CDH1, NOTCH2, MYH9, BRCA2, ERBB4, POLE, FGFR3, ROS1, NOTCH4, LAMA2, EGFR, BRCA1, TP53BP1, ESR1, THBS1, CASP8,* and *NOTCH1.* All genes, except *CDH1* which was less frequently mutated in IBC, were more frequently mutated in IBC compared with non-IBC (Fig. 2). The most frequently mutated genes in IBC were *TP53* (43.0%), *PIK3CA* (29.5%), *MYH9* (8.3%), *NOTCH2* (8.3%), *BRCA2* (7.7%), *ERBB4* (7.1%), *FGFR3* (6.4%), *POLE* (6.4%), *LAMA2* (5.8%), *ARID1A* (5.1%), *NOTCH4* (5.1%), and *ROS1* (5.1%) (Fig. 2). A comparison was made of the mutated genes between IBC and non-IBC according to the four subgroups. Gene mutation frequencies were not significantly different in the triple-negative IBC and non-IBC subgroups (Additional file 3: Figure S1a). In the HR⁻/HER2⁺ subgroup, less mutations on *TP53* were detected in IBC (Additional file 3:

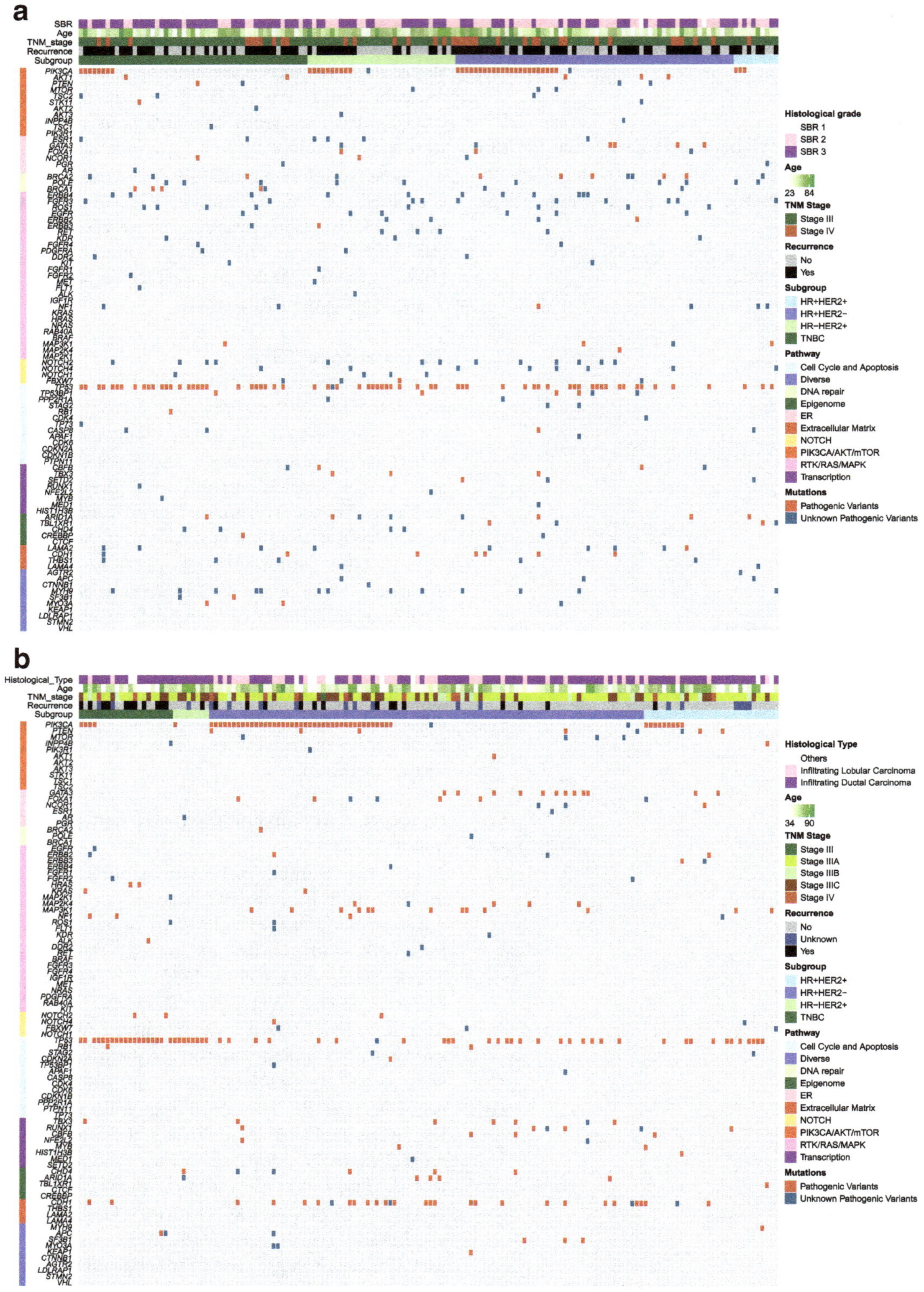

Fig. 1 (See legend on next page.)

Figure S1b). In the HR⁺/HER2⁻ subgroup (Additional file 3: Figure S1c), genes such as *BRCA2, NOTCH2, ERBB4, FGFR3,* and *LAMA2* (all *p* value less than 0.01), and *TP53, NOTCH4, TP53BP1, MYH9,* and *EGFR* (all *p* value less than 0.05) were more frequently mutated in IBC. In the HR⁺/HER2⁺ subgroup (Additional file 3: Figure S1d), *POLE* was found to be more significantly highly mutated in IBC than in non-IBC.

For a better understanding of IBC tumorigenesis, the 91 genes were categorized in 10 different signaling pathways and the pathway was considered altered when at least one gene of the pathway was mutated (Fig. 3). Alteration in DNA repair, RTK/RAS/MAPK, NOTCH, cell cycle and apoptosis, and diverse pathways showed significant differences between the two cohorts ($p < 0.0001$,

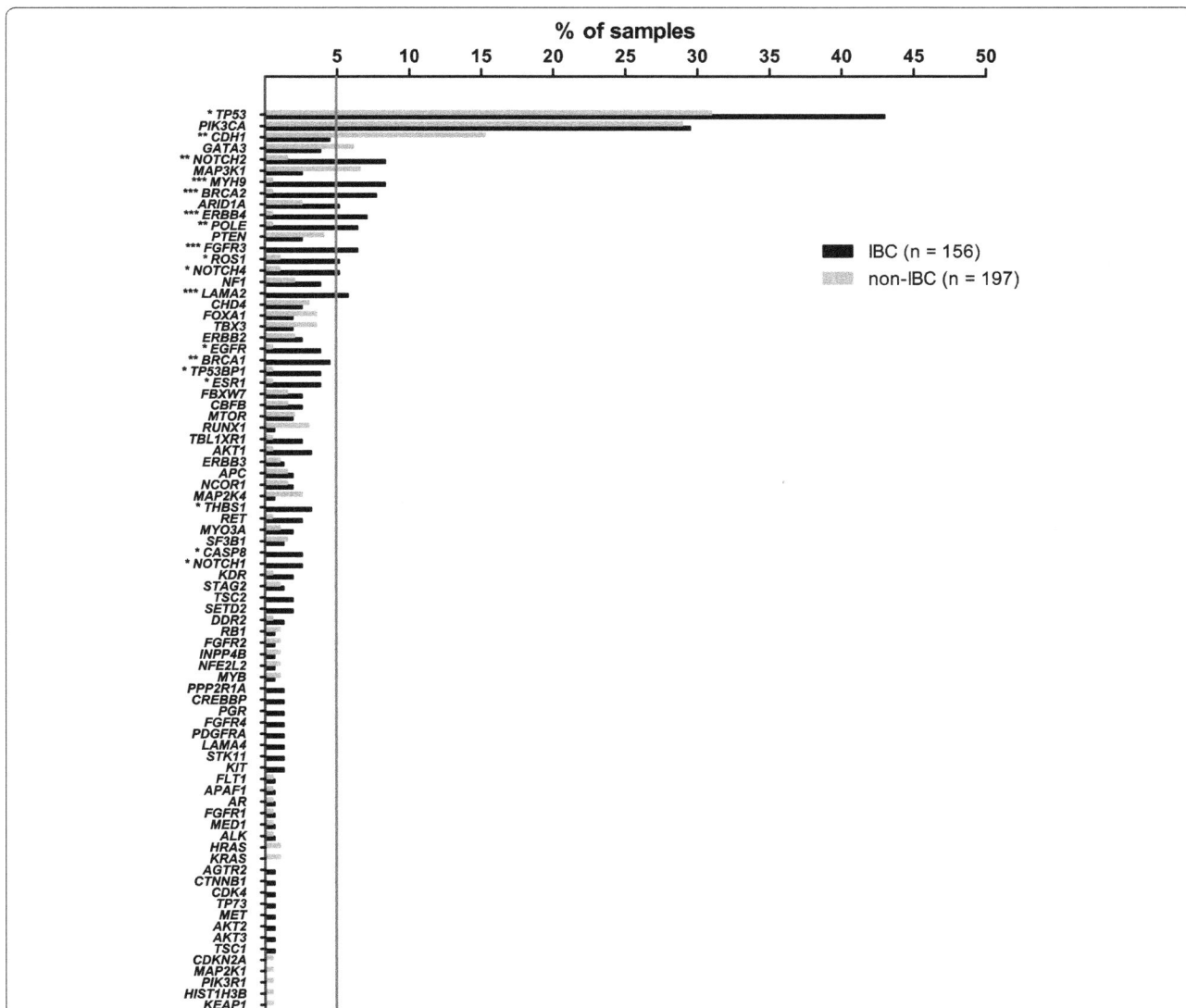

Fig. 2 Comparison of somatic mutation frequency between inflammatory breast cancer (IBC) and non-IBC. Data show the percentage of samples with somatic mutations on our 91 gene panel; the gray bars indicate non-IBC, the black bars indicate IBC; *p < 0.05, **p < 0.01, ***p < 0.001

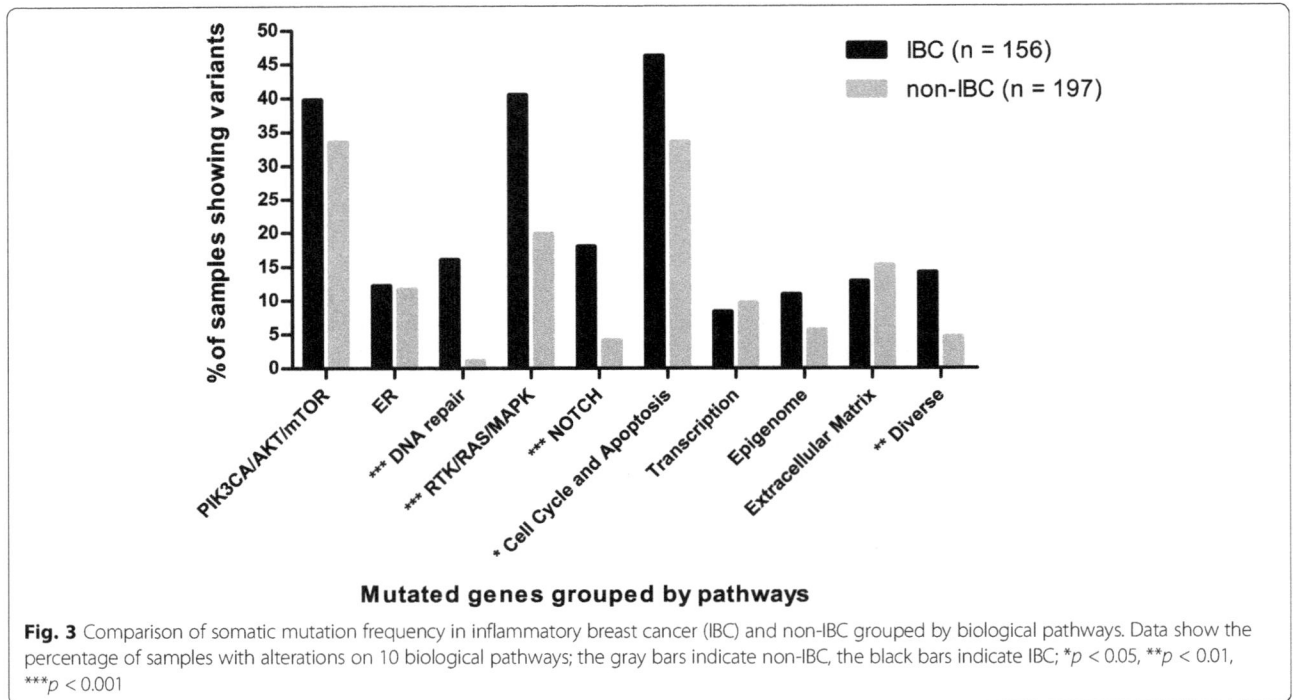

Fig. 3 Comparison of somatic mutation frequency in inflammatory breast cancer (IBC) and non-IBC grouped by biological pathways. Data show the percentage of samples with alterations on 10 biological pathways; the gray bars indicate non-IBC, the black bars indicate IBC; *$p < 0.05$, **$p < 0.01$, ***$p < 0.001$

$p < 0.0001$, $p < 0.0001$, $p = 0.02$, and $p = 0.002$, respectively). Furthermore, we compared alterations of these pathways according to subgroups (Additional file 4: Figure S2). In TNBC, the signaling pathway of DNA repair was more frequently altered in IBC than in non-IBC ($p = 0.02$) (Additional file 4: Figure S2a). In the HR$^-$/HER2$^+$ subgroup, the RTK/RAS/MAPK pathway was significantly more altered in IBC ($p = 0.02$), but the cell cycle and apoptosis pathway was more altered in non-IBC ($p = 0.03$) (Additional file 4: Figure S2b). IBC harbored more mutations in the DNA repair, RTK/RAS/MAPK, NOTCH, and cell cycle pathways in the HR$^+$/HER2$^-$ subgroup than in non-IBC ($p = 0.0001$, $p = 0.003$, $p = 0.001$, and $p = 0.04$, respectively) (Additional file 4: Figure S2c), and DNA repair, epigenome and diverse pathways were also found to be more altered in the HR$^+$/HER2$^+$ subgroup of IBC ($p = 0.007$, $p = 0.02$, and $p = 0.02$, respectively) (Additional file 4: Figure S2d).

Several pathways such as PIK3CA/AKT/mTOR, DNA repair, RTK/RAS/MAPK, NOTCH, and ER include targeted genes. The well-known targeted genes of RTKs and NOTCH families were frequently mutated in IBC. Intriguingly, more unknown pathogenic variants of *ERBB4*, *FGFR3*, *ERBB3*, and *PDGFRA* were detected on the catalytic domain of tyrosine kinase, and we also detected unknown pathogenic variants of *NOTCH4* on the ankyrin repeat domain in several IBC patients (Fig. 1a). Our results thus demonstrated a genomic instability of the IBC cell surface, and we are continuing to explore whether

those frequent unknown pathogenic mutation of RTKs on *ERBB4*, *FGFR3*, *EGFR*, and *ERBB2* are functional and provide potential therapeutic targets in further research.

DNA copy number alterations in IBC

We applied ONCOCNV to calculate the DNA copy number alterations (CNAs) for 156 IBC samples (Additional file 5: Figure S3). In 44 IBC samples with HER2-positive status detected via IHC or FISH, 38 samples were called as having *ERBB2* amplification with ONCOCNV calculation (86.4% concordance was achieved). The rate of *ERBB2* and *MED1* coamplification was 57.1% in IBC, which is similar to that reported in a non-IBC study [19]. The other frequently amplified genes were observed in *FGFR1* in 10.8%, *EGFR* in 4.4%, and *DDR2* in 3.2% of IBC samples. The frequent deletions were found in *RB1* in 5.1%, *STAG2* in 3.8%, and *CDKN2A* and *MAP3K1* in 3.2% of IBC.

Survival analysis of IBC

We compared the gene mutation frequency in 10 pathways between 98 metastatic IBC and 58 non metastatic IBC (Fig. 4). PIK3CA/AKT/mTOR was the only pathway showing a significant difference, which was more frequently altered in metastatic IBC compared with nonmetastatic IBC (48.0% vs. 24.1%, $p = 0.003$). Regarding subgroups, a significant difference was found for this pathway in HR$^+$/HER2$^-$ (58.1% vs. 26.3%, $p = 0.02$). A higher mutation trend is shown in

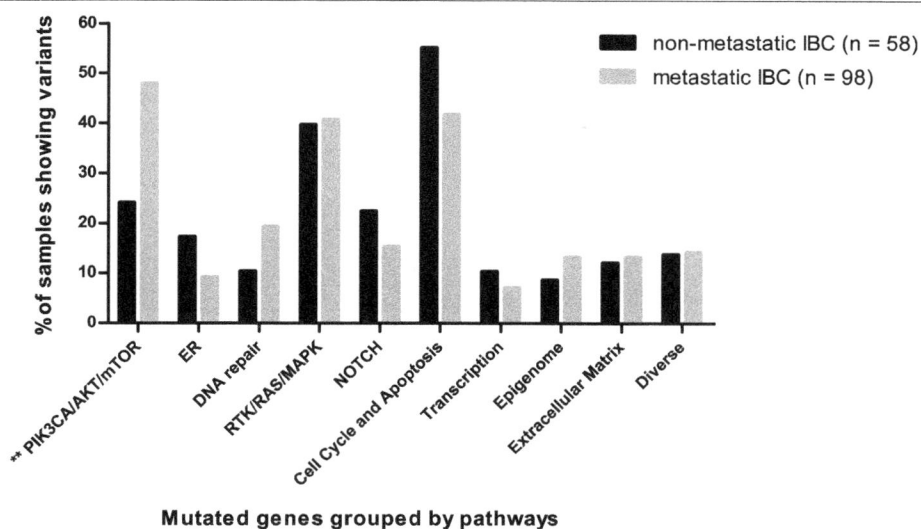

Fig. 4 Comparison of biological pathway between non-metastatic inflammatory breast cancer (IBC) and metastatic IBC. Data show the percentage of samples with alterations on 10 biological pathways; the gray bars indicate metastatic IBC, the black bars indicate non-metastatic IBC; $*p < 0.05$, $**p < 0.01$, $***p < 0.001$

the three other subgroups. Among the 11 genes of the PIK3CA/AKT/mTOR pathway, *PIK3CA* mutations were highly enriched in the metastatic IBC group (38.8% vs. 13.8%, $p = 0.0009$).

Among 120 stage III IBC patients, MFS was available for 115 patients, and one patient was excluded because of disease progression within 6 months. We assessed the relation of *PIK3CA* mutation status with MFS in 114 patients. The median survival was 83.1 months (range 6.2 to 212.1 months). Univariate and multivariate analyses are reported in Table 2. The *PIK3CA* genotype was the only marker significantly associated with MFS in IBC patients (hazard ratio = 2.6, 95% confidence interval (CI) 1.4–4.7, $p = 0.002$; Fig. 5a). The median MFS for the *PIK3CA* mutant-type was 26.0 months and for the *PIK3CA* wild-type it was 101.1 months. Regarding the subgroups, *PIK3CA* mutation was associated with MFS in triple-negative (Fig. 5b) and HR$^-$/HER2$^+$ (Fig. 5c) subgroups, with hazard ratios for *PIK3CA* mutant-type of 5.6 and 12.9, respectively. A high frequency of *PIK3CA* mutation was observed in the HR$^+$/HER2$^-$ IBC subgroup; however, no association between *PIK3CA* mutant-type and MFS was found (hazard ratio = 1.5, 95% CI 0.7–3.6, $p = 0.3$; Fig. 5d). The number of cases was too small to interpret the results for the HR$^+$/HER2$^+$ subgroup. We combined subgroups for further analysis of prognostic impact of *PIK3CA* mutation, and the *PIK3CA* mutant-type was found to significantly associated with worse MFS in HR$^-$ and HER2$^+$ subgroups; no association was found in the HR$^+$ subgroup (Additional file 6: Figure S4).

Table 2 Correlation of *PIK3CA* mutation and classic clinical characteristics with metastasis-free survival (MFS) in primary inflammatory breast cancer (IBC) patients with stage III disease ($n = 114$)

Parameters	n	Univariate analysis		Multivariate analysis	
		HR (95% CI)	p^a	HR (95% CI)	p^b
Age		0.8 (0.5–1.1)	0.6	1.0 (0.5–1.7)	0.9
≤50 years	48				
>50 years	66				
ER status		0.9 (0.6–1.6)	0.8	1.0 (0.5–2.0)	1.0
Negative	67				
Positive	47				
PR status		1.3 (0.8–2.3)	0.3	1.7 (0.8–3.5)	0.1
Negative	82				
Positive	32				
Her2 status		1.7 (1.0–2.8)	0.1	2.0 (1.1–3.8)	0.03
Negative	79				
Positive	35				
SBR grade		1.2 (0.7–2.0)	0.2	1.2 (0.7–2.2)	0.5
III	71				
I and II	43				
PIK3CA		2.6 (1.4–4.7)	0.002	2.7 (1.5–4.7)	0.001
Mut-type	33				
Wild-type	81				

CI confidence interval, *ER* estrogen receptor, *Her2* human epidermal growth factor receptor 2, *HR* hazard ratio, *PR* progesterone receptor, *SBR* Scarf Bloom Richardson classification
[a] Log-rank test
[b] Cox multivariate analyses

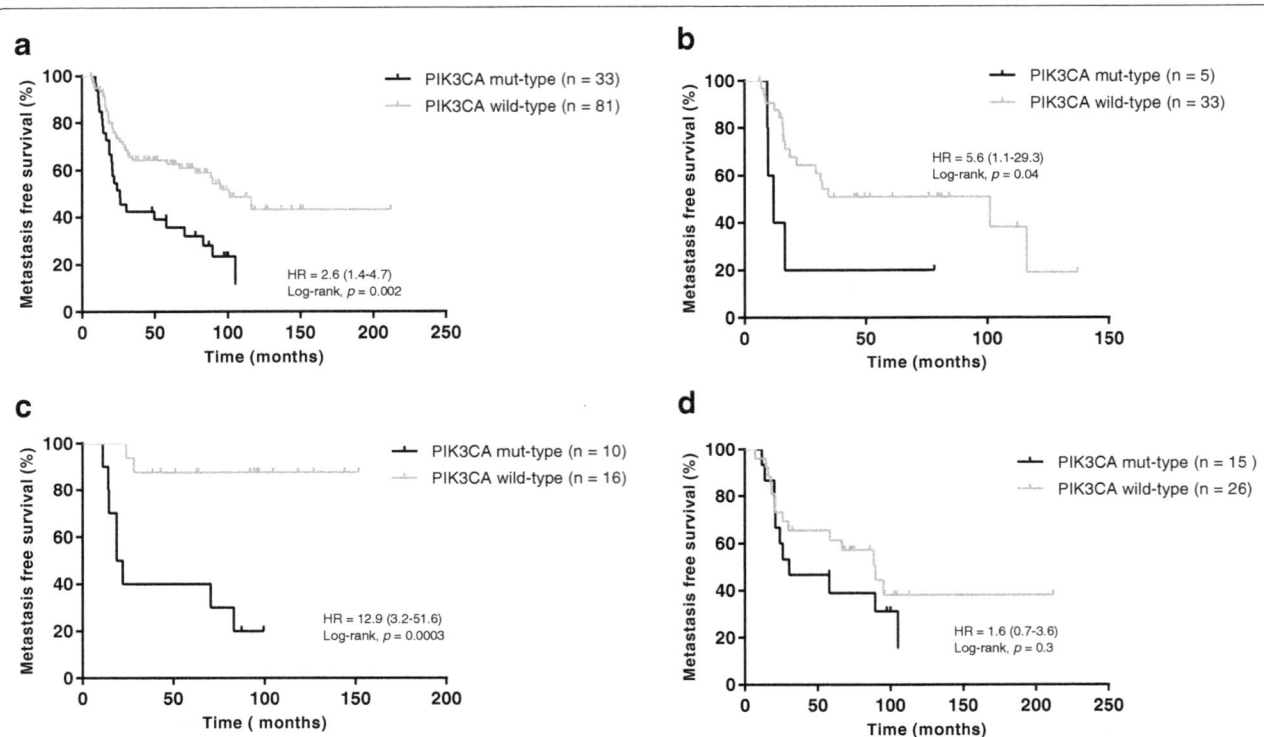

Fig. 5 MFS curves of IBC patients stratified by *PIK3CA* mutation. **a** Kaplan-Meier estimates of MFS according to *PIK3CA* mutations in total IBC patients (*n* = 114); **b** Kaplan-Meier estimates of MFS according to *PIK3CA* mutations in the TNBC subgroup (*n* = 38); **c** Kaplan-Meier estimates of MFS according to *PIK3CA* mutations in the HR⁻/HER2⁺ subgroup (*n* = 26); **d** Kaplan-Meier estimates of MFS according to *PIK3CA* mutations in the HR⁺/HER2⁻ subgroup (*n* = 41). HR hazard ratio

Discussion

A key purpose of precision cancer medicine is to tailor clinical management based on the specific events that are relevant to tumor development and progression. The high frequency of clinically relevant genomic alterations in IBC when sequenced with a targeted NGS raises the possibility that targeted therapies may be developed for patients with this highly aggressive form of breast cancer. First, a heavy mutation burden was found in IBC tumors. This could be the hallmark of increased genomic instability correlating with tumor aggressiveness. *TP53* was the most frequently mutated gene, in accordance with previous studies on IBC [7, 10, 20]. There were 12 genes with more than 5% mutation frequencies in IBC: *TP53, PIK3CA, MYH9, NOTCH2, BRCA2, ERBB4, FGFR3, POLE, LAMA2, ARID1A, NOTCH4,* and *ROS1*. For *TP53, PIK3CA,* and *BRCA2*, high mutation rates in IBC have been also reported by other groups. In contrast, we did not detect higher frequent mutation of *ERBB2, RB1,* or *NOTCH1* [7, 9, 10].

Comparative analysis of biology pathways between IBC and non-IBC revealed high mutation frequencies of genes in DNA repair, NOTCH, and RTK/RAS/MAPK pathways that could be clinically relevant. The alteration of *BRCA1/BRCA2/POLE* genes of the DNA repair

pathway was independent of molecular subtypes, so PARP inhibitor may be especially evaluated in IBC [21]. To the best of our knowledge, this is the first time that *POLE* has been detected frequently mutated in IBC. The correlation of *POLE* mutation with PD1/PD-L1 immunotherapy in colorectal cancer and endometrial cancer [22–24] leads us towards further research to explore whether there is a treatment option for immunotherapy in *POLE*-mutated IBC. Note that POLE-detected variants are not hotspots pathogenic variants that have already been described. *NOTCH1/2/4* and *FBWX7* genes were more frequently mutated in each subgroup of IBC compared with non-IBC. A preclinical study in IBC showed that a gamma secretase inhibitor, RO4929097, was able to block the Notch signaling and to attenuate the stem-like phenotype of IBC cells and regulate the inflammatory environment [25]. Targeting the Notch pathway might be an option for IBC treatment. Receptor tyrosine kinases (RTKs) are frequently activated in cancer cells and therefore have become the target of numerous treatments. The BreastCurie gene panel included most targetable RTK genes and we found that IBC carried higher frequencies of unknown pathogenic variants of RTKs than non-IBC. Higher gene instability due to DNA repair dysfunction may promote variants of unknown significance in IBC but we cannot exclude that other unknown mechanisms are also implicated. Activation of downstream pathways of RTKs, such as ERBB2, EGFR, and IGF1R, has been proven to be related to tumor cell anoikis resistance, and IBC cells have been associated with more evasion of anoikis [26, 27] which is consistent with our findings. We now aim to explore whether the frequent unknown pathogenic mutations of RTKs on *ERBB4*, *FGFR3*, *EGFR*, and *ERBB2* reported in the present study are potential therapeutic targets.

Compared with the breast cancer literature [10, 12, 13, 28], we did not find IBC-specific amplified genes with our gene panel. Unfortunately, some frequent CNAs of breast cancer (e.g., *MYC*, *CCND1* amplification) reported previously were not included in our gene panel. We detected *STAG2* deletion, a tumor suppressor gene coding cohesion protein, in 3.7% of IBC. *STAG2* loss of function was reported in different cancers but not in IBC [29]. However, ONCOCNV did not compute allele frequencies, which may affect the precision of the method in admixed data [15].

Our study demonstrates that *PIK3CA* gene mutations and PIK3CA/AKT/mTOR pathway alteration were very common events in IBC. *PIK3CA* gene mutations were especially observed in luminal and HER2-positive subtypes, and mainly located in hotspots of the helical domain and the catalytic domain, similar to non-IBC in previous reports [13, 30]. Recently, a large pooled analysis of more than 10,000 early-stage breast cancer patients reported that PIK3CA-mutated tumors are associated with a better prognosis [31]. However, this good prognostic effect was observed in $HR^+/HER2^-$ and TNBC subtypes, but not in the $HER2^+$ subtype where *PIK3CA* mutations were associated with a worse overall survival. Interestingly, in our IBC cohort, *PIK3CA* mutation was a poor prognostic factor for MFS for $HER2^+$ and TNBC subtypes, whereas no prognostic value was found in the $HR^+/HER2^-$ subtype. Of note, the prognostic effect was weak in the TNBC subtype of IBC since *PIK3CA* mutations were rare in this subtype and our TNBC cohort was small. For the $HER2^+$ subtype, previous studies reported that *PIK3CA* mutations were associated with adverse prognosis in non-IBC, but results were not conclusive [31–34]. As *PIK3CA* mutation could lead to resistance to anti-HER2 treatments [34, 35], we checked that the percentage of patients in our IBC cohort receiving trastuzumab combined with chemotherapy was balanced in both *PIK3CA* genotypes (71.4% in mutant type, 75.9% in wild type). Therefore, the association between *PIK3CA* mutation and worse MFS in IBC may be reliable. For the $HR^+/HER2^-$ subtype, the prognostic difference regarding *PIK3CA* genotype between IBC and non-IBC may reflect the influence of the PI3K pathway in the two distinct biological environments of

IBC and non-IBC, and we presume interactions between ER and PI3K pathways are different. We know that PI3K inhibitors have been investigated in many breast cancer trials and have shown promising results in ER-positive endocrine therapy-refractory breast cancer [36], but no clinical trials have been performed specifically in IBC to date. The association of *PIK3CA* mutations with worse MFS in IBC should draw our attention to the role of the PI3K pathway in this aggressive and treatment-refractory form of breast cancer. Further experimental research to explore the PI3K pathway in IBC is therefore required.

Conclusions

Overall, IBC is the most aggressive form of breast cancer frequently refractory to conventional therapy and suffers from the lack of a specific treatment. Our study using targeted NGS analysis revealed a high frequency of somatic mutations, in particular in DNA repair, Notch signaling, and RTKs genes, that may guide switching from conventional therapy to targeted agents in IBC. In contrast to non-IBC patients, *PIK3CA* mutation was associated with a poor outcome in IBC patients. These findings encourage clinical trials with targeted therapies that may provide clinical benefit to IBC patients.

Additional files

Additional file 1: Table S1. Pathological and clinical characteristics of non-IBC cohorts. (PDF 169 kb)

Additional file 2: Table S2. BreastCurie gene panel for targeted NGS. (PDF 411 kb)

Additional file 3: Figure S1. Comparison of somatic mutation frequency between IBC and non-IBC in four subgroups. (a) The percentage of samples with somatic mutation in the TNBC subgroup; (b) the percentage of samples with somatic mutation in the $HR^-/HER2^+$ subgroup; (c) the percentage of samples with somatic mutation in the $HR^+/HER2^-$ subgroup; (d) the percentage of samples with somatic mutation in the $HR^+/HER2^+$ subgroup. The gray bars indicate non-IBC, the black bars indicate IBC; *p < 0.05, **p < 0.01, ***p < 0.001. (PDF 52 kb)

Additional file 4: Figure S2. Comparison of biological pathway between IBC and non-IBC in four subgroups. (a) The percentage of samples with alteration on 10 biological pathways in the TNBC subgroup; (b) the percentage of samples with alteration on 10 biological pathways in the $HR^-/HER2^+$ subgroup; (c) the percentage of samples with alteration on 10 biological pathways in the $HR^+/HER2^-$ subgroup; (d) the percentage of samples with alteration on 10 biological pathways in the $HR^+/HER2^+$ subgroup. The gray bars indicate non-IBC, the black bars indicate IBC; *p < 0.05, **p < 0.01, ***p < 0.001. (PDF 41 kb)

Additional file 5: Figure S3. DNA copy number alterations in the IBC cohort. The genes with DNA copy number alterations are grouped along the x axis, the percentage of samples with DNA copy number alterations shown on the y axis, DNA amplifications are indicated by black bars above the x axis, and DNA deletions are indicated by gray bars below the x axis. (PDF 164 kb)

Additional file 6: Figure S4. MFS curves stratified by *PIK3CA* mutation in three subgroups of IBC patients. (a) Kaplan-Meier estimates of MFS according to *PIK3CA* mutations in patients of the HR^- subgroup, (b) Kaplan-Meier estimates of MFS according to *PIK3CA* mutations in patients of the HER2$^+$ subgroup, (c) Kaplan-Meier estimates of MFS according to *PIK3CA* mutations in patients of the HR$^+$ subgroup. (PDF 42 kb)

Abbreviations
BCSS: Breast cancer-specific survival; BRCA1/2: Breast cancer 1/2; ER: Estrogen receptor; FISH: Fluorescence in-situ hybridization; HER2: Human epidermal growth factor receptor 2; HR: Hormone receptor; IHC: Immunohistochemical; MFS: Metastasis-free survival; mTOR: Mammalian target of rapamycin; NGS: Next-generation sequencing; NOTCH1/2/4: Neurogenic locus notch homolog protein 1/2/4; PI3K: Phosphatidylinositol 3-kinase; PIK3CA: Phosphatidylinositol 3-kinase: catalytic: alpha polypeptide gene; POLE: Polymerase (DNA) epsilon; PR: Progesterone receptor; RTK: Receptor tyrosine kinase; SBR: Scarff Bloom Richardson classification; TCGA: The Cancer Genome Atlas; TNBC: Triple-negative breast cancer

Acknowledgments
We thank Odette Mariani from Institut Curie for providing frozen samples.

Funding
This study was supported by l'association pour la recherche de Saint Cloud (ARCS). High-throughput sequencing has been performed by the ICGex NGS platform of the Institut Curie supported by the grants ANR-10-EQPX-03 (Equipex) and ANR-10-INBS-09-08 (France Génomique Consortium) from the Agence Nationale de la Recherche ("Investissements d'Avenir" program), by the Canceropole Ile-de-France, and by the SiRIC-Curie program SiRIC Grant "INCa-DGOS- 4654".

Authors' contributions
XL, FL, IB, and CC made substantial contributions to conception and design, and revising the manuscript, and gave final approval for publication. XL, SV, MB, AB, and CC contributed to acquisition of data, analysis and interpretation of data, and drafted the manuscript. XL, AB, SB, and VB performed data analysis for the study. XL, SV, FL, IB, and CC participated in manuscript preparation and revision. XL, FL, and CC contributed to data collection and database management for the study. All other authors made substantial contributions to the acquisition of data, revising the manuscript, and final approval.

Competing interests
The authors declare that they have no competing interests.

Author details
[1]Department of Breast Oncology, Key Laboratory of Carcinogenesis and Translational Research (Ministry of Education), Peking University Cancer Hospital & Institute, Beijing, China. [2]Pharmacogenomic Unit, Department of Genetics, Curie Institute, PSL Research University, 26 rue d'Ulm, 75005 Paris, France. [3]Clinic bioinformatic Unit, Department of Biopathology, Curie Institute, PSL Research University, Paris, France. [4]Institut Curie Genomics of Excellence (ICGex) Platform, Curie Institute, PSL Research University, Paris, France. [5]EA7331, Paris Descartes University, Sorbonne Paris Cité, Faculty of Pharmaceutical and Biological Sciences, Paris, France. [6]Department of Medical Oncology, Curie Institute, René Huguenin Hospital, Saint-Cloud, France.

References
1. Dawood S, Merajver SD, Viens P, Vermeulen PB, Swain SM, Buchholz TA, et al. International expert panel on inflammatory breast cancer: consensus statement for standardized diagnosis and treatment. Ann Oncol. 2011;22: 515–23. https://doi.org/10.1093/annonc/mdq345.
2. Robertson FM, Bondy M, Yang W, Yamauchi H, Wiggins S, Kamrudin S, et al. Inflammatory breast cancer: the disease, the biology, the treatment. CA Cancer J Clin. 2010;60:351–75. https://doi.org/10.3322/caac.20082.
3. Dawood S, Lei X, Dent R, Gupta S, Sirohi B, Cortes J, et al. Survival of women with inflammatory breast cancer: a large population-based study. Ann Oncol. 2014;25:1143–51. https://doi.org/10.1093/annonc/mdu121.
4. Bertucci F, Finetti P, Rougemont J, Charafe-Jauffret E, Cervera N, Tarpin C, et al. Gene expression profiling identifies molecular subtypes of inflammatory breast cancer. Cancer Res. 2005;65:2170–8. https://doi.org/10.1158/0008-5472.CAN-04-4115.
5. Van Laere S, Van der Auwera I, Van den Eynden G, Van Hummelen P, van Dam P, Van Marck E, et al. Distinct molecular phenotype of inflammatory breast cancer compared to non-inflammatory breast cancer using Affymetrix-based genome-wide gene-expression analysis. Br J Cancer. 2007; 97:1165–74. https://doi.org/10.1038/sj.bjc.6603967.
6. Bertucci F, Ueno NT, Finetti P, Vermeulen P, Lucci A, Robertson FM, et al. Gene expression profiles of inflammatory breast cancer: correlation with response to neoadjuvant chemotherapy and metastasis-free survival. Ann Oncol. 2014;25:358–65. https://doi.org/10.1093/annonc/mdt496.
7. Bertucci F, Finetti P, Vermeulen P, Van Dam P, Dirix L, Birnbaum D, et al. Genomic profiling of inflammatory breast cancer: a review. Breast. 2014;23: 538–45. https://doi.org/10.1016/j.breast.2014.06.008.
8. Van Laere SJ, Ueno NT, Finetti P, Vermeulen P, Lucci A, Robertson FM, et al. Uncovering the molecular secrets of inflammatory breast cancer biology: an integrated analysis of three distinct affymetrix gene expression datasets. Clin Cancer Res. 2013;19:4685–96. https://doi.org/10.1158/1078-0432.CCR-12-2549.
9. Matsuda N, Lim B, Wang Y, Krishnamurthy S, Woodward W, Alvarez RH, et al. Identification of frequent somatic mutations in inflammatory breast cancer. Breast Cancer Res Treat. 2017;163:263–72. https://doi.org/10.1007/s10549-017-4165-0.
10. Ross JS, Ali SM, Wang K, Khaira D, Palma NA, Chmielecki J, et al. Comprehensive genomic profiling of inflammatory breast cancer cases reveals a high frequency of clinically relevant genomic alterations. Breast Cancer Res Treat. 2015;154:155–62. https://doi.org/10.1007/s10549-015-3592-z.
11. Gao J, Aksoy BA, Dogrusoz U, Dresdner G, Gross B, Sumer SO, et al. Integrative analysis of complex cancer genomics and clinical profiles using the cBioPortal. Sci Signal. 2013;6:pl1. https://doi.org/10.1126/scisignal.2004088.
12. Cerami E, Gao J, Dogrusoz U, Gross BE, Sumer SO, Aksoy BA, et al. The cBio cancer genomics portal: an open platform for exploring multidimensional cancer genomics data. Cancer Discov. 2012;2:401–4. https://doi.org/10.1158/2159-8290.CD-12-0095.
13. Cancer Genome Atlas N. Comprehensive molecular portraits of human breast tumours. Nature. 2012;490:61–70. https://doi.org/10.1038/nature11412.
14. Le Tourneau C, Kamal M, Tsimberidou AM, Bedard P, Pierron G, Callens C, et al. Treatment algorithms based on tumor molecular profiling: the essence of precision medicine trials. J Natl Cancer Inst. 2016;108 https://doi.org/10.1093/jnci/djv362.
15. Boeva V, Popova T, Lienard M, Toffoli S, Kamal M, Le Tourneau C, et al. Multi-factor data normalization enables the detection of copy number aberrations in amplicon sequencing data. Bioinformatics. 2014;30:3443–50. https://doi.org/10.1093/bioinformatics/btu436.
16. Lefebvre C, Bachelot T, Filleron T, Pedrero M, Campone M, Soria JC, et al. Mutational profile of metastatic breast cancers: a retrospective analysis. PLoS Med. 2016;13:e1002201. https://doi.org/10.1371/journal.pmed.1002201.
17. Le Tourneau C, Delord JP, Goncalves A, Gavoille C, Dubot C, Isambert N, et al. Molecularly targeted therapy based on tumour molecular profiling versus conventional therapy for advanced cancer (SHIVA): a multicentre, open-label, proof-of-concept, randomised, controlled phase 2 trial. Lancet Oncol. 2015;16:1324–34. https://doi.org/10.1016/S1470-2045(15)00188-6.

18. Andre F, Bachelot T, Commo F, Campone M, Arnedos M, Dieras V, et al. Comparative genomic hybridisation array and DNA sequencing to direct treatment of metastatic breast cancer: a multicentre, prospective trial (SAFIR01/UNICANCER). Lancet Oncol. 2014;15:267–74. https://doi.org/10.1016/S1470-2045(13)70611-9.

19. Lamy PJ, Fina F, Bascoul-Mollevi C, Laberenne AC, Martin PM, Ouafik L, et al. Quantification and clinical relevance of gene amplification at chromosome 17q12-q21 in human epidermal growth factor receptor 2-amplified breast cancers. Breast Cancer Res. 2011;13:R15. https://doi.org/10.1186/bcr2824.

20. Goh G, Schmid R, Guiver K, Arpornwirat W, Chitapanarux I, Ganju V, et al. Clonal evolutionary analysis during HER2 blockade in HER2-positive inflammatory breast cancer: a phase II open-label clinical trial of afatinib +/– vinorelbine. PLoS Med. 2016;13:e1002136. https://doi.org/10.1371/journal.pmed.1002136.

21. Lord CJ, Ashworth A. PARP inhibitors: synthetic lethality in the clinic. Science. 2017;355:1152–8. https://doi.org/10.1126/science.aam7344.

22. Castellucci E, He T, Goldstein DY, Halmos B, Chuy J. DNA polymerase varepsilon deficiency leading to an ultramutator phenotype: a novel clinically relevant entity. Oncologist. 2017;22:497–502. https://doi.org/10.1634/theoncologist.2017-0034.

23. Gargiulo P, Della Pepa C, Berardi S, Califano D, Scala S, Buonaguro L, et al. Tumor genotype and immune microenvironment in POLE-ultramutated and MSI-hypermutated endometrial cancers: new candidates for checkpoint blockade immunotherapy? Cancer Treat Rev. 2016;48:61–8. https://doi.org/10.1016/j.ctrv.2016.06.008.

24. Bourdais R, Rousseau B, Pujals A, Boussion H, Joly C, Guillemin A, et al. Polymerase proofreading domain mutations: new opportunities for immunotherapy in hypermutated colorectal cancer beyond MMR deficiency. Crit Rev Oncol Hematol. 2017;113:242–8. https://doi.org/10.1016/j.critrevonc.2017.03.027.

25. Debeb BG, Cohen EN, Boley K, Freiter EM, Li L, Robertson FM, et al. Pre-clinical studies of notch signaling inhibitor RO4929097 in inflammatory breast cancer cells. Breast Cancer Res Treat. 2012;134:495–510. https://doi.org/10.1007/s10549-012-2075-8.

26. Buchheit CL, Weigel KJ, Schafer ZT. Cancer cell survival during detachment from the ECM: multiple barriers to tumour progression. Nat Rev Cancer. 2014;14:632–41. https://doi.org/10.1038/nrc3789.

27. Buchheit CL, Schafer ZT. BIM-EL localization: the key to understanding anoikis resistance in inflammatory breast cancer cells. Mol Cell Oncol. 2016;3:e1011474. https://doi.org/10.1080/23723556.2015.1011474.

28. Curtis C, Shah SP, Chin SF, Turashvili G, Rueda OM, Dunning MJ, et al. The genomic and transcriptomic architecture of 2,000 breast tumours reveals novel subgroups. Nature. 2012;486:346–52. https://doi.org/10.1038/nature10983.

29. Hill VK, Kim JS, Waldman T. Cohesin mutations in human cancer. Biochim Biophys Acta. 2016;1866:1–11. https://doi.org/10.1016/j.bbcan.2016.05.002.

30. Stemke-Hale K, Gonzalez-Angulo AM, Lluch A, Neve RM, Kuo WL, Davies M, et al. An integrative genomic and proteomic analysis of PIK3CA, PTEN, and AKT mutations in breast cancer. Cancer Res. 2008;68:6084–91. https://doi.org/10.1158/0008-5472.CAN-07-6854.

31. Zardavas D, Te Marvelde L, Milne RL, Fumagalli D, Fountzilas G, Kotoula V, et al. Tumor PIK3CA genotype and prognosis in early-stage breast cancer: a pooled analysis of individual patient data. J Clin Oncol. 2018;36:981–90. https://doi.org/10.1200/JCO.2017.74.8301.

32. Mukohara T. PI3K mutations in breast cancer: prognostic and therapeutic implications. Breast Cancer. 2015;7:111–23. https://doi.org/10.2147/BCTT.S60696.

33. Cizkova M, Susini A, Vacher S, Cizeron-Clairac G, Andrieu C, Driouch K, et al. PIK3CA mutation impact on survival in breast cancer patients and in ERalpha, PR and ERBB2-based subgroups. Breast Cancer Res. 2012;14:R28. https://doi.org/10.1186/bcr3113.

34. Loibl S, Majewski I, Guarneri V, Nekljudova V, Holmes E, Bria E, et al. PIK3CA mutations are associated with reduced pathological complete response rates in primary HER2-positive breast cancer: pooled analysis of 967 patients from five prospective trials investigating lapatinib and trastuzumab. Ann Oncol. 2016;27:1519–25. https://doi.org/10.1093/annonc/mdw197.

35. Bianchini G, Kiermaier A, Bianchi GV, Im YH, Pienkowski T, Liu MC, et al. Biomarker analysis of the NeoSphere study: pertuzumab, trastuzumab, and docetaxel versus trastuzumab plus docetaxel, pertuzumab plus trastuzumab, or pertuzumab plus docetaxel for the neoadjuvant treatment of HER2-positive breast cancer. Breast Cancer Res. 2017;19:16. https://doi.org/10.1186/s13058-017-0806-9.

36. Di Leo A, Johnston S, Lee KS, Ciruelos E, Lonning PE, Janni W, et al. Buparlisib plus fulvestrant in postmenopausal women with hormone-receptor-positive, HER2-negative, advanced breast cancer progressing on or after mTOR inhibition (BELLE-3): a randomised, double-blind, placebo-controlled, phase 3 trial. Lancet Oncol. 2018;19:87–100. https://doi.org/10.1016/S1470-2045(17)30688-5.

14

Exploring the prediction performance for breast cancer risk based on volumetric mammographic density at different thresholds

Chao Wang[1]* [iD], Adam R. Brentnall[1], Jack Cuzick[1], Elaine F. Harkness[2], D. Gareth Evans[3] and Susan Astley[2]

Abstract

Background: The percentage of mammographic dense tissue (PD) defined by pixel value threshold is a well-established risk factor for breast cancer. Recently there has been some evidence to suggest that an increased threshold based on visual assessment could improve risk prediction. It is unknown, however, whether this also applies to volumetric density using digital raw mammograms.

Method: Two case-control studies nested within a screening cohort (ages of participants 46–73 years) from Manchester UK were used. In the first study (317 cases and 947 controls) cases were detected at the first screen; whereas in the second study (318 cases and 935 controls), cases were diagnosed after the initial mammogram. Volpara software was used to estimate dense tissue height at each pixel point, and from these, volumetric and area-based PD were computed at a range of thresholds. Volumetric and area-based PDs were evaluated using conditional logistic regression, and their predictive ability was assessed using the Akaike information criterion (AIC) and matched concordance index (mC).

Results: The best performing volumetric PD was based on a threshold of 5 mm of dense tissue height (which we refer to as VPD5), and the best areal PD was at a threshold level of 6 mm (which we refer to as APD6), using pooled data and in both studies separately. VPD5 showed a modest improvement in prediction performance compared to the original volumetric PD by Volpara with $\Delta AIC = 5.90$ for the pooled data. APD6, on the other hand, shows much stronger evidence for better prediction performance, with $\Delta AIC = 14.52$ for the pooled data, and mC increased slightly from 0.567 to 0.577.

Conclusion: These results suggest that imposing a 5 mm threshold on dense tissue height for volumetric PD could result in better prediction of cancer risk. There is stronger evidence that area-based density with a 6 mm threshold gives better prediction than the original volumetric density metric.

Keywords: Breast density, Thresholding, Digital mammogram, Risk prediction, Breast cancer

* Correspondence: chao.wang@qmul.ac.uk
[1]Centre for Cancer Prevention, Wolfson Institute of Preventive Medicine, Queen Mary University of London, Charterhouse Square, London EC1M 6BQ, UK
Full list of author information is available at the end of the article

Background

The percentage of mammographic density (PD) that appears white in a mammogram and reflects the relative amount of fibroglandular tissue in the breast is a well-established risk factor for breast cancer [1]. PD is the most predictive marker of breast cancer for women after familial causes and polygenic markers when adjusted for age and body mass index (BMI) [2]. For area-based PD, fibroglandular and fatty tissues may be segmented by thresholding, and this is usually achieved by a semi-automatic approach where the threshold is chosen by the investigator using software such as Cumulus [3]. There has been recent evidence that increasing the conventional brightness threshold might better predict breast cancer risk: this has been demonstrated in Korean women with "for presentation" (processed) full-field digital mammograms [4, 5], and Australian women with digitised film mammograms [6].

In addition to subjective visual assessment, another approach for PD estimation using digital mammograms is volumetric density measurement via a fully automated system. Commercial volumetric PD systems including Volpara [7] and Quantra [8] have shown good agreement with semi-automated thresholding and an association with risk of breast cancer [9]. In Volpara, pixel values are calibrated so that the height (amount) of dense tissue at any given point in a mammogram can be estimated, and based on these heights and the estimated breast volume, volumetric density can be determined. By default all dense tissue, regardless of the height at any pixel position, is included to compute the dense volume. However, there appear to be no published studies that have looked at whether applying a threshold to dense tissue heights, effectively excluding some less dense tissue as well as possibly thin sheets or strands of tissue that have similar attenuation coefficients to glandular tissue, could result in better prediction of breast cancer risk.

The aim of this paper is to investigate whether volumetric or area-based PD can be adjusted by varying dense tissue height thresholds so as to better predict breast cancer risk. In previous research [4–6] thresholding was based on pixel brightness from visual assessment, whereas here thresholds on dense tissue heights from volumetric density estimation are used. This allows the calculation of breast density and the application of a chosen threshold to be fully automated (i.e. without manual visual assessment) on digital mammograms. In addition, our thresholding analysis is based on Western women with digital raw mammograms, and to our knowledge this has not been previously examined. An important benefit of using raw images compared to processed images is that it could reduce the discrepancies between different machines due to manufacturers' proprietary processing algorithms.

Methods

Setting and study design

Two case-control studies were designed as a part of the Predicting Risk Of breast Cancer At Screening (PROCAS) cohort, in Manchester, UK [10]. The first case-control study had 317 cases and 947 controls while the second had 318 cases and 935 controls. A detailed description of the data in the two studies has been reported previously [11, 12] (the sample used for analysis differs slightly; see Appendix). Briefly, in the first case-control study, cases comprised women with cancer detected at first screen on entry into the PROCAS cohort, and we refer to this dataset as study 1. As in our previous study [11], the craniocaudal (CC) views of the contralateral breast for cases and the left breast for controls were used. In the second case-control study, each woman had a normal screening mammogram (no cancer detected) on entry into the PROCAS cohort, but an interval or screen-detected cancer arose subsequently, and we refer to this dataset as study 2. Similar to our previous study [11], the CC views of the contralateral breast for cases and the same side for controls were used. The mammograms were obtained on average three years prior to diagnosis of breast cancer and from the same cohort as study 1. In both studies women were matched approximately 3:1 (controls vs cases) by age, BMI, hormone replacement therapy (HRT) use and menopausal status.

Mammograms

All digital raw ("for processing") mammograms were acquired using a GE Senographe system. Volumetric density, especially the height of dense tissue at each point in the mammogram, was assessed using Volpara 1.5.2 (Volpara Health Technologies, Wellington, New Zealand).

Density measurements

One output from the Volpara software is a "density map" - it contains data on dense tissue height at every point in the mammogram, based on an analysis of pixel values and imaging parameters. Whilst no thresholding is applied in the default output of the software, different threshold values can be tested such that only densities with a height greater than a certain threshold value are included for computing total dense volume. For instance, when a threshold level of 5 mm is used, only those density heights greater than 5 mm are employed to calculate the total dense volume. We refer to this approach to computing PD as volumetric PD (VPD) in this paper, and specifically the default volumetric PD output by Volpara as VPD0 (i.e. the threshold level is 0 mm).

The aforementioned approach focuses on percentage of volumetric density as the end point. An alternative approach is to look at the two-dimensional area of dense tissue within the breast: here this is defined as the number of pixels with dense tissue heights greater than a chosen threshold. This is then divided by the total number of pixels in the breast and expressed as a percentage area of dense tissue. As with the volumetric approach, a series of threshold values can be considered. We refer to this as areal PD (APD) in this paper. Note that although APD is an areal measurement, the underlying basis is still volumetric density because dense tissue height (or effectively volume) at each point in the mammogram was used.

Statistical analysis

PDs at various threshold levels, ranging from 0 to 25 mm, were evaluated using conditional logistic regression, based on the pooled data (study 1 and 2 combined) and on study 1 and 2 separately. The Akaike information criterion (AIC) and matched concordance index (mC) [13] were calculated to measure prediction performance. AIC is a likelihood-based statistic derived from the information theory and is a well-established method for model comparison [14]. A lower AIC value indicates better model performance. mC is a modification of the concordance index (or area under the receiving operator characteristic curve, AUC) for matched case-control studies, and gives an average concordance index within matched groups. Bootstrap with 10,000 replications was used to assess whether the difference in mC from different models was statistically significant. All p values are two-sided.

Since biologic phenotypes between screen-detected and interval cancers are different, a further analysis was conducted to test whether there was any significant difference between screen-detected and interval breast cancers. In addition to the fixed threshold level for every woman, sensitivity analysis was conducted by varying the threshold according to a woman's characteristics based on a linear model, using age, BMI, thickness and total volume of the breast to explore the difference between varying and fixed thresholds.

Results

Study characteristics

The demographic characteristics of the women in both studies are presented in Table 1. Age, BMI, menopausal status and HRT use were well-matched between cases and controls in both studies. The median 10-year Tyrer-Cuzick score was higher for cases than controls. The majority of women never used HRT, were postmenopausal, parous and ethnically white.

Results for pooled data

Conditional logistic regression was used to evaluate model fit at various threshold levels using both datasets combined. The resulting AICs for VPDs and APDs are presented in Fig. 1. It can be seen that both VPDs and APDs have their lowest value at the 5–6 mm threshold level, where improvement over original volumetric PD (i.e. VPD0) is clear. APD at the threshold of 6 mm achieved the lowest AIC overall.

Distributions of VPDs and APDs at different threshold levels (0–12 mm) were inspected using box plots as shown in Fig. 2. Correlations between VPD0 and the best performing VPD and APD - VPD5 and APD6, respectively, are presented in Fig. 3. The Spearman statistic was 0.95 for correlation between VPD0 and VPD5, 0.90 for correlation between VPD0 and APD6 and 0.98 for correlation between VPD5 and APD6.

Table 2 compares the results of five modelling schemes using different sets of risk predictors: (1) VPD0; (2) volumetric PD at 5 mm (VPD5); (3) areal PD at 6 mm (APD6); (4) VPD0 + VPD5 and (5) VPD0 + APD6. Each modelling scheme was denoted as M1 to M5, respectively. M1 represents the original volumetric PD estimated by Volpara (i.e. zero or no thresholding) and its model performance was used as the baseline for comparison with other models. M1 was then compared with M2 and M3 which were based on 5 mm and 6 mm thresholds for VPD and APD, respectively, as the best fit was found at these levels of threshold as shown above. M4 was used to explore whether the prediction performance for VPD5 can be further improved by adding the original Volpara estimate (VPD0); similarly, M5 was used to explore whether VPD0 adds information once having already controlled for APD6. The model with the lowest AIC indicates the best modelling approach for breast cancer risk prediction.

As seen in Table 2, M3, the model using only APD at 6 mm, was the best performing in terms of AIC. Compared to M1, the model using original volumetric PD (VPD0), the AIC was substantially improved with $\Delta AIC = 14.52$. mC also increased slightly from M1 to M3 (from 0.567 to 0.577); whilst the change in mC was small it was still statistically significant (p value = 0.019). To show the effect of thresholding, an example is presented in Fig. 4, which shows thresholding of a mammogram at different levels.

Results for study 1 and 2

Following analysis based on pooled data, a series of conditional logistic regression models for study 1 (cancers detected at the first screen on entry into the PROCAS cohort) and study 2 (cancers diagnosed subsequently) were explored, as well as screen-detected vs interval cancers within study 2. Similarly, five modelling schemes (M1–M5) were tested and the results are presented in Tables 3 and 4.

As with the pooled data, M3, the model using only APD at 6 mm, was the preferred model in terms of AIC in study 1 (Table 3). Compared to M1, there was modest

Table 1 Demographics of Study 1 (cancers detected at first screen on entry to the PROCAS study) and Study 2 (cancers detected at a subsequent screen or between screening rounds)

	Study 1			Study 2		
	Controls	Cases	p value	Controls	Cases	p value
	Number (%)	Number (%)		Number (%)	Number (%)	
Age at consent (years)			0.9997			0.9997
< 50	53 (6)	19 (6)		46 (5)	16 (5)	
50–54	242 (26)	79 (25)		194 (21)	64 (20)	
55–59	153 (16)	52 (16)		164 (18)	58 (18)	
60–64	229 (24)	77 (24)		286 (31)	96 (30)	
65–69	196 (21)	66 (21)		198 (21)	68 (21)	
70+	74 (8)	24 (8)		47 (5)	16 (5)	
HRT use			0.0778			0.9320
Unknown	14 (1)	9 (3)		23 (2)	6 (2)	
Never	568 (60)	208 (66)		475 (51)	166 (52)	
Previous	315 (33)	83 (26)		332 (36)	110 (35)	
Current	50 (5)	17 (5)		105 (11)	36 (11)	
BMI (kg/m^2)			0.9954			0.9389
Unknown	1 (0)			1 (0)		
< 25	332 (35)	112 (35)		335 (36)	117 (37)	
25–29	331 (35)	111 (35)		341 (36)	113 (36)	
≥ 30	283 (30)	94 (30)		259 (28)	87 (27)	
Menopausal status			0.4272			0.9889
Unknown	31 (3)	10 (3)		32 (3)	12 (4)	
Premenopausal	92 (10)	32 (10)		67 (7)	22 (7)	
Perimenopausal	112 (12)	38 (12)		134 (14)	46 (14)	
Postmenopausal	712 (75)	237 (75)		702 (75)	238 (75)	
Ethnic origin			0.1880			0.2208
Other/unknown	52 (5)	24 (8)		81 (9)	35 (11)	
White	895 (95)	293 (92)		854 (91)	283 (89)	
Parity			0.7134			0.0399
Unknown	1 (0)			1 (0)	4 (1)	
Nulliparous	112 (12)	40 (13)		91 (10)	44 (14)	
Parous	834 (88)	277 (87)		843 (90)	270 (85)	
Tyrer-Cuzick (10 year risk, % (median, Q1–Q3))	2.74 (2.18–3.58)	2.94 (2.29–3.88)	0.0006	2.67 (2.09–3.55)	2.91 (2.24–4.05)	<.0001
Volumetric PD (median, Q1–Q3)	4.90 (3.63–7.19)	5.43 (4.06–8.13)	0.0034	4.79 (3.58–7.01)	5.51 (3.81–7.98)	0.0044

The p values, from likelihood-ratio chi-square tests, indicate whether there are significant difference between cases and controls

HRT hormone replacement therapy, BMI body mass index, Q1 25th percentile, Q3 75th percentile, PD percent density

improvement in the AIC (ΔAIC = 5.25). Statistically, however, there was little difference in mC between M1 and M3 (p value = 0.60). Adding VPD0 to APD6 (M5) failed to improve model performance in terms of the AIC.

In study 2, M3 was again the best model in terms of the AIC (Table 4). Compared to VPD0 (M1), APD6 (M3) was considerably superior in terms of the AIC (ΔAIC = 9.36). mC for M3 was also significantly higher than for M1 (p value <0.001). VPD0 did not add

statistically significant information after controlling for APD6 (M5 vs M3, p value = 0.24). Indeed, it can be shown that similar to the result shown in Fig. 1, APD6 (M3) was a better predictor than volumetric or other areal PDs at different thresholds both in studies 1 and 2.

A series of likelihood-ratio tests were performed on the aforementioned models to test whether there was any significant difference between screen-detected and interval cancers within study 2. The interaction term

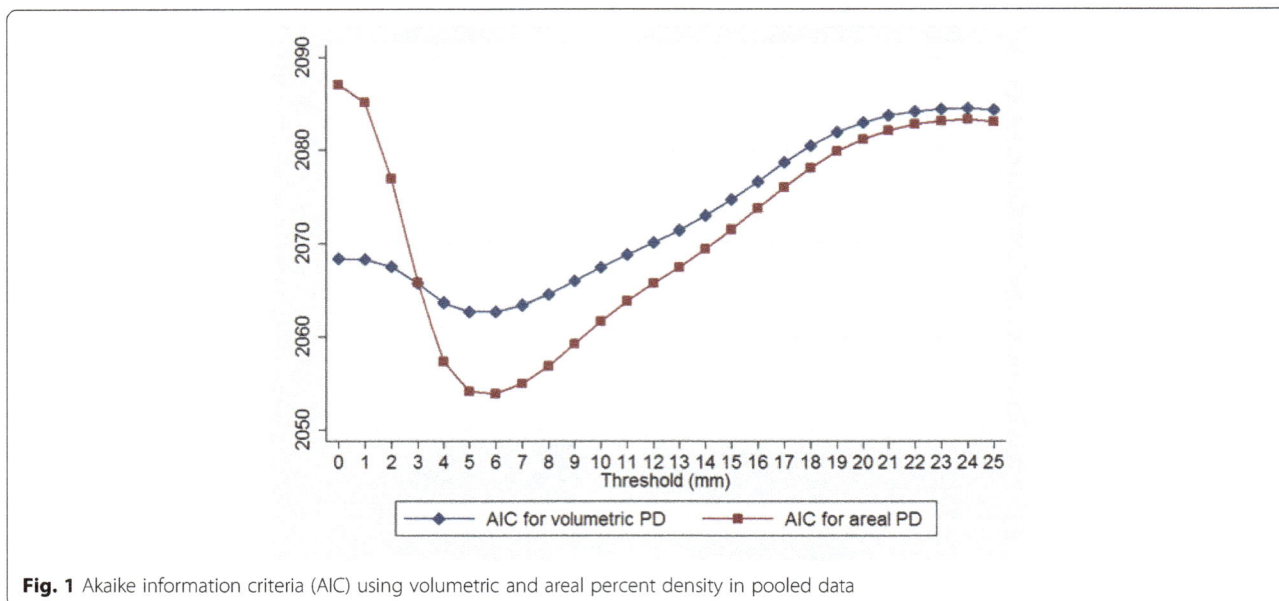

Fig. 1 Akaike information criteria (AIC) using volumetric and areal percent density in pooled data

was found to be statistically significant for APD6 (M3, *p* value = 0.004; M5, *p* value = 0.003). Since VPD0 in M5 did not add information to APD6, the final model for prediction of screen-detected and interval cancers was based on APD at a threshold level of 6 mm (i.e. APD6 with additional interaction term). The resulting standardised odds ratio for APD at the 6 mm threshold was 1.81 for interval cancers (95% CI = 1.42–2.30) and 1.18 for screen-detected cancers (95% CI = 0.99–1.40).

Discussion

This paper explores the impact of various levels of density thresholding on the performance in prediction of breast cancer using digital mammograms. To achieve this, a range of threshold levels from 0 to 25 mm were tested. For VPD, the threshold was varied so that only dense tissue where heights were greater than a given value were included to calculate the total dense volume of the breast. For APD, we counted the number of dense

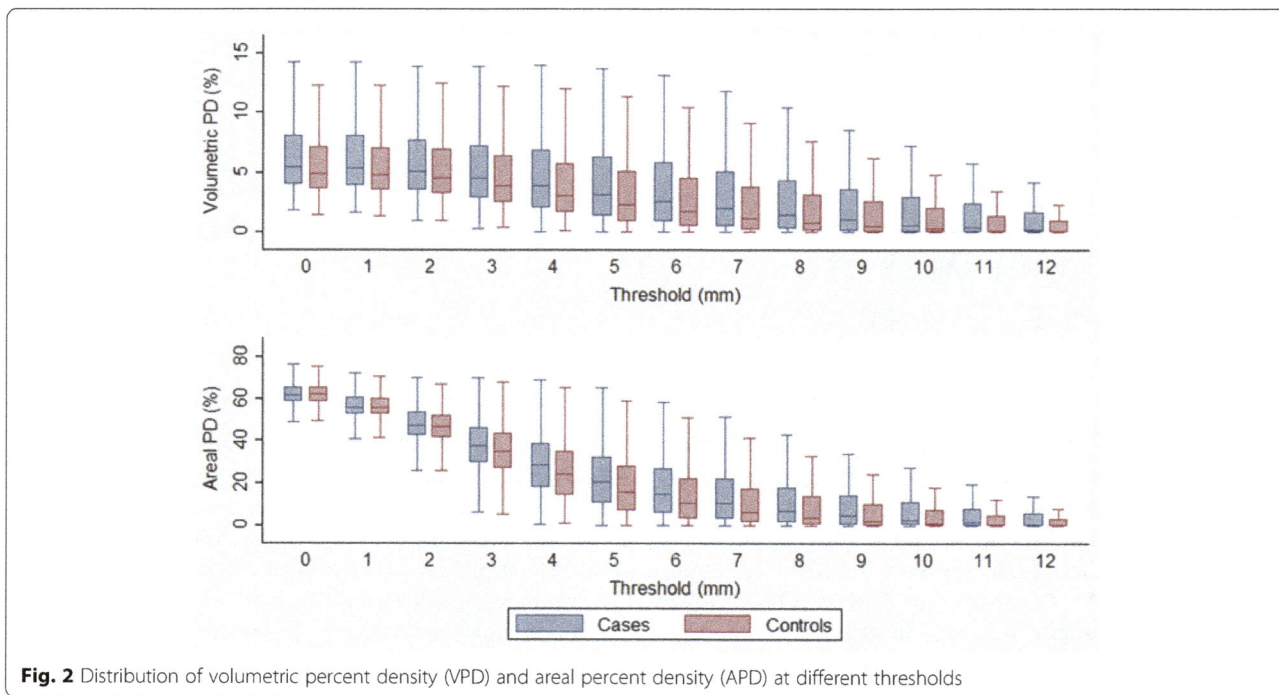

Fig. 2 Distribution of volumetric percent density (VPD) and areal percent density (APD) at different thresholds

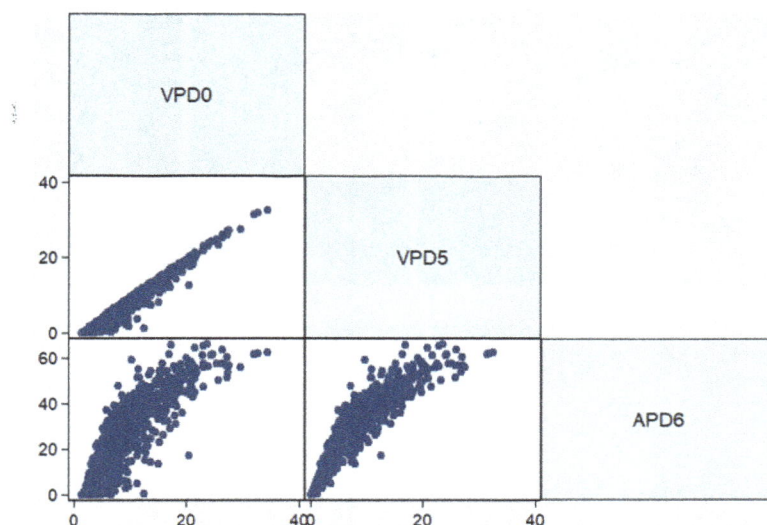

Fig. 3 Correlation between volumetric percent density with a 0 mm threshold (VPD0), VPD with a 5 mm threshold (VPD5) and areal percent density with a 6 mm threshold (APD6)

pixels above the threshold level and compared this with the total number of pixels in the breast to derive the areal PD.

Results from both case-control studies and from the pooled data confirm that a threshold level of 5 mm or 6 mm, either volumetric or areal, improves cancer risk prediction compared to original VPD without thresholding. However, the improvement with VPD at the higher thresholds was relatively small. This is not surprising given the strong correlation between VPD0 and VPD5 (spearman ρ approximately 0.95 in both studies). On the other hand, APD at threshold of 6 mm (APD6) achieved the best results across all models tested, including VPD

and APD at various threshold levels, with $\Delta AIC = 14.52$ for the pooled data compared to VPD0. It is worth noting that APD6 was also highly correlated with VPD0 (spearman ρ approximately 0.90 in both studies), which is not surprising given both APD and VPD measure relative dense tissue albeit from a different perspective. In addition to fixed threshold levels, varying threshold levels were also examined with the level of threshold based on a woman's characteristics such as age, BMI and breast volume; however, the AIC did not improve, so a fixed threshold is preferred.

We also explored the impact of thresholding by visualising mammograms after areas with less dense tissue

Table 2 Modelling results for the pooled data

| | Standardised odds ratio (95% CI) | | | | |
	M1	M2	M3	M4	M5
Volumetric PD (0 mm)	1.26			0.46	0.90
	(1.15, 1.39)			(0.26, 0.82)	(0.74, 1.10)
Volumetric PD (5 mm)		1.29		2.72	
		(1.18, 1.42)		(1.56, 4.74)	
Areal PD (6 mm)			1.34		1.47
			(1.22, 1.47)		(1.21, 1.78)
Model fit statistics					
AIC	1727.15	1721.25	1712.63	1715.81	1713.50
mC	0.567	0.577	0.577	0.583	0.582
	(0.539, 0.596)	(0.548, 0.606)	(0.549, 0.605)	(0.555, 0.611)	(0.553, 0.610)
χ^2	21.98	27.87	36.49	35.32	37.62

Standardized odds ratio is the change in odds for a standard deviation increase in predictors. Confidence intervals (CI) are presented in parentheses for the predictors in each model

M model, *PD* percent density, *AIC* Akaike information criterion, *mC* matched concordance index

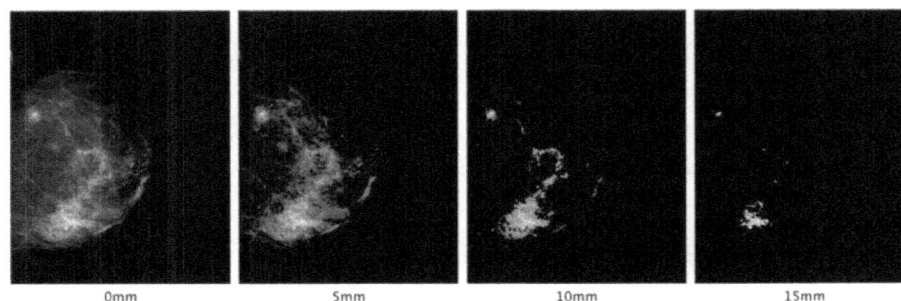

Fig. 4 A visual comparison of "density map" using 0–15 mm threshold levels. Traditional volumetric density such as from the Volpara software uses a 0 mm threshold (no threshold). VPD0, volumetric percent density with a 0 mm threshold; VPD5, VPD with a 5 mm threshold; APD6, areal percent density with a 6 mm threshold

were excluded. As illustrated in Fig. 4, thresholding at 5 mm filtered out a large portion of lower-density areas, and was roughly comparable to *Altocumulus* presented by previous research [6]. Further thresholding at higher levels at 10 and 15 mm seems to exclude too much information, thus no further improvement in prediction was observed at these levels. It appears that by introducing a suitable threshold level (e.g. 5–6 mm), much of the "noise" presented in the mammograms (including fine structures with low attenuation) is removed and hence results in a more predictive PD estimate.

It is also interesting that whilst APD performed much worse than VPD initially when the level of thresholding was low, APD became better than VPD when a threshold level of 4 mm or above was applied, as shown in Fig. 1. This suggests that VPD is relatively insensitive to the "noise" presented in mammograms compared to APD, since VPD is essentially a weighted sum (i.e. if all

dense tissue heights were the same then VPD would be equivalent to APD). However, after exclusion of the noise component, the weights (dense tissue heights) became less relevant, resulting in APD being a better predictor. This is interesting because it suggests that once the density at each point in the mammogram reaches some threshold, the measures are equally informative in terms of cancer risk despite local differences in density.

In terms of the biological plausibility for these findings, the major component of dense breast tissue is stroma [15], and pathways for breast cancer risk associated with dense tissue are likely to involve the stromal cells, extracellular matrix proteins and the epithelial component. It has also been shown that local density is associated with the location where cancer would develop [16]. However, the causal route between dense tissue and breast cancer is unknown, and research is ongoing in this important area [15]. For these reasons we do not

Table 3 Modelling results for study 1 in which cancers were detected at initial screening

	Standardised odds ratio (95% CI)				
	M1	M2	M3	M4	M5
Volumetric PD (0 mm)	1.25			0.51	0.96
	(1.10,1.43)			(0.24,1.09)	(0.73,1.25)
Volumetric PD (5 mm)		1.28		2.44	
		(1.13,1.46)		(1.16,5.14)	
Areal PD (6 mm)			1.31		1.36
			(1.15,1.50)		(1.05,1.78)
Model fit statistics					
AIC	867.80	865.01	862.55	863.87	864.45
mC	0.559	0.564	0.556	0.573	0.560
	(0.518, 0.599)	(0.524, 0.604)	(0.515, 0.595)	(0.533, 0.613)	(0.519, 0.600)
χ^2	10.81	13.60	16.06	16.74	16.16

Standardized odds ratio is the change in odds for a standard deviation increase in predictors. Confidence intervals (CI) are presented in parentheses for the predictors in each model

M model, *PD* percent density, *AIC* Akaike information criterion, *mC* matched concordance index

Table 4 Modelling results for study 2 in which cancers were detected after the initial screening

	Standardised odds ratio (95% CI)				
	M1	M2	M3	M4	M5
Volumetric PD (0 mm)	1.27			0.42	0.84
	(1.11,1.47)			(0.18,0.97)	(0.63,1.12)
Volumetric PD (5 mm)		1.31		3.04	
		(1.14,1.50)		(1.32,6.97)	
Areal PD (6 mm)			1.37		1.58
			(1.19,1.57)		(1.20,2.08)
Model fit statistics					
AIC	861.35	858.24	851.99	855.87	852.61
mC	0.576	0.590	0.599	0.597	0.605
mC	(0.536, 0.616)	(0.551, 0.630)	(0.559, 0.640)	(0.557, 0.636)	(0.565, 0.644)
χ^2	11.17	14.27	20.52	18.64	21.91

Standardized odds ratio is the change in odds for a standard deviation increase in predictors. Confidence intervals (CI) are presented in parentheses for the predictors in each model

M model, *PD* percent density, *AIC* Akaike information criterion, *mC* matched concordance index

speculate further on how this measure of breast density might better capture the biological mechanism for risk due to dense breast tissue. From a measurement accuracy point of view, however, an increased threshold may remove the areas of fat that look slightly grey on the image, which might reduce measurement error. Another possible explanation is that setting an appropriate threshold removes thin sheets or strands of tissue which have similar attenuation coefficients to glandular tissue, and exclusion of this type of tissue might contribute to better density estimation.

Consistent with previous studies [4–6], our results show that once the APD at the optimal threshold level is accounted for, conventional VPD0 no longer adds information - in fact models with multiple PD measurements (M4 and M5) performed worse than the model with only APD6 as a predictor (M3). While the standardised OR and mC, including those based on the original VPD estimated by Volpara (M1), might seem relatively low compared with some previous studies [6, 9], the results are broadly consistent with a body of previous research [4, 17, 18]. For example, Brandt et al. [17] compared VPD with BI-RADS using a large case-control sample (1911 cases and 4170 controls) and identified a similar discriminatory ability for Volpara VPD (AUC = 0.58, 95% CI 0.56–0.59) as in our study. It is also worth noting that the studies that have directly compared VPD by Volpara with established visual-based assessment such as BI-RADS and Cumulus have shown broadly similar ability for risk prediction [12, 17, 19], and so differences in predictive ability between studies might be due to other characteristics of the data. It is plausible that the predictive ability of a density measure differs across different

sub groups of women and types of cancers, such as screen-detected and interval cancers as demonstrated here and by others [18]. This means the predictive ability likely depends on the composition of the study population, which may explain some of the differences between studies.

Previous studies have demonstrated that breast density adds accuracy to established breast cancer risk models such as the Tyrer-Cuzick and Gail models [20, 21], including in combination with single-nucleotide polymorphism risk panels [22]. It is therefore expected that this study will be of clinical importance, as an improved automated density measure is likely to help identify women who require additional screening and to help devise a risk-based screening/prevention strategy.

The strength of our approach, compared to previous studies [4–6], is that the process is fully automated without any human intervention. Also, by using raw ("for processing") digital mammograms, differences due to manufacturers' proprietary processing algorithms are reduced. Our approach, however, would benefit from testing in a wider range of settings. For example, the majority of women in our datasets were white and parous, so it would be important to validate our approach amongst other groups of women. Finally, the mammograms employed in our study are generated from a GE system. Nguyen et al. [5] found that prediction performance may vary considerably between different mammographic machines based on visual assessment. It would be interesting to further explore the impact of thresholding using different systems in which the image properties may differ, and how the method can be calibrated for mammograms from different systems and the resulting discriminatory power in different settings.

Conclusion

This study examined volumetric and areal PDs defined by various thresholds, and found that APD at 6 mm is the best risk predictor of breast cancer in two case-control studies. The results presented in this study confirm findings from previous studies that dense tissue is more important for predicting breast cancer risk. Unlike previous studies where thresholding was based on pixel brightness by visual assessment, the approach adopted in this paper was based on the height of dense tissue calculated from volumetric density estimation, which enables our approach to be fully automated.

Appendix

The number of cases and controls differs from a previous report that compared density measurements using the same women. The reasons are as follows. First, the first case-control study was a subset of one with 317 cases and 952 controls. Three women were excluded due to linkage errors between mammograms and questionnaire data. An additional two women were excluded because the CC view mammograms at the designated side of the breast (i.e. either left or right CC view) were unavailable.

The second case-control study originally had 338 cases and 1014 controls: 23 women were excluded because of unavailability of mammograms at the time of analysis (either no mammograms were provided for some women at the given side; or only mediolateral oblique (MLO) views were available but no CC views). A further 64 women were removed because the side of cancer (left or right) was unknown. A further 12 controls were removed during conditional logistic regression because they had no matched cases as a result of the aforementioned exclusions.

Abbreviations

AIC: Akaike information criterion; APD: Areal percent density; AUC: Area under the receiver operating characteristic curve; BMI: Body mass index; CC: Craniocaudal; CI: Confidence interval; HRT: Hormone replacement therapy; mC: Matched concordance index; PD: Percent density; PROCAS: Predicting Risk Of breast Cancer At Screening; VPD: Volumetric percent density

Funding

This research is partially funded by the Cancer Research UK (grant number C569/A16891). This work was supported by the National Institute for Health Research (NIHR) under its Programme Grants for Applied Research programme (reference number RP-PG-0707-10031: "Improvement in risk prediction, early detection and prevention of breast cancer") and the Genesis Prevention Appeal (references GA09–003 and GA13–006). SA, EH and DGE are funded by the Manchester NIHR Biomedical Research Centre (IS-BRC-1215-20007).The views expressed are those of the author(s) and not necessarily those of Cancer Research UK, the National Health Service (NHS), the NIHR, or the Department of Health.

Authors' contributions

CW developed the codes to estimate VPD and APD after thresholding, performed the statistical analysis, interpreted the results and drafted the manuscript. AB advised on statistical analysis and interpretation and helped to draft the manuscript. EH made substantial contribution to data distribution and helped to draft the manuscript. DGE conceived the PROCAS study. JC and SA conceived the study, interpreted the results and helped to draft the manuscript. All authors read and approved the final manuscript.

Competing interests

The authors declare that they have no competing interests.

Author details

[1]Centre for Cancer Prevention, Wolfson Institute of Preventive Medicine, Queen Mary University of London, Charterhouse Square, London EC1M 6BQ, UK. [2]Centre for Imaging Science, School of Health Sciences, University of Manchester, Stopford Building, Oxford Road, Manchester M13 9PT, UK. [3]Department of Genomic Medicine, University of Manchester, St Mary's Hospital, M13 9WL, Manchester, UK.

References

1. Assi V, Warwick J, Cuzick J, Duffy SW. Clinical and epidemiological issues in mammographic density. Nat Rev Clin Oncol. 2012;9(1):33–40.
2. Hopper JL. Odds per adjusted standard deviation: comparing strengths of associations for risk factors measured on different scales and across diseases and populations. Am J Epidemiol. 2015;182(10):863–7.
3. Byng JW, Boyd NF, Fishell E, Jong RA, Yaffe MJ. The quantitative-analysis of mammographic densities. Phys Med Biol. 1994;39(10):1629–38.
4. Nguyen TL, Aung YK, Evans CF, Yoon-Ho C, Jenkins MA, Sung J, Hopper JL, Song Y-M. Mammographic density defined by higher than conventional brightness threshold better predicts breast cancer risk for full-field digital mammograms. Breast Cancer Res. 2015;17:1–9.
5. Nguyen TL, Choi Y-H, Aung YK, Evans CF, Trinh NH, Li S, Dite GS, Kim MS, Brennan PC, Jenkins MA, et al. Breast cancer risk associations with digital mammographic Density by pixel brightness threshold and mammographic system. Radiology. 2018;286(2):433–42.
6. Nguyen TL, Aung YK, Evans CF, Dite GS, Stone J, MacInnis RJ, Dowty JG, Bickerstaffe A, Aujard K, Rommens JM, et al. Mammographic density defined by higher than conventional brightness thresholds better predicts breast cancer risk. Int J Epidemiol. 2016;46(2):652–61.
7. Highnam R, Brady SM, Yaffe MJ, Karssemeijer N, Harvey J. Robust breast composition measurement - VolparaTM. In: Martí J, Oliver A, Freixenet J, Martí R, editors. Digital mammography: 10th International Workshop, IWDM 2010, Girona, Catalonia, Spain, June 16–18, 2010 Proceedings. Berlin: Springer Berlin Heidelberg; 2010. p. 342–9.
8. Ciatto S, Bernardi D, Calabrese M, Durando M, Gentilini MA, Mariscotti G, Monetti F, Moriconi E, Pesce B, Roselli A, et al. A first evaluation of breast radiological density assessment by QUANTRA software as compared to visual classification. Breast. 2012;21(4):503–6.
9. Eng A, Gallant Z, Shepherd J, McCormack V, Li J, Dowsett M, Vinnicombe S, Allen S, Dos-Santos-Silva I. Digital mammographic density and breast cancer risk: a case-control study of six alternative density assessment methods. Breast Cancer Res. 2014;16:1–12.
10. Evans DGR, Warwick J, Astley SM, Stavrinos P, Sahin S, Ingham S, McBurney H, Eckersley B, Harvie M, Wilson M, et al. Assessing individual breast cancer risk within the U.K. National Health Service Breast Screening Program: a new paradigm for cancer prevention. Cancer Prev Res. 2012;5(7):943–51.
11. Wang C, Brentnall AR, Cuzick J, Harkness EF, Evans DG, Astley S. A novel and fully automated mammographic texture analysis for risk prediction: results from two case-control studies. Breast Cancer Res. 2017;19:1–13.

12. Astley SM, Harkness EF, Sergeant JC, Warwick J, Stavrinos P, Warren R, Wilson M, Beetles U, Gadde S, Lim Y, et al. A comparison of five methods of measuring mammographic density: a case-control study. Breast Cancer Res. 2018;20:1-13.

13. Brentnall AR, Cuzick J, Field J, Duffy SW. A concordance index for matched case-control studies with applications in cancer risk. Stat Med. 2015;34(3): 396–405.

14. Burnham KP, Anderson DR, Huyvaert KP. AIC model selection and multimodel inference in behavioral ecology: some background, observations, and comparisons. Behav Ecol Sociobiol. 2011;65(1):23–35.

15. Ironside AJ, Jones JL. Stromal characteristics may hold the key to mammographic density: the evidence to date. Oncotarget. 2016;7:31550–62.

16. Otsuka M, Harkness EF, Chen X, Moschidis E, Bydder M, Gadde S, Lim YY, Maxwell AJ, Evans GD, Howell A, et al. Local mammographic density as a predictor of breast cancer. In: Proc. SPIE 9414, Medical Imaging 2015: Computer-Aided Diagnosis, 941417 (20 March 2015).

17. Brandt KR, Scott CG, Ma L, Mahmoudzadeh AP, Jensen MR, Whaley DH, Wu FF, Malkov S, Hruska CB, Norman AD, et al. Comparison of clinical and automated breast density measurements: implications for risk prediction and supplemental screening. Radiology. 2016;279(3):710–9.

18. Nickson C, Arzhaeva Y, Aitken Z, Elgindy T, Buckley M, Li M, English DR, Kavanagh AM. AutoDensity: an automated method to measure mammographic breast density that predicts breast cancer risk and screening outcomes. Breast Cancer Res. 2013;15:1-11.

19. Jeffers AM, Sieh W, Lipson JA, Rothstein JH, McGuire V, Whittemore AS, Rubin DL. Breast Cancer risk and mammographic density assessed with semiautomated and fully automated methods and BI-RADS. Radiology. 2017;282(2):348–55.

20. Brentnall AR, Harkness EF, Astley SM, Donnelly LS, Stavrinos P, Sampson S, Fox L, Sergeant JC, Harvie MN, Wilson M, et al. Mammographic density adds accuracy to both the Tyrer-Cuzick and Gail breast cancer risk models in a prospective UK screening cohort. Breast Cancer Res. 2015;17:1-10. https://breast-cancer-research.biomedcentral.com/articles/10.1186/s13058-015-0653-5.

21. Brentnall AR, Cuzick J, Buist DSM, Bowles EJA. Long-term accuracy of breast cancer risk assessment combining classic risk factors and breast density. JAMA Oncol. 2018:e180174. https://jamanetwork.com/journals/jamaoncology/fullarticle/2677301.

22. van Veen EM, Brentnall AR, Byers H, et al. Use of single-nucleotide polymorphisms and mammographic density plus classic risk factors for breast cancer risk prediction. JAMA Oncol. 2018;4(4):476–82.

15

Clonal relatedness in tumour pairs of breast cancer patients

Jana Biermann[1*] , Toshima Z. Parris[1], Szilárd Nemes[2], Anna Danielsson[1], Hanna Engqvist[1], Elisabeth Werner Rönnerman[1,3], Eva Forssell-Aronsson[4], Anikó Kovács[3], Per Karlsson[1†] and Khalil Helou[1†]

Abstract

Background: Molecular classification of tumour clonality is currently not evaluated in multiple invasive breast carcinomas, despite evidence suggesting common clonal origins. There is no consensus about which type of data (e.g. copy number, mutation, histology) and especially which statistical method is most suitable to distinguish clonal recurrences from independent primary tumours.

Methods: Thirty-seven invasive breast tumour pairs were stratified according to laterality and time interval between the diagnoses of the two tumours. In a multi-omics approach, tumour clonality was analysed by integrating clinical characteristics ($n = 37$), DNA copy number ($n = 37$), DNA methylation ($n = 8$), gene expression microarray ($n = 7$), RNA sequencing ($n = 3$), and SNP genotyping data ($n = 3$). Different statistical methods, e.g. the diagnostic similarity index (SI), were used to classify the tumours as clonally related recurrences or independent primary tumours.

Results: The SI and hierarchical clustering showed similar tendencies and the highest concordance with the other methods. Concordant evidence for tumour clonality was found in 46% (17/37) of patients. Notably, no association was found between the current clinical guidelines and molecular tumour features.

Conclusions: A more accurate classification of clonal relatedness between multiple breast tumours may help to mitigate treatment failure and relapse by integrating tumour-associated molecular features, clinical parameters, and statistical methods. Guidelines need to be defined with exact thresholds to standardise clonality testing in a routine diagnostic setting.

Keywords: Tumour clonality, Bilateral breast cancer, Ipsilateral breast cancer, Intertumour heterogeneity, Similarity index, Multiple breast cancer

Background

Approximately 2–15% of women previously diagnosed with breast cancer will develop a second primary carcinoma in the contralateral breast during their lifetime [1, 2]. Interestingly, the risk of developing a breast tumour in the contralateral breast is 2–6-fold higher in breast cancer patients than the risk of developing a first primary breast cancer in the general population [2]. These findings indicate a clonal relationship between bilateral breast cancers as well as a consequence of genetic predisposition and treatment [2, 3]. However, discordance in histologic patterns between bilateral tumours suggests that the majority of bilateral breast cancers have independent tumour origins [4]. Clonality is defined as two tumours deriving from the same progenitor cell that previously underwent malignant changes and gave rise to both of the detected tumours [5]. Consequently, in the early development of the two clones the driver events of the progenitor cell (e.g. copy number alteration (CNA), DNA methylation, mutation, and gene expression profiles) need to have been identical. Due to heterogeneity in subclonal drifts, the variability between the two clones results from the accumulation of diverse molecular changes associated with tumour progression [6]. Nevertheless, similarities in certain tumour features might be due to genetic predisposition and shared environment instead of indicating metastatic spread.

* Correspondence: jana.biermann@gu.se
†Per Karlsson and Khalil Helou contributed equally to this work.
[1]Department of Oncology, Institute of Clinical Sciences, Sahlgrenska Cancer Center, Sahlgrenska Academy at University of Gothenburg, Box 425, SE-405 30 Gothenburg, Sweden
Full list of author information is available at the end of the article

Ipsilateral (unilateral) secondary tumours occur in 10–15% of patients undergoing breast-conserving surgery and radiation therapy [7]. At present, the concordance of hormone receptor status in tumour pairs is the main factor when evaluating potential clonal relatedness of two breast tumours. Clinical characteristics of breast tumours with independent origin are the presence of an in situ component in the second tumour, different degrees of differentiation, different histological subtypes (e.g. invasive carcinoma no special type (NST), invasive lobular carcinoma, tubular, medullary, etc.), absence of locoregional or distant metastases, long time interval between the two tumours, and differences in stage and anatomic location [8, 9]. Determining the concordance of histopathological characteristics between multiple breast carcinomas is insufficient for discerning whether multiple tumours are true recurrences of the primary tumour (clonal) or a new unrelated primary lesion (independent tumour) [10]. Bilateral tumours are currently clinically diagnosed as two different entities, while ipsilateral tumours are classified as local recurrences [1]. Clonal recurrences can represent treatment failure of the first tumour, warranting a change of therapy for the second tumour. Contrastingly, two independent tumours with the same clinical features can be treated similarly since the treatment was successful for the first tumour.

Different techniques in the field of molecular genetics have been used to elucidate tumour clonality, e.g. allelic imbalances [11, 12], CGH (comparative genomic hybridization) [13, 14], array comparative genomic hybridization (aCGH) [15, 16], as well as whole exome and whole genome sequencing [17–19]. In addition, several analytical tools have been proposed to justify the routine clinical use of determining tumour clonality [5, 13, 15, 20–22].

In the present study, 74 invasive breast tumours corresponding to 37 patients were stratified by laterality (bilateral vs. ipsilateral) and the time interval between the diagnosis of the first and second tumour (synchronous vs. metachronous). Both tumours from the same patient were analysed using several genome-wide screening methods and statistical approaches to assess tumour clonality. The level of concordance among the different statistical techniques and molecular data might help to define clonality in multiple tumours and guide treatment decisions for clinicians.

Methods

Patients and clinicopathological data
Fresh-frozen tumour specimens for 74 invasive breast carcinomas, corresponding to 37 patients diagnosed in Western Sweden between 1988 and 1998 with multiple breast cancers, were selected from the tumour bank at the Sahlgrenska University Hospital Oncology Lab

(Gothenburg, Sweden). The patients were stratified into four groups based on the anatomic location of the multiple breast cancers (ipsilateral or bilateral) and time interval between the diagnoses (synchronous or metachronous). Ipsilateral was defined as tumours occurring in the same breast while bilateral was defined as the occurrence of tumours in both breasts. Metachronicity was defined as a time interval greater than 6 months between the diagnoses of the first and second tumours, while synchronicity specified that the two tumours occurred concurrently. Clinicopathological information was obtained from Regional Cancer Centre West (Gothenburg, Sweden) and the Sympathy and Melior databases (Sahlgrenska University Hospital). A part of the dataset was stratified into the molecular breast cancer subtypes (normal-like, basal-like, luminal subtype A, luminal subtype B/human epidermal growth factor receptor 2 (HER2)+, luminal subtype B/HER2-, and HER2/oestrogen receptor (ER)-) as described elsewhere [23, 24]. Luminal subtype B was further stratified according to HER2 status as determined by aCGH; HER2+ was set to $\log_2$ ratio $\geq +0.5$ and HER2- was set to $\log_2$ ratio $< +0.5$ [25]. Routine haematoxylin and eosin-stained slides from formalin-fixed paraffin-embedded (FFPE) blocks were revised by a board-certified breast pathologist. Classification of the subtypes based on immunohistochemistry was not possible due to the lack of information on the Ki-67 status. The patients had an average follow-up time of 7.2 years. None of the patients were diagnosed with distant metastasis at the time of diagnosis of either the first or second tumours. The selection criteria were to use samples from opposite quadrants for ipsilateral cases and no nipple involvement. Representative imprints from each tumour specimen were stained with May-Grünwald Giemsa (Chemicon, Temecula CA, USA) and evaluated for neoplastic cells. Tumour specimens with at least 70% neoplastic cell content were included in downstream analyses.

Array comparative genomic hybridization (aCGH) analysis
aCGH and data pre-processing was performed as previously described [24] and summarised in the Additional file 1: Supplementary Methods. Segmented data for segment analysis were generated using the "GLAD" package [26] in R (v3.4.3) [27]. The "Clonality" package [28] was used to define the likelihood ratio with individual comparisons (LR2) and LR2 p value and required copy number data procession with the "DNAcopy" package [29].

DNA methylation analysis
Sixteen samples were randomly selected to represent each clinical group with four samples corresponding to two patients per group. Purified genomic DNA was processed at the SNP&SEQ technology platform, Uppsala, Sweden,

using Illumina Infinium MethylationEPIC BeadChips (MethylationEPIC_v-1-0; mapped to UCSC Feb 2009 hg19: GRCh37). Raw data (IDAT files) were processed in R using the "RnBeads" package [30]. The probes were normalised with the BMIQ method (beta mixture quantile dilation) [31]. Beta values were obtained with "RnBeads". The intensity values were extracted using the "ChAMP" package to generate segmented copy number data for the segment analysis [32, 33]. The "conumee" package was used to extract unsegmented information of CNAs on the probe level [34]. The unsegmented CNAs were used for the similarity index (SI), the distance measure and the clustering analysis.

Whole transcriptome RNA sequencing (RNA-seq)

Total RNA samples were processed at the Science for Life Laboratory (National Genomics Infrastructure, Stockholm, Sweden). Illumina TruSeq strand-specific RNA libraries (Ribosomal depletion using RiboZero human) containing 125 bp paired-end reads were obtained for each sample on a HiSeq2000 sequencer (Illumina, San Diego, CA, USA). The computations were performed on resources provided by SNIC through Uppsala Multidisciplinary Center for Advanced Computational Science (UPPMAX) [35], as described in the Additional file 1: Supplementary Methods.

Genome-wide single nucleotide polymorphism (SNP) genotyping analysis

Genome-wide SNP genotyping analysis was processed with Illumina Infinium HumanOmni2.5–8 v1.3 Beadchips at the SCIBLU Genomics DNA Microarray Resource Center (SCIBLU), Sweden, as described in the Additional file 1: Supplementary Methods.

Statistical analyses

A p value cut-off of 0.05 was applied in all statistical tests.

Definition of tumour clonality

Tumours derived from a common precursor tumour cell should share certain features, i.e. similar CNAs, genetic variants, shared segments, DNA methylation and gene expression patterns, in addition to non-matching features that were acquired over time. We applied different statistical methods on different types of molecular data to identify similarities between the tumours that classify a tumour pair as clonal and reject the null hypothesis (different features due to independent development of primary tumours).

Similarity index (SI)

The SI assesses whether two tumours identified in the same patient are clonally related or two independent entities by identifying genetic aberrations that are patient-specific and non-recurrent aberrations frequently identified in cancer [21]. In brief, DNA copy number data were normalised and discretized (heterozygous loss (<-0.3); normal; low-level gain (>0.3)) and unique (N_U), shared (N_S), and opposite (N_O) changes were calculated for each tumour pair to obtain the SI:

$$SI = \frac{N_S}{N_S + N_U + N_O}$$

The SI ranges between 0 (completely different) and 1 (identical genomic profiles). The permutation-based P_{SI} gives the percentage of similarities between two tumours that are not due to recurrent chromosomal aberrations or randomness.

The SI remained unchanged for the gene expression microarray data. The normalised $\log_2$ ratios were discretized using a 1.5 fold change cut-off (underexpressed ($\log_2$ ratio < -0.58); neutral; overexpressed ($\log_2$ ratio > 0.58)).

Calculation of the SI was modified for the methylation data (SI_{met}) because the SI for copy number data is based on measuring the amount of alterations from the biologically neutral state (two copies per allele). In DNA methylation, neither methylated nor unmethylated can be defined as the neutral state of a cytosine due to the dynamic of methylation. The SI_{met} uses beta values discretized according to thresholds defined by Du et al. [36], where beta values > 0.8 are defined as methylated, and beta values < 0.2 as unmethylated, while the range from 0.2 to 0.8 is hemi-methylated. The SI_{met} counts the number of all common states between the first and the second tumour per probe and divides it by the total number of probes, giving the percentage of shared methylation states. The main difference is that the SI_{met} uses all probe states while the SI is based on the changes from the neutral state and therefore does not count two tumours that are normal as a shared state.

Hierarchical clustering

Unsupervised hierarchical clustering was applied using single linkage with Euclidean distance [37]. Clustering was performed using the basic "stats" package [27] for the aCGH-derived copy number data (imputed $\log_2$ ratios), the DNA methylation data (beta values and intensity values), the microarray-derived gene expression data (normalised $\log_2$ ratios), and the SNP array data (B allele frequency (BAF) and log R ratio (LRR) values). Two tumours of the same patient were defined as similar (clonal) if they clustered together in the terminal branch of the dendrogram.

Distance measure

The distance measure was used to compute the distance matrix of the Euclidean distances between different tumour samples to evaluate the similarity between two samples. The Euclidean distance was computed using the basic "stats" package [27] for the aCGH-derived copy number data (imputed $\log_2$ ratios), the DNA methylation data (beta values and intensity values), the microarray-derived gene expression data (normalised $\log_2$ ratios), and the SNP array data (LRR values). The distance measure was calculated for true tumour pairs which derive from the same patient and for all artificial combinations of tumour pairs from different patients (permutation). Tumour pairs that are more similar on the probe level will show a shorter distance from each other. Statistical significance for clonality was defined as the distance of a tumour pair of the same patient that is in the lower fifth percentile of the distribution of distances.

Shared segment analysis

In segmented copy number data, the breakpoints and the copy number of each segment was compared between the tumours. A shared segment was defined as an overlap of the exact loci in both ends of the segment where the change in status (loss or gain) occurred with the same direction (increase or decrease in copy numbers). The segment analysis was performed on segmented copy number data derived from aCGH (imputed $\log_2$ ratios), DNA methylation array (intensity values), and SNP array (LRR values). Shared segments were counted for true tumour pairs and all artificial pairs of the respective cohort. Clonality was defined as the number of shared segments above the 95th percentile.

Mutational changes (genetic variants) and fusion transcript analysis

Mutational changes that were identical in both tumours were counted for true tumour pairs and all artificial pairs of the cohort. Clonality was defined as the number of shared mutations above the 95th percentile of the permutation distribution. Shared mutations were counted for genomic and exonic RNA-seq data. In addition, a panel of 254 breast cancer and DNA repair-specific mutation spots proposed by Begg et al. was analysed [38]. The overlap of RNA-seq counts of the genomic and exonic data with the 254-gene panel was used to count the shared mutations of the true and artificial pairs of the cohort. Clonality was defined as the number of shared mutations above the 95th percentile. To test for clonality using profiles of somatic mutations in the "Clonality" package [28], loci-specific probabilities of observing a mutation were obtained from the TCGA breast cancer dataset [39]. Furthermore, fusion transcripts of all tumours were compared and transcripts with identical 5′ and 3′ fusion partner breakpoints were counted.

Cohen's kappa

Cohen's kappa measures the chance-corrected agreement for two observations [40]. Cohen's kappa indices of agreement between different methods applied to estimate clonality were calculated using the R-package "rel" [41].

Results

Tumour synchronicity strongly associated with metastatic spread to the axillary lymph nodes

The 37 breast cancer patients were stratified into four clinical groups based on tumour laterality and the time interval between the diagnoses of the first and second tumours (BM: bilateral-metachronous; BS: bilateral-synchronous; IM: ipsilateral-metachronous; IS: ipsilateral-synchronous). The clinicopathological characteristics are shown in Additional file 2: Table S1. Metastatic spread to the axillary lymph nodes was more prevalent in the synchronous groups (BS: 100%; IS: 85.7%) as compared to the metachronous groups (BM: 61.5%; IM: 14.3%; $P = 0.001$).

Discordances in histopathological characteristics in 32% of the tumour pairs

For the clinical classification of clonality, several histopathological and molecular features were taken into consideration, including histological subtype, the status of ER and HER2, and the molecular subtype (Table 1). While the receptor status was available for most samples, the molecular subtype was only defined for about 40% of the tumours. Thirty-two percent of the patients (12/37) showed discordances between the first and the second tumour, with one-fourth of the 12 patients showing two discordant changes. Most changes were found in the histological subtypes (35%; 6/17 patients), while the molecular subtype differed in 25% (2/8 patients), ER status in 11% (4/35 patients), and HER2 status in 8% (3/37 patients). In patients with metachronous cancer, changes in receptor status from positive to negative were observed for patients BM6 and BM7. The discordant changes were equally distributed between the different clinical groups and showed no significance when stratified by group.

Stratification by laterality revealed differential copy number imbalances

DNA copy number analysis using aCGH was performed to identify recurrent regions of DNA copy number gain (blue) and loss (red) in at least 25% of the tumours in the patient cohort. Recurrent DNA gains were identified on chromosomes 1q, 8q, 16p, 17q, and 20q, while DNA loss was detected on 1p, 8p, 11q, 13q, and 16q (Fig. 1a).

Table 1 Overview of the clinical and histological characteristics of the primary and secondary tumours

Patient	Laterality	Synchronicity	Group	Time interval (days)	Primary tumour				Secondary tumour				Discordance	Clinical classification
					Histology	ER	HER2	Molecular subtype	Histology	ER	HER2	Molecular subtype		
BM1	bilateral	metachronous	BM	346	Invasive carcinoma NST	pos	neg	ND	ND	pos	neg	ND		concordant
BM2	bilateral	metachronous	BM	1694	Invasive carcinoma NST	pos	neg	Luminal B	Invasive lobular carcinoma	pos	neg	ND	Histology	discordant
BM3	bilateral	metachronous	BM	1652	ND	pos	neg	ND	Invasive carcinoma NST	pos	neg	ND		concordant
BM4	bilateral	metachronous	BM	581	Invasive carcinoma NST	neg	neg	Basal-like	Invasive carcinoma NST	neg	neg	ND		concordant
BM5	bilateral	metachronous	BM	1954	Invasive carcinoma NST	pos	neg	ND	Invasive lobular carcinoma	pos	neg	ND	Histology	discordant
BM6	bilateral	metachronous	BM	1417	Invasive lobular carcinoma	pos	neg	ND	Invasive carcinoma NST	neg	neg	HER2/ER-	Histology; ER	discordant
BM7	bilateral	metachronous	BM	456	Invasive carcinoma NST	pos	pos	ND	Invasive carcinoma NST	neg	pos	ND	ER	discordant
BM8	bilateral	metachronous	BM	1152	Invasive lobular carcinoma	pos	neg	ND	Invasive lobular carcinoma	pos	neg	ND		concordant
BM9	bilateral	metachronous	BM	972	Invasive carcinoma NST	neg	neg	ND	Invasive carcinoma NST	neg	neg	ND		concordant
BS1	bilateral	synchronous	BS	0	Invasive carcinoma NST	pos	neg	ND	Invasive carcinoma NST	pos	neg	Luminal B		concordant
BS2	bilateral	synchronous	BS	0	Invasive lobular carcinoma	pos	neg	ND	Invasive carcinoma NST	pos	neg	Luminal B	Histology	discordant
BS3	bilateral	synchronous	BS	14	Invasive carcinoma NST	pos	neg	ND	Invasive carcinoma NST	pos	neg	ND		concordant
BS4	bilateral	synchronous	BS	0	ND	pos	neg	ND	ND	pos	neg	ND		concordant
BS5	bilateral	synchronous	BS	6	Invasive carcinoma NST	pos	neg	ND	Invasive carcinoma NST	pos	neg	ND		concordant
BS6	bilateral	synchronous	BS	0	ND	neg	neg	ND	ND	neg	neg	ND		concordant
BS7	bilateral	synchronous	BS	0	Invasive carcinoma NOS	pos	neg	Luminal B	Invasive lobular carcinoma	neg	neg	ND	Histology; ER	discordant
BS8	bilateral	synchronous	BS	0	Invasive carcinoma NST	pos	neg	ND	Invasive carcinoma NST	pos	neg	ND		concordant
IM1	ipsilateral	metachronous	IM	1855	ND	pos	neg	ND	ND	pos	neg	Luminal B		concordant
IM2	ipsilateral	metachronous	IM	448	ND	neg	neg	ND	ND	neg	neg	ND		concordant
IM3	ipsilateral	metachronous	IM	1944	Invasive carcinoma NST	pos	pos	Luminal B	ND	pos	pos	Luminal B		concordant
IM4	ipsilateral	metachronous	IM	567	Invasive carcinoma NST	pos	neg	Luminal B	ND	pos	neg	HER2/ER-	Subtype	discordant
IM5	ipsilateral	metachronous	IM	712	Invasive carcinoma NST	neg	neg	Basal-like	ND	neg	neg	ND		concordant
IM6	ipsilateral	metachronous	IM	664	ND	pos	neg	ND	ND	pos	neg	ND		concordant
IM7	ipsilateral	metachronous	IM	2454	ND	pos	neg	ND	ND	pos	neg	ND		concordant
IM8	ipsilateral	metachronous	IM	563	Invasive carcinoma NST	pos	neg	Luminal B	Invasive lobular carcinoma	pos	neg	Luminal B	Histology	discordant
IM9	ipsilateral	metachronous	IM	2142	Invasive carcinoma NOS	ND	neg	Luminal B	Invasive carcinoma NOS	pos	neg	Luminal B		concordant
IS1	ipsilateral	synchronous	IS	0	Invasive carcinoma NST	neg	neg	Basal-like	Invasive carcinoma NST	neg	pos	Luminal B	HER2; subtype	discordant
IS2	ipsilateral	synchronous	IS	0	Invasive carcinoma NST	pos	neg	ND	ND	pos	neg	Luminal B		concordant
IS3	ipsilateral	synchronous	IS	0	ND	neg	neg	Basal-like	ND	neg	pos	Basal-like	HER2	discordant
IS4	ipsilateral	synchronous	IS	50	ND	neg	neg	ND	ND	pos	neg	Luminal B	ER	discordant

Table 1 Overview of the clinical and histological characteristics of the primary and secondary tumours *(Continued)*

Patient	Laterality	Synchronicity	Group	Time interval (days)	Primary tumour Histology	ER	HER2	Molecular subtype	Secondary tumour Histology	ER	HER2	Molecular subtype	Discordance	Clinical classification
IS5	ipsilateral	synchronous	IS	0	Invasive carcinoma NST	pos	neg	Luminal B	Invasive carcinoma NST	pos	neg	Luminal B		concordant
IS6	ipsilateral	synchronous	IS	0	Invasive carcinoma NST	pos	neg	ND	ND	pos	neg	ND		concordant
IS7	ipsilateral	synchronous	IS	0	Invasive carcinoma NOS	pos	neg	ND	ND	pos	neg	ND		concordant
IS8	ipsilateral	synchronous	IS	0	Invasive carcinoma NST	pos	neg	Luminal B	ND	pos	neg	ND		concordant
IS9	ipsilateral	synchronous	IS	0	ND	neg	pos	Basal-like	ND	neg	neg	ND	HER2	discordant
IS10	ipsilateral	synchronous	IS	0	Invasive carcinoma NST	pos	neg	Luminal B	ND	pos	neg	Luminal B		concordant
IS11	ipsilateral	synchronous	IS	0	Invasive carcinoma NOS	neg	pos	HER2/ER-	ND	neg	pos	HER2/ER-		concordant

ER oestrogen receptor status, *HER2* human epidermal growth factor receptor 2 status, *ND* not determined, *NOS* not otherwise specified, *NST* no special type

These results were in line with DNA gains and losses frequently identified in breast cancer [42–44]. There was very little difference in the DNA copy number profiles when stratified by synchronicity (excluding copy number variations (CNVs) and probes from sex chromosomes) with 59 significantly different genomic regions displaying DNA copy number imbalances (Fig. 1b). Most noticeable were losses of the entire chromosome 14 and the long arm of chromosome 11 in the metachronous subgroup. In contrast, stratification by laterality yielded 134 statistically significant minimal common regions of copy number imbalances, including more fractions of genome altered in the ipsilateral subgroup with prominent losses on 8p and 11p (Fig. 1c).

DNA methylation showed higher variability in synchronous tumours

The variability of the beta values was the highest in the bilateral and synchronous groups and consequently in the BS group, which was in line with patients BS7 and BS8 having the highest variability in methylation patterns between the two respective tumour pairs (Additional file 3: Table S2).

Principal component analysis of the methylation data showed a statistically significant association with synchronicity ($P = 0.007$), while no further associations to other variables were found. Kruskal's non-metric multidimensional scaling (MDS) demonstrated that most of the synchronous samples were further away from each other, while the metachronous samples formed a distinct cluster, suggesting a higher variability of beta values in synchronous samples (Fig. 2).

Strong consensus in clonality could be found for the tumours of patients BM7, BS8, and IS1, while the tumour pairs for patients BS7 and IS4 were determined to be independent primary tumours (Table 2). In general, DNA methylation intensity values were a more liberal method for clonality classification, in particular the clustering analysis, and frequently classified tumour pairs as similar in comparison with other types of molecular data.

Ipsilateral synchronous tumours showed similar gene expression by microarray

The gene expression cohort consisted of seven patients with ipsilateral tumours (three metachronous and four

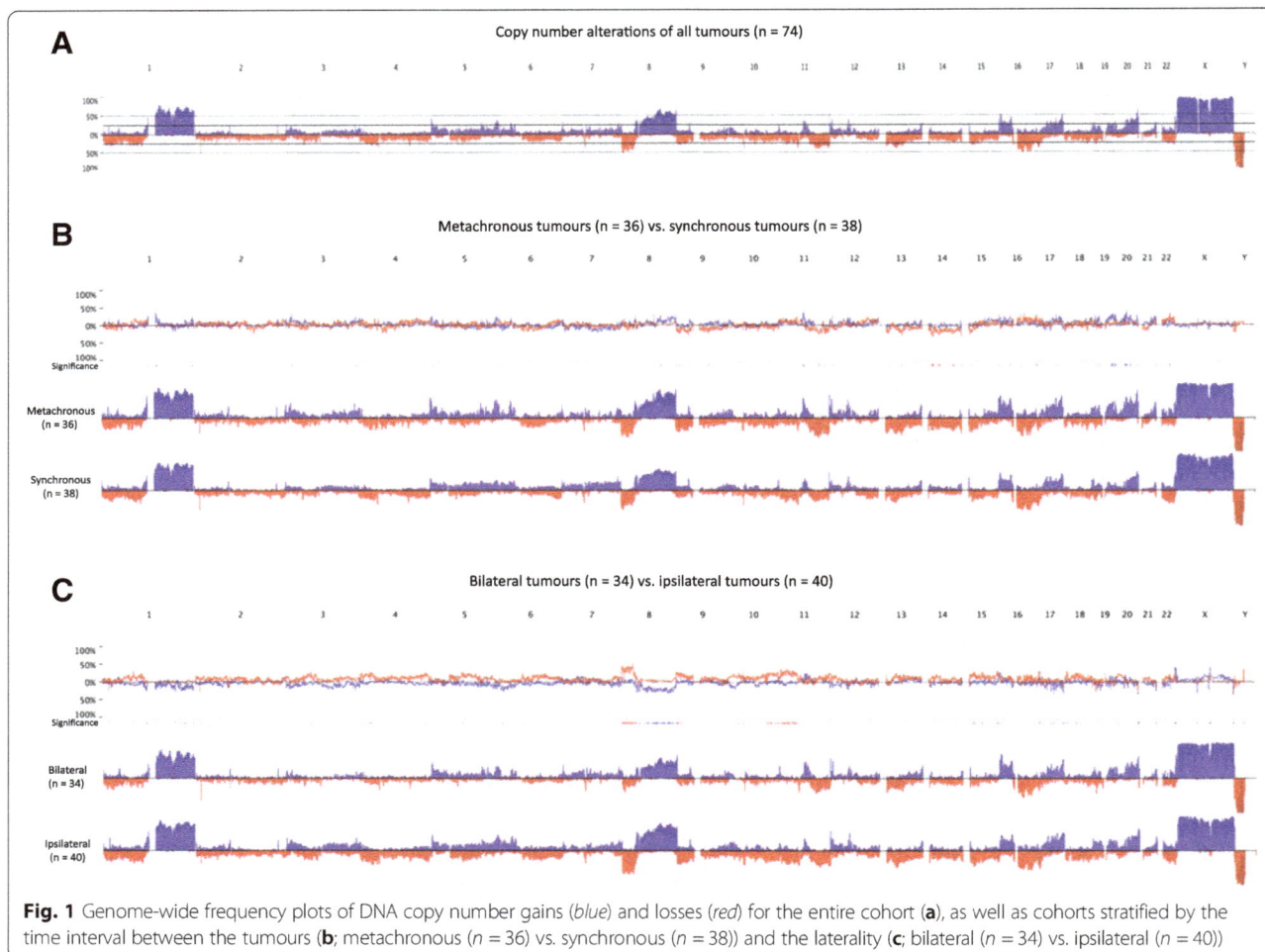

Fig. 1 Genome-wide frequency plots of DNA copy number gains (*blue*) and losses (*red*) for the entire cohort (**a**), as well as cohorts stratified by the time interval between the tumours (**b**; metachronous (*n* = 36) vs. synchronous (*n* = 38)) and the laterality (**c**; bilateral (*n* = 34) vs. ipsilateral (*n* = 40))

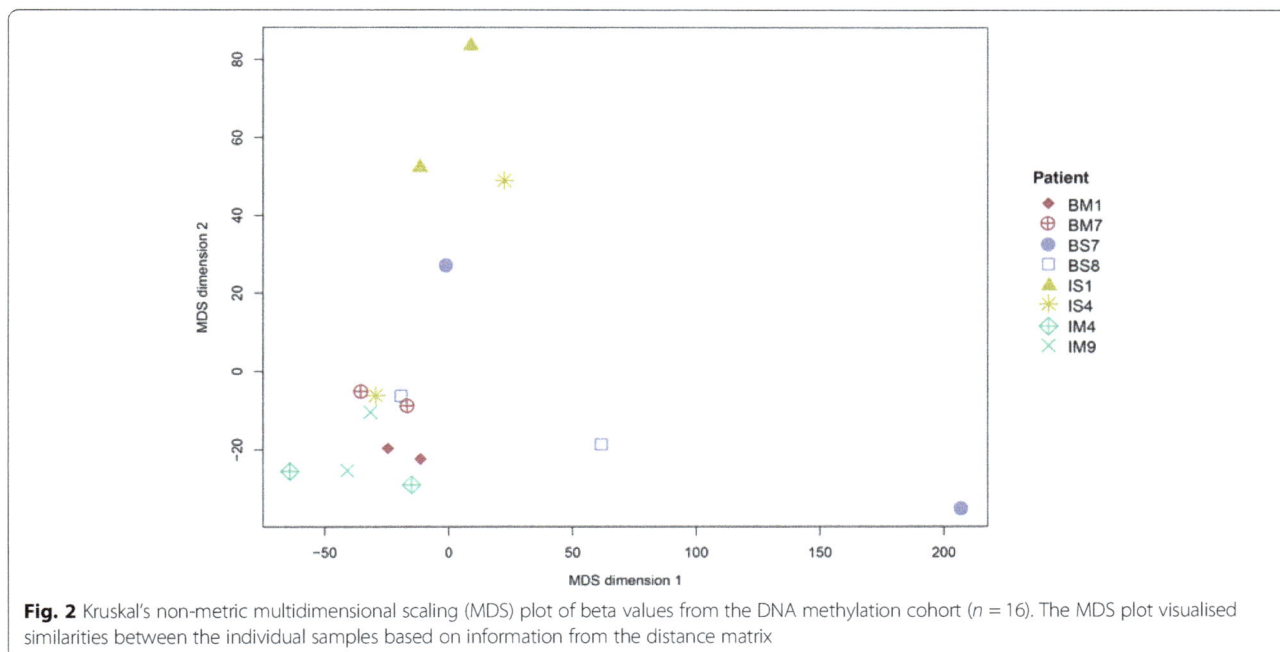

Fig. 2 Kruskal's non-metric multidimensional scaling (MDS) plot of beta values from the DNA methylation cohort ($n = 16$). The MDS plot visualised similarities between the individual samples based on information from the distance matrix

synchronous). The clonality analyses based on gene expression microarray data showed strong concordance to the clinical groups with all four synchronous cases being similar for all analyses while 2/3 metachronous cases were classified as different entities (Additional file 4: Table S3). All analyses of the gene expression cohort were in line with the aCGH results except for patient IM4, whom was classified as independent in the gene expression analysis and equivocal in the aCGH data set. MDS demonstrated similar gene expression patterns between the tumour pairs of the patients IM3, IS3, and IS10 (Additional file 5: Figure S1A).

Varying tendencies for clonality within RNA-seq and SNP data

RNA-seq and SNP genotyping were performed for both tumours of patients IM4, IS10, and IS11. A total of 64 fusion transcripts were detected in the two tumours of patient IM4, with five fusion transcripts (7.8%) containing the same fusion breakpoints in the 5′- and 3′-gene partners in both tumours (Additional file 6: Table S4). For patients IS10 and IS11, 1/836 (0.1%) and 5/153 (3.3%) fusion transcripts were identical between the two tumours, respectively. No other shared fusion transcripts were found between different tumours. The RNA-seq data was then evaluated to identify shared genetic variants in genomic and exonic (coding) regions. Shared genomic variants (genome-wide and the 254-gene panel) showed similar tendencies that were in line with the aCGH distance measure and SNP shared segment (LRR) data (Additional file 7: Table S5). The shared exonic variants in the 254-gene panel only found two shared

mutations in patient IM4, which contradicted most other RNA-seq results. The shared segment and clustering analyses of the SNP array data classified patient IS10 as clonal, which was in line with the aCGH results but contradicted the distance measure and MDS, which classified the LRRs of the tumour pair IM4 as most similar (Additional file 5: Figure S1B). The "Clonality" package applied on the exonic variants classified all tumour pairs as clonal. A circos plot summarising the results of patient IM4 visualised the similarities in copy number profiles of both aCGH-derived $\log_2$ ratio and SNP array-derived LRR and fusion transcripts (Fig. 3).

Tumour clonality defined in 46% of the patients

Calculation of Cohen's kappa indices was applied to detect the highest agreement between the different statistical methods used to estimate clonality. For the aCGH data, hierarchical clustering and the similarity index (SI) were identified as the most appropriate (0.659 and 0.630, respectively). Since the SI is easier to interpret as a measure and independent of the cohort, it presented the most reasonable definition of clonality and determined 46% (17/37) of the tumour pairs as clonal (Fig. 4). No statistical significance was found to associate the tumour clonality defined by the SI with the clinical classification (Wilcoxon rank sum test: $P_{Laterality} = 0.247$; $P_{Synchronicity} = 0.095$; Analysis of variance (ANOVA): $P_{Clinical\ groups} = 0.229$), highlighting the alarming reality that there is very little connection between current clinical guidelines and the biology underlying tumour clonality.

The majority of the analyses conducted were in agreement with the SI except for patients BM1, IM4, IM7,

Table 2 Summary of clonality tests for the methylation cohort ($n = 8$)

	Patients	BM1	BM7	BS7	BS8	IM4	IM9	IS1	IS4
	Laterality	Bilateral	Bilateral	Bilateral	Bilateral	Ipsilateral	Ipsilateral	Ipsilateral	Ipsilateral
	Synchronicity	Metachronous	Metachronous	Synchronous	Synchronous	Metachronous	Metachronous	Synchronous	Synchronous
	Group	BM	BM	BS	BS	IM	IM	IS	IS
aCGH data	**Similarity Index**								
	SI	0.261	0.580	0.323	0.571	0.402	0.237	0.217	0.200
	P_{SI}	25.600	66.450	39.810	65.930	51.650	17.890	10.510	2.710
	P	0.183	**0.005**	0.087	**0.005**	**0.032**	0.269	0.359	0.434
	Clustering (Euclidean distance, single linkage)								
	Clustering	different	similar	different	similar	similar	different	different	different
	Distance measure								
	Euclidean	46.801	19.823	59.036	16.362	43.821	60.220	63.932	66.099
	5th percentile	not sign.	significant	not sign.	significant	not sign.	not sign.	not sign.	not sign.
	Shared segments								
	Segments	34	37	10	32	24	3	53	38
	95th percentile	significant	significant	not sign.	significant	significant	not sign.	significant	significant
	Clonality package								
	LR2	0.044	135.409	0.011	34,945,440	0.008	0.006	0.000	0.001
	P	0.262	**0.009**	0.455	**0.000**	0.519	0.552	0.912	0.879
Methylation data Beta values	**Similarity Index for methylation**								
	SI_{met}	0.879	0.880	0.685	0.815	0.868	0.871	0.911	0.833
	P_{SI}	8.510	8.610	0.000	1.240	7.350	7.660	11.710	3.410
	P	**0.018**	**0.018**	0.947	0.526	**0.018**	**0.018**	**0.018**	0.333
	Clustering (Euclidean distance, single linkage)								
	Clustering	similar	different	different	different	similar	different	similar	different
	Distance measure								
	Euclidean	87.969	86.972	228.809	125.860	92.508	90.574	71.300	134.247
	5th percentile	significant	significant	not sign.	not sign.	not sign.	not sign.	significant	not sign.
Methylation data Intensity values	**Similarity Index**								
	SI	0.578	0.573	0.439	0.594	0.517	0.565	0.648	0.467
	P_{SI}	20.360	19.770	0.000	22.520	11.010	18.650	29.070	1.410
	P	**0.018**	**0.018**	0.737	**0.018**	0.088	**0.018**	**0.018**	0.456
	Clustering (Euclidean distance, single linkage)								
	Clustering	similar	similar	different	similar	similar	similar	similar	similar

Table 2 Summary of clonality tests for the methylation cohort ($n = 8$) (Continued)

Patients	BM1	BM7	BS7	BS8	IM4	IM9	IS1	IS4
Laterality	Bilateral	Bilateral	Bilateral	Bilateral	Ipsilateral	Ipsilateral	Ipsilateral	Ipsilateral
Synchronicity	Metachronous	Metachronous	Synchronous	Synchronous	Metachronous	Metachronous	Synchronous	Synchronous
Group	BM	BM	BS	BS	IM	IM	IS	IS
Distance measure								
Euclidean	148.829	130.060	194.202	158.604	160.988	147.229	124.268	171.320
5th percentile	**significant**	**significant**	not sign.	**significant**	**significant**	**significant**	**significant**	not sign.
Shared segments								
Segments	64	14	9	18	6	11	47	7
95th percentile	**significant**	**significant**	not sign.	**significant**	not sign.	not sign.	**significant**	not sign.
Clonality package								
LR2	4.53	28.46	0.00	241,461,300	300,802.20	1.63	34,907,040,000,000	0.15
P	0.080	**0.036**	0.795	**0.000**	**0.009**	0.107	**0.000**	0.241
Consensus in clonality:	7/13	12/13	0/13	10/13	8/13	4/13	9/13	2/13

P_{SI} percentage of similarities between two tumours that are not due to recurrent chromosomal aberrations or randomness, *LR2* final likelihood ratio with individual comparisons. Statistically significant variables ($P < 0.05$) are displayed in bold text

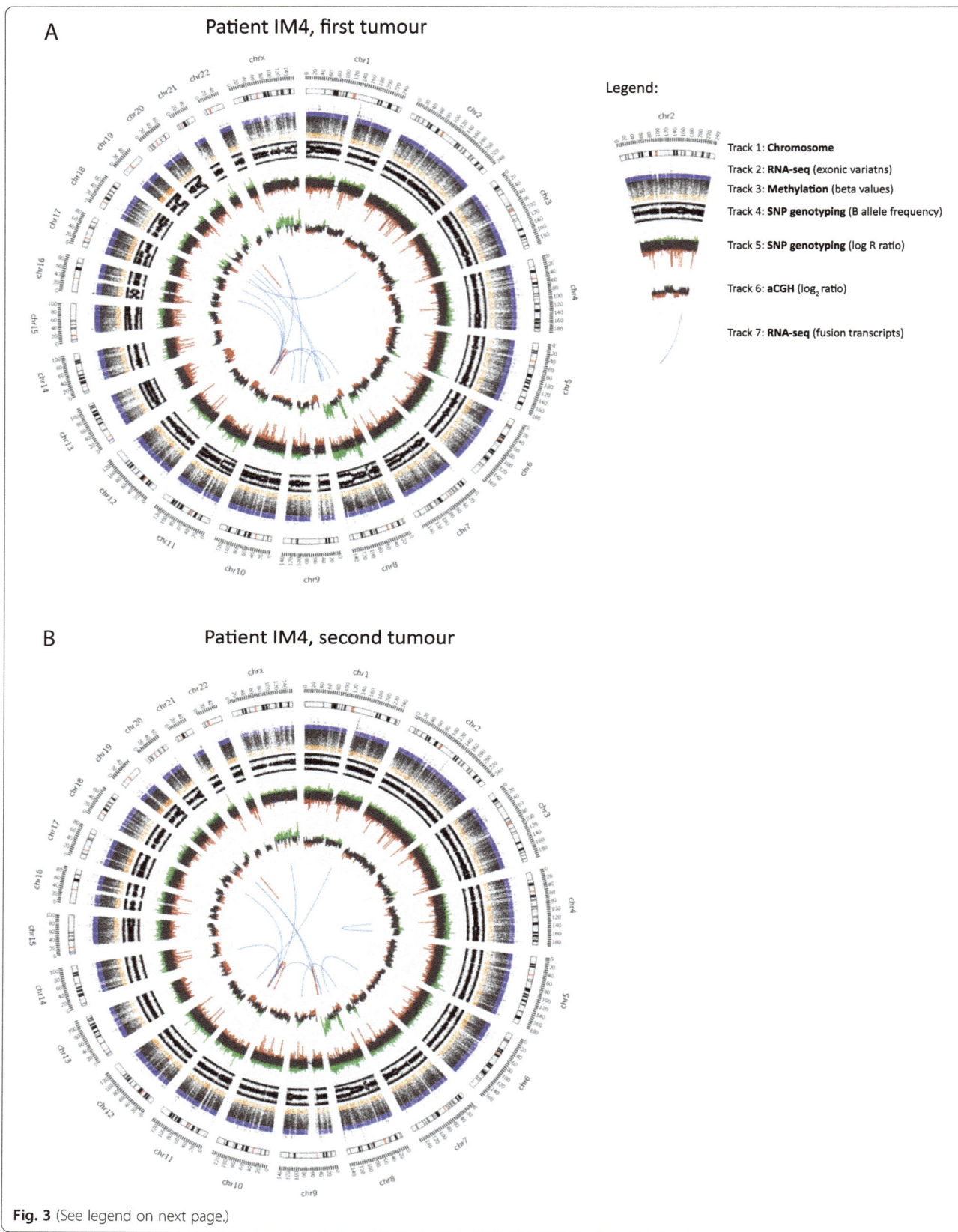

A Patient IM4, first tumour

B Patient IM4, second tumour

Legend:

Track 1: **Chromosome**

Track 2: **RNA-seq** (exonic variatns)

Track 3: **Methylation** (beta values)

Track 4: **SNP genotyping** (B allele frequency)

Track 5: **SNP genotyping** (log R ratio)

Track 6: **aCGH** (log$_2$ ratio)

Track 7: **RNA-seq** (fusion transcripts)

Fig. 3 (See legend on next page.)

(See figure on previous page.)
Fig. 3 Circos plots depicting aCGH-derived DNA copy number profiles, genome-wide SNP genotyping, DNA methylation beta values, and RNA-seq data in the first (**a**) and second (**b**) tumour of breast carcinoma patient IM4. Circos plot *Track 1:* Chromosome cytobands from pter to qter. The centromere is shown as a *red bar. Track 2:* Mutations in exonic regions (exonic variants) identified with RNA-seq data are shown as *dark grey bars. Track 3:* Beta values of DNA methylation data. *Track 4:* B allele frequency of SNP genotyping data. *Track 5:* Log R ratio of SNP genotyping data, where copy number gains and losses are depicted in *green* and *red*, respectively. *Track 6:* Log$_2$ ratio of aCGH data, where copy number gains and losses are depicted in *green* and red, respectively. *Track 7:* Gene fusions identified with RNA-seq data. Intrachromosomal and interchromosomal gene fusions are shown in *red* and *blue lines*, respectively

IS1, and IS7 (Fig. 4). Interestingly, the histopathological concordances often showed opposite tendencies compared to the aCGH analysis. The different methods applied to the DNA methylation, gene expression and SNP array data sets displayed strong homogeneity within their type of data regardless of the method applied. The results for the SI and hierarchical clustering were consistent in most data sets. The distance measure also overlapped with these results but seemed to be a more conservative measure since fewer tumour pairs were classified as clonal. The shared segment analysis with the aCGH data clearly favoured the clonality hypothesis with defining 21/37 tumour pairs as clonal along with 4/8 cases in the methylation intensity data and 1/3 in the LRR data. The shared segment analysis was in most cases consistent between the different types of data.

Discussion

Here, we show that molecular and statistical analyses are powerful tools for classifying clonal recurrences and independent primary tumours. This study provides valuable insight into which molecular technologies were most informative for investigating clonal relatedness in tumour pairs. Although tumour clonality should govern the choice of treatment, bilateral breast tumours are generally treated as different primary tumours and not as potential failure of the previous treatment. Tumour characteristics such as histological subtype, molecular subtype, presence of ductal carcinoma in situ (DCIS), and receptor status are currently used to choose treatment strategies for patients with multiple breast tumours. However, to fully comprehend the association between multiple tumours, routine clinical and diagnostic

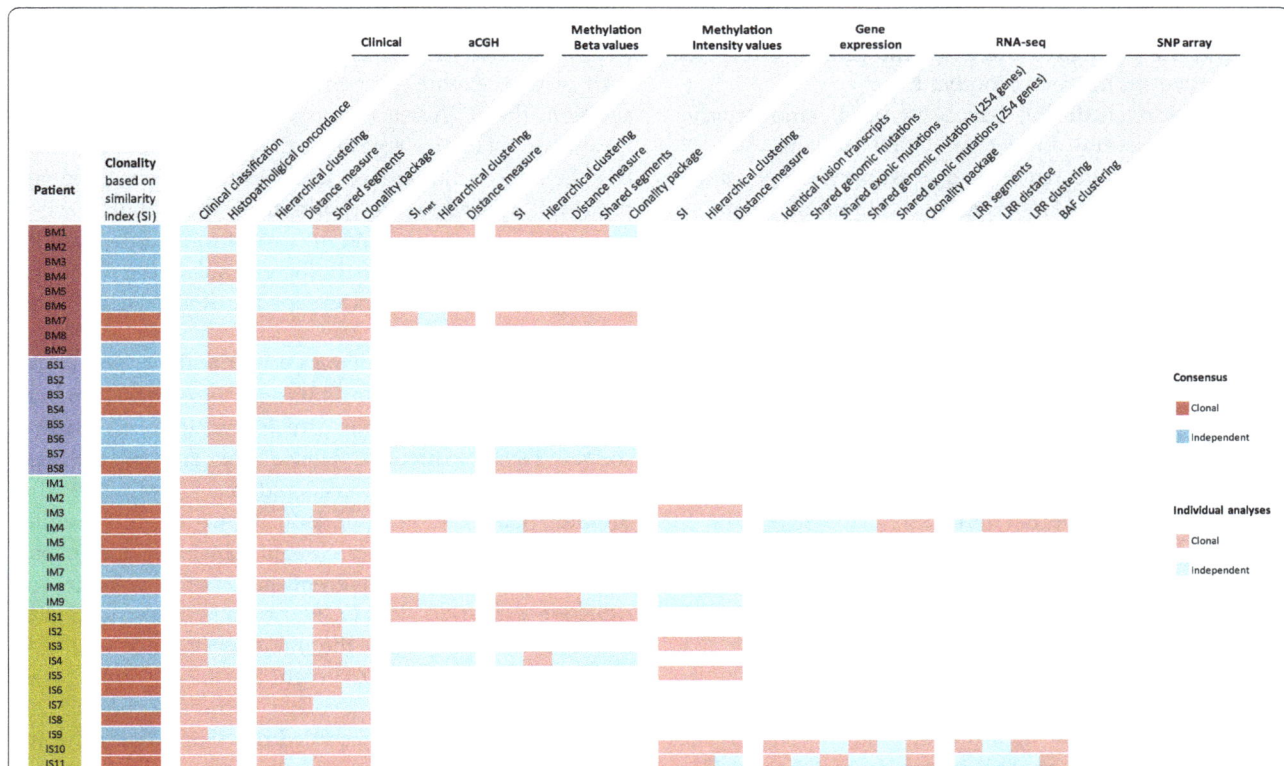

Fig. 4 Overview of the different statistical methods applied sorted by the type of data. *Red boxes* indicate that the analysis defined the tumour pair as clonal and *blue boxes* indicate independence of the tumours. *BAF* B allele frequency, *BM* bilateral-metachronous, *BS* bilateral-synchronous, *IM* ipsilateral-metachronous, *IS* ipsilateral-synchronous, *LRR* log R ratio, *SI* similarity index, *SI$_{met}$* modified SI for methylation data

testing needs to be conducted in conjunction with molecular and bioinformatics methods.

In the majority of the analyses, the type of molecular data analysed had a stronger impact on clonality determination than the analytical method used. This raises the question of which biological phenomenon provides the most stable evidence for clonality. DNA methylation and gene expression are more dynamic than DNA mutations and CNAs, and might therefore be more similar due to environmental factors. CNAs are acquired at early stages of tumourigenesis [45, 46] making them the most stable type of biological data in this study. An overlap of tendencies in clonality between the aCGH and DNA methylation data was seen for only 50% of the cohort (BM7, BS7, BS8, and IS4), giving a less optimistic view on using DNA methylation as a clonality tool compared to results from other reported studies [47, 48]. In the DNA methylation data, synchronicity accounted for more variation than metachronicity, providing further evidence that synchronous tumours are more different from each other with regard to DNA methylation patterns. However, the small cohort size limited the conclusions that can be drawn. The overlap of results between gene expression and copy number data was surprisingly high since gene expression is more unstable than DNA alterations. Gene expression-based analyses defined all IS cases as clonal indicating that gene expression patterns are very similar for tumour cells arising in the same breast at the same time, possibly due to their adjacent microenvironment.

Hierarchical clustering has been used, among other methods, in several studies to define clonality [15, 47, 49]. Clustering is designed as an unsupervised classification tool to discover underlying structures of a data set under the assumption that the number of clusters and their members are unknown. The disadvantage of clustering is that clonality depends on the relationship between individual tumours and the linkage between tumour clusters. Using Euclidean distance with single linkage is the only way to circumvent these disadvantages [37]. The results from the SI and hierarchical clustering analyses exhibited a strong overlap in their classification. Calculation of Cohen's kappa showed the highest agreement of the different analyses for the SI and the clustering. Thus, the SI represented the most suitable approach in defining clonality since it is a specialised technique specifically developed for this purpose and provides easy interpretation.

In the DNA methylation cohort, clustering of the intensity values classified 7/8 tumour pairs as clonal and therefore did not provide a precise segregation between clonally related tumours and independent tumours. The aCGH, DNA methylation intensity and LRR data should biologically refer to the same phenomenon (CNAs) and consequently show the same tendencies for different genomic loci. Therefore, it was unexpected that the results of the clustering and shared segment analysis for those data sets did not show stronger concordance. Furthermore, it was anticipated that the results from the clustering and the distance measure were more in agreement since the first step of clustering is the Euclidean distance. In most cases, the distance measure seemed to be a stricter method than the SI and clustering.

In comparison with genomic variants, mutation analyses based on exonic variants or gene panels represent a subset of the full picture. The different tendencies between the methods represent a drawback for potential applications of sequencing panels in the clinic. The fusion transcript analysis was the only method that did not show any overlaps between patients. Moreover, unspliced fusion transcripts provide the transcribed level of CNAs, which highlights the functional consequences of CNAs and makes them an important tool to assess tumour clonality. Our RNA-seq-based mutation approach had several limitations starting with the lack of matched normal samples to exclude germline mutations and normal DNA nucleotide variations. However, common genetic variants found in the human population were removed. Furthermore, our approach did not account for the frequency of mutations in breast cancer since rare mutations give much stronger evidence for clonality than common mutations [22]. In the frequency-based approach of the "Clonality" package, a further limitation was that RNA-seq data was compared with whole exome sequencing data from TCGA. In addition, the RNA-seq cohort was too small to perform meaningful statistics regarding the 95th percentile, which is a general limitation of using permutation-based approaches. Therefore, the results from this cohort have to be viewed with caution and in context to the other results. Tumours from patient IS10, for example were clonal regarding all other analyses except the RNA-seq and SNP genotyping array.

Whole genome sequencing (WGS) is the more appropriate method to evaluate mutations in comparison with RNA-seq, which does not give information on untranscribed DNA sequences. Hence, the lack of common mutations cannot be considered as a guarantee that tumour pairs are independent. However, intratumour heterogeneity complicates clonality analyses due to biological differences in different parts of a tumour and subclone evolution. In aCGH, contamination with normal cells could diminish the intensity of detected CNAs and small cell populations might not be detected. However, by using only samples that showed a tumour cell content of at least 70%, we ruled out that a lack of clonal relatedness could be due to a lack of tumour cells.

Few studies based on molecular approaches have been conducted to define clonality in multiple breast tumours and there is no consensus on which type of data and analysis method provides the most stable definition of clonality. A direct comparison of these studies to the findings presented here might, however, not be justified due to differences in the study set-up, methods and statistics. In a study on a contralateral cohort using low-coverage WGS, Alkner et al. demonstrated clonal relatedness in 10% (1/10) of the patients [19], which was lower than the clonal relatedness of bilateral tumours in our study (29%, 5/17 patients). Klevebring et al. found 12% (3/25) of their BM cohort to be clonally related using whole exome sequencing (WES) [18], which was also lower than the clonal relatedness of BM tumours in our study (22%, 2/9 patients). Desmedt et al. studied IS tumours and defined 67% (24/36) of the patients as clonal using a targeted mutation screening and 100% (8/8) of the patients as clonal using low-coverage WGS [50]. Our IS cohort showed clonality in 64% (7/11) of the patients, which is surprisingly closer to the mutational approach than the copy number-based approach. Our report is the first, to our knowledge, to compare different approaches (type of molecular data and statistical method) and clinical groups (BM, BS, IM, and IS) between each other.

Conclusions

There are many studies published on tumour clonality using different types of data and statistical methods. Most studies defined their own methods and cohort-specific cut-offs. Currently, there is no consensus about which type of data and especially which statistical analysis is the most suitable and there are surprisingly few studies that compare and evaluate the feasibility of these different approaches. Nonetheless, extremely similar or different tumour pairs (BM7, BS7, IM3, IS4, and IS5) showed consistent results regardless of the statistical analysis or biological data used, but clinic guidelines need to be defined with exact thresholds in order to standardise clonality testing in a routine diagnostic setting. In metachronous cancer, clonality between the first and second tumour may indicate an insufficient effect of the treatment for the first tumour and the patient could benefit from a change in treatment. An independent new primary tumour would indicate a more favourable prognosis than a recurrence. Hence, the discrimination between a clonal and independent origin of the second tumour is of high importance for the patient. In our study, the distance measure proved to be the most conservative method for defining clonality and the shared segment analysis the most liberal. Gene expression data classified all ipsilateral-synchronous cases as clonal, demonstrating that gene expression strongly depends on the nearby tumour microenvironment. The SI using aCGH data was found to be the most suitable method to classify tumour clonality, as it had the highest concordance

with all results and can be easily integrated into clinic routine using FFPE samples to obtain copy number data. But most importantly, the definition of tumour clonality based on the current clinicopathological markers needs to be revised due to the limited intersects between current clinical guidelines and the underlying biology of tumour clonality.

Additional files

Additional file 1: Supplementary Methods. Description of nucleic acid isolation and purification, aCGH gene expression microarray, RNA-seq and SNP array analysis. (DOCX 37 kb)

Additional file 2: Table S1. Overview of clinical characteristics of the patient and tumour information stratified by the clinical groups (BM, BS, IM, and IS). (XLSX 16 kb)

Additional file 3: Table S2. Variabilities of the studied sample groups with the variability spanning between 5th and 95th percentile of the beta values. (XLSX 10 kb)

Additional file 4: Table S3. Summary of clonality tests for the gene expression microarray cohort ($n = 7$). (XLSX 14 kb)

Additional file 5: Figure S1. Non-metric multidimensional scaling (MDS) plot of (**A**) normalised $\log_2$ ratios from gene expression data, and (**B**) LRR values from SNP array data. The MDS plot visualised similarities between the individual samples based on information from the distance matrix. (TIF 1784 kb)

Additional file 6: Table S4. Overview of the shared fusion transcripts in patient IM4, IS10, and IS11. (XLSX 13 kb)

Additional file 7: Table S5. Summary of clonality tests for the RNA-seq and SNP genotyping cohort ($n = 6$). (XLSX 14 kb)

Abbreviations
aCGH: Array comparative genomic hybridization; ANOVA: Analysis of variance; BAF: B allele frequency; BM: bilateral-metachronous; BS: bilateral-synchronous; CGH: Comparative genomic hybridization; CNA: Copy number alteration; CNV: Copy number variation; DCIS: Ductal carcinoma in situ; ER: Oestrogen receptor status; FFPE: Formalin-fixed paraffin-embedded; HER2: Human epidermal growth factor receptor 2 status; IM: Ipsilateral-metachronous; IS: Ipsilateral-synchronous; LR2: Likelihood ratio with individual comparisons; LRR: Log R ratio; MDS: Kruskal's non-metric multidimensional scaling; NOS: Not otherwise specified; NST: No special type; RNA-seq: RNA sequencing; SI: Similarity index; SI_{met}: Modified SI for methylation data; SNP: Single nucleotide polymorphism; WES: Whole exome sequencing; WGS: Whole genome sequencing

Acknowledgements
We are grateful to BILS (Bioinformatics Infrastructure for Life Sciences) and NBIS (National Bioinformatics Infrastructure Sweden) for their bioinformatics support.

Funding
This work was supported by grants from the Stiftelsen Assar Gabrielssons Fond (FB 17–09; JB), the Swedish Cancer Society (CAN 2012/406; CAN 2015/311; K H), the King Gustav V Jubilee Clinic Cancer Research Foundation (2016:65; KH), and the LUA/ALF-agreement in West of Sweden healthcare region (PK).

Authors' contributions

KH and PK were responsible for overall study concept. JB, TZP, and AD were responsible for the design of experiments. PK, AD, JB, AK, and EWR collected the clinical data. TZP, and HE contributed to the bioinformatics analyses. SN contributed to the statistical analyses. EWR and EFA provided technical and material support. AD, TZP and JB performed the experiments. JB analysed the data, performed the statistical analyses, and wrote the manuscript. All authors reviewed, edited, and approved the final manuscript.

Authors' information

KH and PK share last author status.

Competing interests

The authors declare that they have no competing interests.

Author details

[1]Department of Oncology, Institute of Clinical Sciences, Sahlgrenska Cancer Center, Sahlgrenska Academy at University of Gothenburg, Box 425, SE-405 30 Gothenburg, Sweden. [2]Swedish Hip Arthroplasty Register, 405 30 Gothenburg, Sweden. [3]Department of Clinical Pathology and Genetics, Sahlgrenska University Hospital, 413 45 Gothenburg, Sweden. [4]Department of Radiation Physics, Institute of Clinical Sciences, Sahlgrenska Cancer Center, Sahlgrenska Academy at University of Gothenburg, 405 30 Gothenburg, Sweden.

References

1. Raymond JS, Hogue CJ. Multiple primary tumours in women following breast cancer, 1973-2000. Br J Cancer. 2006;94(11):1745–50.
2. Chen Y, Thompson W, Semenciw R, Mao Y. Epidemiology of contralateral breast cancer. Cancer Epidemiol Biomark Prev. 1999;8(10):855–61.
3. Vaittinen P, Hemminki K. Risk factors and age-incidence relationships for contralateral breast cancer. Int J Cancer. 2000;88(6):998–1002.
4. Dawson PJ, Maloney T, Gimotty P, Juneau P, Ownby H, Wolman SR. Bilateral breast cancer: one disease or two? Breast Cancer Res Treat. 1991;19(3):233–44.
5. Begg CB, Eng KH, Hummer AJ. Statistical tests for clonality. Biometrics. 2007; 63(2):522–30.
6. Nowell PC. The clonal evolution of tumor cell populations. Science. 1976; 194(4260):23–8.
7. Lannin DR, Haffty BG. End results of salvage therapy after failure of breast-conservation surgery. Oncology (Williston Park). 2004;18(3):272–9. discussion 280–272, 285–276, 292
8. Chaudary MA, Millis RR, Hoskins EO, Halder M, Bulbrook RD, Cuzick J, Hayward JL. Bilateral primary breast cancer: a prospective study of disease incidence. Br J Surg. 1984;71(9):711–4.
9. Noguchi S, Motomura K, Inaji H, Imaoka S, Koyama H. Differentiation of primary and secondary breast cancer with clonal analysis. Surgery. 1994; 115(4):458–62.
10. Intra M, Rotmensz N, Viale G, Mariani L, Bonanni B, Mastropasqua MG, Galimberti V, Gennari R, Veronesi P, Colleoni M, et al. Clinicopathologic characteristics of 143 patients with synchronous bilateral invasive breast carcinomas treated in a single institution. Cancer. 2004;101(5):905–12.
11. Imyanitov EN, Suspitsin EN, Grigoriev MY, Togo AV, Kuligina E, Belogubova EV, Pozharisski KM, Turkevich EA, Rodriquez C, Cornelisse CJ, et al. Concordance of allelic imbalance profiles in synchronous and metachronous bilateral breast carcinomas. Int J Cancer. 2002;100(5):557–64.
12. Saad RS, Denning KL, Finkelstein SD, Liu Y, Pereira TC, Lin X, Silverman JF. Diagnostic and prognostic utility of molecular markers in synchronous bilateral breast carcinoma. Mod Pathol. 2008;21(10):1200–7.
13. Waldman FM, DeVries S, Chew KL, Moore DH 2nd, Kerlikowske K, Ljung BM. Chromosomal alterations in ductal carcinomas in situ and their in situ recurrences. J Natl Cancer Inst. 2000;92(4):313–20.
14. Park SC, Hwang UK, Ahn SH, Gong GY, Yoon HS. Genetic changes in bilateral breast cancer by comparative genomic hybridisation. Clin Exp Med. 2007;7(1):1–5.
15. Bollet MA, Servant N, Neuvial P, Decraene C, Lebigot I, Meyniel JP, De Rycke Y, Savignoni A, Rigaill G, Hupe P, et al. High-resolution mapping of DNA breakpoints to define true recurrences among ipsilateral breast cancers. J Natl Cancer Inst. 2008;100(1):48–58.
16. Brommesson S, Jonsson G, Strand C, Grabau D, Malmstrom P, Ringner M, Ferno M, Hedenfalk I. Tiling array-CGH for the assessment of genomic similarities among synchronous unilateral and bilateral invasive breast cancer tumor pairs. BMC Clin Pathol. 2008;8:6.
17. Castellarin M, Milne K, Zeng T, Tse K, Mayo M, Zhao Y, Webb JR, Watson PH, Nelson BH, Holt RA. Clonal evolution of high-grade serous ovarian carcinoma from primary to recurrent disease. J Pathol. 2013;229(4):515–24.
18. Klevebring D, Lindberg J, Rockberg J, Hilliges C, Hall P, Sandberg M, Czene K. Exome sequencing of contralateral breast cancer identifies metastatic disease. Breast Cancer Res Treat. 2015;151(2):319–24.
19. Alkner S, Tang MH, Brueffer C, Dahlgren M, Chen Y, Olsson E, Winter C, Baker S, Ehinger A, Ryden L, et al. Contralateral breast cancer can represent a metastatic spread of the first primary tumor: determination of clonal relationship between contralateral breast cancers using next-generation whole genome sequencing. Breast Cancer Res. 2015;17:102.
20. Ostrovnaya I, Seshan VE, Begg CB. Comparison of properties of tests for assessing tumor clonality. Biometrics. 2008;64(4):1018–22.
21. Nemes S, Danielsson A, Parris TZ, Jonasson JM, Bulow E, Karlsson P, Steineck G, Helou K. A diagnostic algorithm to identify paired tumors with clonal origin. Genes Chromosomes Cancer. 2013;52(11):1007–16.
22. Ostrovnaya I, Seshan VE, Begg CB. Using somatic mutation data to test tumors for clonal relatedness. Ann Appl Stat. 2015;9(3):1533–48.
23. Hu H, Li J, Plank A, Wang H, Daggard G. Comparative Study of Classification Methods for Microarray Data Analysis. In: Proceedings of the Fifth Australasian Conference on Data Mining and Analystics: 2006; Sydney, Australia edn, vol. 2006: Inc: Australian Computer Society. 2006;61:33–37.
24. Parris TZ, Danielsson A, Nemes S, Kovacs A, Delle U, Fallenius G, Mollerstrom E, Karlsson P, Helou K. Clinical implications of gene dosage and gene expression patterns in diploid breast carcinoma. Clin Cancer Res. 2010; 16(15):3860–74.
25. Goldhirsch A, Wood WC, Coates AS, Gelber RD, Thurlimann B, Senn HJ. Strategies for subtypes--dealing with the diversity of breast cancer: highlights of the St. Gallen international expert consensus on the primary therapy of early breast Cancer 2011. Ann Oncol. 2011;22(8):1736–47.
26. Hupe P, Stransky N, Thiery JP, Radvanyi F, Barillot E. Analysis of array CGH data: from signal ratio to gain and loss of DNA regions. Bioinformatics. 2004; 20(18):3413–22.
27. R Core Team. R: A Language and Environment for Statistical Computing: R Foundation for Statistical Computing; 2018.
28. Ostrovnaya I, Seshan VE, Olshen A, Begg CB. Clonality: an R package for testing clonal relatedness of two tumors from the same patient based on their genomic profiles. Bioinformatics. 2011;27:1698–9.
29. Seshan and Olshen: DNAcopy: A Package for Analyzing DNA Copy Data. 2010.
30. Assenov Y, Muller F, Lutsik P, Walter J, Lengauer T, Bock C. Comprehensive analysis of DNA methylation data with RnBeads. Nat Meth. 2014;11(11): 1138–40.
31. Teschendorff AE, Marabita F, Lechner M, Bartlett T, Tegner J, Gomez-Cabrero D, Beck S. A beta-mixture quantile normalization method for correcting probe design bias in Illumina Infinium 450 k DNA methylation data. Bioinformatics. 2013;29(2):189–96.
32. Feber A, Guilhamon P, Lechner M, Fenton T, Wilson GA, Thirlwell C, Morris TJ, Flanagan AM, Teschendorff AE, Kelly JD, et al. Using high-density DNA methylation arrays to profile copy number alterations. Genome Biol. 2014; 15(2):R30.
33. Morris TJ, Butcher LM, Feber A, Teschendorff AE, Chakravarthy AR, Wojdacz TK, Beck S. ChAMP: 450k Chip analysis methylation pipeline. Bioinformatics. 2014;30(3):428–30.

34. Hovestadt V, Zapatka M. conumee: Enhanced copy-number variation analysis using Illumina DNA methylation arrays. In: R package version 1.9.0 edn; 2017.

35. Lampa S, Dahlo M, Olason PI, Hagberg J, Spjuth O. Lessons learned from implementing a national infrastructure in Sweden for storage and analysis of next-generation sequencing data. Gigascience. 2013;2(1):9.

36. Du P, Zhang X, Huang C-C, Jafari N, Kibbe WA, Hou L, Lin SM. Comparison of Beta-value and M-value methods for quantifying methylation levels by microarray analysis. BMC Bioinformatics. 2010;11:587.

37. Ostrovnaya I, Begg CB. Testing clonal relatedness of tumors using Array comparative genomic hybridization: a statistical challenge. Clin Cancer Res. 2010;16(5):1358.

38. Begg CB, Ostrovnaya I, Geyer FC, Papanastasiou AD, Ng CKY, Sakr RA, Bernstein JL, Burke KA, King TA, Piscuoglio S, et al. Contralateral breast cancers: independent cancers or metastases? Int J Cancer. 2018;142(2):347–56. https://doi.org/10.1002/ijc.31051.

39. TCGA. The Cancer Genome Atlas (TCGA). https://cancergenome.nih.gov/.

40. Cohen J. A coefficient of agreement for nominal scales. Educ Psychol Meas. 1960;20(1):37–46.

41. Lo Martire R. rel: Reliability Coefficients. version 1.3.1 ed; 2017.

42. Hicks J, Krasnitz A, Lakshmi B, Navin NE, Riggs M, Leibu E, Esposito D, Alexander J, Troge J, Grubor V, et al. Novel patterns of genome rearrangement and their association with survival in breast cancer. Genome Res. 2006;16(12):1465–79.

43. Fridlyand J, Snijders AM, Ylstra B, Li H, Olshen A, Segraves R, Dairkee S, Tokuyasu T, Ljung BM, Jain AN, et al. Breast tumor copy number aberration phenotypes and genomic instability. BMC Cancer. 2006;6(1):96.

44. Haverty PM, Fridlyand J, Li L, Getz G, Beroukhim R, Lohr S, Wu TD, Cavet G, Zhang Z, Chant J. High-resolution genomic and expression analyses of copy number alterations in breast tumors. Genes Chromosomes Cancer. 2008; 47(6):530–42.

45. Gao R, Davis A, McDonald TO, Sei E, Shi X, Wang Y, Tsai PC, Casasent A, Waters J, Zhang H, et al. Punctuated copy number evolution and clonal stasis in triple-negative breast cancer. Nat Genet. 2016;48(10):1119–30.

46. Wang Y, Waters J, Leung ML, Unruh A, Roh W, Shi X, Chen K, Scheet P, Vattathil S, Liang H, et al. Clonal evolution in breast cancer revealed by single nucleus genome sequencing. Nature. 2014;512(7513):155–60.

47. Moarii M, Pinheiro A, Sigal-Zafrani B, Fourquet A, Caly M, Servant N, Stoven V, Vert JP, Reyal F. Epigenomic alterations in breast carcinoma from primary tumor to locoregional recurrences. PLoS One. 2014;9(8):e103986.

48. Huang KT, Mikeska T, Li J, Takano EA, Millar EK, Graham PH, Boyle SE, Campbell IG, Speed TP, Dobrovic A, et al. Assessment of DNA methylation profiling and copy number variation as indications of clonal relationship in ipsilateral and contralateral breast cancers to distinguish recurrent breast cancer from a second primary tumour. BMC Cancer. 2015;15:669.

49. Song F, Li X, Song F, Zhao Y, Li H, Zheng H, Gao Z, Wang J, Zhang W, Chen K. Comparative genomic analysis reveals bilateral breast cancers are genetically independent. Oncotarget. 2015;6(31):31820–9.

50. Desmedt C, Fumagalli D, Pietri E, Zoppoli G, Brown D, Nik-Zainal S, Gundem G, Rothe F, Majjaj S, Garuti A, et al. Uncovering the genomic heterogeneity of multifocal breast cancer. J Pathol. 2015;236(4):457–66.

16

SNAI2 upregulation is associated with an aggressive phenotype in fulvestrant-resistant breast cancer cells and is an indicator of poor response to endocrine therapy in estrogen receptor-positive metastatic breast cancer

Carla L. Alves[1]*, Daniel Elias[1], Maria B. Lyng[1], Martin Bak[2] and Henrik J. Ditzel[1,3,4]*

Abstract

Background: Endocrine resistance in estrogen receptor-positive (ER+) breast cancer is a major clinical problem and is associated with accelerated cancer cell growth, increased motility and acquisition of mesenchymal characteristics. However, the specific molecules and pathways involved in these altered features remain to be detailed, and may be promising therapeutic targets to overcome endocrine resistance.

Methods: In the present study, we evaluated altered expression of epithelial-mesenchymal transition (EMT) regulators in ER+ breast cancer cell models of tamoxifen or fulvestrant resistance, by gene expression profiling. We investigated the specific role of increased SNAI2 expression in fulvestrant-resistant cells by gene knockdown and treatment with a SNAIL-p53 binding inhibitor, and evaluated the effect on cell growth, migration and expression of EMT markers. Furthermore, we evaluated SNAI2 expression by immunohistochemical analysis in metastatic samples from two cohorts of patients with breast cancer treated with endocrine therapy in the advanced setting.

Results: SNAI2 was found to be significantly upregulated in all endocrine-resistant cells compared to parental cell lines, while no changes were observed in the expression of other EMT-associated transcription factors. SNAI2 knockdown with specific small interfering RNA (siRNA) converted the mesenchymal-like fulvestrant-resistant cells into an epithelial-like phenotype and reduced cell motility. Furthermore, inhibition of SNAI2 with specific siRNA or a SNAIL-p53 binding inhibitor reduced growth of cells resistant to fulvestrant treatment. Clinical evaluation of SNAI2 expression in two independent cohorts of patients with ER+ metastatic breast cancer treated with endocrine therapy in the advanced setting ($N = 86$ and $N = 67$) showed that high SNAI2 expression in the metastasis correlated significantly with shorter progression-free survival on endocrine treatment ($p = 0.0003$ and $p = 0.004$).

(Continued on next page)

* Correspondence: calves@health.sdu.dk; hditzel@health.sdu.dk
[1]Department of Cancer and Inflammation Research, Institute of Molecular Medicine, University of Southern Denmark, J.B. Winsløwsvej 25, 5000 Odense C, Denmark
Full list of author information is available at the end of the article

(Continued from previous page)

Conclusions: Our results suggest that SNAI2 is a key regulator of the aggressive phenotype observed in endocrine-resistant breast cancer cells, an independent prognostic biomarker in ER+ advanced breast cancer treated with endocrine therapy, and may be a promising therapeutic target in combination with endocrine therapies in ER+ metastatic breast cancer exhibiting high SNAI2 levels.

Keywords: Endocrine resistance, Epithelial-mesenchymal transition, Estrogen receptor-positive breast cancer, Fulvestrant, SNAI2

Background

Approximately 80% of all breast tumors are positive for estrogen receptor (ER+), which is an indicator of potential responsiveness to endocrine therapy both in the adjuvant and advanced settings [1]. Despite the efficacy of endocrine therapy for treatment of ER+ breast cancer, a significant number of patients develop resistance to these drugs. There is considerable evidence suggesting that acquisition of endocrine resistance is accompanied by accelerated tumor growth and increased metastatic propensity, and is associated with morphological changes characteristic of cells undergoing epithelial-mesenchymal transition (EMT) [2]. However, key questions remain regarding the central molecules controlling the EMT process during development of endocrine resistance, which may be promising therapeutic targets in combination with endocrine therapy.

EMT is a complex process characterized by loss of epithelial features, such as downregulation of the E-cadherin and occludins, and acquisition of mesenchymal properties, including upregulation of vimentin and fibronectin, and cytoskeleton reorganization [3]. EMT has been associated with increased cell migration capacity and invasiveness, and is a prominent hallmark of cancer progression [4, 5]. Epithelial tumor cells may acquire a mesenchymal-like phenotype to facilitate migration and invasion and then possibly reverse to an epithelial state through mesenchymal-epithelial transition (MET) to form organized tumorigenic nodules at the lodgment sites [6]. EMT and MET are regulated by signals from the stroma associated with tumors, such as transforming growth factor (TGF)-β, and by a series of EMT-inducing transcription factors, including SNAI1, SNAI2, TWIST, ZEB1 and ZEB2 [7].

The role of EMT in endocrine resistance was first reported in studies on ER-depleted breast cancer cells, which were found to convert the non-invasive epithelial features into a mesenchymal-like phenotype with invasive characteristics [6, 8]. Moreover, EMT has been shown to mediate endocrine resistance through the action of EMT transcription factors. SNAI family members were found to directly repress ER [9, 10] and enhance the anti-apoptotic behavior of cancer cells, contributing to resistance to therapy [11]. A large body of evidence supports the importance of EMT in sustaining cancer stem cells (CSCs), which can be intrinsically resistant to treatment [12].

Furthermore, several growth factor receptors, such as epidermal growth factor receptor (EGFR), insulin-like growth factor 1 receptor (IGF-1R) and fibroblast growth factor 1 receptor (FGFR1), which are involved in the EMT process, are highly expressed in ER- breast tumor cells, supporting the link between EMT and insensitivity to endocrine therapy [2]. The emerging role of EMT as a mediator of endocrine resistance in breast cancer has raised interest in therapeutic strategies based on reversing EMT to prevent tumor progression and re-sensitizing tumor cells to endocrine therapy [13]. One promising pharmacological approach involves the development of specific inhibitors of EMT-associated transcription factors to therapeutically inhibit EMT induction or target the mesenchymal cell type [14].

In this study, we investigated the altered expression of various EMT regulators in MCF-7-based breast cancer cell models of endocrine resistance by gene array. We observed upregulation of SNAI2 in fulvestrant-resistant and tamoxifen-resistant cells compared to the parental cell lines, while other EMT-associated transcription factors were not altered. Inhibition of SNAI2 induced epithelial characteristics, reduced cell motility, and impaired growth of fulvestrant-resistant breast cancer cells. High levels of SNAI2 in ER+ metastatic tumor samples from two cohorts of patients treated with endocrine therapy in the advanced setting correlated significantly with poor clinical outcome. Our findings indicated SNAI2 as an independent prognosis biomarker in ER+ metastatic breast cancer patients treated with endocrine therapy and a potential novel therapeutic target that may contribute to reversing EMT and re-sensitizing breast cancer cells to endocrine therapy.

Methods

Cell lines and culture conditions

The original MCF-7 cell line was obtained from the Breast Cancer Task Force Cell Culture Bank, Mason Research Institute. MCF-7 cells were gradually adapted to grow in low serum concentration [15], and this subline, MCF-7/S0.5, was used to establish two fulvestrant-resistant cell models, MCF-7/182R (including 182R-1 and 182R-6 cell lines) and MCF-7/164R (including 164R-1 and 164R-4 cell lines), by extended treatment with 100 nM of fulvestrant

(ICI 182,780) or ICI 164,384, respectively [16]. Tamoxifen-resistant (TamR) cell lines, including TamR-1, TamR-4, TamR-7 and TamR-8 cells, were established from MCF-7/S0.5 by long-term treatment with 1 μM of tamoxifen [17]. The MCF-7/S0.5 cell line was routinely propagated in phenol red-free Dulbecco's modified Eagle medium (DMEM)/F12 (Gibco) supplemented with 1% glutamine (Gibco), 1% heat-inactivated fetal bovine serum (FBS; Gibco) and 6 ng/ml insulin (Sigma-Aldrich). Fulvestrant-resistant and tamoxifen-resistant cell lines were maintained in the same growth medium as MCF-7/S0.5 supplemented with 100 nM fulvestrant (Tocris) or 1 μM tamoxifen (Sigma-Aldrich), respectively. Cells were grown in a humidified atmosphere of 5% CO_2 at 37 °C and the growth medium was renewed every second or third day. To reduce variability between experiments, cells were maintained at low passage numbers (< 10 passages) throughout the experiments. All cell lines underwent DNA authentication using Cell ID™ System (Promega) before the described experiments to ensure consistent cell identity.

Global gene expression profiling
MCF-7/S0.5, tamoxifen-resistant and fulvestrant-resistant cell lines were grown to 70–80% confluence for total RNA purification using a RNA kit (Qiagen) and arrayed separately in Affymetrix Gene Chip® Human Genome U133 plus 2.0 arrays (Affymetrix), as described [18]. Data were analyzed using Partek Genomic Suite (Partek Inc.). Genes from the data set that exhibited twofold or greater alteration in expression and false discovery rate (FDR) cutoff < 0.05 were considered as significantly altered regulated.

RNA isolation and reverse transcription (RT)-quantitative (q)PCR (RT-qPCR)
Total RNA was extracted using Isol-Lysis Reagent, TRIzol® (Life technologies) followed by chloroform and isopropyl alcohol (Sigma-Aldrich) for separation and precipitation of RNA. Concentration and purity were measured using the NanoDrop-1000 spectrophotometer (Saveen). Complementary DNA (cDNA) was synthesized using RevertAid Premium Reverse Transcriptase kit (Fermentas). Relative quantification of gene expression was performed using SYBR® Green PCR Mastermix (Applied Biosystems) according to manufacturer's instructions. The following primers purchased from Qiagen were used: SNAI2 (QT00044128), CDH1 (QT00080143), and PUM1 (QT00029421) QuantiTect® Primer. PUM1 was used as the reference gene for normalization. RT-qPCR reactions were performed on a StepOnePlus™ Real-Time PCR system from Applied Biosystems and data were obtained from StepOne Software Version 2.1. Relative

expression levels were calculated using the comparative threshold method [19].

Western blotting
Whole cell extracts were obtained using radioimmunoprecipitation assay (RIPA) buffer (50 mM Tris HCl (pH 8), 150 mM NaCl (pH 8), 1% IgePAL 630, 0.5% sodium dioxycholate, 0.1% SDS) containing protease and phosphatase inhibitors (Roche). The protein concentration of the lysate samples was determined using Pierce bicinchoninic acid (BCA) Protein Assay Kit (Thermo Fisher Scientific) and the optical density (OD) was measured at 562 nm in the microplate reader Sunrise™ 500 ELISA-reader (Tecan). 10–20 μg of total protein lysate was loaded on a 4–20% SDS-PAGE gel (Biorad) under reducing conditions and electroblotted onto a polyvinylidene difluoride (PVDF) transfer membrane. Prior to primary antibody incubation, membranes were blocked in Tris-buffered saline (TBS), 0.1% Tween-20 (Sigma-Aldrich) containing 5% non-fat dry milk powder (Sigma-Aldrich) or 5% bovine serum albumin (Sigma-Aldrich). The following antibodies were used according to the manufacturer's protocol: anti-E-cadherin (#3195, Cell Signaling), anti-SNAI2 (#9585, Cell Signaling); anti-vimentin (#6630, Sigma-Aldrich); anti-ERα antibody (#9101, Thermo Fisher Scientific); anti-SOX2 (#AF2018, R&D Systems); anti-β-actin (#6276, Abcam) as loading control; horseradish peroxidase (HRP)-conjugated goat anti-mouse (#P0447, Dako); HRP-conjugated goat anti-rabbit (#P0448, Dako); HRP-conjugated donkey anti-goat (#sc-2020, Santa Cruz Biotechnology). The membrane was developed with Enhanced Chemiluminescence (ECL) Prime Western Blotting Detection Reagents (GE Healthcare) and visualized using the Fusion-Fx7–7026 WL/26MX instrument (Vilbaer).

siRNA-mediated gene knockdown
Cells were transfected with siRNA against SNAI2 (s13127; Life Technologies) or SOX2 (D-011778-01; Dharmacon) using an Electroporation Ingenio kit (Mirus Bio) in a Nucleofector™ II device (Amaxa, Lonza) or Lipofectamine 3000 reagent (Thermo Fischer Scientific), respectively, according to manufacturers' instructions. Mission siRNA Universal Negative Control (SIC001) (Sigma-Aldrich) was used as control. Transfected cells were seeded in 24-well plates (5×10^4 cells/well) to evaluate gene knockdown efficiency 48 h following transfection, by RT-qPCR. Transfected cells were seeded in T25 flasks (5×10^5 cells) and incubated for 96 h to assess protein expression by western blotting.

Cell growth assay
Transfected cells were seeded ($2.5–5 \times 10^4$ cells/well) in 24-well plates and incubated for 24 and 96 h at 37 °C in

5% CO_2 for evaluation of cell growth using crystal violet-based colorimetric assay [20]. For growth assays with the chemical inhibitor, cells were seeded (3×10^4 cells/well) in 24-well plates in the presence of 3 μM SNAIL-p53 binding inhibitor GN25 (Millipore) or its solvent (DMSO, Sigma-Aldrich), and cell growth was measured 72 h after seeding using crystal violet-based colorimetric assay. The OD was analyzed at 570 nm in a Sunrise™ 500 absorbance reader (Tecan).

Cell migration assay

A total of 1×10^5 cells, starved overnight, were harvested in serum-free medium and seeded in the upper chamber of 8-μm-pore polystyrene membrane chamber-insert Transwell® apparatus (Corning, Costar) in 24-well plates with 10% FBS medium, according to the manufacturer's instructions. Cells were incubated for 96 h at 37 °C in 5% CO_2. Cells on the top surface of the insert were removed with a cotton swab, and cells that migrated to the bottom face of the insert were fixed and stained with crystal violet in methanol solution. To determine the number of migrated cells, five random fields were used to count cells at the microscope. To determine the total number of cells that migrated in one insert, the average number of cells counted was divided by the area of the microscope viewing field and then multiplied by the entire area of the Transwell insert (0.3 cm^2). Normalization of migration according to growth rate was performed using crystal violet staining.

Cell invasion assay

Cell invasion was evaluated using a QCM ECMatrix 24-well kit (Chemicon ECM550) according to the manufacturer's instructions. Cells were seeded in serum-free medium in the upper chamber of an insert in 24-well plates with 10% FBS medium, and incubated for 96 h at 37 °C in 5% CO_2. Invading cells were detached, lysed, stained with dye, and measured by fluorescent light emission (480 nm/520 nm) using a Victor3™ 1420 counter (Perkin Elmer Wallac). Fluorescent measurements were reported as relative fluorescent unit (RFU) values. Light emission was normalized to cell growth rate measured by crystal violet colorimetric assay.

Immunocytochemical analysis

MCF-7/S0.5 and fulvestrant-resistant cells were fixed in 4% formalin, paraffin-embedded, and mounted in 4-μm sections on glass slides. Antigen retrieval was performed by boiling sections in T-EG solution/TRS buffer (Dako). Sections were incubated with anti-SOX2 antibody (#AF2018, R&D Systems) for one hour at room temperature. PowerVision Poly-HRP was used as the detection system. Microscopy of cells was performed using a Leica DMLB microscope (×100 or ×200/numerical aperture (NA) 1.25, Leica Microsystems) using LasV3.6 acquisition software.

Clinical samples

Formalin-fixed, paraffin-embedded (FFPE) metastatic tumor samples from patients with ER+ breast cancer treated with endocrine therapy in the advanced setting were selected by database extraction from the archives of the Department of Pathology at Odense University Hospital (OUH) encompassing the period 2004–2013 ($N = 165$; cohort 1) and 2013–2016 ($N = 128$; cohort 2). Patients eligible for inclusion were those with ER+ breast cancer with metastatic disease, who had undergone surgery or biopsy at OUH, and for whom complete clinical information and pathological verification that the metastatic lesion was of breast cancer origin were available. Exclusion criteria were competing cancer(s), cytological biopsies, or insufficient material in the FFPE block. These parameters yielded 86 (cohort 1) and 67 (cohort 2) metastatic lesions from patients with advanced breast cancer treated with endocrine therapy. The metastatic biopsies used for evaluation of SNAI2 expression were obtained prior to treatment with endocrine therapy. Tumors were defined as ER+ if ≥ 1% of the tumor cells stained positive.

Immunohistochemical staining

Whole FFPE sections of metastatic lesions were incubated with anti-SNAI2 (#sc-15391, Santa Cruz Biotechnology) and immunostained using the HRP-conjugated PowerVision+™ system on the autostainer TechMateTM 500 (Dako), as described [21]. A Leica DMLB microscope (×100/numerical aperture 1.25, Leica Microsystems) and LasV3.6 acquisition software were used for tissue microscopy. Evaluation of the staining was performed by an experienced breast pathologist in a blinded setup. SNAI2 expression was observed in the cell nucleus and cytoplasm and tumors were scored based on the staining intensity score (0–3). The cutoff value for high versus low SNAI2 (intensity score = 2) was determined and optimized in cohort 1 employing the web-based tool Cutoff Finder [22] with the "survival significance" function, and the same cutoff was then applied to cohort 2.

Clinical endpoints

Progression-free survival (PFS) was defined as the time from the date of initiation of endocrine treatment until disease progression within 5 years. Patients without progression within a 5-year period were censored at the date of database retrieval from the registry or 5 years from the date of endocrine treatment initiation, whichever came first.

Statistical analysis

One-way analysis of variance (ANOVA) was used based on twofold or greater change in expression and a FDR of < 0.05 to select genes differentially expressed between MCF-7-based endocrine-resistant and endocrine-sensitive cell lines. The two-tailed t test was used to compare data between groups from RT-qPCR, cell growth and migration assays. Association between SNAI2 expression and patient clinicopathological parameters was determined by Fisher's exact and the chi-square (χ^2) test. Multivariate analysis was performed using a Cox proportional hazard regression model to assess the adjusted hazard ratio (HR) of PFS by SNAI2 expression and clinicopathological characteristics, including age at metastasis, site of relapse and human epidermal growth factor receptor 2 (HER2) status. Survival curves were generated using Kaplan-Meier estimates from the log-rank test to evaluate the correlation between SNAI2 expression and PFS. STATA v14.0 (STATACorp) and GraphPad Prism v5.0 (GraphPad Software, Inc.) were used for statistical analysis. P values < 0.05 were considered statistically significant.

Results

The EMT transcription regulator SNAI2 is upregulated in endocrine-resistant breast cancer cells

To identify EMT-associated genes involved in the endocrine-resistant phenotype of breast cancer cells, we evaluated whether several EMT regulators exhibited altered expression in our gene expression profiling data from MCF-7-based fulvestrant-resistant and tamoxifen-resistant cell lines [18, 23]. Among the transcription factors involved in the regulation of EMT, SNAI2 was found to be significantly upregulated in fulvestrant-resistant (FulvR) and tamoxifen-resistant (TamR) cells compared to their parental cell lines (twofold or greater alteration in expression, $p < 0.05$) (Fig. 1a and b). Altered expression of SNAI2 was verified in two fulvestrant-resistant cell line models (182R and 164R), each containing two cell lines, and four tamoxifen-resistant cell lines, at messenger RNA (mRNA) (Fig. 1c and d) and protein levels (Fig. 1e and f) using RT-qPCR and western blotting, respectively. We previously demonstrated the functional importance of SNAI2 in tamoxifen resistance [24], therefore the present study focused on the role of this EMT-associated transcription factor in the mechanisms of resistance to fulvestrant.

Fulvestrant-resistant cells show increased motility and higher expression of mesenchymal markers compared to fulvestrant-sensitive cell lines

To investigate whether SNAI2 upregulation in fulvestrant-resistant cells is associated with a mesenchymal phenotype, we evaluated cell migration, invasion, and

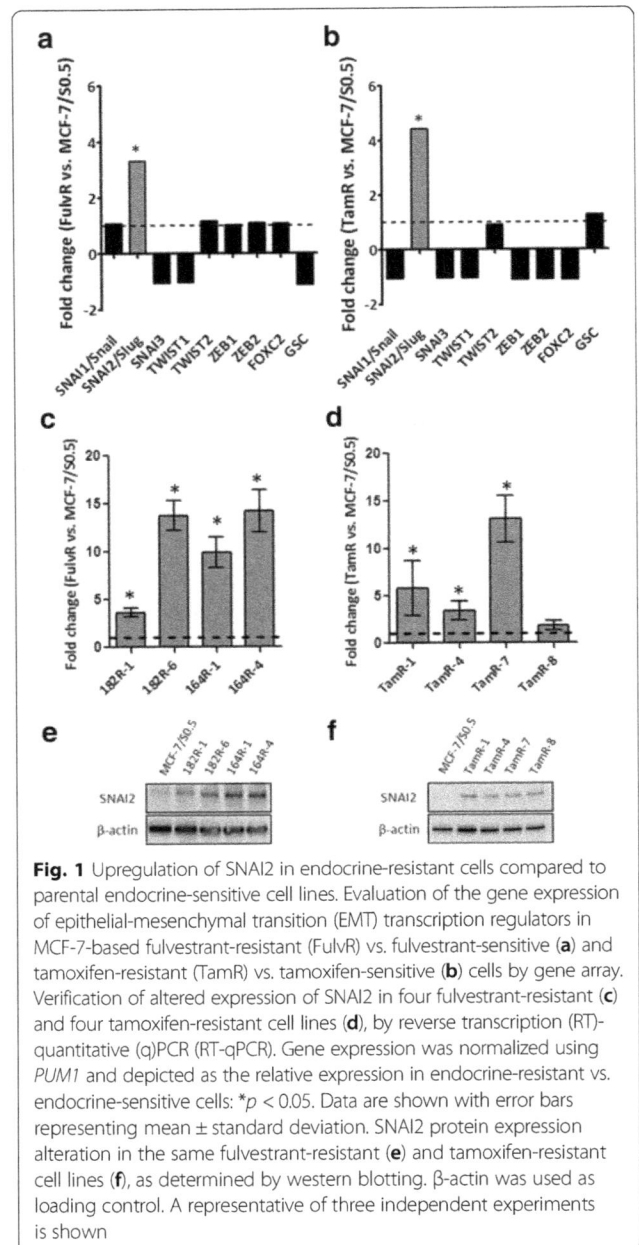

Fig. 1 Upregulation of SNAI2 in endocrine-resistant cells compared to parental endocrine-sensitive cell lines. Evaluation of the gene expression of epithelial-mesenchymal transition (EMT) transcription regulators in MCF-7-based fulvestrant-resistant (FulvR) vs. fulvestrant-sensitive (a) and tamoxifen-resistant (TamR) vs. tamoxifen-sensitive (b) cells by gene array. Verification of altered expression of SNAI2 in four fulvestrant-resistant (c) and four tamoxifen-resistant cell lines (d), by reverse transcription (RT)-quantitative (q)PCR (RT-qPCR). Gene expression was normalized using PUM1 and depicted as the relative expression in endocrine-resistant vs. endocrine-sensitive cells: *$p < 0.05$. Data are shown with error bars representing mean ± standard deviation. SNAI2 protein expression alteration in the same fulvestrant-resistant (e) and tamoxifen-resistant cell lines (f), as determined by western blotting. β-actin was used as loading control. A representative of three independent experiments is shown

expression of EMT markers in the two fulvestrant-resistant models. All four fulvestrant-resistant cell lines had significantly greater ability to migrate compared with fulvestrant-sensitive cell lines (Fig. 2a and b). However, neither fulvestrant-resistant nor fulvestrant-sensitive cells were able to invade extracellular matrix (ECM)-coated membrane (data not shown). Further, fulvestrant-resistant cells exhibited higher expression of vimentin and lower expression of E-cadherin, consistent with a mesenchymal phenotype, whereas parental fulvestrant-sensitive cells exhibited epithelial-like features, including high E-cadherin

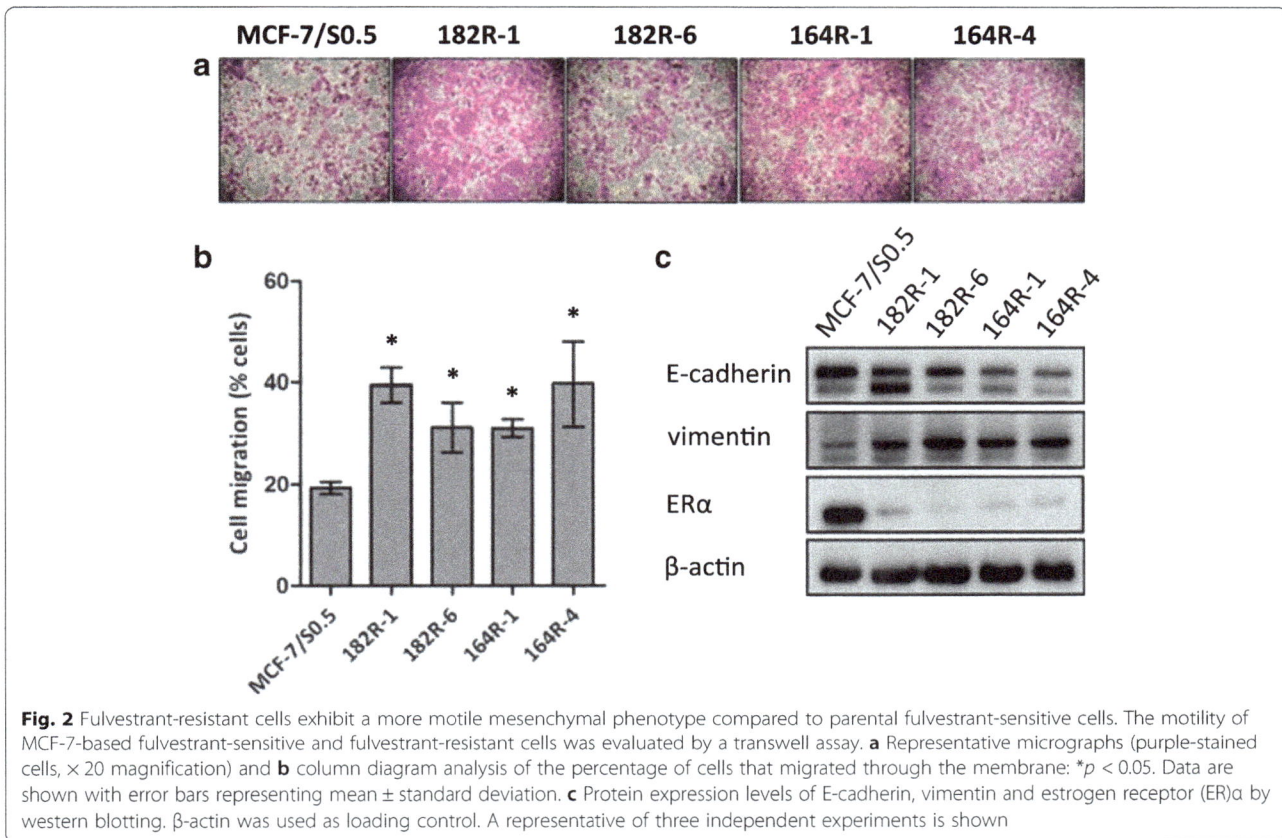

Fig. 2 Fulvestrant-resistant cells exhibit a more motile mesenchymal phenotype compared to parental fulvestrant-sensitive cells. The motility of MCF-7-based fulvestrant-sensitive and fulvestrant-resistant cells was evaluated by a transwell assay. **a** Representative micrographs (purple-stained cells, × 20 magnification) and **b** column diagram analysis of the percentage of cells that migrated through the membrane: *$p < 0.05$. Data are shown with error bars representing mean ± standard deviation. **c** Protein expression levels of E-cadherin, vimentin and estrogen receptor (ER)α by western blotting. β-actin was used as loading control. A representative of three independent experiments is shown

and low vimentin expression (Fig. 2c). The expression of ER was markedly reduced, but still present, in all fulvestrant-resistant cells compared to the parental cell line (Fig. 2c).

SNAI2 knockdown restores epithelial-like features and impairs growth of fulvestrant-resistant breast cancer cells

To evaluate the role of SNAI2 in the control of EMT characteristics and resistance to fulvestrant, we performed gene knockdown studies with specific siRNA targeting SNAI2 in the two fulvestrant-resistant breast cancer cell models. Transient transfection of siRNA against SNAI2 led to efficient downregulation of SNAI2 in both fulvestrant-resistant cells and the parental MCF-7 cell line, as determined by RT-qPCR (Fig. 3a). Protein levels of SNAI2 following SNAI2 knockdown were determined by western blotting and are shown in Additional file 1: Figure S1A. Migration of fulvestrant-resistant cells following SNAI2 downregulation was significantly reduced compared with cells transfected with control siRNA (Fig. 3b and c). Furthermore, E-cadherin mRNA expression was increased in fulvestrant-resistant cells following SNAI2 knockdown, as determined by RT-qPCR (Fig. 3d), supporting that there is alteration to a more epithelial-like phenotype. Protein levels of E-cadherin following SNAI2 knockdown were determined

by western blotting and are shown in Additional file 1: Figure S1B. Additionally, inhibition of SNAI2 by siRNA-mediated knockdown or treatment with SNAIL-p53 binding inhibitor (GN25) reduced growth of fulvestrant-resistant cells (Fig. 3e and f, respectively). The effect of SNAI2 inhibition in reducing fulvestrant-sensitive cell growth was comparable to that of fulvestrant treatment alone (Fig. 3e and f).

As SNAI2 has been implicated in breast CSCs by controlling SOX2 transcription [25], we evaluated SOX2 levels in FFPE fulvestrant-resistant and parental sensitive cell lines and found that SOX2 was upregulated in fulvestrant-resistant compared to fulvestrant-sensitive cells (Fig. 3g). Next, we evaluated the effect of SNAI2 knockdown in SOX2 levels and observed a marked reduction in SOX2 protein expression in three of the four fulvestrant-resistant cell lines (Fig. 3h), suggesting that upregulation of SOX2 in fulvestrant-resistant cells may be mediated by SNAI2. Finally, we evaluated the relevance of SOX2 in fulvestrant resistance by siRNA-mediated knockdown (Additional file 2: Figure S2). We found that reduction of SOX2 expression resulted in decreased fulvestrant-resistant cell growth comparable to the effect of SNAI2 inhibition, which suggests that the role of SNAI2 in controlling growth of resistant cells might be dependent on regulation of SOX2 expression.

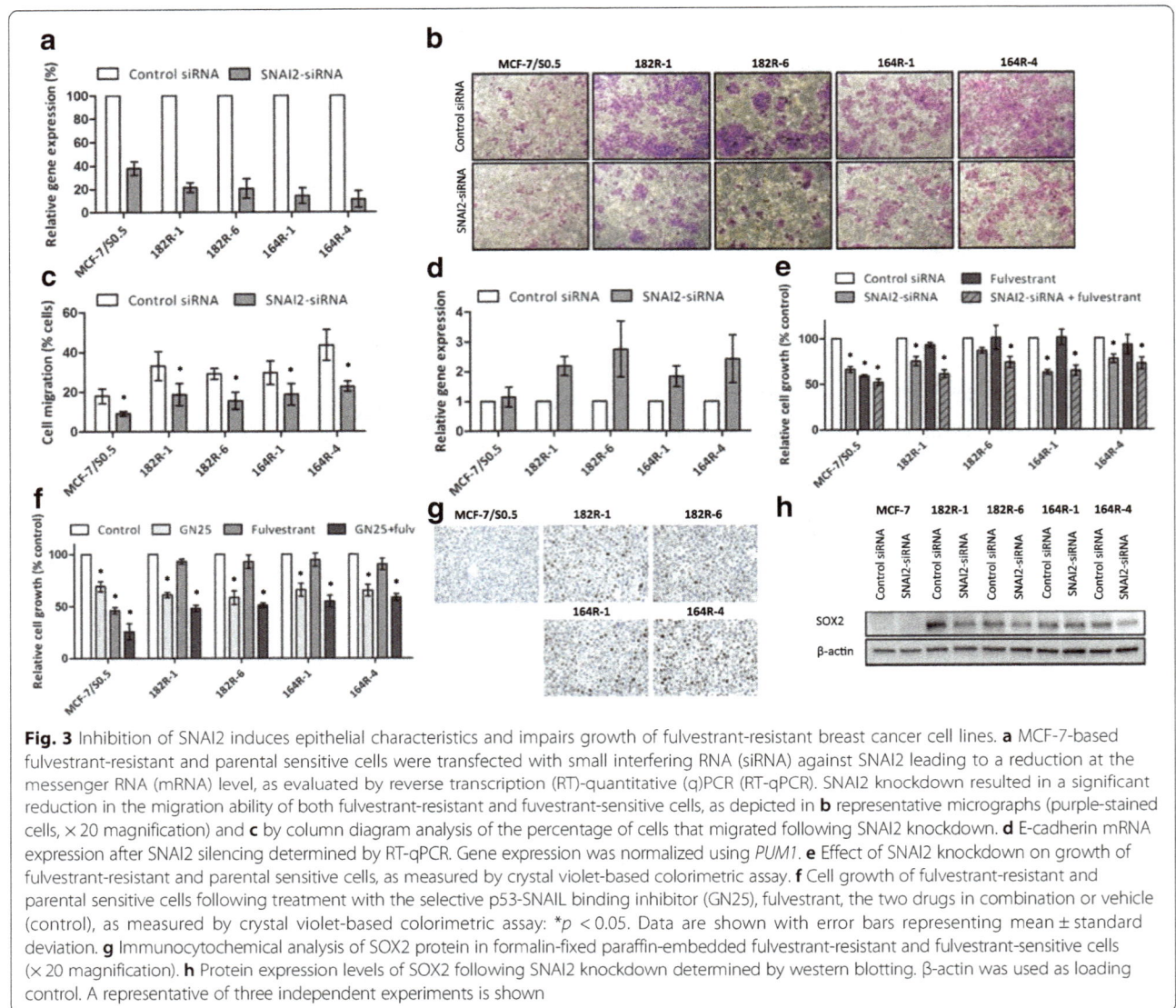

Fig. 3 Inhibition of SNAI2 induces epithelial characteristics and impairs growth of fulvestrant-resistant breast cancer cell lines. **a** MCF-7-based fulvestrant-resistant and parental sensitive cells were transfected with small interfering RNA (siRNA) against SNAI2 leading to a reduction at the messenger RNA (mRNA) level, as evaluated by reverse transcription (RT)-quantitative (q)PCR (RT-qPCR). SNAI2 knockdown resulted in a significant reduction in the migration ability of both fulvestrant-resistant and fuvestrant-sensitive cells, as depicted in **b** representative micrographs (purple-stained cells, × 20 magnification) and **c** by column diagram analysis of the percentage of cells that migrated following SNAI2 knockdown. **d** E-cadherin mRNA expression after SNAI2 silencing determined by RT-qPCR. Gene expression was normalized using *PUM1*. **e** Effect of SNAI2 knockdown on growth of fulvestrant-resistant and parental sensitive cells, as measured by crystal violet-based colorimetric assay. **f** Cell growth of fulvestrant-resistant and parental sensitive cells following treatment with the selective p53-SNAIL binding inhibitor (GN25), fulvestrant, the two drugs in combination or vehicle (control), as measured by crystal violet-based colorimetric assay: *$p < 0.05$. Data are shown with error bars representing mean ± standard deviation. **g** Immunocytochemical analysis of SOX2 protein in formalin-fixed paraffin-embedded fulvestrant-resistant and fulvestrant-sensitive cells (× 20 magnification). **h** Protein expression levels of SOX2 following SNAI2 knockdown determined by western blotting. β-actin was used as loading control. A representative of three independent experiments is shown

SNAI2 expression strongly correlates with clinical outcome in patients with ER+ advanced breast cancer

To investigate the clinical relevance of SNAI2, we evaluated the expression of this protein by immunohistochemical analysis in full sections of ER+ metastatic lesions from an initial cohort of postmenopausal patients treated with endocrine treatment in the advanced setting ($N = 86$), including patients treated with fulvestrant, tamoxifen, and aromatase inhibitors. Clinical and pathological characteristics of this cohort are shown in Table 1. Survival analysis showed that patients with tumors expressing high levels of SNAI2 exhibited significantly shorter PFS on endocrine therapy (median time to progression 4.41 months vs. 9.90 months, $p = 0.0003$) (Fig. 4a). To validate the results from the initial cohort, we analyzed a second cohort of postmenopausal patients with ER+ metastatic breast cancer treated with endocrine treatment in the advanced setting

($N = 67$), including patients treated with fulvestrant, tamoxifen, and aromatase inhibitors. Clinical and pathological characteristics of the second cohort are also shown in Table 1. Analysis of the data from this cohort confirmed significant correlation between high SNAI2 expression and shorter PFS in patients on endocrine therapy (6.57 months vs. 18.67 months, $p = 0.004$) (Fig. 4b). Furthermore, we tested the correlation between SNAI2 expression in metastasis and PFS in patients treated with fulvestrant, from cohort 1 ($N = 45$) and cohort 2 ($N = 44$) (Additional file 3: Figure S3A and B, respectively). Although there were no statistically significant results, likely due to the small number of patients in individual analysis of the two cohorts, there was separation of the Kaplan-Meier curves and the median time to progression was shorter in patients with SNAI2-high than with SNAI2-low metastasis in both cohorts (cohort 1,

Table 1 Clinical and pathological characteristics of patients with estrogen receptor (ER)+ advanced breast cancer according to SNAI2 level

Parameters	Cohort 1				Cohort 2			
	SNAI2 low	SNAI2 high	Number	p^a	SNAI2 low	SNAI2 high	Number	p^a
Age at primary tumor								
≤ 50 years	8	6	14	0.86	14	7	21	0.11
> 50 years	43	29	72		20	26	46	
Age at metastatic disease								
≤ 50 years	3	1	4	0.64	7	1	8	0.05
> 50 years	48	34	82		27	32	59	
Size (mm) of primary tumor								
≤ 20	18	12	30	0.24	12	10	22	0.34
> 20 to ≤ 50	18	13	31		11	17	28	
> 50	1	4	5		2	2	4	
Unknown	14	6	20		9	4	13	
Nodal status of primary tumor Number of positive lymph nodes								
0	11	10	21	0.46	7	6	13	0.37
1–3	16	10	26		8	10	18	
> 3	12	11	23		7	11	18	
Unknown	12	4	16		12	6	18	
Grade of primary tumor								
I	8	9	17	0.06	6	6	12	0.06
II	12	15	27		7	16	23	
III	9	2	11		5	1	6	
Unknown	22	9	31		16	10	26	
HER2 status of metastasis								
Normal	41	30	71	0.62	29	31	60	0.11
Amplified	4	1	5		1	2	3	
Unknown	6	4	10		4	0	4	
Dominant site of relapse								
Soft tissue	38	23	61	0.65	15	17	32	0.17
Bone	8	8	16		15	8	23	
Viscera	5	4	9		4	8	12	
Total number	51	35	86		34	33	67	

HER2 human epidermal growth factor receptor 2
[a] χ2 or Fisher's exact test

median time to progression 4.16 vs. 7.56 months, respectively, $p = 0.07$; cohort 2, median time to progression of 3.35 vs. 8.12 months, respectively, $p = 0.14$). To increase the sample size, we performed Kaplan-Meier estimates and the log-rank test in fulvestrant-treated patients from both cohorts combined ($N = 89$), which showed shorter PFS in patients with metastasis exhibiting high SNAI2 compared with those with metastasis expressing low SNAI2 (median time to progression of 3.52 vs. 7.56 months, respectively, $p = 0.03$) (Fig. 4c). Representative micrographs of breast cancer sections showing low SNAI2 expression (staining intensity score 0 and 1) or high SNAI2 expression (staining intensity score 2 and 3) are presented in Fig. 4d–g. None of the available clinicopathological characteristics of either primary or metastatic tumors correlated significantly with SNAI2 levels (Table 1). Cox proportional hazard regression analysis of PFS according to SNAI2 level and clinicopathological characteristics of the metastatic disease, including age, site of relapse and HER2 status (Table 2), showed that SNAI2 was independently prognostic of PFS on endocrine therapy in both cohorts (cohort 1, HR 2.11, 95% CI of the ratio,

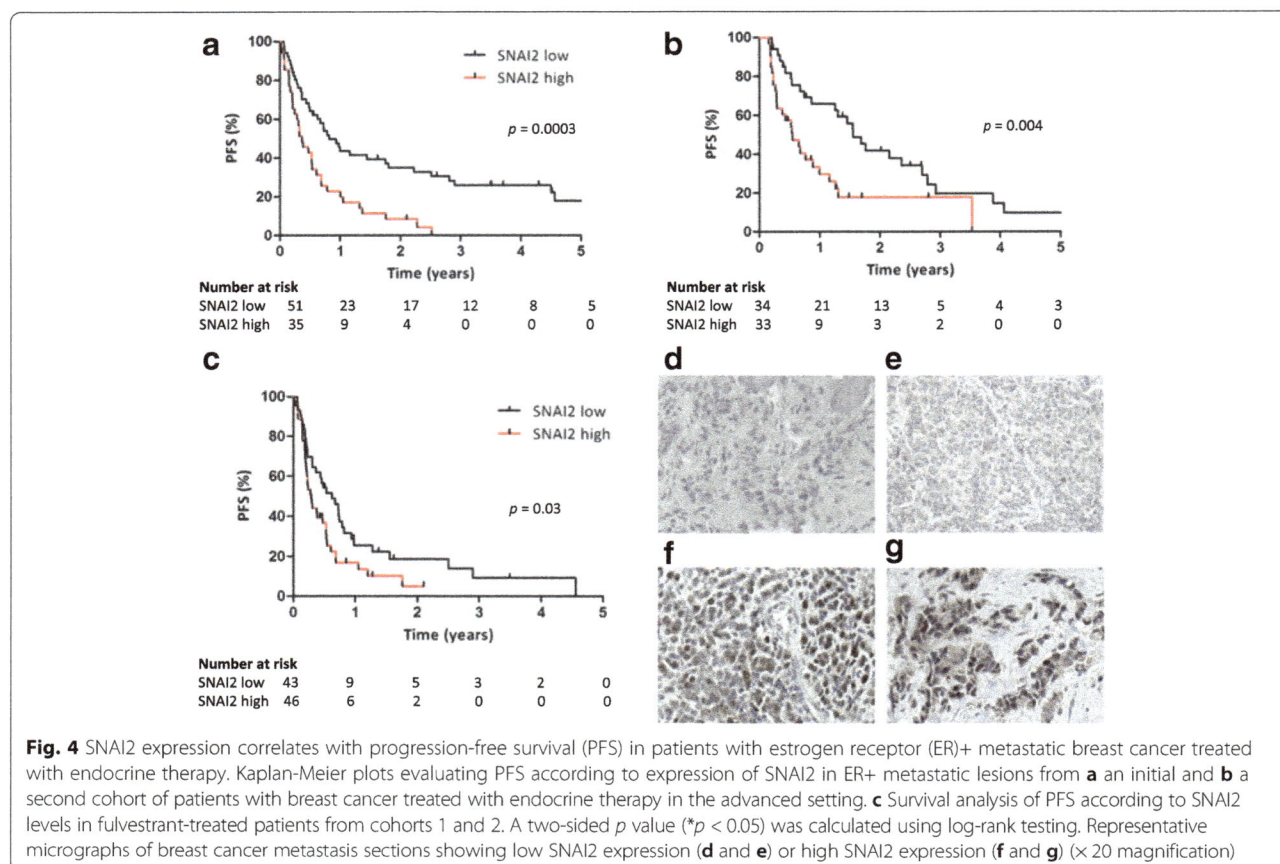

Fig. 4 SNAI2 expression correlates with progression-free survival (PFS) in patients with estrogen receptor (ER)+ metastatic breast cancer treated with endocrine therapy. Kaplan-Meier plots evaluating PFS according to expression of SNAI2 in ER+ metastatic lesions from **a** an initial and **b** a second cohort of patients with breast cancer treated with endocrine therapy in the advanced setting. **c** Survival analysis of PFS according to SNAI2 levels in fulvestrant-treated patients from cohorts 1 and 2. A two-sided p value (*p < 0.05) was calculated using log-rank testing. Representative micrographs of breast cancer metastasis sections showing low SNAI2 expression (**d** and **e**) or high SNAI2 expression (**f** and **g**) (× 20 magnification)

1.21–3.66, p = 0.008; cohort 2, HR 1.92, 95% CI of the ratio, 1.03–3.59, p = 0.04).

Discussion

The development of resistance to endocrine therapy involves alteration of multiple pathways that may be targeted with novel therapeutic agents. Inhibition of growth factor receptor pathways that cross-talk with ER and blockage of cell cycle progression have been shown to be promising strategies in ER+ breast cancer treatment. A growing body of evidence implicating enrichment of EMT markers in breast cancer cells resistant to endocrine treatment supports the use of novel pharmacological strategies targeting EMT for breast cancer. By inhibiting EMT, tumor cells could maintain, or reverse to, an epithelial

state with reduced migratory capacity and re-sensitization to endocrine therapy. However, the specific molecules involved in the regulation of EMT that should be targeted to overcome endocrine resistance remain to be defined.

In this study, we show that SNAI2, a mediator of EMT highly expressed in triple-negative breast cancer [26], is upregulated in endocrine-resistant cells, whereas other EMT-associated transcription factors, such as SNAI1/3, TWIST1/2, ZEB1/2, FOXC2, and GSC, are unaltered. We previously reported that miRNA-593, which is predicted to target SNAI2, is downregulated in tamoxifen-resistant cell lines, implicating SNAI2 in tamoxifen resistance [24]. We also showed that this EMT-inducing transcription factor is a key molecule in the control of tamoxifen-resistant cell growth [24]. In the present study, we focused on the

Table 2 Regression analysis of progression-free survival according to SNAI2 level and clinicopathological characteristics

Variable	Cohort 1		Cohort 2	
	Hazard ratio (95% CI)	p	Hazard ratio (95% CI)	p
SNAI2 level	2.11 (1.21–3.66)	0.008	1.92 (1.03–3.59)	0.04
Age at metastasis	2.19 (0.37–12.95)	0.39	0.90 (0.33–2.49)	0.85
Site of relapse	1.47 (0.98–2.21)	0.07	0.85 (0.56–1.31)	0.47
HER2 status of metastasis	1.46 (0.50–4.28)	0.49	1.49 (0.34–6.52)	0.60

HER2 human epidermal growth factor receptor 2

possible role of SNAI2 in fulvestrant resistance and showed that fulvestrant-resistant cells, which express high levels of SNAI2, exhibit increased migration, higher expression of the mesenchymal marker vimentin, and reduced levels of the epithelial marker E-cadherin compared with the parental fulvestrant-sensitive cell line. Our data concur with previous studies showing that tamoxifen-resistant MCF-7 breast cancer cells display enhanced motile and invasive behavior and EM-like properties compared with tamoxifen-sensitive MCF-7 cells [27, 28].

Previous investigations have demonstrated that silencing of ER in ER+ MCF-7 breast cancer cells leads to acquisition of endocrine resistance and mesenchymal features, which contribute to tumor aggressiveness and metastatic ability [6, 29]. Studies have also reported that ER and SNAI2 levels are inversely correlated and that ER directly suppresses SNAI2 transcription, thus regulating EMT [30, 31]. Despite decreased ER levels in our fulvestrant-resistant cells expressing high SNAI2, these cells remain ER+ and are growth-stimulated by estrogen and inhibited by tamoxifen treatment [16]. Although overexpression of SNAIL in ER+ breast cancer cell lines has been shown to induce resistance to tamoxifen accompanied by reduced ER levels, ectopic expression of ER in these cells did not restore sensitivity to tamoxifen, suggesting that SNAIL might promote resistance to anti-estrogens independent of ER signaling [32].

We observed that reduction of SNAI2 expression impaired cell migration and increased E-cadherin levels in two fulvestrant-resistant breast cancer cell models, confirming a key role for SNAI2 in the control of cell motility and maintenance of a mesenchymal phenotype in resistant cells. These findings are in line with previous reports showing increased mesenchymal characteristics by ectopic expression of SNAI2 in ER+ MCF-7 cells [10]. Additionally, it has been shown that SNAI1/SNAI2 can induce drug resistance in breast cancer cells via alteration of cell survival signaling pathways [24, 32]. We demonstrated that siRNA-mediated knockdown of SNAI2 impairs growth of fulvestrant-resistant cells, which exhibit a high level of SNAI2. In contrast, growth of SNAI2-low breast cancer cells was significantly inhibited by fulvestrant alone, and downregulation of SNAI2 had no additional effect on decreasing the growth of these cells compared to standard endocrine therapy. The role of SNAI2 in controlling the growth of resistant cell lines was further supported by the observation that treatment with a chemical agent interfering with SNAIL binding to p53 (GN25) markedly decreased their growth. Although it is not clear that the growth inhibitory effect of GN25 was due to specific inhibition of SNAI2, as the agent targets other SNAI proteins such as SNAI1 and SNAI3, it seems plausible since SNAI2 was the only SNAI-family member that exhibited increased expression

in fulvestrant-resistant cells. These findings suggest that tumor cells exhibiting high levels of SNAI2 may benefit from inhibition of SNAI2 in combination with standard fulvestrant treatment, while tumors with low SNAI2 expression can be treated with fulvestrant alone. Previous studies have demonstrated that SNAI2 increases stemness in breast cancer cells when co-expressed with SOX9 [33] or through regulation of stem cell markers, including c-Myc, SOX2 and Oct4 [10], possibly contributing to drug resistance. Interestingly, we found upregulation of SOX2 in MCF-7-based fulvestrant-resistant cells compared to fulvestrant-sensitive cells, and SNAI2 knockdown decreased SOX2 expression in three of the four fulvestrant-resistant cell lines, suggesting that SNAI2 might be involved in the mechanism of regulation of this stem marker in fulvestrant resistance.

Finally, we evaluated the clinical relevance of SNAI2 expression in metastatic lesions from two independent cohorts of patients with ER+ breast cancer treated with endocrine therapy in the advanced setting and showed that high SNAI2 levels correlated significantly with shorter PFS in patients on endocrine therapy, including fulvestrant. Correlation between high SNAI2 expression in primary breast tumors and shorter relapse-free survival has been previously demonstrated in ER+ breast cancer [34]. Studies have also shown that high SNAI2 expression in primary ER- breast tumors correlates with poor prognosis in those patients [35, 36]. Nevertheless, our study is the first to our knowledge to report the prognostic value of SNAI2 in patients with ER+ advanced breast cancer treated with endocrine therapy.

Conclusions
In summary, our data support SNAI2 as a key regulator of the aggressive phenotype observed in endocrine-resistant breast cancer cells and a prognostic biomarker in ER+ advanced breast cancer treated with endocrine therapy. These findings highlight the role of SNAI2 as a potential target for therapeutic strategies against EMT and endocrine resistance.

Additional files

Additional file 1: Figure S1. SNAI2 and E-cadherin protein levels following siRNA-mediated SNAI2 knockdown. MCF-7-based fulvestrant-resistant and parental-sensitive cells were transfected with siRNA against SNAI2 and SNAI2 (A) and E-cadherin (B) protein levels were evaluated 96 h following transfection, by Western blotting. β-actin was used as loading control. (TIF 357 kb)

Additional file 2: Figure S2. SOX2 knockdown reduces growth of fulvestrant-resistant breast cancer cells. (A) 182R-1 fulvestrant-resistant cells were transfected with siRNA against SOX2 leading to a reduction at the mRNA level, as evaluated by RT-qPCR. Gene expression was normalized using PUM1. (B) SOX2 knockdown resulted in decreased growth of fulvestrant-resistant cells as measured by crystal violet-based colorimetric assay. Cells were grown in medium containing fulvestrant.

Experiment was performed in technical triplicates and results are shown with error bars representing mean ± standard deviation. (TIF 313 kb)

Additional file 3: Figure S3. Correlation between SNAI2 expression and PFS in patients with ER+ metastatic breast cancer from cohort 1 and 2 treated with fulvestrant. Kaplan-Meier plots evaluating PFS according to expression of SNAI2 in ER+ metastatic lesions from fulvestrant-treated patients from cohort 1 (A) and cohort 2 (B). A two-sided p value (*$p < 0.05$) was calculated using log-rank testing. (TIF 351 kb)

Abbreviations
CI: Confidence interval; CSCs: Cancer stem cells; ECM: Extracellular matrix; EMT: Epithelial-mesenchymal transition; ER +: Estrogen receptor-positive breast cancer; FBS: Fetal bovine serum; FDR: False discovery rate; FFPE: Formalin-fixed paraffin-embedded; FulvR: Fulvestrant-resistant cells; HER2: Human Epidermal growth factor Receptor 2; HR: Hazard ratio; HRP: Horseradish peroxidase; MET: Mesenchymal-epithelial transition; OD: Optical density; OUH: Odense University Hospital; PFS: Progression-free survival; RT-qPCR: Reverse transcription (RT)-quantitative (q)PCR; siRNA: Small interfering RNA; TamR: Tamoxifen-resistant cells

Acknowledgements
We would like to thank Anne E. Lykkesfeldt for providing the tamoxifen-resistant and fulvestrant-resistant cell lines, Lisbet Mortensen and Ole Nielsen at the Department of Pathology, Odense University Hospital, for excellent technical assistance with the immunocytochemical and immunohistochemical staining, and M. Kat Occhipinti for editorial assistance.

Funding
This work was supported by the Danish Cancer Society (H.J. Ditzel), Danish Cancer Research Foundation (C.L. Alves), A Race Against Breast Cancer (H.J. Ditzel), Region of Southern Denmark Research Foundation (H.J. Ditzel), Odense University Hospital Research Council (H.J. Ditzel), Region of Southern Denmark Research Council (H.J. Ditzel), Academy of Geriatric Cancer Research (AgeCare) (H.J. Ditzel), and National Experimental Therapy Partnership (NEXT) Innovation Fund Denmark (H.J. Ditzel).

Authors' contributions
CLA, DE, and HJD participated in the study design, analysis, and interpretation of data and writing of the manuscript. DE and HJD supervised the study. CLA, MBL, MB, and HJD contributed to data acquisition. All authors read and approved the final manuscript.

Competing interests
The authors declare that they have no competing interests.

Author details
[1]Department of Cancer and Inflammation Research, Institute of Molecular Medicine, University of Southern Denmark, J.B. Winsløwsvej 25, 5000 Odense C, Denmark. [2]Department of Pathology, Odense University Hospital, 5000 Odense, Denmark. [3]Department of Oncology, Odense University Hospital, 5000 Odense, Denmark. [4]Academy of Geriatric Cancer Research (AgeCare), Odense University Hospital, 5000 Odense, Denmark.

References
1. Keen JC, Davidson NE. The biology of breast carcinoma. Cancer. 2003;97:825–33.
2. Luqmani YA, Alam-Eldin N. Overcoming resistance to endocrine therapy in breast cancer: new approaches to a nagging problem. Med Princ Pract. 2016;25(Suppl 2):28–40.
3. Sarrio D, Rodriguez-Pinilla SM, Hardisson D, Cano A, Moreno-Bueno G, Palacios J. Epithelial-mesenchymal transition in breast cancer relates to the basal-like phenotype. Cancer Res. 2008;68:989–97.
4. Gupta GP, Massague J. Cancer metastasis: building a framework. Cell. 2006;127:679–95.
5. Thiery JP. Epithelial-mesenchymal transitions in tumour progression. Nat Rev Cancer. 2002;2:442–54.
6. Al Saleh S, Al Mulla F, Luqmani YA. Estrogen receptor silencing induces epithelial to mesenchymal transition in human breast cancer cells. PLoS One. 2011;6:e20610.
7. Polyak K, Weinberg RA. Transitions between epithelial and mesenchymal states: acquisition of malignant and stem cell traits. Nat Rev Cancer. 2009;9:265–73.
8. Luqmani YA, Al Azmi A, Al Bader M, Abraham G, El Zawahri M. Modification of gene expression induced by siRNA targeting of estrogen receptor alpha in MCF7 human breast cancer cells. Int J Oncol. 2009;34:231–42.
9. Dhasarathy A, Kajita M, Wade PA. The transcription factor snail mediates epithelial to mesenchymal transitions by repression of estrogen receptor-alpha. Mol Endocrinol. 2007;21:2907–18.
10. Li Y, Wu Y, Abbatiello TC, Wu WL, Kim JR, Sarkissyan M, et al. Slug contributes to cancer progression by direct regulation of ERalpha signaling pathway. Int J Oncol. 2015;46:1461–72.
11. Voutsadakis IA. Epithelial-mesenchymal transition (EMT) and regulation of EMT Factors by steroid nuclear receptors in breast cancer: a review and in silico investigation. J Clin Med. 2016;5:11.
12. Dave B, Mittal V, Tan NM, Chang JC. Epithelial-mesenchymal transition, cancer stem cells and treatment resistance. Breast Cancer Res. 2012;14:202.
13. Al Saleh S, Sharaf LH, Luqmani YA. Signalling pathways involved in endocrine resistance in breast cancer and associations with epithelial to mesenchymal transition (Review). Int J Oncol. 2011;38:1197–217.
14. Davis FM, Stewart TA, Thompson EW, Monteith GR. Targeting EMT in cancer: opportunities for pharmacological intervention. Trends Pharmacol Sci. 2014;35:479–88.
15. Briand P, Lykkesfeldt AE. Effect of estrogen and antiestrogen on the human breast cancer cell line MCF-7 adapted to growth at low serum concentration. Cancer Res. 1984;44:1114–9.
16. Lykkesfeldt AE, Larsen SS, Briand P. Human breast cancer cell lines resistant to pure anti-estrogens are sensitive to tamoxifen treatment. Int J Cancer. 1995;61:529–34.
17. Lykkesfeldt AE, Madsen MW, Briand P. Altered expression of estrogen-regulated genes in a tamoxifen-resistant and ICI 164,384 and ICI 182,780 sensitive human breast cancer cell line, MCF-7/TAMR-1. Cancer Res. 1994;54:1587–95.
18. Elias D, Vever H, Laenkholm AV, Gjerstorff MF, Yde CW, Lykkesfeldt AE, et al. Gene expression profiling identifies FYN as an important molecule in tamoxifen resistance and a predictor of early recurrence in patients treated with endocrine therapy. Oncogene. 2015;34:1919–27.
19. Livak KJ, Schmittgen TD. Analysis of relative gene expression data using real-time quantitative PCR and the 2(−Delta Delta C(T)) method. Methods. 2001;25:402–8.
20. Lundholt BK, Briand P, Lykkesfeldt AE. Growth inhibition and growth stimulation by estradiol of estrogen receptor transfected human breast epithelial cell lines involve different pathways. Breast Cancer Res Treat. 2001;67:199–214.
21. Leth-Larsen R, Lund R, Hansen HV, Laenkholm AV, Tarin D, Jensen ON, et al. Metastasis-related plasma membrane proteins of human breast cancer cells identified by comparative quantitative mass spectrometry. Mol Cell Proteomics. 2009;8:1436–49.
22. Budczies J, Klauschen F, Sinn BV, Gyorffy B, Schmitt WD, Darb-Esfahani S, et al. Cutoff Finder: a comprehensive and straightforward Web application enabling rapid biomarker cutoff optimization. PLoS One. 2012;7:e51862.

23. Alves CL, Elias D, Lyng M, Bak M, Kirkegaard T, Lykkesfeldt AE, et al. High CDK6 protects cells from fulvestrant-mediated apoptosis and is a predictor of resistance to fulvestrant in estrogen receptor-positive metastatic breast cancer. Clin Cancer Res. 2016;22:5514–26.

24. Joshi T, Elias D, Stenvang J, Alves CL, Teng F, Lyng MB, et al. Integrative analysis of miRNA and gene expression reveals regulatory networks in tamoxifen-resistant breast cancer. Oncotarget. 2016;7:57239–53.

25. Samanta S, Sun H, Goel HL, Pursell B, Chang C, Khan A, et al. IMP3 promotes stem-like properties in triple-negative breast cancer by regulating SLUG. Oncogene. 2016;35:1111–21.

26. Proia TA, Keller PJ, Gupta PB, Klebba I, Jones AD, Sedic M, et al. Genetic predisposition directs breast cancer phenotype by dictating progenitor cell fate. Cell Stem Cell. 2011;8:149–63.

27. Hiscox S, Jiang WG, Obermeier K, Taylor K, Morgan L, Burmi R, et al. Tamoxifen resistance in MCF7 cells promotes EMT-like behaviour and involves modulation of beta-catenin phosphorylation. Int J Cancer. 2006;118:290–301.

28. Ward A, Balwierz A, Zhang JD, Kublbeck M, Pawitan Y, Hielscher T, et al. Re-expression of microRNA-375 reverses both tamoxifen resistance and accompanying EMT-like properties in breast cancer. Oncogene. 2013;32:1173–82.

29. Bouris P, Skandalis SS, Piperigkou Z, Afratis N, Karamanou K, Aletras AJ, et al. Estrogen receptor alpha mediates epithelial to mesenchymal transition, expression of specific matrix effectors and functional properties of breast cancer cells. Matrix Biol. 2015;43:42–60.

30. Ye Y, Xiao Y, Wang W, Yearsley K, Gao JX, Barsky SH. ERalpha suppresses slug expression directly by transcriptional repression. Biochem J. 2008;416:179–87.

31. Ye Y, Xiao Y, Wang W, Yearsley K, Gao JX, Shetuni B, et al. ERalpha signaling through slug regulates E-cadherin and EMT. Oncogene. 2010;29:1451–62.

32. Jiang Y, Zhao X, Xiao Q, Liu Q, Ding K, Yu F, et al. Snail and Slug mediate tamoxifen resistance in breast cancer cells through activation of EGFR-ERK independent of epithelial-mesenchymal transition. J Mol Cell Biol. 2014;6:352–4.

33. Guo WJ, Keckesova Z, Donaher JL, Shibue T, Tischler V, Reinhardt F, et al. Slug and Sox9 Cooperatively Determine the Mammary Stem Cell State. Cell. 2012;148:1015–28.

34. Chimge NO, Baniwal SK, Little GH, Chen YB, Kahn M, Tripathy D, et al. Regulation of breast cancer metastasis by Runx2 and estrogen signaling: the role of SNAI2. Breast Cancer Res. 2011;13:R127.

35. Liu T, Zhang XY, Shang M, Zhang YX, Xia BS, Niu M, et al. Dysregulated expression of Slug, vimentin, and E-cadherin correlates with poor clinical outcome in patients with basal-like breast cancer. J Surg Oncol. 2013;107:188–94.

36. Storci G, Sansone P, Trere D, Tavolari S, Taffurelli M, Ceccarelli C, et al. The basal-like breast carcinoma phenotype is regulated by SLUG gene expression. J Pathol. 2008;214:25–37.

17

Monitoring Src status after dasatinib treatment in HER2+ breast cancer with ^{89}Zr-trastuzumab PET imaging

Brooke N. McKnight and Nerissa T. Viola-Villegas[*] (iD)

Abstract

Background: De novo or acquired resistance in breast cancer leads to treatment failures and disease progression. In human epidermal growth factor receptor 2 (HER2)-positive (HER2+) breast cancer, Src, a non-receptor tyrosine kinase, is identified as a major mechanism of trastuzumab resistance, with its activation stabilizing aberrant HER2 signaling, thus making it an attractive target for inhibition. Here, we explored the causal relationship between Src and HER2 by examining the potential of ^{89}Zr-trastuzumab as a surrogate imaging marker of Src activity upon inhibition with dasatinib in HER2+ breast cancer.

Methods: HER2+ primary breast cancer cell lines BT-474 and trastuzumab-resistant JIMT-1 were treated with dasatinib and assessed for expression and localization of HER2, Src, and phosphorylated Src (pSrc) (Y416) through western blots and binding assays. Mice bearing BT-474 or JIMT-1 tumors were treated for 7 or 14 days with dasatinib. At the end of each treatment, tumors were imaged with ^{89}Zr-trastuzumab. The results of ^{89}Zr-trastuzumab positron emission tomography (PET) was compared against tumor uptake of fluorodeoxyglucose (^{18}F-FDG) obtained the day before in the same group of mice. Ex vivo western blots and immunohistochemical staining (IHC) were performed for validation.

Results: In BT-474 and JIMT-1 cells, treatment with dasatinib resulted in a decrease in internalized ^{89}Zr-trastuzumab. Confirmation with immunoblots displayed abrogation of pSrc (Y416) signaling; binding assays in both cell lines demonstrated a decrease in cell surface and internalized HER2-bound tracer. In xenograft models, dasatinib treatment for 7 days (BT-474, 11.05 ± 2.10 % injected dose per gram of tissue %(ID)/g; JIMT-1, 3.88 ± 1.47 %ID/g)) or 14 days (BT-474, 9.20 ± 1.85 %ID/g; JIMT-1, 4.45 ± 1.23 %ID/g) resulted in a significant decrease in ^{89}Zr-trastuzumab uptake on PET compared to untreated control (BT-474, 17.88 ± 2.18 %ID/g; JIMT-1, 8.04 ± 1.47 %ID/g). No difference in ^{18}F-FDG uptake was observed between control and treated cohorts. A parallel decrease in membranous HER2 and pSrc (Y416) staining was observed in tumors post treatment on IHC. Immunoblots further validated the ^{89}Zr-trastuzumab-PET readout. Positive correlation was established between ^{89}Zr-trastuzumab tumor uptake versus tumor regression, pSrc and pHER2 expression.

Conclusions: ^{89}Zr-trastuzumab can potentially assess tumor response to dasatinib in HER2+ breast cancer and could be used as a surrogate tool to monitor early changes in Src signaling downstream of HER2.

Keywords: Src, pSrc, pHER2, HER2, Dasatinib, PET, Trastuzumab, Breast cancer

* Correspondence: villegan@karmanos.org
Department of Oncology, Karmanos Cancer Institute, 4100 John R Street, Detroit, MI 48201, USA

Background

The human epidermal growth factor receptor 2 (HER2) has become a critical therapeutic target with trastuzumab as the mainstream, first-in-line standard of care in patients with HER2-positive breast cancer [1, 2]. Unfortunately, response rates to HER2-targeted therapy remain dismal due to acquired and de novo resistance, which in part can be attributed to alterations in receptor tyrosine kinases (RTKs) [3], and downstream signaling transduction pathways, such as Src [4, 5].

Src is a non-receptor tyrosine kinase expressed ubiquitously that interacts with several RTKs [6]. Its activation enhances cellular migration and survival [7]. Elevated Src has been shown to stabilize HER2 and vice versa [6, 8–10], establishing a functional relationship between the two oncogenes [8]. This was reported in a study by Fan et al. wherein Src abrogation concomitantly led to decreased HER2 levels within 7–14 days of treatment with a Src inhibitor, PP2, in vitro [9]. Thus, Src is implicated as one of the key molecules driving resistance to trastuzumab therapy, making this signaling axis an attractive target for inhibition.

Dasatinib (Sprycel®) is a Src and BCR/ABL tyrosine kinase inhibitor, which was approved by the Food and Drug Administration (FDA) for treatment of leukemia in 2006 [11]. Preclinical data reported by Seoane et al. demonstrated the synergistic effects of dasatinib with trastuzumab as evidenced by attenuated phosphorylated levels of Src, extracellular signal-related protein kinase (ERK) and protein kinase B (Akt) in HER2+ breast cancer [12]. These preclinical findings were validated in a prospective phase I–II trial exploring the combined efficacy and safety of dasatinib, trastuzumab and paclitaxel in patients with breast cancer [13]. Monitoring of tumor response to this drug cocktail was conducted through immunohistochemical analysis (IHC) of patients' skin samples. However, better ways to non-invasively monitor tumor response can be achieved by exploring the direct causal relationship between HER2 and Src.

In this study, we investigated the potential of ^{89}Zr (half-life $(t_{1/2})$ ~ 3.27 days) labeled trastuzumab (Herceptin®) as a surrogate tool to monitor biologic effects of dasatinib treatment in HER2-positive (HER2+) breast cancer. We first evaluated the specificity of ^{89}Zr-trastuzumab in both HER2+ and Src-active breast cancer cell lines, BT-474 and JIMT-1, which are trastuzumab-sensitive and trastuzumab-resistant, respectively. MDA-MB-468 triple-negative breast cancer cell line was used as a control. We next examined the utility of fluorodeoxyglucose (^{18}F-FDG) and ^{89}Zr-trastuzumab as a predictive imaging tool using the same group of mice bearing either BT-474 or JIMT-1 tumors treated with dasatinib. After imaging, a correlation was tested between ^{89}Zr-trastuzumab positron emission

tomography (PET) uptake and changes in tumor volume, immunoblots, and IHC analysis.

Methods

Cell lines, reagents, and xenografts

BT-474 and JIMT-1 cells were a generous gift from Prof. Jason S. Lewis at Memorial Sloan Kettering Cancer Center (MSKCC). MDA-MB-468 cells were provided by the Karmanos Cancer Institute (KCI) Biobanking and Correlative Sciences (BCS) Core. BT-474 cells were grown in 1:1 DMEM:F12 (VWR) + 5% FBS + 1% Pen-Strep + 1% non-essential amino acids (NEAA) (Corning); JIMT-1 and MDA-MB-468 cells were grown in DMEM + 1% Pen-strep + 5% FBS (Sigma). All cells were grown at 37 °C with 5% CO_2 and routinely tested for mycoplasma with MycoAlert Mycoplasma Detection Kit (Lonza). The cell lines were further authenticated by the Biobanking and Correlative Services Core at Wayne State University. Dasatinib (Selleckchem) was prepared as a 50-mM stock concentration in dimethyl sulfoxide (DMSO) and serially diluted to the desired concentration with cell culture medium for in vitro assays. Trastuzumab was obtained from the Karmanos Cancer Center pharmacy. Primary antibodies for western blots and IHC are commercially available and are detailed in Additional file 1: Table S1. Anti-rabbit and anti-mouse HRP-linked secondary antibodies were purchased from GE (NA934, NA931).

All animal handling and manipulations were conducted in accordance with the guidelines set by Wayne State University Institutional Animal Use and Care Committee. For imaging experiments, female athymic nu/nu mice (6–8 weeks old, Envigo) were subcutaneously (s.c.) injected with 5×10^6 MDA-MB-468 or 5×10^6 JIMT-1 breast cancer cells. For BT-474 xenografts, mice were implanted s.c. with 0.72 mg slow-release 60-day 17-β Estradiol pellets (SE-121, Innovative Research of America) on the nape of the neck for 2–3 days before 10×10^6 cells were injected. All cells were injected as a suspension in 150 μL 1:1 medium:Matrigel® (BD Biosciences, Bedford, MA, USA) on the right shoulder. Monitoring of tumor growth was performed weekly with calipers. The tumor volume was calculated using the formula: length × width × height × π/6. Mice with tumor volumes ranging from 150 to 250 mm^3 were utilized.

Radiosynthesis of ^{89}Zr-trastuzumab

p-Benzyl-isothiocyanate-desferrioxamine (DFO, Macrocylics, Inc.) was conjugated to trastuzumab and a non-specific human IgG isotype (14506, Sigma-Aldrich) according to published protocols [14, 15]. The synthesis was performed using 4:1 mol equivalence of DFO-Bz-SCN to trastuzumab or IgG, respectively in 0.9% saline, pH ~ 9 at 37 °C for 1 h. Pure, monoclonal antibody DFO-conjugates were obtained by passing through a spin column filter with a molecular weight cutoff of 30 kDa (GE Vivaspin 500) using sterile saline as eluting buffer.

Approximately 1 mCi (37 MBq) of ^{89}Zr-oxalate (3D Imaging, LLC) was neutralized to pH 7.0–7.2 using 1 M NaOH. Trastuzumab-DFO (200 μg) was added to the ^{89}Zr solution. The reaction was quenched after 1–1.5 h incubation at room temperature upon addition of 5 μL of 50 mM EDTA (pH ~ 7) to eliminate any non-specifically bound ^{89}Zr. Radiolabeling efficiency > 95% was determined by radio-instant thin layer chromatography (iTLC) using silica gel-impregnated iTLC strip (Agilent Technologies, Santa Clara, CA, USA) and 50 mM EDTA as the solid and mobile phase, respectively. Pure ^{89}Zr-trastuzumab was obtained through spin column centrifugation (GE Vivaspin 500, MWCO: 30 kDa) with saline used for eluting unbound radiometal. Radiochemical purity > 99% was achieved based on iTLC analysis. ^{89}Zr-trastuzumab was assessed for immunoreactivity as previously described [16]. Radiolabeling and purification of a non-specific human IgG monoclonal antibody was performed as aforementioned.

IC$_{50}$ Calculations

Half-maximal inhibitory concentration (IC$_{50}$) values were obtained for BT-474 and JIMT-1 breast cancer cell lines. Wells were seeded with ~ 1×10^4 cells and incubated overnight at 37 °C in 5% CO$_2$. Cells were treated with increasing concentrations of dasatinib (1 nM to 1 mM) and incubated for 72 h then analyzed for viability using alamar blue assay (Life Technologies). After 4 h incubation with alamar blue, absorbance was read at 570 nm on an Infinite M200 plate reader (Tecan). IC$_{50}$ was calculated in GraphPad Prism (v. 7.02) using a non-linear dose response plotting the log(concentration) versus % viable cells.

Internalization assay

Wells were seeded with 50,000 cells and incubated overnight. Cells were treated with the established IC$_{50}$ for dasatinib in complete medium for 0–48 h. After incubation, radiolabeled protein (100 ng, 0.30 μCi, 111 kBq) in 1 mL of medium was added to each well. The plates were incubated at 37 °C for 2 h. Following the incubation period, the medium was collected and the cells were rinsed with 1× PBS twice. Surface-bound activity was removed by washing the cells in 100 mM acetic acid + 100 mM glycine (1:1, pH 3.5) at 4 °C. The cells were then lysed with 1 M NaOH. All washes (medium plus PBS, acid and alkaline) were collected in separate tubes and measured for bound activity using a gamma counter (Perkin Elmer). The percentage of internalized activity was calculated as the ratio of the activity of the lysate and the total activity collected from the medium plus PBS, and base washes, normalized to

50,000 cells counted using a Countess II Automated Cell Counter (Thermo Fisher).

In vitro competitive binding assay

Binding of ^{89}Zr-trastuzumab was evaluated in all three cell lines. Wells were seeded with 10,000 cells and incubated overnight. After incubation, radiolabeled protein (1 μCi/mL, 37 kBq/mL, 0.25 μg) in 1 mL of medium was added to each well with or without 10-fold excess unlabeled trastuzumab (1 μg). The plates were incubated at 4 °C for 1 h. Following the incubation period, the medium was collected and the cells were rinsed with 1 mL 1 × PBS twice. The cells were then lysed with 1 mL 1 M NaOH. All washes (medium including PBS and alkaline wash) were collected in separate tubes and measured for counts using a gamma counter (Perkin Elmer). The percentage of bound activity was calculated as the ratio of the activity of the lysate and the total activity collected from the medium plus PBS, and base washes, and was normalized to cell count using a Countess II Automated Cell Counter (Thermo Fisher).

Immunoblots

After dasatinib treatment, cells were lysed on ice using 1 × RIPA buffer (Pierce) supplemented with HALT protease and phosphatase inhibitor cocktail (Pierce). Tumors were mechanically lysed using a handheld homogenizer Polytron PE 1200E (VWR) in the same buffer. Total protein was measured using a Pierce BCA Protein Assay Kit (Thermo Fisher).

Proteins were separated on a 4–12% bis-tris NuPAGE gel (Invitrogen) before transferring to an Immobilon-P polyvinylidene di fluoride (PVDF) membrane (Millipore Sigma). Membranes were blocked in 5% non-fat dry milk in Tris-buffered saline and Tween 20 (TBST) buffer for 1 h at room temperature. Primary antibodies (Additional file 1: Table S1) were diluted in TBST with 0.02% sodium azide and incubated at 4 °C before blotting with HRP-linked secondary antibodies in 5% milk-TBST for 2 h at room temperature. Proteins were visualized using Amersham ECL (GE) with images collected and analyzed using a ChemiDoc (BioRad) system with Image Lab (Bio-Rad) software. Densitometry was calculated using ImageJ.

Mouse treatment studies

Dasatinib (75 mg/kg body weight in 150 μL 1:1 sterile water:glycerol) was administered to BT-474 and JIMT-1 tumor-bearing mice by oral gavage for 7 and 14 days. Untreated control mice were given a 1:1 mix of water and glycerol (150 μL total volume via oral gavage) as placebo. Food and water were given *ad libitum*. Tumor volumes were recorded 2–3 times per week. Percent change in tumor volume was analyzed using measurements obtained before the start of treatment and at the time of imaging.

PET imaging and distribution

On the last day of treatment, mice bearing BT-474 or JIMT-1 tumors ($n = 3$–4) were fasted 8 h before intravenously (i.v.) administering ^{18}F-FDG (150–200 µCi, 5.55–7.4 MBq). The mice were anesthetized with 1–2% isoflurane immediately after tracer injections. PET scans were acquired 1 h post-injection (p.i.). After 24 h, ^{89}Zr-trastuzumab (200–240 µCi, 7.40–8.88 MBq, 67–80 µg, 40–50 nmol) in sterile saline was administered i.v. in the same group of mice. Small-animal PET scans were acquired at 48 h p.i. using a microPET-R4 scanner (Concorde Microsystems). All mice were fully anesthetized with 1–2% isoflurane (Baxter, Deerfield, IL, USA) during each scan acquisition. Images were reconstructed via filter back projection. ASIPro VM™ software (Concorde Microsystems) was used to analyze volumes of interest (VOI) on various planar sections from the acquired image by manually drawing on the tumor site and on select organs. The average VOI was calculated and expressed as the percentage of injected dose per gram of tissue (%ID/g). Mice were euthanized after imaging via CO_2 asphyxiation and cervical dislocation. Tumors were removed and immediately snap frozen in liquid nitrogen and stored at – 80 °C until decayed (~ 35 days).

^{89}Zr-trastuzumab biodistribution was performed at 48 h p.i. of the tracer (20–30 µCi, 0.74–1.11 MBq, 336–504 nmol, 5–7 µg) in mice bearing BT-474 or JIMT-1 tumors. ^{89}Zr-IgG (20–30 µCi, 0.74–1.11 MBq, 5-7 µg, 336–504 nmol) was injected in a separate group of tumor-bearing mice to assess non-specific accumulation of the tracer. Mice were sacrificed as stated above. Bound activity was measured on tissues of interest using a gamma counter (Perkin Elmer Wizard2) and is expressed as the percentage of injected dose per gram of tissue (wet weight).

Immunohistochemical analysis

Tumors embedded in optimal cutting temperature (OCT) blocks were sliced into 5-µm sections (Leica CM 1850), mounted on positively charged slides (Fisher) and dried overnight at room temperature. Slides were fixed in pre-cooled acetone for 10 min and allowed to evaporate ~20 min. Endogenous activity was blocked with 0.3% H_2O_2 for 10 min, before incubation with 10% FBS in PBS for 1 h in a humidified chamber at room temperature. Tissues were immunostained for HER2 and pSrc (Y416) (Additional file 1: Table S1) using a Histomouse Max broad spectrum 3,3-diaminobenzidine (DAB) kit (Invitrogen). Slides were scanned using a Leica SCN 400 slide scanner with image viewer software.

Statistical analysis

Statistical analysis was performed by two-way analysis of variance (ANOVA) using GraphPad Prism v. 7.02. A value of $p < 0.05$ was considered statistically significant. Data were expressed as the mean ± S.D.

Results

Characterization of ^{89}Zr-trastuzumab

High radiolabeling yields (> 95%) were obtained with > 97% purity after purification via spin column. Specific activity of 3.0 ± 0.2 mCi/mg (111 ± 7.4 Bq/µmol) was established. The labeled antibody retained immunoreactivity towards HER2 with 85% retention (Additional file 2: Figure S1, $n = 3$).

In vitro treatment studies with dasatinib

BT-474 (Fig. 1a) and JIMT-1 (Fig. 1b) cells were treated with increasing concentrations of dasatinib to achieve IC_{50} values of 1.3 ± 0.12 µM, and 0.22 ± 0.09 µM, respectively, 72 h post-treatment. Treated and control groups of cells were lysed and analyzed by western blot. In BT-474 cells (Fig. 1c), total abrogation of pSrc (Y416, directly associated with full tyrosine kinase activity) [17, 18] and pHER2 (Y1221/1222, autophosphorylation site) were observed after 6 h of exposure. While in JIMT-1 cells (Fig. 1d), attenuation of pSrc (Y416) activity after 6 h and pHER2 (Y1221/1222) at 24 h was displayed post dasatinib treatment. No changes in total HER2 or Src protein levels were observed for either cell line as shown by densitometry.

Src treatment lowers ^{89}Zr-trastuzumab internalization

We next interrogated the ability of HER2 to internalize ^{89}Zr-trastuzumab after dasatinib treatment over time (Fig. 2a). A steady decrease in ^{89}Zr-trastuzumab internalization was exhibited by both cell lines. Internalization of ^{89}Zr-trastuzumab in untreated BT-474 was measured at 10.37 ± 1.62%; however, internalized fractions decreased after 6 h and 24 h of dasatinib treatment with ~ 7.68 ± 0.53% ($p = 0.02$), and 7.42 ± 0.74% ($p = 0.03$), respectively. At 48 h, only ~ 4.78 ± 0.42% ($p = 0.006$) of the radiotracer was found intracellularly. JIMT-1 cells also showed a reduction in internalization upon treatment, albeit after extended drug exposure. From 2.6 ± 0.25% internalized in untreated cells, no significant internalized fractions were observed at 6 h (1.96 ± 0.46%, $p = 0.10$). At prolonged treatment times, a reduction in internalized activity was observed (24 h, 1.22 ± 0.10%, $p = 0.009$ and 48 h, 0.17 ± 0.5%, $p < 0.0001$).

Membrane-bound levels of ^{89}Zr-trastuzumab displayed a similar trend to internalized fractions of the imaging probe during dasatinib treatment (Fig. 2a). Compared to untreated BT-474 cells with 14.10 ± 1.22% surface-bound radiotracer, a decrease was observed in treated groups

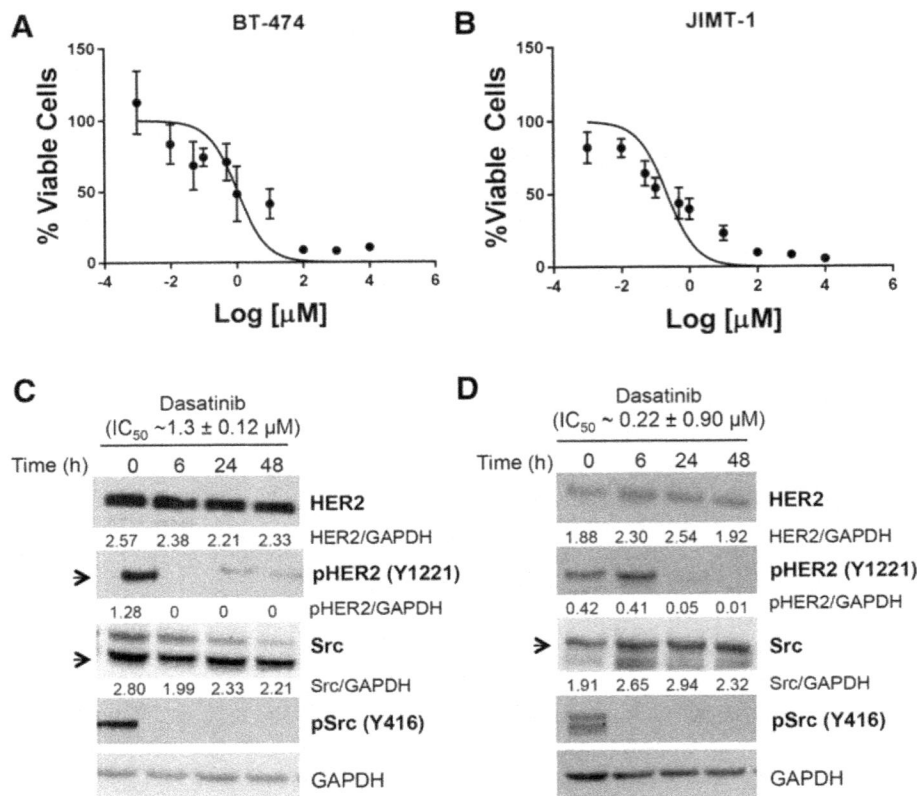

Fig. 1 Dasatinib treatment decreases phosphorylated Src (pSrc) (Y416) and phosphorylated human epidermal growth factor receptor 2 (pHER2) (Y-1221) protein levels in vitro. BT-474 (**a**) or JIMT-1 (**b**) cells were treated with increasing concentrations of dasatinib for 72 h to achieve half maximal inhibitory concentration (IC$_{50}$) values of 1.3 ± 0.12 μM and 0.22 ± 0.09 μM, respectively. BT-474 cells (**c**) and JIMT-1 (**d**) were treated with the IC$_{50}$ dasatinib up to 48 h and western blots were performed for HER2, Src, pSrc (Y416), and pHER2 (Y1221/1222). Densitometry results are shown as the ratio of target protein/glyceraldehyde-3-phosphate dehydrogenase (GAPDH)

after 24 h (11.42 ± 2.04%, $p = 0.038$) and 48 h (8.88 ± 1.44%, $p = 0.0002$) of treatment. Concurrent lower tracer binding was observed in JIMT-1 cells but at longer incubation with dasatinib (48 h, 0.34 ± 0.21%, $p = 0.028$) relative to untreated cells at 3.16 ± 0.50%.

These findings are in good agreement with the western blot results wherein abrogation of pHER2 (Y1221/1222) after treatment over 6 h in BT-474 and 24 h in JIMT-1 corresponded to reduced internalization of the tracer at these time points. Collectively, this study suggests an association between decreased cell-surface binding and functional internalization of [89]Zr-trastuzumab (percentage bound and internalized) and response to dasatinib treatment.

Validation of [89]Zr-trastuzumab specificity to HER2

In the in vitro studies using BT-474, JIMT-1, and MDA-MB-468 cells, co-administration of 25-fold unlabeled trastuzumab exhibited lower binding of [89]Zr-trastuzumab in HER2+ cell lines (BT-474, 1.07 ± 0.24% vs. 6.64 ± 1.14%, $p < 0.0001$; JIMT-1, 0.65 ± 0.18 vs.

1.46 ± 0.24, $p = 0.0007$). No change in probe uptake was observed in the HER2- MDA-MB-468 cells (0.71 ± 0.40 vs. 1.11 ± 0.56, $p = 0.34$) (Additional file 3: Figure S2A).

Mice bearing BT-474, JIMT-1, or MDA-MB-468 xenografts were imaged with [89]Zr-trastuzumab at 48 h p.i. (Additional file 3: Figure S2B, C). MDA-MB-468 tumors exhibited the lowest uptake with 3.9 ± 0.6 %ID/g, compared to BT-474 (17.9 ± 2.2 %ID/g, $p < 0.001$) and JIMT-1 (7.7 ± 0.6 %ID/g, $p < 0.001$) tumors. There was significantly less [89]Zr-trastuzumab uptake in JIMT-1 tumors compared to BT-474 ($p < 0.0001$).

The specificity of the HER2-specific tracer was further challenged using [89]Zr-IgG through distribution studies. In BT-474 tumors, [89]Zr-trastuzumab uptake was 16.01 ± 3.78 %ID/g, compared to the non-specific probe (1.02 ± 0.87 %ID/g, $p = 0.0002$) (Additional file 4: Figure S3, Additional file 5: Table S2). Accumulation of [89]Zr-trastuzumab (4.13 ± 2.36 %ID/g) in JIMT-1 xenografts of (Additional file 4: Figure S3, Additional file 6: Table S3) was significantly higher than [89]Zr-IgG with 0.79 ± 0.24 %ID/g ($p = 0.034$).

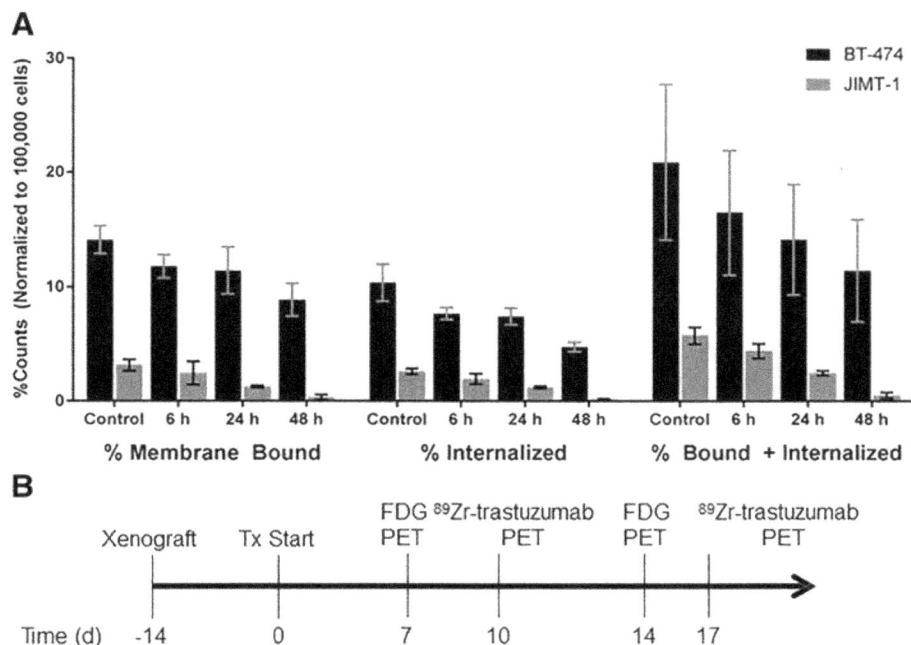

Fig. 2 [89]Zr-trastuzumab binding and uptake decreases upon dasatinib treatment. Internalization and binding assays of [89]Zr-trastuzumab on BT-474 and JIMT-1 cells treated with dasatinib half maximal inhibitory concentration (IC$_{50}$) from 0 to 48 h showed a decrease in probe internalization and binding over time (**a**). Treatment and imaging scheme illustrates treatment of tumors for 7 days and/or 14 days with dasatinib followed by positron emission tomography (PET) with fluorodeoxyglucose (^{18}F-FDG). [89]Zr-trastuzumab was administered a day after with imaging acquired 48 h post injection (**b**). Tx, treatment; d, days

In vivo monitoring of tumor response to dasatinib

Mice bearing palpable BT-474 tumors were dosed with dasatinib for 7 and 14 days and imaged with ^{18}F-FDG 24 h prior to administration of [89]Zr-trastuzumab (Fig. 2b). Tumor uptake of ^{18}F-FDG was not statistically different between untreated mice (3.60 ± 1.51% ID/g) and treated cohorts at 7 days (3.86 ± 0.59 %ID/g, $p = 0.99$) and 14 days (4.63 ± 0.21 %ID/g, $p = 0.80$) (Fig. 3a). In comparison, [89]Zr-trastuzumab exhibited a significant decrease in tumor accumulation in both treated groups (7 days, 11.05 ± 2.10 %ID/g, $p < 0.0001$; 14 days, 9.2 ± 1.85 %ID/g, $p < 0.0001$) compared to untreated tumors (17.88 ± 2.18 %ID/g) (Fig. 3b). No significant difference in probe uptake was observed between 7-day and 14-day treatments ($p = 0.39$) (Fig. 3c). A significant positive correlation was achieved (Fig. 3d, Additional file 7: Table S4) wherein a decrease in tumor volume, measured prior and after treatment, matched a reduction in PET tumor VOI ($r = 0.85$, $p = 0.001$).

In JIMT-1 tumor-bearing mice, FDG-PET did not distinguish between tumors in untreated groups (3.81 ± 0.78 %ID/g) and dasatinib-treated groups (7 days, 3.36 ± 0.89 %ID/g, $p = 0.73$; 14 days, 3.20 ± 1.37 %ID/g, $p = 0.61$) (Fig. 4a). In the same mice imaged with [89]Zr-trastuzumab, tumor uptake displayed VOIs of 8.04 ± 0.71 %ID/g in the control, whereas there was a two-fold decrease in uptake

in the treated groups at 7 days (3.88 ± 1.47 %ID/g, $p < 0.0001$) and 14 days (4.45 ± 1.23 %ID/g, $p < 0.0001$) (Fig. 4b). Tracer accumulation did not differ between 7-day and 14-day treatment ($p = 0.71$) (Fig. 4c). A strong association between [89]Zr-trastuzumab PET uptake and tumor volume regression was recapitulated in this tumor model ($r = 0.82$, $p = 0.0002$) (Fig. 4d, Additional file 8: Table S5). Collectively, these results suggest that [89]Zr-trastuzumab can effectively delineate tumors responsive to dasatinib treatment.

Ex vivo analysis of JIMT-1 or BT-474 tumors

After imaging, tumors were removed for ex vivo validation of the PET readout. From the immunoblot analysis, BT-474 tumors had moderately decreased levels of total Src upon treatment with dasatinib, whereas its activity was mitigated 2.6-fold as displayed by pSrc (Y416) levels in both 7-day and 14-day treated cohorts (Fig. 5a). Additionally, there was a decrease in total HER2 as assessed by densitometry after 7-day and 14-day treatments (Fig. 5a). A positive correlation was observed between tumor VOI values and pSrc (Y416) ($r = 0.70$, $p = 0.025$) (Fig. 5b) and pHER2 ($r = 0.64$, $p = 0.046$) (Fig. 5c) (measured by densitometry) for BT-474.

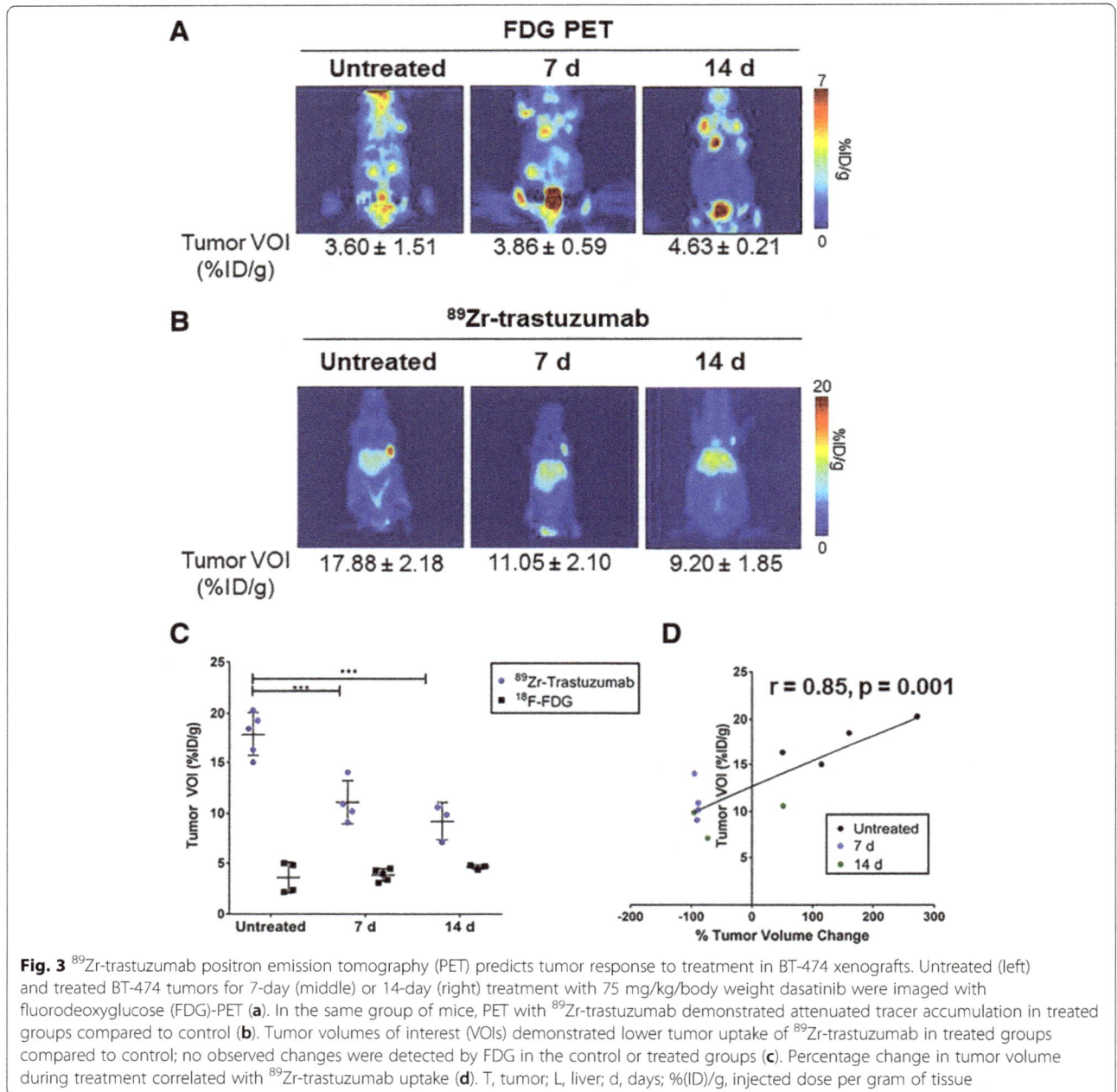

Fig. 3 [89]Zr-trastuzumab positron emission tomography (PET) predicts tumor response to treatment in BT-474 xenografts. Untreated (left) and treated BT-474 tumors for 7-day (middle) or 14-day (right) treatment with 75 mg/kg/body weight dasatinib were imaged with fluorodeoxyglucose (FDG)-PET (**a**). In the same group of mice, PET with [89]Zr-trastuzumab demonstrated attenuated tracer accumulation in treated groups compared to control (**b**). Tumor volumes of interest (VOIs) demonstrated lower tumor uptake of [89]Zr-trastuzumab in treated groups compared to control; no observed changes were detected by FDG in the control or treated groups (**c**). Percentage change in tumor volume during treatment correlated with [89]Zr-trastuzumab uptake (**d**). T, tumor; L, liver; d, days; %(ID)/g, injected dose per gram of tissue

Treated and control JIMT-1 tumors did not show a difference in total HER2 or Src expression; however, a noticeable decrease in both pSrc and pHER2 after 7-day and 14-day treatments was displayed (Fig. 5d). Moreover, there was significant, positive association between pSrc (Y416) ($r = 0.68$, $p = 0.022$) and [89]Zr-trastuzumab tumor VOI (Fig. 5e). A direct relationship between dephosphorylated HER2 and tracer uptake in the tumor was also demonstrated ($r = 0.63$, $p = 0.037$) (Fig. 5f).

IHC was performed to visualize subcellular localization of HER2 and pSrc (Y416) in excised tumors. Untreated BT-474 tumors showed strong, positive membranous HER2 staining (Fig. 6a, top left panel), whereas, predominant cytoplasmic HER2 localization was exhibited in tumors treated for 14 days. (Fig. 6a, top right). Less pSrc (Y416) staining was observed in treated tumors (Fig. 6a, bottom right) compared to control (Fig. 6a, bottom left). Control JIMT-1 tumors exhibited lower expression of membrane-localized HER2 (Fig. 6b, top left) compared to BT-474 but translocation to cytoplasmic regions was observed in treated sections (Fig. 6b, top right). Higher pSrc (Y416) staining waas displayed in control (Fig. 6b, bottom right) versus dasatinib-treated tumor sections (Fig. 6b, bottom left).

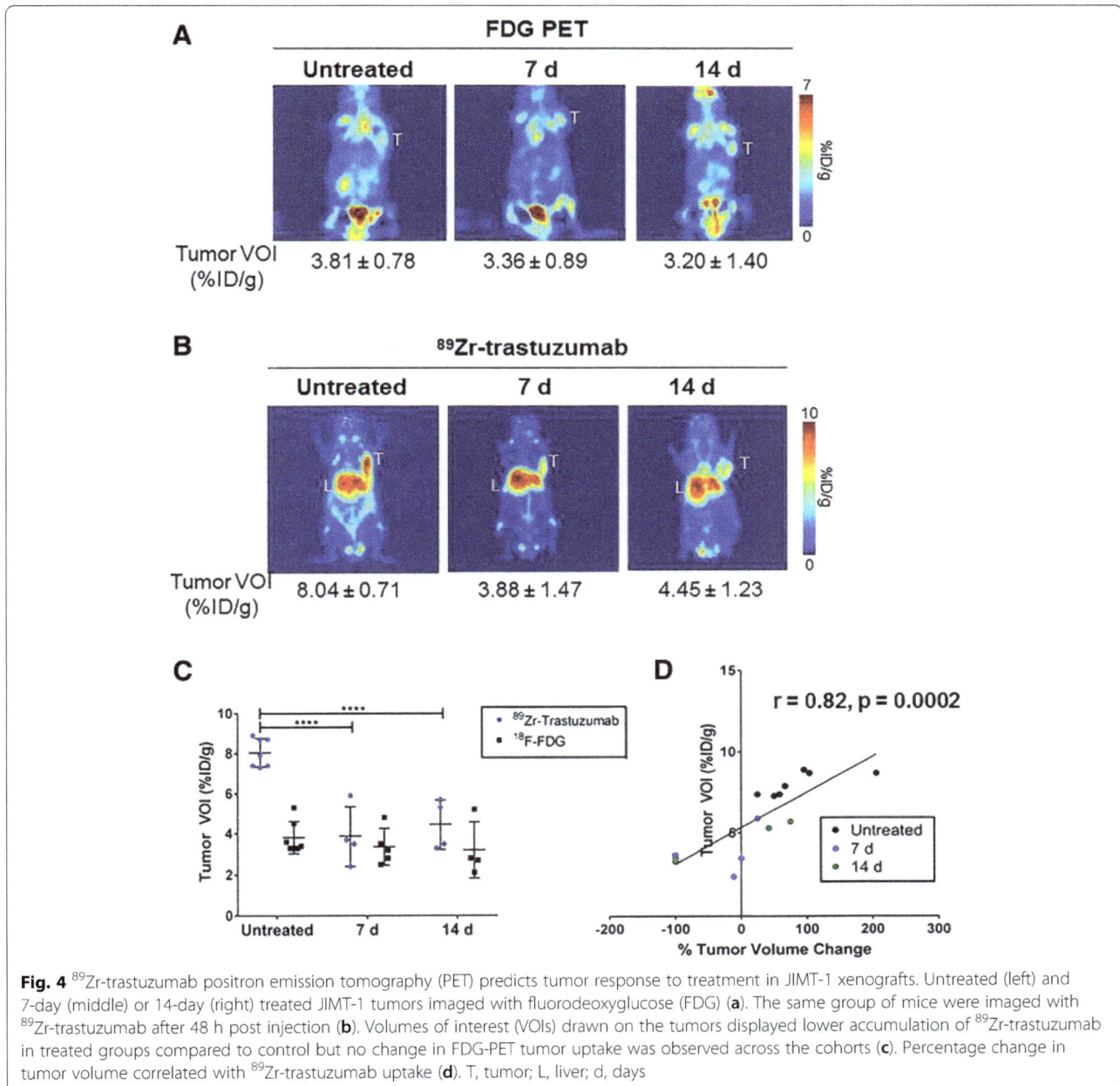

Fig. 4 89Zr-trastuzumab positron emission tomography (PET) predicts tumor response to treatment in JIMT-1 xenografts. Untreated (left) and 7-day (middle) or 14-day (right) treated JIMT-1 tumors imaged with fluorodeoxyglucose (FDG) (**a**). The same group of mice were imaged with 89Zr-trastuzumab after 48 h post injection (**b**). Volumes of interest (VOIs) drawn on the tumors displayed lower accumulation of 89Zr-trastuzumab in treated groups compared to control but no change in FDG-PET tumor uptake was observed across the cohorts (**c**). Percentage change in tumor volume correlated with 89Zr-trastuzumab uptake (**d**). T, tumor; L, liver; d, days

Discussion

Trastuzumab has been the standard of care in HER2+ breast cancer for two decades [19]. Unfortunately, about half of patients with HER2-overexpressing breast cancer do not respond to trastuzumab due to de novo and acquired resistance mechanisms [20]. The non-receptor tyrosine kinase Src was shown to be one of the key modulators of trastuzumab response, and is an important downstream node of multiple trastuzumab resistance pathways [5–7, 18, 20]. Targeting Src with dasatinib in vitro re-sensitized trastuzumab-resistant cell lines, suggesting this pathway as a strategy to overcome resistance

[6]. Using the Src inhibitor PP2, Fan et al. demonstrated that in vitro cellular Src modulation of trastuzumab-sensitive HER2+/estrogen receptor (ER)-negative SKBr3 cells decreased HER2 levels after 7 days and abrogated the expression completely after 14 days of treatment [9]. Further evidence identified improved anti-tumor effects in trastuzumab-resistant gastric xenografts compared to parental implants upon treatment with bosutinib, a Src-specific drug [21].

These preclinical findings were substantiated in patient studies implicating Src hyperactivity with trastuzumab resistance [6, 10]. In fact, tumors with high levels of

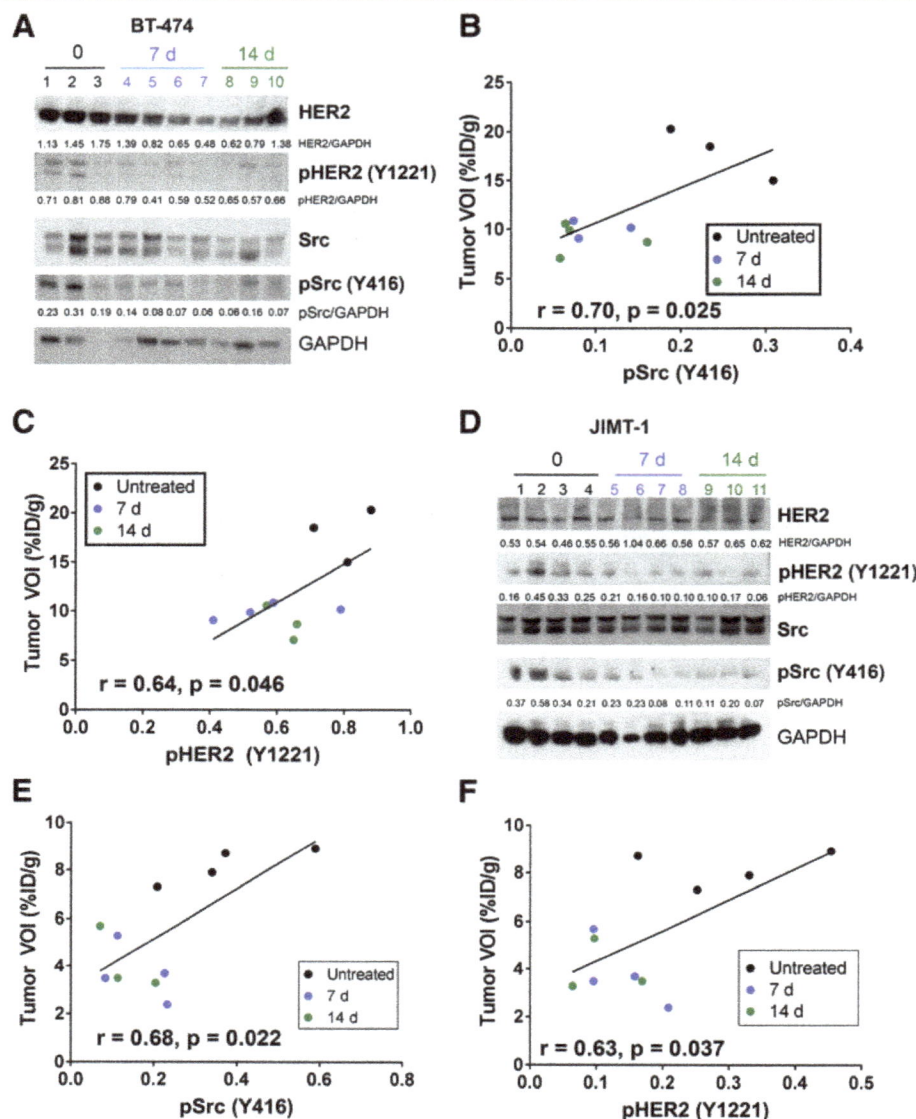

Fig. 5 Ex vivo validation on excised BT-474 and JIMT-1 tumors confirm positron emission tomography (PET) uptake. Western blots were performed for human epidermal growth factor receptor 2 (HER2), Src, and phosphorylated Src (pSrc) (Y416) expression using BT-474 tumor lysates (**a**); a plot of the pSrc (Y416) densitometry showed a linear relationship with [89]Zr-trastuzumab PET uptake (**b**). A plot of the pHER2 (Y1221) densitometry showed a linear relationship with [89]Zr-trastuzumab PET uptake (**c**). Similarly, JIMT-1 tumors obtained after PET was lysed and analyzed for protein expression using western blots (**d**). pSrc (Y416) also demonstrated a direct linear correlation with [89]Zr-trastuzumab PET uptake in JIMT-1 tumors (**e**). A plot of the pHER2 (Y1221) densitometry showed a linear relationship with [89]Zr-trastuzumab PET uptake (**f**). All densitometry values were obtained as the ratio of total protein to glyceraldehyde-3-phosphate dehydrogenase (GAPDH)

phosphorylated Src at the Y416 residue presented with a lower clinical response rates, higher progressive disease, and shorter survival rates after trastuzumab treatment, compared to those with lower phosphorylated Src (Y416) levels [6, 10]. With this strong body of evidence, Src has become an appealing therapeutic target in the clinic. The GEICAM 2010/04 study (NCT01306942), in particular, initiated a safety and proof-of-concept synergistic study, which included dasatinib in combination with standard-of-care trastuzumab and paclitaxel [13].

Through pathology of sequential patient skin biopsies, reduction of pSrc was observed post-dasatinib treatment, with lower expression found with combined trastuzumab treatment [13]. The main concern with pSrc (Y416) as a biomarker of response lies in utilizing invasive sequential biopsies, which does not provide real-time information on the status of the tyrosine kinase.

Recently, Veach et al. reported the development and in vitro biological and in vivo pharmacologic activity of a ^{18}F-labeled analog of dasatinib [22]. Dosimetric and

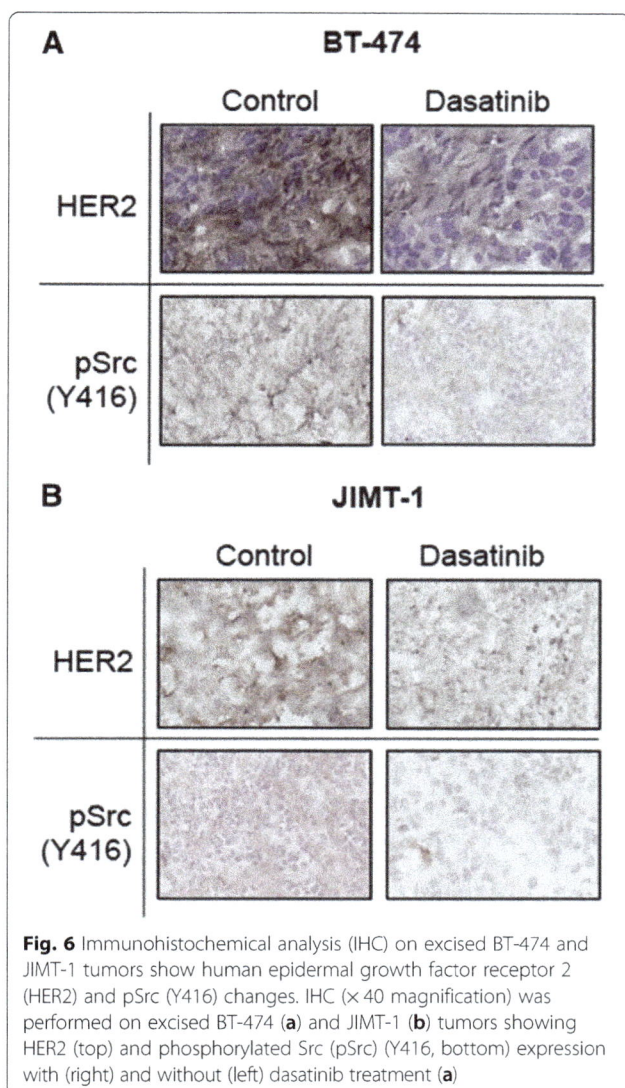

Fig. 6 Immunohistochemical analysis (IHC) on excised BT-474 and JIMT-1 tumors show human epidermal growth factor receptor 2 (HER2) and pSrc (Y416) changes. IHC (× 40 magnification) was performed on excised BT-474 (**a**) and JIMT-1 (**b**) tumors showing HER2 (top) and phosphorylated Src (pSrc) (Y416, bottom) expression with (right) and without (left) dasatinib treatment (**a**)

pharmacokinetic profiles were investigated in preclinical studies [23] and are currently being investigated in clinical trials (NCT01916135). This method has its limitations since this can potentially miss functional effects upstream or downstream of the Src signaling pathway. The underlying relationship between Src and aberrant HER2 signaling provided us the impetus to examine ^{89}Zr-trastuzumab PET as a surrogate predictive marker of dasatinib treatment.

Using ^{89}Zr-trastuzumab as a surrogate marker of targeted inhibition of effector molecules downstream of the HER2 signaling pathway has been conceptually proven, for example, with Hsp90 inhibition [24]. Currently, this imaging probe is investigated in the clinic not only for diagnostic and staging purposes but also as a marker of response to other targeted treatments (NCT01081600 for AUY922 HSP90 inhibitor, NCT01565200 for T-DM1) [25]. To the best of our knowledge, this is the first study

that demonstrated the potential of ^{89}Zr-trastuzumab PET to monitor Src response to dasatinib treatment in trastuzumab-sensitive and trastuzumab-refractory breast cancer xenografts with proven Src activity. Specifically, we have shown that ^{89}Zr-trastuzumab detects reduced functional HER2 through a concomitant decrease in internalization of the tracer after 6 h (BT-474) or 48 h (JIMT-1) of dasatinib treatment. The lower 89Zr-trastuzumab internalization was coupled with lower total HER2 present on the membrane, confirmed by ^{89}Zr-trastuzumab binding experiments and western blots of pHER2(Y1221/1222). To date, limited information is known about the association between HER2 receptor internalization and dephosphorylation, which requires further study [26]. From our in vivo studies, a strong positive correlation was demonstrated between ^{89}Zr-trastuzumab tumor uptake and tumor regression, changes in pSrc at the Y416 residue, and autophosphorylated HER2 at the Y1221/1222 residue. Importantly, the HER2-specific tracer detected these molecular events, where FDG, the gold standard PET imaging agents, has failed. Our histology studies encompassing decreased pSrc (Y416) with concomitant lower membranous HER2 further support and validate the ^{89}Zr-trastuzumab PET readout. Taken together, ^{89}Zr-trastuzumab can potentially be explored and utilized to assess dasatinib therapy in HER2+ breast cancer patients with elevated Src activity. However, it is worth noting that our studies are limited to single-agent Src inhibition; the utility of ^{89}Zr-trastuzumab PET in combined therapies including dasatinib in HER2+ breast cancer still warrants further investigation.

Conclusions
^{89}Zr-trastuzumab can potentially delineate changes in Src activity and status in HER2+ breast cancer in both trastuzumab-sensitive and trastuzumab-resistant phenotypes.

Additional files

Additional file 1: Table S1. Antibodies and dilutions used for each study. (JPG 425 kb)

Additional file 2: Figure S1. ^{89}Zr-trastuzumab retains immunoreactivity in BT-474. Immunoreactivity of ^{89}Zr-trastuzumab showed retained reactivity with $r^2 = 0.96$. (JPG 173 kb)

Additional file 3: Figure S2. ^{89}Zr-trastuzumab is specific for HER2 in vitro and in vivo. BT-474, JIMT-1 and MDA-MB-468 cells were incubated with 100 ng ^{89}Zr-trastuzumab alone or co-incubated with 25-fold unlabeled trastuzumab before being lysed and radioactivity was measured using a gamma counter. (A) Nude mice bearing MDA-MB-468, BT-474 or JIMT-1 tumors were imaged with ^{89}Zr-trastuzumab 48 h p.i. (B) Tumor VOIs showing significant uptake in HER2+ tumors, but no uptake in MDA-MB-468 (HER2-) tumors (C). (TIF 4980 kb)

Additional file 4: Figure S3. ^{89}Zr-trastuzumab tumor uptake compared to isotype matched control. Mice bearing BT-474 and JIMT-1 tumors were injected with ^{89}Zr-IgG or ^{89}Zr-trastuzumab and tumors were removed 48 h p.i. and measured using a gamma counter. In both cell lines, specific

[89]Zr-trastuzumab uptake was significantly higher than isotype control IgG. (JPG 267 kb)

Additional file 5: Table S2. [89]Zr-trastuzumab and [89]Zr-IgG biodistribution in BT-474 tumors. (JPG 117 kb)

Additional file 6: Table S3. [89]Zr-trastuzumab and [89]Zr-IgG biodistribution in JIMT-1 tumors. (JPG 116 kb)

Additional file 7: Table S4. [89]Zr-trastuzumab tumor VOI, pSrc (416) densitometry, and pHER2 (Y1221/1222) densitometry values for BT-474. (JPG 64 kb)

Additional file 8: Table S5. [89]Zr-trastuzumab tumor VOI, pSrc (416) densitometry, and pHER2 (Y1221/1222) densitometry values for JIMT-1. (JPG 68 kb)

Abbreviations

DFO: p-Benzyl-isothiocyanate-desferrioxamine; DMEM: Dulbecco's modified Eagle's medium; DMSO: Dimethyl sulfoxide; FBS: Fetal bovine serum; ^{18}F-FDG: [18]Fluorine-Fluorodeoxyglucose; GAPDH: Glyceraldehyde-3-phosphate dehydrogenase; HER2: Human epidermal growth factor receptor 2; HRP: Horseradish peroxidase; IC_{50}: Half maximal inhibitory concentration; IHC: Immunohistochemical analysis; iTLC: Instant thin layer chromatography; i.v.: Intravenously; kDa: KiloDalton; PBS: Phosphate-buffered saline; PET: Positron emission tomography; p.i.: Post-injection; pSrc: Phosphorylated Src; RTKs: Receptor tyrosine kinases; s.c.: Subcutaneously; TBST: Tris-buffered saline and Tween 20; VOI: Volume of interest

Acknowledgements

We would like to thank Julie Boerner, PhD and Lisa Polin, PhD for technical discussions, Agnes Malysa for assistance on the IHC studies and Kirk Douglas and Xin Lu for assistance with the μPET machine.

Funding

Acknowledgements are extended to the following National Institutes of Health (NIH) grant-funding support: R00 CA181492 (NTV) and T32 CAA09531 (BNM). The authors further acknowledge the Microscopy, Imaging and Cytometry Resources Core and the Animal Model and Therapeutic Evaluation Core (AMTEC), which are supported, in part, by NIH Center grant P30 CA022453 to the Karmanos Cancer Institute at Wayne State University, and the Perinatology Research Branch of the National Institutes of Child Health and Development at Wayne State University.

Authors' contributions

NTV is the principal investigator of the project, conceptualized and designed the study and oversaw the experimental planning and data analysis. BNM performed all of the experiments and statistical analysis and assisted in experimental planning and experimental design. Both authors edited, read and approved the final manuscript.

Competing interests

The authors declare that they have no competing interests.

References

1. Ryan Q, Ibrahim A, Cohen MH, Johnson J, Ko CW, Sridhara R, et al. FDA drug approval summary: lapatinib in combination with capecitabine for previously treated metastatic Breast cancer that overexpresses HER-2. Oncologist. 2008;13:1114–9. https://doi.org/10.1634/theoncologist.2008-0816.
2. Hortobagyi GN. Trastuzumab in the treatment of breast cancer. N Engl J Med. 2005;353:1734–6. https://doi.org/10.1056/NEJMe058196.
3. Neves H, Kwok HF. Recent advances in the field of anti-cancer immunotherapy. BBA Clinical. 2015;3:280–8.
4. Gonzalez-Angulo AM, Morales-Vasquez F, Hortobagyi GN. Overview of resistance to systemic therapy in patients with breast cancer. Adv Exp Med Biol. 2007;608:1–22.
5. Muthuswamy SK. Trastuzumab resistance: All roads lead to SRC. Nat Med. 2011;17:416–8.
6. Zhang S, Huang WC, Li P, Guo H, Poh SB, Brady SW, et al. Combating trastuzumab resistance by targeting SRC, a common node downstream of multiple resistance pathways. Nat Med. 2011;17:461–9. https://doi.org/10.1038/nm.2309.
7. Mayer EL, Krop IE. Advances in targeting Src in the treatment of breast cancer and other solid malignancies. Clin Cancer Res. 2010;16:3526–32.
8. Tan M, Li P, Klos KS, Lu J, Lan KH, Nagata Y, et al. ErbB2 promotes Src synthesis and stability: novel mechanisms of Src activation that confer breast cancer metastasis. Cancer Res. 2005;65:1858–67.
9. Fan P, McDaniel RE, Kim HR, Clagett D, Haddad B, Craig Jordan V. Modulating therapeutic effects of the c-Src inhibitor via oestrogen receptor and human epidermal growth factor receptor 2 in breast cancer cell lines. Eur J Cancer. 2012;48:3488–98.
10. Peiró G, Ortiz-Martínez F, Gallardo A, Pérez-Balaguer A, Sánchez-Payá J, Ponce JJ, et al. Src, a potential target for overcoming trastuzumab resistance in HER2-positive breast carcinoma. Br J Cancer. 2014;111:689–95.
11. Talpaz M, Shah NP, Kantarjian H, Donato N, Nicoll J, Paquette R, et al. Dasatinib in imatinib-resistant Philadelphia chromosome–positive leukemias. N Engl J Med. 2006;354:2531–41. https://doi.org/10.1056/NEJMoa055229.
12. Seoane S, Montero JC, Ocaña A, Pandiella A. Effect of multikinase inhibitors on caspase-independent cell death and DNA damage in HER2-overexpressing breast cancer cells. J Natl Cancer Inst. 2010;102:1432–46.
13. Ocana A, Gil-Martin M, Martín M, Rojo F, Antolín S, Guerrero Á, et al. A phase I study of the SRC kinase inhibitor dasatinib with trastuzumab and paclitaxel as first line therapy for patients with HER2-overexpressing advanced breast cancer. GEICAM/2010-04 study. Oncotarget. 2017. https://doi.org/10.18632/oncotarget.17113.
14. Viola-Villegas NT, Sevak KK, Carlin SD, Doran MG, Evans HW, Bartlett DW, et al. Noninvasive imaging of PSMA in prostate tumors with89Zr-labeled huJ591 engineered antibody fragments: the faster alternatives. Mol Pharm. 2014;11:3965–73.
15. Janjigian YY, Viola-Villegas N, Holland JP, Divilov V, Carlin SD, Gomes-DaGama EM, et al. Monitoring afatinib treatment in HER2-positive gastric cancer with 18F-FDG and 89Zr-Trastuzumab PET. J Nucl Med. 2013;54:936–43. https://doi.org/10.2967/jnumed.112.110239.
16. Lindmo T, Boven E, Cuttitta F, Fedorko J, Bunn PA. Determination of the immunoreactive function of radiolabeled monoclonal antibodies by linear extrapolation to binding at infinite antigen excess. J Immunol Methods. 1984;72:77–89.
17. Boerner RJ, Kassel DB, Barker SC, Ellis B, DeLacy P, Knight WB. Correlation of the phosphorylation states of pp60(c-src) with tyrosine kinase activity: the intramolecular pY530-SH2 complex retains significant activity if Y419 is phosphorylated. Biochemistry. 1996;35:9519–25.
18. Belsches-Jablonski AP, Biscardi JS, Peavy DR, D a T, D a R, Parsons SJ. Src family kinases and HER2 interactions in human breast cancer cell growth and survival. Oncogene. 2001;20:1465–75. https://doi.org/10.1038/sj.onc.1204205.
19. Hudis CA. Trastuzumab–mechanism of action and use in clinical practice. N Engl J Med. 2007;357:39–51. https://doi.org/10.1056/NEJMra043186.
20. Lan KH, Lu CH, Yu D. Mechanisms of trastuzumab resistance and their clinical implications: Annals of the New York Academy of Sciences; 2005. p. 70–5.

21. Jin MH, Nam A-R, Park JE, Bang J-H, Bang Y-J, Oh D-Y. Resistance mechanism against trastuzumab in HER2-positive cancer cells and its negation by Src inhibition. Mol Cancer Ther. 2017;16:1145–54. https://doi.org/10.1158/1535-7163.MCT-16-0669.

22. Veach DR, Namavari M, Pillarsetty N, Santos EB, Beresten-Kochetkov T, Lambek C, et al. Synthesis and biological evaluation of a fluorine-18 derivative of dasatinib. J Med Chem. 2007;50:5853–7.

23. Dunphy MPS, Zanzonico P, Veach D, Somwar R, Pillarsetty N, Lewis J, et al. Dosimetry of 18F-labeled tyrosine kinase inhibitor SKI-249380, a dasatinib-tracer for PET imaging. Mol Imaging Biol. 2012;14:25–31.

24. Holland JP, Caldas-Lopes E, Divilov V, V a L, Taldone T, Zatorska D, et al. Measuring the pharmacodynamic effects of a novel Hsp90 inhibitor on HER2/neu expression in mice using Zr-DFO-trastuzumab. PLoS One. 2010;5:e8859. https://doi.org/10.1371/journal.pone.0008859.

25. Massicano AVF, Marquez-Nostra BV, Lapi SE. targeting her2 in nuclear medicine for imaging and therapy. Mol Imaging. 2018;17.

26. Dong H, Ma L, Gan J, Lin W, Chen C, Yao Z, et al. PTPRO represses ERBB2-driven breast oncogenesis by dephosphorylation and endosomal internalization of ERBB2. Oncogene. 2017;36(3):410–22.

18

Molecular patterns of cancer colonisation in lymph nodes of breast cancer patients

Gaurav Chatterjee[1,2,3†], Trupti Pai[1,2,3†], Thomas Hardiman[1,2], Kelly Avery-Kiejda[4], Rodney J. Scott[4], Jo Spencer[5], Sarah E. Pinder[2] and Anita Grigoriadis[1,2,6*] [iD]

Abstract

Lymph node (LN) metastasis is an important prognostic parameter in breast carcinoma, a crucial site for tumour–immune cell interaction and a gateway for further dissemination of tumour cells to other metastatic sites. To gain insight into the underlying molecular changes from the pre-metastatic, via initial colonisation to the fully involved LN, we reviewed transcriptional research along the evolving microenvironment of LNs in human breast cancers patients. Gene expression studies were compiled and subjected to pathway-based analyses, with an emphasis on immune cell-related genes. Of 366 studies, 14 performed genome-wide gene expression comparisons and were divided into six clinical-biological scenarios capturing different stages of the metastatic pathway in the LN, as follows: metastatically involved LNs are compared to their patient-matched primary breast carcinomas (scenario 1) or the normal breast tissue (scenario 2). In scenario 3, uninvolved LNs were compared between LN-positive patients and LN-negative patients. Scenario 4 homed in on the residual uninvolved portion of involved LNs and compared it to the patient-matched uninvolved LNs. Scenario 5 contrasted uninvolved and involved LNs, whilst in scenario 6 involved (sentinel) LNs were assessed between patients with other either positive or negative LNs (non-sentinel). Gene lists from these chronological steps of LN metastasis indicated that gene patterns reflecting deficiencies in dendritic cells and hyper-proliferation of B cells parallel to tumour promoting pathways, including cell adhesion, extracellular matrix remodelling, cell motility and DNA repair, play key roles in the changing microenvironment of a pro-metastatic to a metastatically involved LN. Similarities between uninvolved LNs and the residual uninvolved portion of involved LNs hinted that LN alterations expose systemic tumour-related immune responses in breast cancer patients. Despite the diverse settings, gene expression patterns at different stages of metastatic colonisation in LNs were recognised and may provide potential avenues for clinical interventions to counteract disease progression for breast cancer patients.

Keywords: Expression, Lymph node, Premetastatic niche, Breast cancer

Introduction

The lymph nodes (LNs) are functional units of the immune system that act as immunological hubs supporting the complex interactions between T cells, B cells, antigen-presenting cells and stromal cells. LNs receive cells and potential immunogenic substances via the afferent lymphatics that drain the tissues and enter the LNs at the peripheral subcapsular sinus and also via the high endothelial venules, which support lymphocyte entry from the blood [1, 2]. The LN is a dynamic organ capable of undergoing dramatic remodelling, in terms of both architecture and function, in response to pathological conditions such as inflammation or cancer [3]. Many solid cancers spread through the lymphatic system to distant organs, with the LNs typically serving as a first site of seeding outside primary tumour [4–6]. For these tumours, the presence and extent of LN metastasis are markers of aggressive phenotype, often having an inverse linear relationship with prognosis [7–9]. In breast carcinoma patients, metastasis to LN is an important factor for staging the tumour and routine assessment for invasive

* Correspondence: anita.grigoriadis@kcl.ac.uk
†Gaurav Chatterjee and Trupti Pai contributed equally to this work.
[1]Cancer Bioinformatics, King's College London, Innovation Hub, Cancer Centre at Guy's Hospital, Great Maze Pond, London SE1 9RT, UK
[2]School of Cancer & Pharmaceutical Sciences, CRUK King's Health Partners Centre, King's College London, Innovation Hub, Comprehensive Cancer Centre at Guy's Hospital, Great Maze Pond, London SE1 9RT, UK
Full list of author information is available at the end of the article

breast carcinoma patients includes histopathological assessment of the presence of metastasis, the number of involved LNs and the presence or absence of extra-nodal extension [10].

Although the LN is a functional organ for tumour–immune system interaction and may be a read-out for systemic immune responses, studies of the molecular characteristics of LNs have centred around mutational alterations and structural genome rearrangements, whereas transcriptional research has been limited in both human and pre-clinical models [11]. Most studies have aimed to identify molecular signatures associated with good and bad prognosis in primary breast tumours, and gene sets consistently predicting the development of LN metastasis have yet to be determined [12–17], while the genomes of relapsed or secondary breast cancers have revealed that metastases and primary tumours are clonally related, share several driver mutations and often acquire additional novel variants that are not present in the primary lesion [18].

In the metastatic LN, a multitude of factors play important roles in tilting the balance between pro-metastatic immunosuppression and anti-tumoural immune response [19–21]. Given the significant implication of LN metastasis for systemic cancer burden, surprisingly little emphasis has been given to elucidate the underlying molecular signals and cellular alterations of the evolving LN microenvironment between the uninvolved (cancer-free) and the involved (metastatic) LNs in breast cancer patients. Some of these changes include lymphangiogenesis and increased lymph flow [22], recruitment and expansion of immunosuppressive cells (including myeloid-derived suppressor cells and regulatory T cells) [23], upregulation of chemokines and cytokines, blood vessel remodelling [24, 25] and a lower percentage of effector T cells [26]. We recently comprehensively histologically characterised diverse immune and stromal features in primary tumours and their associated involved and uninvolved axillary LNs in a cohort of 309 invasive breast cancer patients (143/309 LN positive) [27] and observed that architectural alterations of the uninvolved LN are significant predictors for distant metastases. A similar finding of prognostic information from examination of the LN architecture was observed in melanoma [28]. In preclinical mouse models, the involvement of innate lymphoid RORγt+ ILC3 cells, fibroblast reticular cells and cancer-associated fibroblasts in the induction of an immunosuppressive and pro-metastatic microenvironment in tumour-draining LNs was reported [29–31], while uninvolved regional LNs in rats with prostate tumours displayed varying degrees of genetic changes depending on prostate tumour groups and their metastatic capacity [32].

With regards to emerging immunotherapy approaches, the LN microenvironment and the nature of the immune response have been identified as potent indicators of response to therapeutic interventions [33, 34]. With the central position of the LN as an immune organ and as a gateway for further dissemination of tumour cells to other metastatic sites, we conducted a comprehensive review of existing gene expression-based research performed on LNs in human breast cancers. We categorised these gene expression studies along the evolving microenvironment of axillary metastases. By starting with early colonisation to the replacement of the entire LN with metastasis, these expression patterns capture information on the molecular mechanisms and changes in immune composition that allow the exploration of LNs as a pro-metastatic niche. Since patients with locoregional breast cancer typically have a high risk of developing distant metastasis and thus poor overall survival, it is particularly important to establish whether transcriptomic patterns indicative of metastasis might translate into new therapeutic strategies, including the successful implementation of immunotherapy.

Materials and methods
Literature search and data collection
A review of the English literature was performed, focusing on gene expression data derived from human LN tissue and the primary lesion in breast cancer patients (if matched LN tissue was interrogated), using the combination of the following keywords: "breast cancer", "metastasis", "lymph nodes" and "gene expression" in "all fields" in PUBMED and Ovid MEDLINE ® (accessed on 13th October 2017 and revised on 5th June 2018). All abstracts were manually screened and their methodologies were reviewed. Papers were selected if genome-wide (i.e. microarray or RNA-sequencing based) gene expression analyses of LNs of breast cancer patients were performed (*n* = 14). Studies of primary breast tumours and distant metastatic sites which reported only the LN status of the patients were excluded (see consort diagram in Fig. 1). The review was conducted according to the preferred reporting items for systematic reviews and meta-analyses (PRISMA) statement [35].

Data analysis
Of a total 366 papers screened, 14 studies were included in the review: Calvo et al. [36], Feng et al. [37], Hao et al. [38], Lähdesmäki et al. [39], Weigelt et al. [40], Ellsworth et al. [41], Vecchi et al. [42], Suzuki et al. [43], Mathe et al. [44], Zuckerman et al. [45], Blackburn et al. [46], Valente et al. [47], Rizwan et al. [48] (all of which performed microarray-based gene expression analyses); and Liang et al. [49], which used 18–27 million paired-end riboZero RNA-sequencing. Genes with differential expression between the respective scenarios were obtained directly from the publications; no cut-offs were applied (Table 1). Using the biomaRt R package [50, 51], either gene names or microarray features

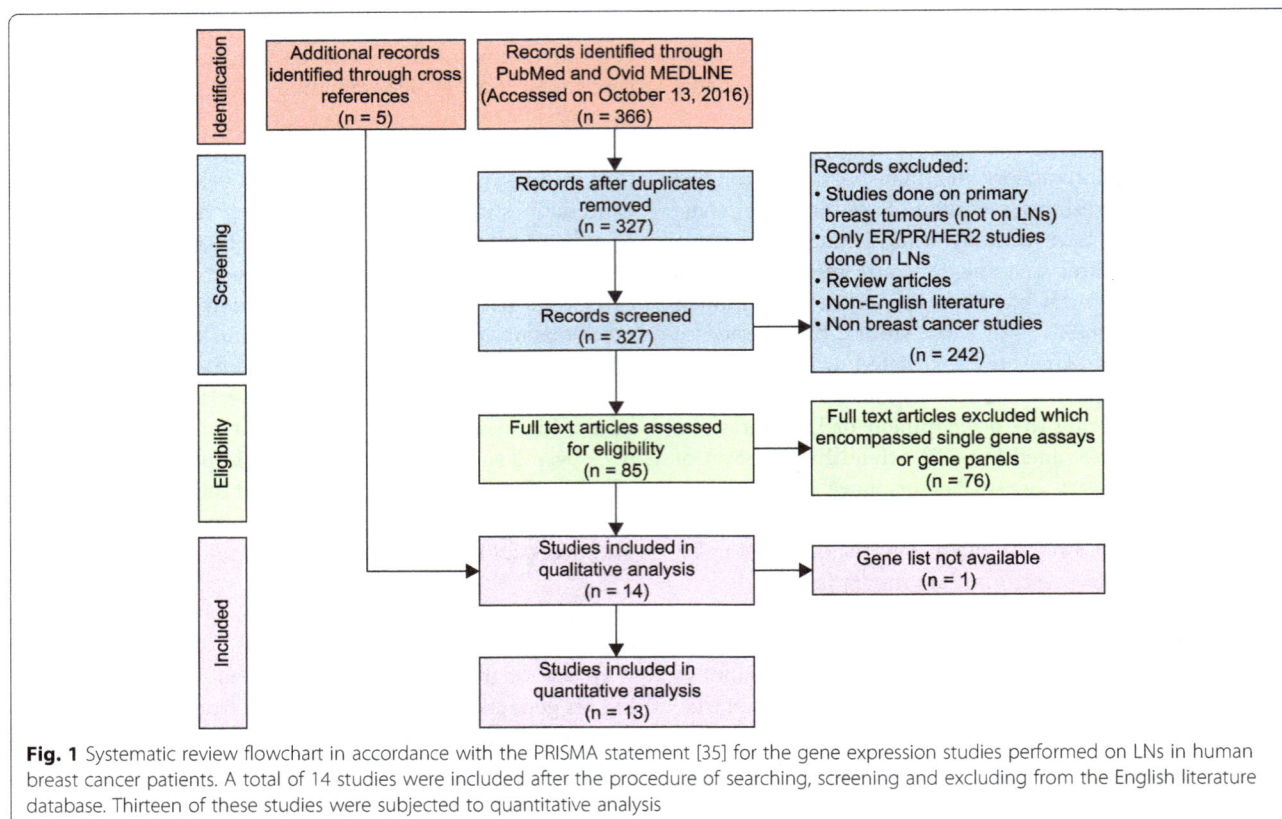

Fig. 1 Systematic review flowchart in accordance with the PRISMA statement [35] for the gene expression studies performed on LNs in human breast cancer patients. A total of 14 studies were included after the procedure of searching, screening and excluding from the English literature database. Thirteen of these studies were subjected to quantitative analysis

were converted to ENSEMBL ID (ENSEMBL GRCh37.p13) [52] (Additional files 1, 2 and 3: Tables S1–S3). If microarray features could not be mapped, assuming that their sequences are retired (i.e are not present in any current sequence database), they were excluded from further studies. Once an ENSEMBL ID list was created, HGNC symbols, genomic location and their common gene ontology terms were recorded. From these ENSEMBL gene lists, pathway analyses were conducted on de-regulated genes using the WebGestalt tool [53] (Additional file 4: Table S4). The over-representation analysis (ORA) was applied based on the *Homo sapiens* Gene Ontology (GO) biological processes database. The whole genome was used as a reference; all GO terms < 0.05 FDR were extracted. To remove redundant GO terms, the Revigo tool with parameter "small" was used [54]. The resultant GO terms and differentially expressed genes were compared between the groups. To capture genes representative for specific immune cell populations, the gene lists compounded from the studies were cross-referenced with published immune metagenes [55].

Results and discussion

Overview of expression profiling studies on LNs in breast cancer

A total of 14 genome-wide transcriptomic studies on LN samples were selected to decipher the molecular features of the evolving LN microenvironment as a locoregional metastatic site [36–49]. Each article published lists of genes specifically transcriptionally activated or repressed in LNs, ranging from cancer-free to metastatic settings. The cohorts were of mixed-receptor (Estrogen (ER), Progesterone (PR) and Human epidermal growth factor receptor (HER2)) invasive breast carcinomas, including two studies of invasive carcinomas of ductal/no special type only and one exclusively examining triple negative breast carcinomas (TNBC). To paint a chronological picture of the changing microenvironment of the evolving metastatic LN, the studies were grouped into six "scenarios", described below in detail (Table 1, Fig. 2).

Scenario 1: Comparison between involved LN and primary breast carcinoma, the drivers of metastasis

With the common aims of searching for drivers of metastatic progression, developing metastatic signatures predictive of distant metastasis [37, 42] and identifying molecular targets for metastasis-specific therapy or markers of resistance, eight of 14 studies captured transcriptional alterations between involved LNs and their patient-matched primary carcinoma. Expression patterns and gene regulatory pathways potentially driving metastatic dissemination were determined, while the point of acquiring metastatic efficiency in a primary tumour's

Table 1 Genome-wide expression studies of LNs of breast carcinoma patients

Clinical question	Study	Breast carcinoma	Sample cohort	Results
Scenario 1 Involved lymph node (ILN) versus primary tumours (PT)	Calvo et al. [36], 2013	IDC	18 PT vs matching ILN	Infrequent loss of luminal differentiation in metastatic LN
	Feng et al. [37], 2007	IDC	26 PT vs matching ILN	79 DEG
	Hao et al. & Lähdesmäki et al. [38, 39], 2004	Invasive BC	9 PT vs matching ILN	280 DEG
	Weigelt et al [40], 2005	Invasive BC	15 PT vs matching ILN	No classifier or single gene could discriminate
	Ellsworth et al. [41], 2009	Invasive BC	20 PT vs matching ILN	51 DEG
	Vecchi et al. [42], 2008	Invasive BC	26 PT vs matching ILN	270 DEG
	Suzuki et al. [43], 2007	Invasive BC	10 PT vs matching ILN	84 DEG
Scenario 2 Involved LN versus normal adjacent breast tissue (NAT)	Mathe et al. [44], 2015	TNBC	15 ILN vs 17 NAT	83 genes were significantly associated with LN metastasis
Scenario 3 Uninvolved LN in LN-positive versus LN-negative patients	Zuckerman et al. [45], 2013	Invasive BC	11 PT, 30 LN, 21 PB	116/219 DEG (SLN/NSLN, respectively)
	Blackburn et al. [46], 2017	Invasive BC	24 LN from NP vs 40 LN from NN	No genes were differentially expressed with stringent FDR
Scenario 4 Uninvolved residual portion of involved LN versus uninvolved LN	Valente et al. [47], 2014	Invasive BC	20 matched pairs of involved and uninvolved LN	22 DEG
	Zuckerman et al. [45], 2013	Invasive BC	11 PT, 30 LN, 21 PB	103 DEG
Scenario 5 Involved LN versus uninvolved LN	Rizwan et al. [48], 2015	Invasive BC	16 involved vs 3 uninvolved LN	13 DEG
Scenario 6 Positive sentinel LNs in patients with additional, non-sentinel, positive LNs to patients with additional, non-sentinel, negative LNs	Liang et al. [49], 2015	Invasive BC	3 NSLN+ SLN vs 3 NSLN− SLN	160 DEG

BC breast carcinoma, DEG differentially expressed genes, IDC invasive ductal carcinoma (no special type), ILN involved LN, LN lymph node, NAT normal adjacent breast tissue, NN node-negative patients, NP node-positive patients, NSLN non-sentinel lymph node, PT primary tumour, SLN sentinel lymph node

timeline was intended to be revealed. These studies focussed on the cancerous tissue itself rather than the LN microenvironment; thus, the material selected for analyses had at least 70% tumour tissue, or laser microdissection was performed.

Although high transcriptomic similarity between primary carcinoma and its corresponding LN metastasis was consistently observed [36, 39–41, 43], genes exclusively expressed in either of these two cancerous tissues was reported. Taking into consideration the diversity of the clinical characteristics of these cohorts, we asked whether any commonalities among activated or repressed genes could be established, potentially pointing collectively to deregulated biological themes. Among the eight studies, a total of 88 genes were found to be differentially expressed between the involved LN and the primary tumour in at least two studies, while the downregulation of 21 genes associated with cell–extracellular matrix (ECM) interaction, ECM remodelling, epithelial–mesenchymal transition (EMT) and loss of basement membrane function [56, 57] was common to three studies (Additional files 1 and 2: Tables S1 and S2).

Downregulation of EMT-associated genes in the involved LN might suggest that, as the metastasis becomes established, reversal of EMT and restoration to epithelial phenotype are essential for the successful colonisation [47]. Stromal cells play a significant part in this process, particularly matrix metalloproteinases MMP2 and MMP7, as these proteins are associated with the breakdown of the ECM, as well as innate immune response [58]. CD10, a membrane metalloendopeptidase, is present at various stages of B-cell maturation and of particular importance in LNs, where it is strongly expressed by germinal centre B cells, the most highly proliferative lymphocyte subset in LNs [59]. CD10 was less abundant in involved LNs compared to the primary lesions in three studies [36, 41, 42], potentially pointing to a lack of differentiation potential of B cells.

Three genes, namely those encoding collagenase 11A1 (COL11A1), Asporin (ASPN) and Periostin (POSTN), were reported in four studies as having lower abundance in involved LNs compared to primary tumour tissue [37, 38, 41–43]. All three genes function in remodelling ECM and ECM-associated protein degradation of

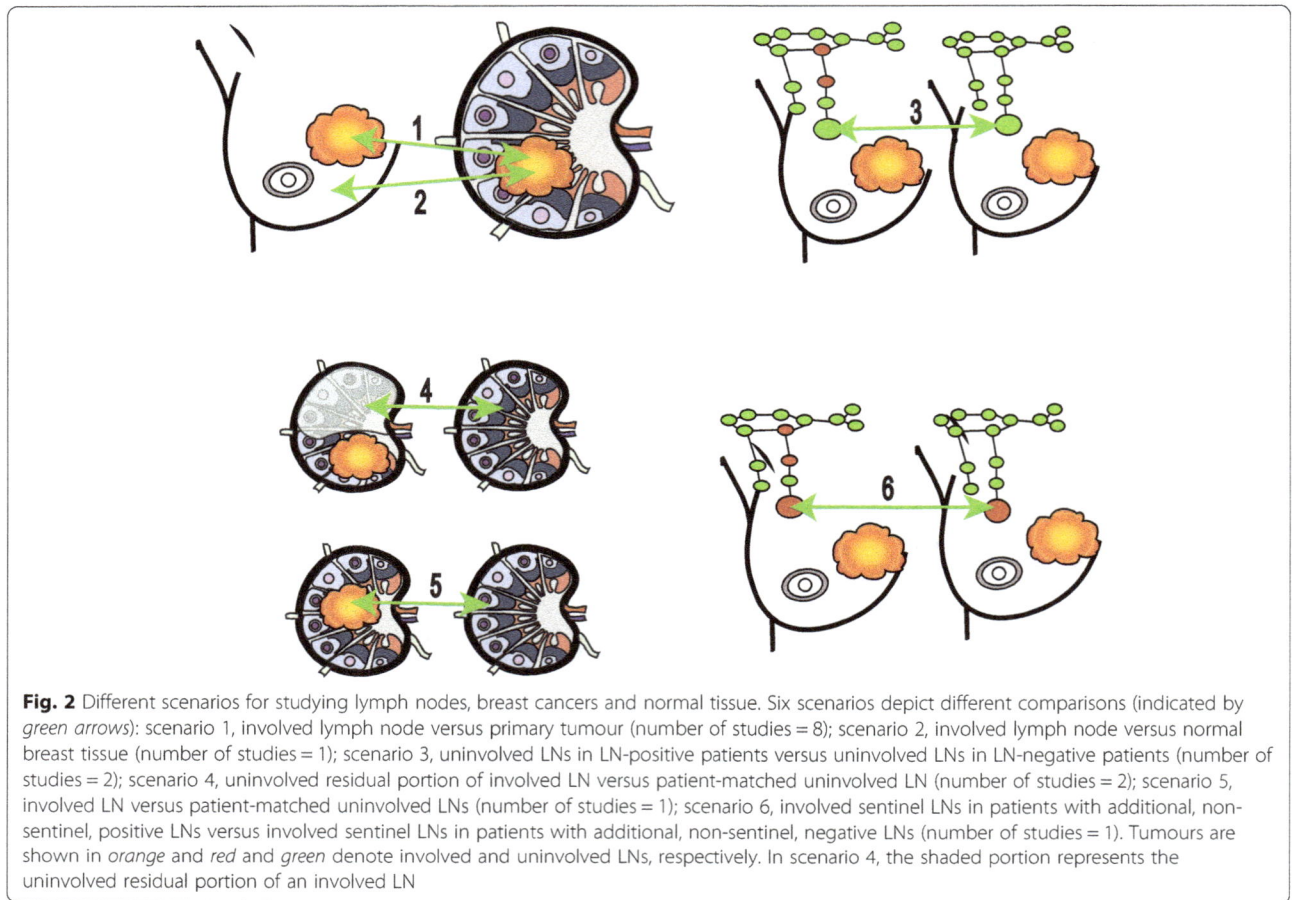

Fig. 2 Different scenarios for studying lymph nodes, breast cancers and normal tissue. Six scenarios depict different comparisons (indicated by *green arrows*): scenario 1, involved lymph node versus primary tumour (number of studies = 8); scenario 2, involved lymph node versus normal breast tissue (number of studies = 1); scenario 3, uninvolved LNs in LN-positive patients versus uninvolved LNs in LN-negative patients (number of studies = 2); scenario 4, uninvolved residual portion of involved LN versus patient-matched uninvolved LN (number of studies = 2); scenario 5, involved LN versus patient-matched uninvolved LNs (number of studies = 1); scenario 6, involved sentinel LNs in patients with additional, non-sentinel, positive LNs versus involved sentinel LNs in patients with additional, non-sentinel, negative LNs (number of studies = 1). Tumours are shown in *orange* and *red* and *green* denote involved and uninvolved LNs, respectively. In scenario 4, the shaded portion represents the uninvolved residual portion of an involved LN

the basement membrane. ECM remodelling is a well-established mechanistic prerequisite for dissemination of the primary cancer and genes involved in ECM are frequently part of metastatic gene sets in several other solid tumours [60]. *COL11A1* promotes cell proliferation, migration and tumourigenesis of many human malignancies [61]. This gene is currently being investigated as a diagnostic marker for non-small cell lung carcinoma (NSCLC) and, by targeting *COL11A1*, chemoresistance might be overruled [62]. The stromal expression of *ASPN* and *POSTN* has been shown to be associated with aggressive tumour phenotypes and poor prognosis in prostate and colorectal cancers, respectively [63, 64]. Whether their lack of expression in involved LNs provides additive risk information for disease progression warrants further investigation.

Complement component 7 (C7), a protein involved in the innate immune system, and part of the membrane attack complex that mediates lysis of pathogens, was the only gene of higher abundance in involved LNs reported in four studies [37, 41–43]. Since C7 may be related to processing and responding to different tumour neo-antigens present in involved LNs, its presence might reflect attempts

of the involved LN to counterattack the metastatic colonisation.

Besides the malignant epithelial component, the transcriptional profiles of involved LNs almost always still harbour significant signals of immune and stroma cells. Among all eight studies, a total of 64 immune cell-related genes were identified (Fig. 3a, b, Additional file 5: Table S5), including those associated with the upregulation of chemokines, ligands and receptors, cytotoxic CD8+ T cells, both immature and activated B cells, T-cell receptor (TCR) activation, MHC class II, Th1 and Th2 cells in involved LNs. Conversely, genes downregulated in involved LNs were associated with dendritic cells (DCs), mast cells and monocytes. DCs are antigen-presenting cells that enter the LNs via the afferent lymphatics and that prime the effector T cells to initiate adaptive immune responses. Germinal centre responses are dependent on T cells activated by DCs. A depletion of DCs could represent a major immune escape mechanism in cancers [65] due to lymphangiogenic responses in the metastatic node [66]. A previous study found that not only the number but also the spatial clustering of dendritic cells in tumour-draining LNs affects clinical outcome of breast and other cancer patients [67]. In

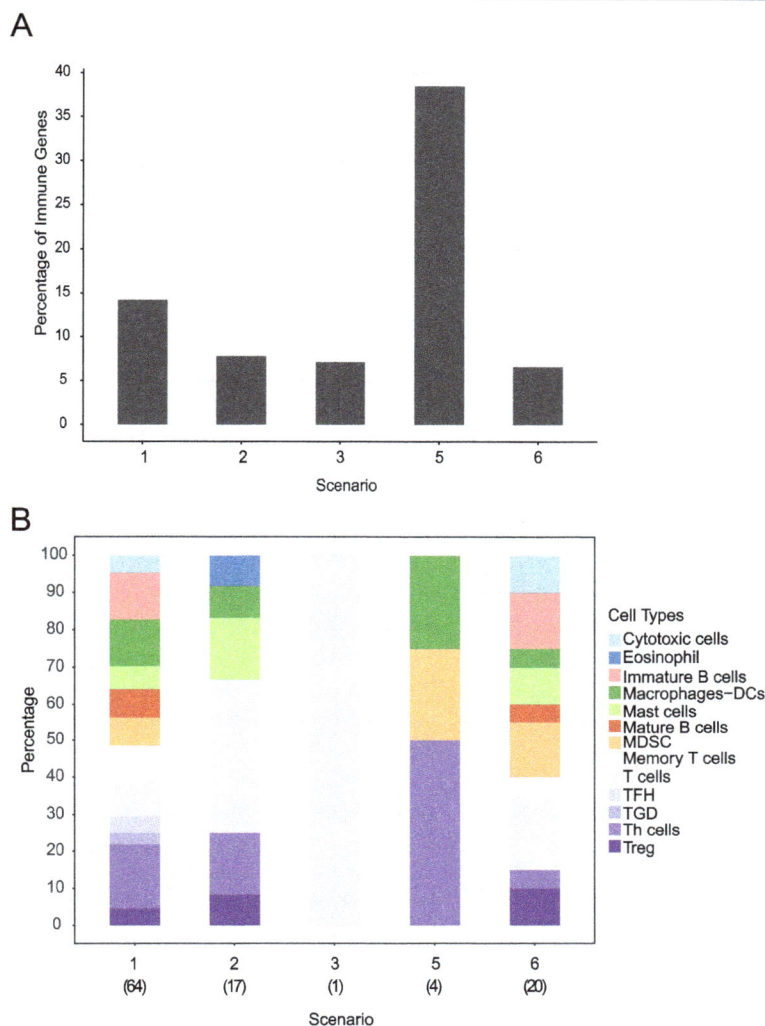

Fig. 3 Immune cell composition in different scenarios. **a** The percentage of genes representing specific immune cell populations in each of the scenarios. **b** The proportion of different immune cell populations among all the immune-related genes in each scenario. (Scenario 4 was omitted as the reported 103 differentially expressed genes could not be retrieved from the original study)

melanoma, for example, decreased numbers of plasmacytoid DCs (pDC) in peripheral blood had independent negative prognostic value mainly linked to stage IV disease and with associated gradual decline in pDC levels just before relapse [68]. Indeed, a multitude of factors, including number, spatial organisation, migration and maturation status of DCs, play a pivotal role in determining the anti-tumour immune response/pro-tumour immunosuppression balance [69, 70]. Conventional dendritic cell type 1 (cDC1) is the key player in stimulating CD8+ T cells and inducing antitumor T-cell responses [71], and various subtypes of blood derived LN-resident DCs (pDC, Clec9A+ DCs, BDCA+ DCs) can induce both Th1 and Th2 cytokines [72]. Thus, a dynamic interplay with the modulation of humoral and cellular immune responses, histologically

corroborated by the reactive nodal changes with follicular, paracortical and sinusoidal hyperplasia, is present in these involved LNs [27].

Overall, our unifying analyses repeatedly demonstrated a consistent plasticity in ECM and immune cells in metastatic LN tissue, despite the underlying molecular similarities between the primary carcinomas and patient-matched involved LNs. Cancer genomes reflect clonal persistence and clonal extinction during cancer evolution [18]. A recent comprehensive single cell analysis of chemoresistant TNBC supported an evolutionary model in which an adaptive selection in the cancer genome is paralleled by an acquired transcriptional program, including ECM degradation and EMT [73]. Given the remarkable molecular similarities between primary lesions and involved LNs, the metastatic genetic programme may be activated at an early stage during breast cancer development [15, 74], some cancerous cells may acquire their metastatic proficiency late due to clonal evolution [75], and as a sum are continually reshaping the metastatic molecular expression profile [43]. In parallel, as the metastatic potential of these cells evolves and increases over time, and the local microenvironment, through the interaction with endothelial, stromal and immune cells, carries significant determinants for successful colonisation in the LN.

Scenario 2: Comparison with normal breast tissue, pinpointing the changes in metastasis

To decipher the remarkable similarities between a breast primary tumour and its LN metastasis, Mathe and colleagues [44] made multiple comparisons between normal breast tissue, LN-positive primary tumours, LN-negative primary tumours and LN metastases. Their hypothesis for identifying genes crucial for metastatic spread relied on: (i) genes differentially expressed between primary tumour versus normal, tumour-adjacent breast tissue (NAT) in a LN-positive patient, followed by (ii) genes expressed in involved LN compared to normal breast tissue, and then (iii) selecting only those genes which were absent in primary tumours versus normal breast tissue in LN-negative patients. Through this step-wise approach, 14 genes were found commonly as downregulated in involved LNs (*APOD, MME, OMD, F2RL2, DCN, PTN, SFRP2, FMO1, OGN, SRPX, SPARCL1, MMP16, LRRC1, HMCN1*; Additional file 3: Table S3). *SPRX, SPARCL1, MMP16* and *HMCN1* are again involved in cell adhesion, ECM breakdown and organisation. *DCN* influences regulatory T cell (Treg)-mediated immunosuppression, while *CD10*, as noted above, is essential for highly proliferative and pro-apoptotic germinal centre B cells [59, 76].

Performing an overrepresentation analysis using the GO database [53], pathways frequently deregulated in involved LNs in both scenarios 1 and 2 included ossification, cell adhesion, ECM organisation, cell proliferation, cell motility, apoptotic process and development of vasculature. Remodelling of the ECM and vascular proliferation are corroborated by the histological alterations in stromal architecture seen in LNs when metastasis manifests itself (Additional file 4: Table S4) and have previously been linked to metastasis in multiple solid tumours [77].

In parallel, a delicate balance between helper and regulatory T cells seems to create a pro-metastatic immunosuppressive niche in the LN, as identified by seven downregulated (*EGR1, RBMS3, CD34, IGF1, MEIS2, CMA1, DLC1*) and five upregulated (*MAD2L1, STAT1, KIF11, ANLN, DLGAP5*) genes associated with specific

immune cell populations, especially T-cell function including helper (*RBMS3, DLC1*) activated (*MAD2L1, KIF11, ANLN, DLGAP5*) and regulatory T cells. Different subsets of helper T cells, including Th17 and the heterogeneity of Tregs, are critical for cancer progression and metastasis [78, 79], again emphasising that the balance between different subsets of helper and regulatory T cells is a crucial factor in successful colonisation.

Gene expression patterns across different phenotypical LN groups By exclusively studying the involved LNs, key questions of "when" does the LN microenvironment develop signals to potentially attract cancer cells and when, why and how these cancer cells can home in in such an immune cell-dominant environment are omitted. LNs at different stages of colonisation provide the opportunity to obtain insight into the underlying biology of the evolving pre-metastatic setting. The following four scenarios adopted the diverse approaches across nodes of different status (Fig. 2):

Scenario 3: By comparing uninvolved LNs in LN-positive and LN-negative breast cancer patients, the premetastatic niche and early genetic aberrations were interrogated for changes in immune response, vasculature and cellular proliferation, which are potentially measureable even before detectable metastasis has occurred. Here, molecular changes specific for a node-to-node manner and alterations systemically affecting the regional nodes can be determined [45–47].

Scenario 4: Comparison between the uninvolved, residual portion of a LN bearing a metastatic carcinoma with patient-matched negative nodes allowed identification of late-stage alterations in the secondary microenvironment, which may indirectly support metastatic growth [45, 47].

Scenario 5: By comparing involved LNs with uninvolved LNs, alterations of immune and stromal cells within similar secondary microenvironments are captured [48].

Scenario 6: By relating positive sentinel LNs in patients with additional, non-sentinel, positive LNs to patients with additional, non-sentinel, negative LNs, gene patterns conferring increased risk of developing metastasis in other LNs might be delineated [49].

Scenario 3: The uninvolved LN, the first step towards metastasis

The first step in the colonisation of the LN by tumour cells is potentially the preparation of the LN microenvironment, even before the tumour cells arrive. Blackburn et al. [46] and Valente et al. [47] investigated the transcriptomic profiles of uninvolved LNs in LN-positive and LN-negative patients to identify early preparatory changes in the LN microenvironment. Both studies did not observe significant differences in gene expression patterns between the uninvolved LNs of LN-positive versus uninvolved LNs of LN-negative breast cancer patients [46, 47], leading the authors conclude that (a) the physical presence of metastatic tumour cells may be crucial to elicit a pro-metastatic niche in the LNs and (b) these pro-metastatic changes occur in a LN-to-LN manner and are not reflected systematically in uninvolved LNs in an otherwise LN-positive patient.

Studying the early metastatic changes, Zuckerman et al. [45] followed a different approach by purifying immune cells from uninvolved sentinel and non-sentinel LNs. In uninvolved LNs (of entirely LN-negative patients), gene patterns were associated with immune cell regulation and signalling pathways such as antigen presentation (HLA-DQA, HLA-A, HLA-DRB3), lymphocyte activation (HLA-DOA, IL23A, IL4, PLCG2, TICAM1), cytokine–cytokine receptor interaction (IL12RB2, IL4, CCR8, TNFRSF21, IL23A, IL3RA) and pro-inflammatory TREM1 and IL-17 signalling [80, 81], indicating an effective antigen-processing and anti-tumour response. TREM1 signalling activates monocyte-macrophage and neutrophil-mediated immune responses. The IL-17 pathway stimulates Th17 cells to respond to a variety of foreign antigens and is involved in autoimmune diseases [82]. Activation of such pro-inflammatory immune pathways in a LN-negative patient's LNs may facilitate an effective tumour response that prevents successful further spreading and colonisation of metastatic cells. In this context, breast cancer cells have been shown to hinder the functioning of dendritic cells and other antigen-processing cells [83]. In contrast, the uninvolved LNs of LN-positive patients had higher levels of genes involved in relaxin signalling, which attracts mononuclear cells to create an immunosuppressive environment [84]. The lack of effective immune responses, including antigen presentation, together with tumour promoting factors may all synergise to establish the necessary immunosuppressive pre-metastatic niche in the uninvolved LN of LN-positive patients. These

molecular alterations may cause various architectural changes, including changes in size and location of germinal centres in uninvolved LNs of LN-positive breast cancer patients, as we have observed previously [27].

Scenario 4: Residual portion of an involved LN, a surviving immune microenvironment

A reflection of the vanishing immune cell microenvironment from the uninvolved to the involved LN is provided by assessment of the residual portion of a LN where some colonisation by tumour cells has started (Figs. 2 and 4). The uninvolved, 'normal' residual portion of an otherwise involved LN offers a unique snapshot of direct interaction between LN stromal and immune cells with tumour cells. To study the gene expression exclusively from this area of the LN, Valente et al. [47] confirmed the absence of tumour cells with AE1/AE3 immunohistochemical staining and laser microdissected the cancer-free tissue for RNA extraction. Similarly, Zuckerman and colleagues carefully selected, with flow cytometry-based sorting, only immune cells from residual LN materials [45]. Most genes downregulated in the residual parts of involved LNs, when compared to completely uninvolved LNs, were involved in regulation of immune response (HPGDS, STAB2, CLEC4M, PROS1, TFPI), advocating a pro-metastatic immunosuppressive microenvironment. STAB2, a scavenger receptor, is known to regulate leukocyte trafficking in LNs through lymphatic endothelial cells [85], theoretically maintaining defence and tissue homeostasis, and in parallel spreading neoplastic cells. Similarly, in uninvolved LNs of otherwise LN-positive patients, pathways downregulated in the residual portion of positive LNs were pro-inflammatory immune-related pathways like TREM1 signalling (NOD2, TLR5), whilst the upregulated pathways were associated with cell cycle (RAD51, KIF23, PLK4), DNA repair (RFC2, BRIP1) and tumour-promoting angiopoietin signalling (RASA1, BRIP1). In residual LN tissue (from nodes with metastatic tumour) compared to uninvolved LNs, B-cell-related genes (AICDA, IGKC, IGKV1-5, IGKV3-

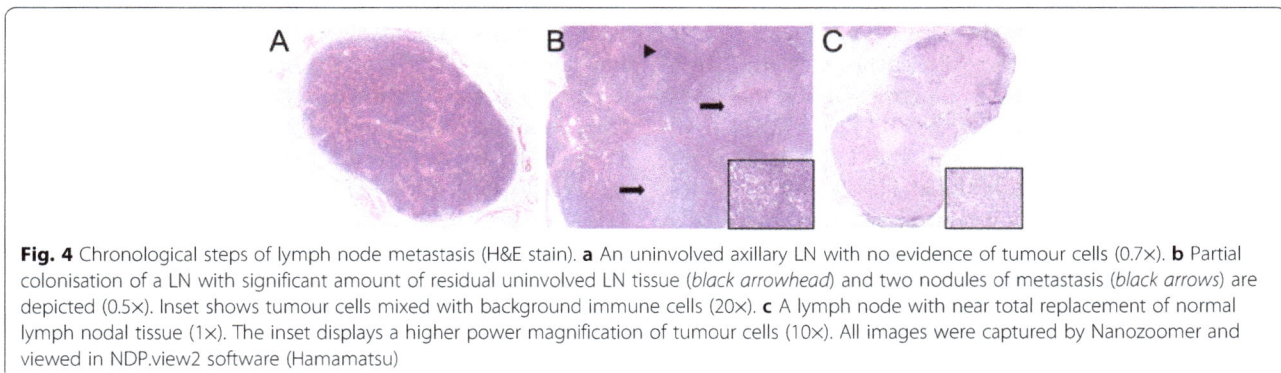

Fig. 4 Chronological steps of lymph node metastasis (H&E stain). **a** An uninvolved axillary LN with no evidence of tumour cells (0.7×). **b** Partial colonisation of a LN with significant amount of residual uninvolved LN tissue (*black arrowhead*) and two nodules of metastasis (*black arrows*) are depicted (0.5×). Inset shows tumour cells mixed with background immune cells (20×). **c** A lymph node with near total replacement of normal lymph nodal tissue (1×). The inset displays a higher power magnification of tumour cells (10×). All images were captured by Nanozoomer and viewed in NDP.view2 software (Hamamatsu)

20), many of them specifically expressed in germinal centres, were highly active. B cells and ectopic germinal centres have previously been linked to chronic inflammation and tumour promotion [86, 87] and may represent prognostic indicators for developing distant metastases (Figs. 2 and 4) [27, 28]. The upregulation of cell cycle and DNA repair pathway genes can further be linked to germinal centres, as these are zones of high proliferation. One might hypothesise that, in uninvolved LNs of LN-positive patients and in the residual 'normal' part of an involved LN, the upregulation of germinal centre B cell genes, in parallel to the dampening of antigen presentation and T-cell priming, results in an altered tumour-promoting response, primarily mediated by B cells. Defective immune regulation in which B-cell proliferation or humoral response is activated, in spite of the dampening of the antigen presentation and leukocyte activation, through some alternative pathways could create a prometastatic environment. Furthermore, the abundance of kappa light chain genes as overexpressed in residual LN tissue point to an alternative B-cell activation pathway biased towards B cells expressing kappa light chains and of oligoclonal nature. In the presence of B-cell proliferation, it is essential to study markers such as PD-1, a negative regulator of B-cell differentiation and expressed by the majority of T cells in germinal centres. B cells can both positively and negatively regulate T-cell-mediated antitumor immune responses; however, their function in generating a specific pre-metastatic niche has yet to be established [66].

Scenario 5: From an uninvolved to an involved LN status

To study the penultimate step in the evolving LN microenvironment one can look at the extreme endpoints, i.e. to capture transcriptional changes in the involved LN as a whole and compare with the uninvolved LN. Rizwan and colleagues mainly focussed on change in collagen density in LNs in a murine metastatic breast cancer model, and examined expression patterns derived from publicly available microarray-based data (GSE4408), in which 16 involved and three uninvolved human LNs from breast cancer patients were compared [48]. Ten of the 14 genes transcriptionally activated in involved LNs were fibronectin (*FN1*), three collagen genes (*COL1A2, COL1A1, COL3A1*) and six integrin family members (*ITGB5, ITGA2, ITGA9, ITGB7, ITGA2B, ITGA4*). All are key players in cell adhesion, cell–ECM interaction and ECM modulation (Additional files 3 and 4: Tables S3 and S4). Involved LNs displayed increased collagen I and basement membrane density in this murine metastatic breast cancer model. Increased collagen can promote tumour spread, not only by augmenting cell motility and regulating tumour promoting cell–ECM interactions, but also by altering immune responses, including switching the phenotypes of macrophages to a tumour-promoting M2 type [88] as well as a reduction of B-cell follicles [48].

Scenario 6: The final step—can involved LNs send signals to other uninvolved LNs to promote tumour dissemination?

The number of involved LNs in breast cancer is associated with the risk of developing distant metastasis [7]. The prediction of the extent and number of involved non-sentinel LNs by assessing the sentinel LN(s) would potentially have practical clinical importance, as axillary LN dissection in a group of sentinel LN-positive patients could be avoided [89, 90]. The study by Liang and colleagues, although performed on only six patients, addressed the question of whether completely replaced LNs, especially the sentinel LNs, could send 'signals' to uninvolved LNs in preparation to disseminate the tumour cells [50]. By comparing involved sentinel LNs in patients with additional metastasis in non-sentinel LNs to those with otherwise negative axillary (non-sentinel) LNs, tumour-promoting pathways were represented in the non-sentinel LN-positive group, indicated by the expression of kallikrein subfamily members (*KLK10, KLK11, KLK12, KLK13*), proteolysis and steroid receptor signalling. In contrast, genes involved in plasma membrane and B cell receptor signalling, including *CD22, CD72, Igα, Igβ, CD19* and *CD21*, were depleted in parallel with *SYK, LYN, BTK* and *PTPN6*. In the group of patients with additional positive LNs, specific gene fusions were noted, especially involving *IGLL5*, a surrogate light chain involved in B-cell development [91]. Using immune metagenes denoting specific immune cell populations [55], an overlap between immature and activated B cells (*FCRLA, FAM129C, CD22, PAX5*), helper T cells (*SIGLEC10*), MDSCs (*CEACAM8, FCER2*), mast cells (*CLC, SIGLEC14*) and regulatory T cells (*CD72, IL9R*) (Additional file 5: Table S5) was observed. Taken together, a recurrent theme for further tumour cell spreading emerges in these gene expression patterns, pointing strongly to a key role of B cells and germinal centres in LNs. Accumulating evidence supports a role for B cells in breast cancer immunology [92], and therapeutic approaches targeting B cells may before long demonstrate their relevance. Already in 2015, Sagiv-Barif and colleagues reported substantial enhanced anti-tumour responses in the 4T1 TNBC mouse model when treated with a combination of anti-PDL-1 with ibrutinib, an inhibitor of Bruton's tyrosin kinase (*BTK*) [93], an essential kinase for B cell maturation, signalling, and graft-versus-host disease [94]. Clinical trials (e.g. ClinicalTrials.gov NCT02403271) are currently evaluating B-cell depletion or *BTK* inhibition along with checkpoint inhibition and will soon expose whether such combination therapies enhance anti-tumour immunity and potentially even reduce checkpoint inhibitor-associated treatment-related toxicities in breast cancers [95].

LN, a read-out for the systemic immune response?

Being an early site of tumour dissemination, the LN hosts a variety of tumour–immune system interactions. The ultimate question remains whether certain patterns in LNs of breast cancer patients' mirror changes in the systemic immune response to the tumour in the organism. Valente et al. [46] and Blackburn et al. [47] argued that the physical presence of cancer cells in the LN is crucial for pre-metastatic niche development and that the changes are therefore not systemic. However, recent research, such as the presence of similar immune gene sets in the uninvolved LNs in LN-positive patients and the residual tissue of involved LNs [45], in addition to peripheral blood and to some extent in the immune compartment of the primary tumour [45], identified changes most likely indicative of a systemic effect in LN-positive patients. In keeping with this hypothesis, work on systemic immune responses to effective immunotherapies in preclinical murine breast cancer models has proven experimentally that changes in the immune composition persist in primary tumours, regional LNs, peripheral blood, bone marrow and other lymphoid organs [34].

Limitations

Despite the scarcity of expression data from LN tissue of breast cancer patients, together these data expose snapshots of the steps of the molecular transitions that occur, starting from the uninvolved LN in LN-positive patients, to uninvolved residual tissue of involved LNs, to fully involved LNs, and finally the pro-disseminating signals in involved LNs. Ideally, all these comparisons should be examined within an individual patient's samples to exclude patient-to-patient heterogeneity. Genome-wide studies of whole LN samples mask effects in this highly spatially organised immune organ. Using sophisticated imaging technologies or single cell -omics analyses to capture the earliest stages of LN metastasis, i.e. when tumour cells enter through the afferent lymphatic vessels and colonise in the subcapsular sinus [96], would provide valuable biological and potentially clinically relevant information.

Conclusion

The prognostic relevance of changes in uninvolved LNs is tantalising as it highlights the need to study the interconnected roles of immune, stromal and endothelial cells within this small immune organ as well as the whole immune system [27, 28]. With the recent findings of the systemic orchestration of immune cells with effective immunotherapy [34], examination of local plus systemic tumour–immune cell interactions might hold the key for successful immunotherapeutic strategies. Although some patterns are evident from close scrutiny of existing literature, the 'premetastatic' LN represents an unmet knowledge gap; comprehensive cellular and molecular studies focusing on changes in different immune cell compartments at different time-points during the development of metastasis are needed to unlock this complicated biological process, from both a mechanistic and therapeutic point of view.

Additional files

Additional file 1: Table S1. Gene list compiled from all the studies included in scenario 1 (involved LN versus primary breast tumour). (PDF 75 kb)

Additional file 2: Table S2. Genes found to be differentially expressed in multiple studies included in scenario 1 (involved LN versus primary breast tumour). (PDF 18 kb)

Additional file 3: Table S3. Fully compiled gene list across all scenarios. (PDF 75 kb)

Additional file 4: Table S4. Pathway-based analysis of the differentially expressed genes across all the scenarios. (PDF 33 kb)

Additional file 5: Table S5. Differentially expressed genes representing specific immune cell populations across all the scenarios. (PDF 21 kb)

Acknowledgments
We thank Patrycja Gazinska for providing the H&E images.

Funding
AT is supported by Breast Cancer Now, Breast Cancer Research Trust and Cancer Research UK King's Health Partners Centre at King's College London. TH is funded by the MRC-DTP at King's College London. GC and TP have been recipients of scholarships from Tata Memorial Centre.

Authors' contributions
Concept and design: GC, TP, AG. Data acquisition: GC, TG, TH, AM, RJS, AG. Data analysis and interpretation: GC, TP, TH, JS, SP, AG. Wrote the manuscript: GC, TP, SP, AG. Critically reviewed the manuscript: GC, TP, JS, SP, AG. All authors read and approved the final manuscript.

Competing interests
The authors declare that they have no competing interests.

Author details
[1]Cancer Bioinformatics, King's College London, Innovation Hub, Cancer Centre at Guy's Hospital, Great Maze Pond, London SE1 9RT, UK. [2]School of Cancer & Pharmaceutical Sciences, CRUK King's Health Partners Centre, King's College London, Innovation Hub, Comprehensive Cancer Centre at Guy's Hospital, Great Maze Pond, London SE1 9RT, UK. [3]Department of Pathology, Tata Memorial Centre, 8th Floor, Annexe Building, Mumbai, India. [4]Priority Research Centre for Cancer, School of Biomedical Sciences and Pharmacy, Faculty of Health, University of Newcastle, Newcastle, NSW 2308, Australia. [5]Peter Gorer Department of Immunobiology, King's College London, Guy's Hospital, 2nd Floor, Borough Wing, London SE1 9RT, UK. [6]Breast Cancer Now Research Unit, Innovation Hub, Cancer Centre at Guy's Hospital, King's College London, Faculty of Life Sciences and Medicine, London SE1 9RT, UK.

References

1. Ji R-C. Lymph nodes and cancer metastasis: new perspectives on the role of intranodal lymphatic sinuses. Int J Mol Sci. 2017;18(1):51.
2. Ruddle NH. Lymphatic vessels and tertiary lymphoid organs. J Clin Invest. 2014;124(3):953–9.
3. Zhu M, Fu YX. The role of core TNF/LIGHT family members in lymph node homeostasis and remodeling. Immunol Rev. 2011;244(1):75–84.
4. Lund AW, Wagner M, Fankhauser M, Steinskog ES, Broggi MA, Spranger S, et al. Lymphatic vessels regulate immune microenvironments in human and murine melanoma. J Clin Invest. 2016;126(9):3389–402.
5. Tauchi Y, Tanaka H, Kumamoto K, Tokumoto M, Sakimura C, Sakurai K, et al. Tumor-associated macrophages induce capillary morphogenesis of lymphatic endothelial cells derived from human gastric cancer. Cancer Sci. 2016;107(8):1101–9.
6. Ji RC. Lymph node lymphangiogenesis: a new concept for modulating tumor metastasis and inflammatory process. Histol Histopathol. 2009;24(3):377–84.
7. Amin MB, Greene FL, Edge SB, Compton CC, Gershenwald JE, Brookland RK, et al. The eighth edition AJCC cancer staging manual: Continuing to build a bridge from a population-based to a more "personalized" approach to cancer staging. CA Cancer J Clin. 2017;67(2):93–9.
8. Dickson PV, Gershenwald JE. Staging and prognosis of cutaneous melanoma. Surg Oncol Clin N Am. 2011;20(1):1–17.
9. Carter CL, Allen C, Henson DE. Relation of tumor size, lymph node status, and survival in 24,740 breast cancer cases. Cancer. 1989;63(1):181–7.
10. The Royal College of Pathologists. available from: https://www.rcpath.org/resourceLibrary/g148-breastdataset-hires-jun16-pdf.html. Accessed 5 June 2018.
11. Kroigard AB, Larsen MJ, Thomassen M, Kruse TA. Molecular concordance between primary breast cancer and matched metastases. Breast J. 2016; 22(4):420–30.
12. Ellsworth RE, Field LA, Love B, Kane JL, Hooke JA, Shriver CD. Differential gene expression in primary breast tumors associated with lymph node metastasis. Int J Breast Cancer. 2011;2011:142763.
13. Sotiriou C, Neo SY, McShane LM, Korn EL, Long PM, Jazaeri A, et al. Breast cancer classification and prognosis based on gene expression profiles from a population-based study. Proc Natl Acad Sci U S A. 2003;100(18):10393–8.
14. Sotiriou C, Pusztai L. Gene-expression signatures in breast cancer. N Engl J Med. 2009;360(8):790–800.
15. van de Vijver MJ, He YD, van't Veer LJ, Dai H, Hart AA, Voskuil DW, et al. A gene-expression signature as a predictor of survival in breast cancer. N Engl J Med. 2002;347(25):1999–2009.
16. van't Veer LJ, Dai H, van de Vijver MJ, He YD, Hart AA, Mao M, et al. Gene expression profiling predicts clinical outcome of breast cancer. Nature. 2002; 415(6871):530–6.
17. Zhang Z, Yamashita H, Toyama T, Sugiura H, Ando Y, Mita K, et al. ATBF1-a messenger RNA expression is correlated with better prognosis in breast cancer. Clin Cancer Res. 2005;11(1):193–8.
18. Yates LR, Knappskog S, Wedge D, Farmery JHR, Gonzalez S, Martincorena I, et al. Genomic evolution of breast cancer metastasis and relapse. Cancer Cell. 2017;32(2):169–84.e7.
19. Jones D, Pereira ER, Padera TP. Growth and immune evasion of lymph node metastasis. Front Oncol. 2018;8:36.
20. Liu Y, Cao X. Characteristics and significance of the pre-metastatic niche. Cancer Cell. 2016;30(5):668–81.
21. Sleeman JP. The lymph node pre-metastatic niche. J Mol Med (Berl). 2015; 93(11):1173–84.
22. Harrell MI, Iritani BM, Ruddell A. Tumor-induced sentinel lymph node lymphangiogenesis and increased lymph flow precede melanoma metastasis. Am J Pathol. 2007;170(2):774–86.
23. Ogawa F, Amano H, Eshima K, Ito Y, Matsui Y, Hosono K, et al. Prostanoid induces premetastatic niche in regional lymph nodes. J Clin Invest. 2014; 124(11):4882–94.
24. Chung MK, Do IG, Jung E, Son YI, Jeong HS, Baek CH. Lymphatic vessels and high endothelial venules are increased in the sentinel lymph nodes of patients with oral squamous cell carcinoma before the arrival of tumor cells. Ann Surg Oncol. 2012;19(5):1595–601.
25. Qian CN, Berghuis B, Tsarfaty G, Bruch M, Kort EJ, Ditlev J, et al. Preparing the "soil": the primary tumor induces vasculature reorganization in the sentinel lymph node before the arrival of metastatic cancer cells. Cancer Res. 2006;66(21):10365–76.
26. Kohrt HE, Nouri N, Nowels K, Johnson D, Holmes S, Lee PP. Profile of immune cells in axillary lymph nodes predicts disease-free survival in breast cancer. PLoS Med. 2005;2(9):e284.
27. Grigoriadis A, Gazinska P, Pai T, Irhsad S, Wu Y, Millis R, et al. Histological scoring of immune and stromal features in breast and axillary lymph nodes is prognostic for distant metastasis in lymph node-positive breast cancers. J Pathol Clin Res. 2018;4(1):39–54.
28. Abbott J, Buckley M, Taylor LA, Xu G, Karakousis G, Czerniecki BJ, et al. Histological immune response patterns in sentinel lymph nodes involved by metastatic melanoma and prognostic significance. J Cutan Pathol. 2018;45(6):377–86.
29. Riedel A, Shorthouse D, Haas L, Hall BA, Shields J. Tumor-induced stromal reprogramming drives lymph node transformation. Nat Immunol. 2016; 17(9):1118–27.
30. Costa A, Kieffer Y, Scholer-Dahirel A, Pelon F, Bourachot B, Cardon M, et al. Fibroblast heterogeneity and immunosuppressive environment in human breast cancer. Cancer Cell. 2018;33(3):463–479.e10.
31. Irshad S, Flores-Borja F, Lawler K, Monypenny J, Evans R, Male V, et al. RORgammat(+) innate lymphoid cells promote lymph node metastasis of breast cancers. Cancer Res. 2017;77(5):1083–96.
32. Strömvall K, Thysell E, Halin Bergström S, Bergh A. Aggressive rat prostate tumors reprogram the benign parts of the prostate and regional lymph nodes prior to metastasis. PLoS One. 2017;12(5):e0176679.
33. Chen J, Wang L, Yao Q, Ling R, Li K, Wang H. Drug concentrations in axillary lymph nodes after lymphatic chemotherapy on patients with breast cancer. Breast Cancer Res. 2004;6(4):R474.
34. Spitzer MH, Carmi Y, Reticker-Flynn NE, Kwek SS, Madhireddy D, Martins MM, et al. Systemic immunity is required for effective cancer immunotherapy. Cell. 2017;168(3):487–502 e15.
35. Moher D, Liberati A, Tetzlaff J, Altman DG. Preferred reporting items for systematic reviews and meta-analyses: the PRISMA statement. PLoS Med. 2009;6(7):e1000097.
36. Calvo J, Sanchez-Cid L, Munoz M, Lozano JJ, Thomson TM, Fernandez PL. Infrequent loss of luminal differentiation in ductal breast cancer metastasis. PLoS One. 2013;8(10):e78097.
37. Feng Y, Sun B, Li X, Zhang L, Niu Y, Xiao C, et al. Differentially expressed genes between primary cancer and paired lymph node metastases predict clinical outcome of node-positive breast cancer patients. Breast Cancer Res Treat. 2007;103(3):319–29.
38. Hao X, Sun B, Hu L, Lahdesmaki H, Dunmire V, Feng Y, et al. Differential gene and protein expression in primary breast malignancies and their lymph node metastases as revealed by combined cDNA microarray and tissue microarray analysis. Cancer. 2004;100(6):1110–22.
39. Lahdesmaki H, Hao X, Sun B, Hu L, Yli-Harja O, Shmulevich I, et al. Distinguishing key biological pathways between primary breast cancers and their lymph node metastases by gene function-based clustering analysis. Int J Oncol. 2004;24(6):1589–96.
40. Weigelt B, Wessels LF, Bosma AJ, Glas AM, Nuyten DS, He YD, et al. No common denominator for breast cancer lymph node metastasis. Br J Cancer. 2005;93(8):924–32.
41. Ellsworth RE, Seebach J, Field LA, Heckman C, Kane J, Hooke JA, et al. A gene expression signature that defines breast cancer metastases. Clin Exp Metastasis. 2009;26(3):205–13.
42. Vecchi M, Confalonieri S, Nuciforo P, Vigano MA, Capra M, Bianchi M, et al. Breast cancer metastases are molecularly distinct from their primary tumors. Oncogene. 2008;27(15):2148–58.
43. Suzuki M, Tarin D. Gene expression profiling of human lymph node metastases and matched primary breast carcinomas: clinical implications. Mol Oncol. 2007;1(2):172–80.
44. Mathe A, Wong-Brown M, Morten B, Forbes JF, Braye SG, Avery-Kiejda KA, et al. Novel genes associated with lymph node metastasis in triple negative breast cancer. Sci Rep. 2015;5:15832.
45. Zuckerman NS, Yu H, Simons DL, Bhattacharya N, Carcamo-Cavazos V, Yan N, et al. Altered local and systemic immune profiles underlie lymph node metastasis in breast cancer patients. Int J Cancer. 2013;132(11):2537–47.
46. Blackburn HL, Ellsworth DL, Shriver CD, Ellsworth RE. Breast cancer metastasis to the axillary lymph nodes: are changes to the lymph node "soil" localized or systemic? Breast Cancer. 2017;11:1178223417691246.
47. Valente AL, Kane JL, Ellsworth DL, Shriver CD, Ellsworth RE. Molecular response of the axillary lymph node microenvironment to metastatic colonization. Clin Exp Metastasis. 2014;31(5):565–72.

48. Rizwan A, Bulte C, Kalaichelvan A, Cheng M, Krishnamachary B, Bhujwalla ZM, et al. Metastatic breast cancer cells in lymph nodes increase nodal collagen density. Sci Rep. 2015;5:10002.

49. Liang F, Qu H, Lin Q, Yang Y, Ruan X, Zhang B, et al. Molecular biomarkers screened by next-generation RNA sequencing for non-sentinel lymph node status prediction in breast cancer patients with metastatic sentinel lymph nodes. World J Surg Oncol. 2015;13(1):258.

50. Durinck S, Moreau Y, Kasprzyk A, Davis S, De Moor B, Brazma A, et al. BioMart and Bioconductor: a powerful link between biological databases and microarray data analysis. Bioinformatics. 2005;21(16):3439–40.

51. Durinck S, Spellman PT, Birney E, Huber W. Mapping Identifiers for the Integration of Genomic Datasets with the R/Bioconductor package biomaRt. Nat Protoc. 2009;4(8):1184–91.

52. Flicek P, Amode MR, Barrell D, Beal K, Brent S, Carvalho-Silva D, et al. Ensembl 2012. Nucleic Acids Res. 2012;40(Database issue):D84–90.

53. Wang J, Vasaikar S, Shi Z, Greer M, Zhang B. WebGestalt 2017: a more comprehensive, powerful, flexible and interactive gene set enrichment analysis toolkit. Nucleic Acids Res. 2017;45(W1):W130–W7.

54. Supek F, Bošnjak M, Škunca N, Šmuc T. REVIGO summarizes and visualizes long lists of gene ontology terms. PLoS One. 2011;6(7):e21800.

55. Angelova M, Charoentong P, Hackl H, Fischer ML, Snajder R, Krogsdam AM, et al. Characterization of the immunophenotypes and antigenomes of colorectal cancers reveals distinct tumor escape mechanisms and novel targets for immunotherapy. Genome Biol. 2015;16(1):64.

56. Pickup MW, Mouw JK, Weaver VM. The extracellular matrix modulates the hallmarks of cancer. EMBO Rep. 2014;15(12):1243–53.

57. Holle AW, Young JL, Spatz JP. In vitro cancer cell–ECM interactions inform in vivo cancer treatment. Adv Drug Deliv Rev. 2016;97:270–9.

58. Edman K, Furber M, Hemsley P, Johansson C, Pairaudeau G, Petersen J, et al. The Discovery of MMP7 inhibitors exploiting a novel selectivity trigger. ChemMedChem. 2011;6(5):769–73.

59. Höller S, Horn H, Lohr A, Mäder U, Katzenberger T, Kalla J, et al. A cytomorphological and immunohistochemical profile of aggressive B-cell lymphoma: high clinical impact of a cumulative immunohistochemical outcome predictor score. J Hematop. 2009;2(4):187–94.

60. Kondoh N, Ishikawa T, Ohkura S, Arai M, Hada A, Yamazaki Y, et al. Gene expression signatures that classify the mode of invasion of primary oral squamous cell carcinomas. Mol Carcinog. 2008;47(10):744–56.

61. Li A, Li J, Lin J, Zhuo W, Si J. COL11A1 is overexpressed in gastric cancer tissues and regulates proliferation, migration and invasion of HGC-27 gastric cancer cells in vitro. Oncol Rep. 2017;37(1):333–40.

62. Shen L, Yang M, Lin Q, Zhang Z, Zhu B, Miao C. COL11A1 is overexpressed in recurrent non-small cell lung cancer and promotes cell proliferation, migration, invasion and drug resistance. Oncol Rep. 2016;36(2):877–85.

63. Rochette A, Boufaied N, Scarlata E, Hamel L, Brimo F, Whitaker HC, et al. Asporin is a stromally expressed marker associated with prostate cancer progression. Br J Cancer. 2017;116(6):775–84.

64. Oh HJ, Bae JM, Wen XY, Cho NY, Kim JH, Kang GH. Overexpression of POSTN in tumor stroma is a poor prognostic indicator of colorectal cancer. J Pathol Transl Med. 2017;51(3):306–13.

65. Kusume A, Sasahira T, Luo Y, Isobe M, Nakagawa N, Tatsumoto N, et al. Suppression of dendritic cells by HMGB1 is associated with lymph node metastasis of human colon cancer. Pathobiology. 2009;76(4):155–62.

66. Balsat C, Blacher S, Herfs M, Van de Velde M, Signolle N, Sauthier P, et al. A specific immune and lymphatic profile characterizes the pre-metastatic state of the sentinel lymph node in patients with early cervical cancer. Oncoimmunology. 2017;6(2):e1265718.

67. Chang AY, Bhattacharya N, Mu J, Setiadi AF, Carcamo-Cavazos V, Lee GH, et al. Spatial organization of dendritic cells within tumor draining lymph nodes impacts clinical outcome in breast cancer patients. J Transl Med. 2013;11:242.

68. Chevolet I, Speeckaert R, Schreuer M, Neyns B, Krysko O, Bachert C, et al. Clinical significance of plasmacytoid dendritic cells and myeloid-derived suppressor cells in melanoma. J Transl Med. 2015;13:9.

69. Tran Janco JM, Lamichhane P, Karyampudi L, Knutson KL. Tumor-infiltrating dendritic cells in cancer pathogenesis. J Immunol. 2015;194(7):2985–91.

70. Ma Y, Shurin GV, Peiyuan Z, Shurin MR. Dendritic cells in the cancer microenvironment. J Cancer. 2013;4(1):36–44.

71. Gardner A, Ruffell B. Dendritic cells and cancer immunity. Trends Immunol. 2016;37(12):855–65.

72. Segura E, Valladeau-Guilemond J, Donnadieu M-H, Sastre-Garau X, Soumelis V, Amigorena S. Characterization of resident and migratory dendritic cells in human lymph nodes. J Exp Med. 2012;209(4):653.

73. Kim C, Gao R, Sei E, Brandt R, Hartman J, Hatschek T, et al. Chemoresistance evolution in triple-negative breast cancer delineated by single-cell sequencing. Cell. 2018;173(4):879–93 e13.

74. Ramaswamy S, Ross KN, Lander ES, Golub TR. A molecular signature of metastasis in primary solid tumors. Nat Genet. 2003;33(1):49–54.

75. Montel V, Huang TY, Mose E, Pestonjamasp K, Tarin D. Expression profiling of primary tumors and matched lymphatic and lung metastases in a xenogeneic breast cancer model. Am J Pathol. 2005;166(5):1565–79.

76. Oh E, Choi IK, Hong J, Yun CO. Oncolytic adenovirus coexpressing interleukin-12 and decorin overcomes Treg-mediated immunosuppression inducing potent antitumor effects in a weakly immunogenic tumor model. Oncotarget. 2017;8(3):4730–46.

77. Cox TR, Erler JT. Remodeling and homeostasis of the extracellular matrix: implications for fibrotic diseases and cancer. Dis Model Mech. 2011;4(2):165–78.

78. Ward-Hartstonge KA, Kemp RA. Regulatory T-cell heterogeneity and the cancer immune response. Clin Transl Immunol. 2017;6:e154.

79. Marshall EA, Ng KW, Kung SH, Conway EM, Martinez VD, Halvorsen EC, et al. Emerging roles of T helper 17 and regulatory T cells in lung cancer progression and metastasis. Mol Cancer. 2016;15(1):67.

80. Gibot S, Cravoisy A, Levy B, Bene M-C, Faure G, Bollaert P-E. Soluble triggering receptor expressed on myeloid cells and the diagnosis of pneumonia. N Engl J Med. 2004;350(5):451–8.

81. Qian Y, Kang Z, Liu C, Li X. IL-17 signaling in host defense and inflammatory diseases. Cell Mol Immunol. 2010;7:328.

82. Liu CJ, Tsai CY, Chiang SH, Tang SJ, Chen NJ, Mak TW, et al. Triggering receptor expressed on myeloid cells-1 (TREM-1) deficiency augments BAFF production to promote lupus progression. J Autoimmun. 2017;78:92–100.

83. Tourkova IL, Shurin GV, Ferrone S, Shurin MR. Interferon regulatory factor 8 mediates tumor-induced inhibition of antigen processing and presentation by dendritic cells. Cancer Immunol Immunother. 2009;58(4):567–74.

84. Figueiredo KA, Mui AL, Nelson CC, Cox ME. Relaxin stimulates leukocyte adhesion and migration through a relaxin receptor LGR7-dependent mechanism. J Biol Chem. 2006;281(6):3030–9.

85. Ji RC. Lymph nodes and cancer metastasis: new perspectives on the role of intranodal lymphatic sinuses. Int J Mol Sci. 2016;18(1):51.

86. de Visser KE, Korets LV, Coussens LM. De novo carcinogenesis promoted by chronic inflammation is B lymphocyte dependent. Cancer Cell. 2005;7(5):411–23.

87. William J, Euler C, Christensen S, Shlomchik MJ. Evolution of autoantibody responses via somatic hypermutation outside of germinal centers. Science. 2002;297(5589):2066–70.

88. Fang M, Yuan J, Peng C, Li Y. Collagen as a double-edged sword in tumor progression. Tumour Biol. 2014;35(4):2871–82.

89. Hwang RF, Krishnamurthy S, Hunt KK, Mirza N, Ames FC, Feig B, et al. Clinicopathologic factors predicting involvement of nonsentinel axillary nodes in women with breast cancer. Ann Surg Oncol. 2003;10(3):248–54.

90. Van Zee KJ, Manasseh DM, Bevilacqua JL, Boolbol SK, Fey JV, Tan LK, et al. A nomogram for predicting the likelihood of additional nodal metastases in breast cancer patients with a positive sentinel node biopsy. Ann Surg Oncol. 2003;10(10):1140–51.

91. Pridans C, Holmes ML, Polli M, Wettenhall JM, Dakic A, Corcoran LM, et al. Identification of Pax5 target genes in early B cell differentiation. J Immunol. 2008;180(3):1719–28.

92. Tsou P, Katayama H, Ostrin EJ, Hanash SM. The emerging role of B cells in tumor immunity. Cancer Res. 2016;76(19):5597–601.

93. Sagiv-Barfi I, Kohrt HEK, Czerwinski DK, Ng PP, Chang BY, Levy R. Therapeutic antitumor immunity by checkpoint blockade is enhanced by ibrutinib, an inhibitor of both BTK and ITK. Proc Natl Acad Sci U S A. 2015;112(9):E966–E72.

94. Miklos D, Cutler CS, Arora M, Waller EK, Jagasia M, Pusic I, et al. Ibrutinib for chronic graft-versus-host disease after failure of prior therapy. Blood. 2017;130(21):2243–50.

95. Liudahl SM, Coussens LM. B cells as biomarkers: predicting immune checkpoint therapy adverse events. J Clin Invest. 2018;128(2):577–9.

96. Pereira ER, Jones D, Jung K, Padera TP. The lymph node microenvironment and its role in the progression of metastatic cancer. Semin Cell Dev Biol. 2015;38:98–105.

19

Loss of amphiregulin reduces myoepithelial cell coverage of mammary ducts and alters breast tumor growth

Serena P. H. Mao[1], Minji Park[1], Ramon M. Cabrera[1], John R. Christin[2], George S. Karagiannis[1,3,4], Maja H. Oktay[1,3,4], Dietmar M. W. Zaiss[5], Scott I. Abrams[6], Wenjun Guo[2], John S. Condeelis[1,3,4], Paraic A. Kenny[7] and Jeffrey E. Segall[1,3]* [ID]

Abstract

Background: Amphiregulin (AREG), a ligand of the epidermal growth factor receptor, is not only essential for proper mammary ductal development, but also associated with breast cancer proliferation and growth. In the absence of AREG, mammary ductal growth is stunted and fails to expand. Furthermore, suppression of AREG expression in estrogen receptor-positive breast tumor cells inhibits in-vitro and in-vivo growth.

Methods: We crossed AREG-null (AREG$^{-/-}$) mice with the murine luminal B breast cancer model, MMTV-PyMT (PyMT), to generate spontaneous breast tumors that lack AREG (AREG$^{-/-}$ PyMT). We evaluated tumor growth, cytokeratin-8 (K8)-positive luminal cells, cytokeratin-14 (K14)-positive myoepithelial cells, and expression of AREG, Ki67, and PyMT. Primary myoepithelial cells from nontumor-bearing AREG$^{+/+}$ mice underwent fluorescence-activated cell sorting and were adapted to culture for in-vitro coculture studies with AT-3 cells, a cell line derived from C57Bl/6 PyMT mammary tumors.

Results: Intriguingly, PyMT-induced lesions progress more rapidly in AREG$^{-/-}$ mice than in AREG$^{+/+}$ mice. Quantification of K8$^+$ luminal and K14$^+$ myoepithelial cells in non-PyMT AREG$^{-/-}$ mammary glands showed fewer K14$^+$ cells and a thinner myoepithelial layer. Study of AT-3 cells indicated that coculture with myoepithelial cells or exposure to AREG, epidermal growth factor, or basic fibroblast growth factor can suppress PyMT expression. Late-stage AREG$^{-/-}$ PyMT tumors are significantly less solid in structure, with more areas of papillary and cystic growth. Papillary areas appear to be both less proliferative and less necrotic. In The Cancer Genome Atlas database, luminal-B invasive papillary carcinomas have lower AREG expression than luminal B invasive ductal carcinomas.

Conclusions: Our study has revealed a previously unknown role of AREG in myoepithelial cell development and PyMT expression. AREG expression is essential for proper myoepithelial coverage of mammary ducts. Both AREG and myoepithelial cells can suppress PyMT expression. We find that lower AREG expression is associated with invasive papillary breast cancer in both the MMTV-PyMT model and human breast cancer.

Keywords: Amphiregulin, Mammary ductal development, MMTV-PyMT, Breast cancer

* Correspondence: Jeffrey.segall@einstein.yu.edu
[1]Department of Anatomy and Structural Biology, Albert Einstein College of Medicine, 1301 Morris Park Avenue, Bronx, NY 10461, USA
[3]Gruss Lipper Biophotonics Center, Albert Einstein College of Medicine, Bronx, NY 10461, USA
Full list of author information is available at the end of the article

Background

Breast cancer remains the most common form of cancer among women in the USA. In the most recent estimates, there are over 250,000 new cases and 40,000 new deaths predicted in 2018 alone [1]. Overexpression of epidermal growth factor receptor (EGFR) has been shown to be an important predictor of early recurrence and death in breast cancer [2, 3]. Historically, patients with positive EGFR status were associated with shorter relapse-free and overall survival. However, therapies targeting EGFR in breast cancer have been met with many challenges and little success [4–6]. Amphiregulin (AREG), a ligand of EGFR, has been found to be overexpressed in estrogen receptor (ER)-positive breast cancer [7]. Further evidence shows that loss of AREG in breast cancer cells can stunt tumor proliferation, growth, and invasiveness in vitro and in vivo [8–10]. In addition to breast cancer, AREG has been shown to play an important role in mammary gland development. During puberty, AREG is the only EGFR ligand that is transcriptionally activated by estrogen receptor signaling in the mammary gland [11]. In the absence of AREG, the mammary ductal tree fails to expand and remains as a rudimentary tree throughout adulthood. In mammary gland transplant studies, epithelial AREG expression and stromal EGFR expression have been identified as critical for proper mammary gland development [12]. Interestingly, when AREG-null epithelial cells are transplanted into a cleared mammary gland, regardless of EGFR status in the stroma, the resultant gland shows a lack of cytokeratin-14 (K14) protein, a marker for myoepithelial cells [13]. While it is unknown whether AREG supports development and maintenance of myoepithelial cells, some evidence suggests that under low EGFR signaling conditions, mammary stem cells (MaSCs) preferentially differentiate into luminal, not myoepithelial, cells [14]. In the same study, it was shown that in the presence of AREG, but not EGF, normal ductal development occurred. Therefore, it is possible that AREG is not only important for the expansion of the ductal tree, but also for proper differentiation of epithelial progenitor cells into luminal and myoepithelial cells.

Little is known about how AREG expression alters breast cancer initiation and progression. In our studies, we sought to better understand the role of AREG in breast cancer using the MMTV-PyMT (PyMT) mouse model. The PyMT model is a widely used murine model of breast cancer due to its similarities in tumor progression stages to human breast cancer [15, 16]. Furthermore, activation of PyMT drives many oncogenic pathways involving key signaling molecules, such as Src, Ras, and PI3K that are overexpressed in many different human cancers [17–19]. By crossing PyMT mice with AREG-null mice, we have evaluated the properties of the spontaneous PyMT breast tumor model in the absence of AREG.

In the studies described, we show for the first time novel functions of AREG in mammary gland development, PyMT expression, and breast cancer growth.

Methods

Mice

All animal studies were conducted with approval by the Albert Einstein College of Medicine Institutional Animal Care and Use Committee (IACUC). All husbandry was provided by the Institute of Animal Studies (IAS) under the supervision of veterinarians at the institution. Mice were maintained in a pathogen-free facility under controlled light cycles and temperatures. In our animal experiments, we used transgenic mice expressing the polyoma middle-T antigen (PyMT) controlled by the mammary tumor virus (MMTV) in the C57Bl/6 background as our murine breast cancer model. These animals were provided by Dr Jeffrey W. Pollard at our institution, bred in-house, and maintained on the C57Bl/6 background. To explore the role of amphiregulin (AREG) in breast cancer, we used AREG-knockout (AREG$^{-/-}$) mice in the same background [20]. Genotypes of offspring were identified by quantitative PCR (qPCR) via Transnetyx (Cordova, TN, USA).

Lesion growth and histological measurements

Palpable lesion growth was evaluated three times weekly using a digital caliper. Animals were sacrificed once the largest lesion reached 1 cm in diameter. Animals whose lesions ruptured prior to reaching the appropriate size were excluded from our analyses. AREG$^{-/-}$ lesions had a greater tendency to be cystic and may have ruptured more easily than AREG$^{+/+}$ lesions as they grew bigger. Lesions were excised and fixed in 10% formalin for 72 h. Tissues were then embedded in paraffin and serially sectioned for immunohistochemistry and immunofluorescence studies. Tumor progression was evaluated by a breast cancer pathologist (MHO) for presence of hyperplasia, ductal carcinoma in situ, and adenocarcinoma in a blinded fashion. All IHC and H&E staining was performed by the Histology and Comparative Pathology core facility at Albert Einstein College of Medicine. Slides were scanned using the 3DHISTECH Pannoramic 250 flash II digital whole slide scanner. Cystic evaluation was completed by examining 1-cm lesions for the presence of cysts. If a lesion had at least one cyst, it was considered cystic in our analysis.

Necrosis analysis

H&E stains of 1-cm AREG$^{+/+}$ PyMT ($N = 32$) and AREG$^{-/-}$ PyMT ($N = 22$) tumors were evaluated for the presence of necrosis. Quantification of the percentage of necrosis per tumor was determined by averaging the percentage of necrosis in individual 5× fields. The fields used in the analysis were determined randomly using a grid placed over the tissue image in Pannoramic Viewer so as to select unbiased areas. Solid and papillary areas were analyzed separately to determine the amount of necrosis in each type of histological structure. Statistical analysis was performed using the Mann–Whitney test.

Circulating tumor cell measurement

The in-vivo intravasation assay for circulating tumor cells (CTCs) was performed as described previously [21–24]. A 25-gauge needle and syringe coated with heparin was inserted into the right ventricle of the heart of anesthetized mice and up to 1 ml of blood was collected from the heart puncture and transferred to a 15-ml tube with 10 ml of 1× RBC lysis buffer (cat. 00-4300-54; Affymetrix). After a 10-min incubation at room temperature, the cell suspension was pelleted by centrifugation at 200 x g for 5 min. The cell pellet was reconstituted in 10 ml of Dulbecco's modified Eagle medium DMEM/F12 (cat. 11320–033; Gibco), supplemented with 20% fetal bovine serum (FBS)-premium select (cat. S11510; Atlanta Biologicals) and plated in a 10-cm tissue culture-treated Petri dish. Media were changed after 48 h. After a 1-week incubation, single tumor cells attached on the dish were counted. Finally, the cell count was normalized to 1 ml of blood.

Metastasis measurements

After mice were sacrificed, the lungs were inflated with 10% formalin and fixed for 72 h. After fixation, the samples were embedded in paraffin and sectioned. Lungs were stained with hematoxylin and eosin (H&E). The number of metastatic foci was counted and their area was measured.

Carmine staining

The mammary fat pads were evaluated using carmine staining as described previously [25]. Briefly, glands were fixed in Carnoy's fixative overnight at 4 °C. Glands were rehydrated in serial dilutions of ethanol and rinsed once with water followed by staining with 0.2% carmine alum solution overnight at room temperature. The next day, glands were incubated in 1% HCl/70% EtOH solution for 4 h to remove the excess carmine stain. Glands were then dehydrated in increasing concentrations of ethanol. A 1-h xylene incubation was used to clear the tissue. Cleared glands were mounted in Permount (cat. SP15–500; Fisher Scientific). Finally, the slides were scanned using a conventional digital scanner.

Immunofluorescence

Slides were deparaffinized and stained as described previously [24]. The following primary antibodies were used: PyMT (cat. NB100-2749; Novus Biologicals), IBA1 (cat. NB100-1028; Novus Biologicals), CD31 (cat. 77699; Cell Signaling), KRT8 (cat. TROMA-I; Developmental Studies Hybridoma Bank), and KRT14 (cat. 905304; Biolegend). After deparaffinization, slides were placed in a 1× target retrieval solution (cat. S169984-2; Agilent Technologies) and incubated overnight in the Retriever 220 V (cat. 62700-20; Electron Microscopy Sciences) for antigen retrieval. Slides were washed in 1× PBS and incubated with blocking buffer (10% donkey serum/ 0.1% Triton-X100) for 1 h at 4 °C. Primary antibodies were diluted in 1× PBS-T at the following concentrations: PyMT 1:100, IBA1 1:100, CD31 1:250, KRT8 1:30, and KRT14 1:1000. Samples were incubated with primary antibody solutions overnight at 4 °C. Before secondary antibody incubation, slides were washed three times in 1× PBS-T for 5 min each. The secondary antibodies used were Alexa Fluor 647 donkey anti-rabbit IgG (cat. A31573; Life Technologies), Alexa Fluor 488 donkey anti-Rat IgG (cat. A21208; Life Technologies), and Alexa Fluor 568 donkey anti-goat (cat. A11077; Life Technologies). Secondary antibodies were diluted in 1× PBS-T at 1:250. Secondary antibody incubation was performed at room temperature for 1 h. Slides were mounted using Dapi-Fluoromount-G (cat. OB010020; Southern Biotech) and stored at 4 °C. Slides were scanned using the 3DHISTECH Pannoramic 250 flash II digital whole slide scanner. The 20 × 0.8 NA objective lens was used for all scans.

PyMT expression quantitation and analysis

Three to five fields per sample were chosen for analysis. Images were taken in Pannoramic Viewer and opened in ImageJ. All images were converted to 8-bit and the same threshold was applied to all images. After the threshold was designated, the region of interest (ROI) covered only the mammary ducts or lesions. The surrounding vessels, fat, and stroma were excluded. The PyMT immunofluorescence intensity was analyzed only within the ROIs.

In-situ hybridization

In-situ hybridization experiments were performed using the manufacturer's protocol for the BaseScope™ Assay (cat. 322971; ACD). After the signal was detected, the slides were blocked with 4% donkey serum (cat. D9663-10ML; Sigma-Aldrich) in 0.1% 1× PBS-T for 1 h at room temperature. Slides were stained for PyMT using the protocol described earlier.

Mammary epithelial cell counting and myoepithelial cell layer thickness measurement

Mammary ducts were immunostained for K8 and K14 to visualize luminal (K8+) and myoepithelial (K14+) cells. The ratio of myoepithelial cells to total mammary epithelial cells was counted manually and calculated for five ducts per mammary fat pad. At least three AREG$^{+/+}$ mice and three AREG$^{-/-}$ mice were used for this analysis. In cases of uncertainty, a confocal microscope was utilized to differentiate the different cell layers. The outlines of myoepithelial cells were traced to calculate the thickness of the myoepithelial cells.

Mammary epithelial cell isolation

Methods used to retrieve mammary epithelial cells (MECs) from mice were described previously [26]. Excised mammary glands were placed in ice-cold PBS. Glands were finely minced on a bacterial Petri dish and resuspended in 3 ml/mouse DMEM/F12 (cat. 11320-033; Gibco). Then 300 units/ml collagenase III (cat. LS004182; Worthington), 50 µg/ml DNase I (cat. LS002139; Worthington), and 5 µM Y-27632 (cat. Y-5301; LC Labs) were added and incubated at 37 °C for 2 h under constant rotation. Afterward, the digestion mixture was thoroughly mixed and PBS was added to 15 ml. The mixture was centrifuged at 300 × g for 5 min. To remove the erythrocytes, the cell pellet was resuspended with 1 ml RBC lysis buffer (8.3 g/L ammonium acetate, 10 mM Tris–HCl pH 7.5) and incubated on ice for 1 min. The cell mixture was thoroughly mixed, PBS was added to 15 ml, and the mixture was centrifuged again. The cell pellet was resuspended in 1 ml 0.05% Trypsin–EDTA (cat. MT25052CI; Corning) and incubated at 37 °C for 5 min. Trypsin was diluted with 10% FBS in DMEM/F12 and the cell mixture was centrifuged. To dissociate the luminal and myoepithelial cells, the cell pellet was resuspended in 1 ml DMEM/F12, 1 U/ml Dispase (cat. LS02109; Worthington), and 100 µg/ml DNase. The cell mixture was incubated at 37 °C for 5 min and passed through a 40-µm cell strainer. Then 5 ml of PBS was added to the final cell suspension. The cell number was determined using a hemocytometer. The cells were centrifuged and resuspended in FACS buffer (1 ml FBS, 31 ml PBS, 8 ml 10 mM EDTA) at 1 million cells/100 µl.

Fluorescence-activated cell sorting

To isolate myoepithelial cells from the cell suspension, the cells were labeled with 1:100 biotin TER-119 (cat. 116204; Biolegend), biotin CD45 (cat. 103104; Biolegend), biotin CD31 (cat. 102404; Biolegend), APC EpCAM (cat. 17–5791-80; Affymetrix), and PerCP-Cy5.5 CD49f (cat. 562475; BD Biosciences). After a 15-min incubation on ice, streptavidin v450 (cat. 560797; BD Biosciences) and 1 µg/ml DAPI (cat. 422801; Biolegend) were added for another 15-min incubation. Cells were washed once and resuspended in fluorescence-activated cell sorting (FACS) buffer. The lineage-negative

(TER-119$^-$CD45$^-$CD31$^-$) EpCAM$^-$CD49f$^+$ cells were identified as myoepithelial cells.

Cell lines and cell culture

Sorted myoepithelial cells were centrifuged and resuspended in 1:20 Matrigel (cat. 354234; Corning) and cultured in advanced-DMEM/F12 (cat. 12634010; Life Technologies) supplemented with 10 ng/ml EGF (cat. 585506; Biolegend), 20 ng/ml bFGF (cat. 710304; Biolegend), 4 µg/ml heparin (cat. H3149-10KU; Sigma-Aldrich), 5% newborn calf serum (cat. SH3011803; HyClone), and 5 µM Y-27632.

AT-3 cells, a murine breast cancer cell line derived from MMTV-PyMT tumors in the C57Bl/6 background, were cultured at 7% CO_2 in DMEM high glucose (cat. MT-10-013-CV; Corning) supplemented with 10% FBS premium-select, penicillin–streptomycin (cat. MT30002CI; Corning), 15 mM HEPES (cat. 15630080; Life Technologies), 2 mM L-glutamine (cat. SH3003401; HyClone), NEAA (cat. SH3023801; HyClone), 1 mM sodium pyruvate (cat. 13-115E; Lonza Walkersville), and 1:250,000 2-mercaptoethanol (cat. M6250-100ML; Sigma Aldrich).

In-vitro experiments

For the coculture experiments, 300,000 primary myoepithelial cells and 300,000 AT-3 cells were plated together in a six-well tissue culture plate overnight. In the control well, 300,000 AT-3 cells were plated. Cells were lysed on the following day using Buffer RLT Plus (cat. 1053393; Qiagen) and RNA was extracted using the RNeasy Plus Mini Kit (cat. 74134; Qiagen). Subsequently, cDNA was synthesized and amplified using the Superscript II system (cat. 11904-018; Thermofisher Scientific).

For the stimulation experiments, 300,000 AT-3 cells were plated overnight. On the following day, the media were switched to those containing either 10 ng/ml EGF, 10 ng/ml bFGF, 100 ng/ml AREG (cat. 989-AR-100; R&D Systems), or both EGF and bFGF. Cells were lysed after a 24-h incubation period.

Quantitative RT-PCR

The gene expression level of PyMT was measured in the coculture and stimulation experiments using a SYBR Green Real-Time Master Mix and PyMT primers. The PyMT primer sequences were TTCGATCCGATCCT AGATGC and TGCCGGGAACGTTTTATTAG. PyMT expression was normalized to GAPDH expression. The GAPDH primer sequences were CTGGAGAAACCTGC CAAGTA and TGTTGCTGTAGCCGTATTCA. Each experiment was done in triplicate and repeated at least three independent times. Relative PyMT expression levels were derived from the GAPDH mean cycle threshold (Ct) values subtracted by the PyMT Ct values.

Myoepithelial cells and AT-3 cells had similar levels of GAPDH. In coculture experiments, ΔCt values were adjusted to compensate for a twofold dilution in PyMT expression level. Changes in relative PyMT expression levels between experiment and control were measured as the fold change (ΔΔCt).

TCGA analysis

The Cancer Genome Atlas (TCGA) Research Network (http://cancergenome.nih.gov/) provided a database of human breast cancer patient data which we analyzed for AREG expression and histological subtype. Since the MMTV-PyMT model was characterized as most similar to the luminal B subtype in human breast cancer, we chose our sample population from patient tumors that were identified as luminal B subtype. With the final sample of 123 patient samples, 115 were nonpapillary invasive ductal cancer (IDC) and eight were invasive papillary breast cancer (IPC). AREG RNAseq expression data provided by TCGA for these patient samples were then evaluated [27, 28].

Statistical analyses

All statistical analyses were carried out using GraphPad Prism 7 software. Statistical analyses were performed using tests as indicated in the figure legends.

Results

Expansion and progression of tumorigenic lesions is accelerated in the absence of AREG

We examined the role of AREG in breast cancer using the MMTV-PyMT (PyMT) model in AREG$^{-/-}$ mice. The appearance of lesions by carmine staining was visible in the mammary fat pads (MFPs) of both AREG$^{+/+}$ PyMT (Fig. 1a) and AREG$^{-/-}$ PyMT (Fig. 1b) females as early as 6 weeks of age. Lesions were larger in AREG$^{-/-}$ PyMT mice at 6 weeks, and by 12 weeks the difference in size of the lesions was even more dramatic (Fig. 1c–e). Interestingly, the lesions in AREG$^{+/+}$ PyMT mice were found in distinct regions in the ductal tree while in AREG$^{-/-}$ PyMT mice much of the ductal tree appeared to convert into the growing lesion. The appearance of multiple lesions in the AREG$^{+/+}$ PyMT ductal tree is consistent with previous reports [16]. We measured the growth of palpable lesions in

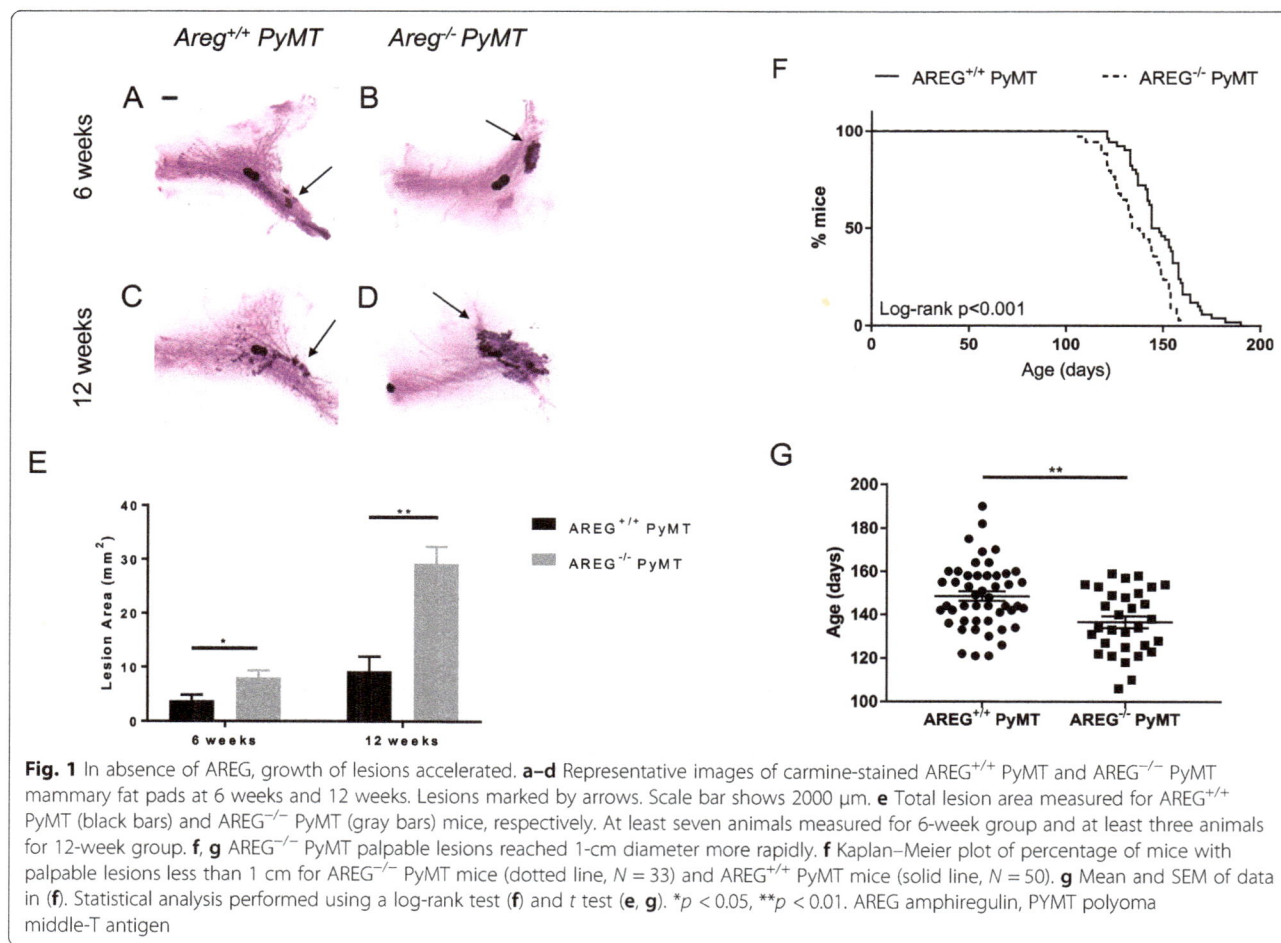

Fig. 1 In absence of AREG, growth of lesions accelerated. **a–d** Representative images of carmine-stained AREG$^{+/+}$ PyMT and AREG$^{-/-}$ PyMT mammary fat pads at 6 weeks and 12 weeks. Lesions marked by arrows. Scale bar shows 2000 μm. **e** Total lesion area measured for AREG$^{+/+}$ PyMT (black bars) and AREG$^{-/-}$ PyMT (gray bars) mice, respectively. At least seven animals measured for 6-week group and at least three animals for 12-week group. **f, g** AREG$^{-/-}$ PyMT palpable lesions reached 1-cm diameter more rapidly. **f** Kaplan–Meier plot of percentage of mice with palpable lesions less than 1 cm for AREG$^{-/-}$ PyMT mice (dotted line, N = 33) and AREG$^{+/+}$ PyMT mice (solid line, N = 50). **g** Mean and SEM of data in (**f**). Statistical analysis performed using a log-rank test (**f**) and t test (**e, g**). *p < 0.05, **p < 0.01. AREG amphiregulin, PYMT polyoma middle-T antigen

AREG$^{+/+}$ PyMT and AREG$^{-/-}$ PyMT mice three times per week using a digital caliper until the largest palpable lesion reached a diameter of 1 cm (Additional file 1: Figure S1). The largest lesion reached the 1-cm endpoint significantly faster in AREG$^{-/-}$ PyMT mice (Fig. 1f). The average ages at which AREG$^{+/+}$ PyMT mice and AREG$^{-/-}$ PyMT mice reached the endpoint were 144 days and 134 days, respectively (Fig. 1g).

Consistent with the growth data, tumor progression was also accelerated in the AREG$^{-/-}$ PyMT mice. Histology of the lesions was evaluated by a breast cancer pathologist (MHO). Based on these assessments, the lesions of 12-week-old AREG$^{+/+}$ PyMT mice were found to be predominantly at the stage of hyperplasia, with some limited areas of DCIS and invasive carcinoma (Fig. 2a, c). However, lesions of age-matched AREG$^{-/-}$ PyMT mice showed more areas that had progressed to DCIS and invasive carcinoma (Fig. 2b, d, e).

To determine whether AREG-associated effects in tumor growth and progression were associated with changes in intravasation and metastasis, we examined metastases in the lungs as well as circulating tumor cells (CTCs) in these animals. Overall, we found no difference

in metastasis as measured by the number of foci or total area in the lungs (Additional file 2: Figure S2A, B) or number of CTCs (Additional file 2: Figure S2C). In summary, loss of AREG appears to enhance expansion of tumorigenic lesions and accelerate tumor progression, but does not have an effect on intravasation and metastasis.

Using in-situ hybridization, we confirmed that AREG is expressed in AREG$^{+/+}$ animals in the ductal cells and TEBs, consistent with previous studies (Fig. 3a) [13], with no expression in AREG$^{-/-}$ animals. We then compared the localization of AREG and PyMT expression in AREG$^{+/+}$ PyMT animals and found that they were inversely related. PyMT expression was absent in ducts and TEBs where AREG was expressed, while AREG expression was rare in hyperplastic and tumor structures in which PyMT staining was present (Fig. 3a, PyMT panel).

In both AREG$^{+/+}$ PyMT and AREG$^{-/-}$ PyMT mammary glands, all lesions express PyMT (Fig. 3b). Interestingly, the intensity of PyMT fluorescence in these lesions is similar in AREG$^{+/+}$ PyMT and AREG$^{-/-}$ PyMT mammary glands (Fig. 3c). Since the lesions are larger in AREG$^{-/-}$ PyMT

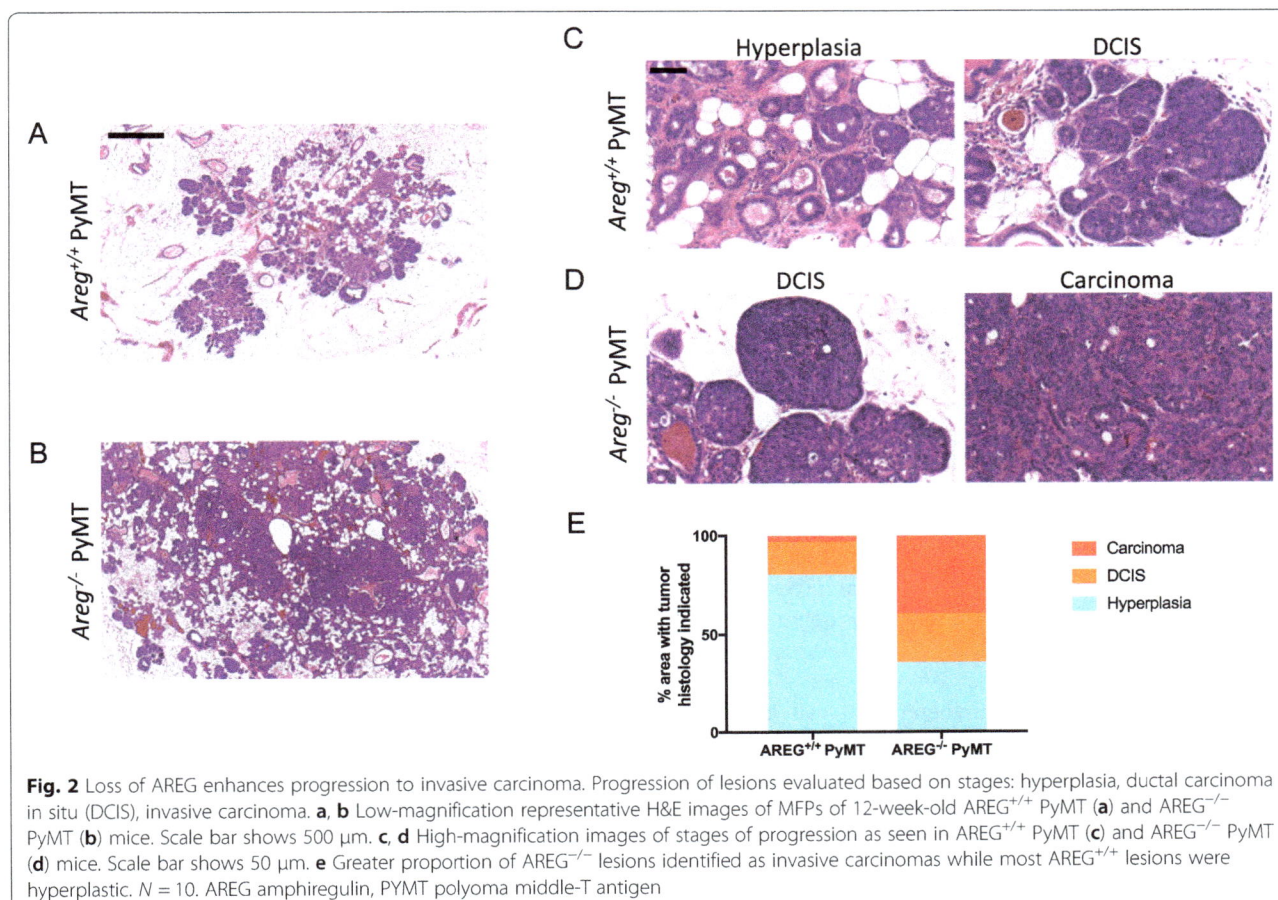

Fig. 2 Loss of AREG enhances progression to invasive carcinoma. Progression of lesions evaluated based on stages: hyperplasia, ductal carcinoma in situ (DCIS), invasive carcinoma. a, b Low-magnification representative H&E images of MFPs of 12-week-old AREG$^{+/+}$ PyMT (a) and AREG$^{-/-}$ PyMT (b) mice. Scale bar shows 500 μm. c, d High-magnification images of stages of progression as seen in AREG$^{+/+}$ PyMT (c) and AREG$^{-/-}$ PyMT (d) mice. Scale bar shows 50 μm. e Greater proportion of AREG$^{-/-}$ lesions identified as invasive carcinomas while most AREG$^{+/+}$ lesions were hyperplastic. $N = 10$. AREG amphiregulin, PYMT polyoma middle-T antigen

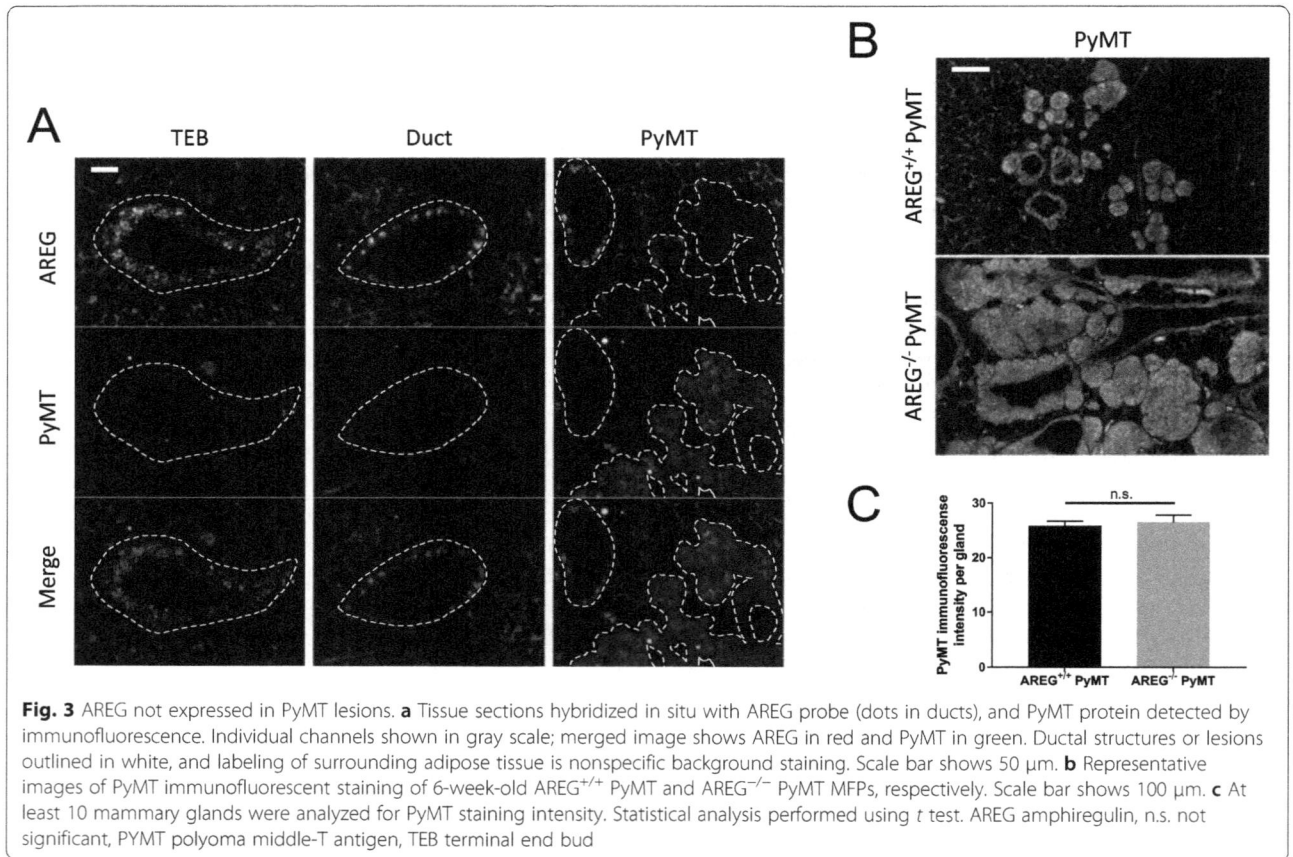

Fig. 3 AREG not expressed in PyMT lesions. **a** Tissue sections hybridized in situ with AREG probe (dots in ducts), and PyMT protein detected by immunofluorescence. Individual channels shown in gray scale; merged image shows AREG in red and PyMT in green. Ductal structures or lesions outlined in white, and labeling of surrounding adipose tissue is nonspecific background staining. Scale bar shows 50 μm. **b** Representative images of PyMT immunofluorescent staining of 6-week-old AREG$^{+/+}$ PyMT and AREG$^{-/-}$ PyMT MFPs, respectively. Scale bar shows 100 μm. **c** At least 10 mammary glands were analyzed for PyMT staining intensity. Statistical analysis performed using t test. AREG amphiregulin, n.s. not significant, PYMT polyoma middle-T antigen, TEB terminal end bud

MFPs, this suggests that PyMT is expressed in more areas in AREG$^{-/-}$ PyMT mammary glands. However, the level of expression does not differ in the absence of AREG.

Absence of AREG results in reduced myoepithelial cell number, coverage, and thickness

Even though the ductal tree is much smaller than in the wildtype, lesion growth in AREG$^{-/-}$ PyMT mice was significantly greater. We examined the mammary ducts of 6-week-old and 12-week-old AREG$^{+/+}$ and AREG$^{-/-}$ mice in the absence of PyMT to determine whether differences in the mammary ducts may explain the enhanced lesion growth in AREG$^{-/-}$ mice. We used cytokeratin-8 (K8) and cytokeratin-14 (K14) staining to visualize the luminal and myoepithelial layers of the mammary duct, respectively. The myoepithelial cell layer in the AREG$^{-/-}$ mice was often discontinuous (Fig. 4a, arrow) and K14 staining cells could be seen also in the luminal layer. Overall, the myoepithelial cell layer was thinner (Fig. 4b, d) and the proportion of K14$^+$ myoepithelial cells was smaller (Fig. 4c, e) in both 6-week-old and 12-week-old AREG$^{-/-}$ mice. Since it is possible that PyMT tumors initiate from mature duct termini in AREG$^{+/+}$ mice, we compared the proportion of myoepithelial cells in ducts and terminal acini in AREG$^{+/+}$

mammary glands and found that there were fewer myoepithelial cells in the acini as well (Fig. 4f).

Because myoepithelial cells are recognized to be tumor suppressors [29], we hypothesized that myoepithelial cells might be able to suppress PyMT expression. A reduction in myoepithelial cells in the AREG$^{-/-}$ mammary ducts might lead to induction of PyMT expression in more ductal cells, resulting in more lesion formation in AREG$^{-/-}$ PyMT mice. To test this hypothesis, we cocultured primary myoepithelial cells with AT-3 cells, a breast tumor cell line derived from C57Bl/6 MMTV-PyMT mammary tumors [30]. When cocultured with primary myoepithelial cells, PyMT expression in AT-3 cells was significantly reduced (Fig. 4g).

In addition, AREG and FGFR signaling are critical for proper mammary gland elongation and branching [31]. We therefore examined PyMT expression in AT-3 cells cultured in the presence of the EGFR ligands EGF and AREG, as well as FGFR ligand bFGF. In the presence of AREG, EGF, or bFGF, PyMT expression in AT-3 cells was reduced (Fig. 4h). Therefore, a loss of AREG expression in vivo could contribute to the broader expression of PyMT seen in the AREG$^{-/-}$ mice through both a reduction in myoepithelial cells as well as reduced EGFR and FGFR signaling.

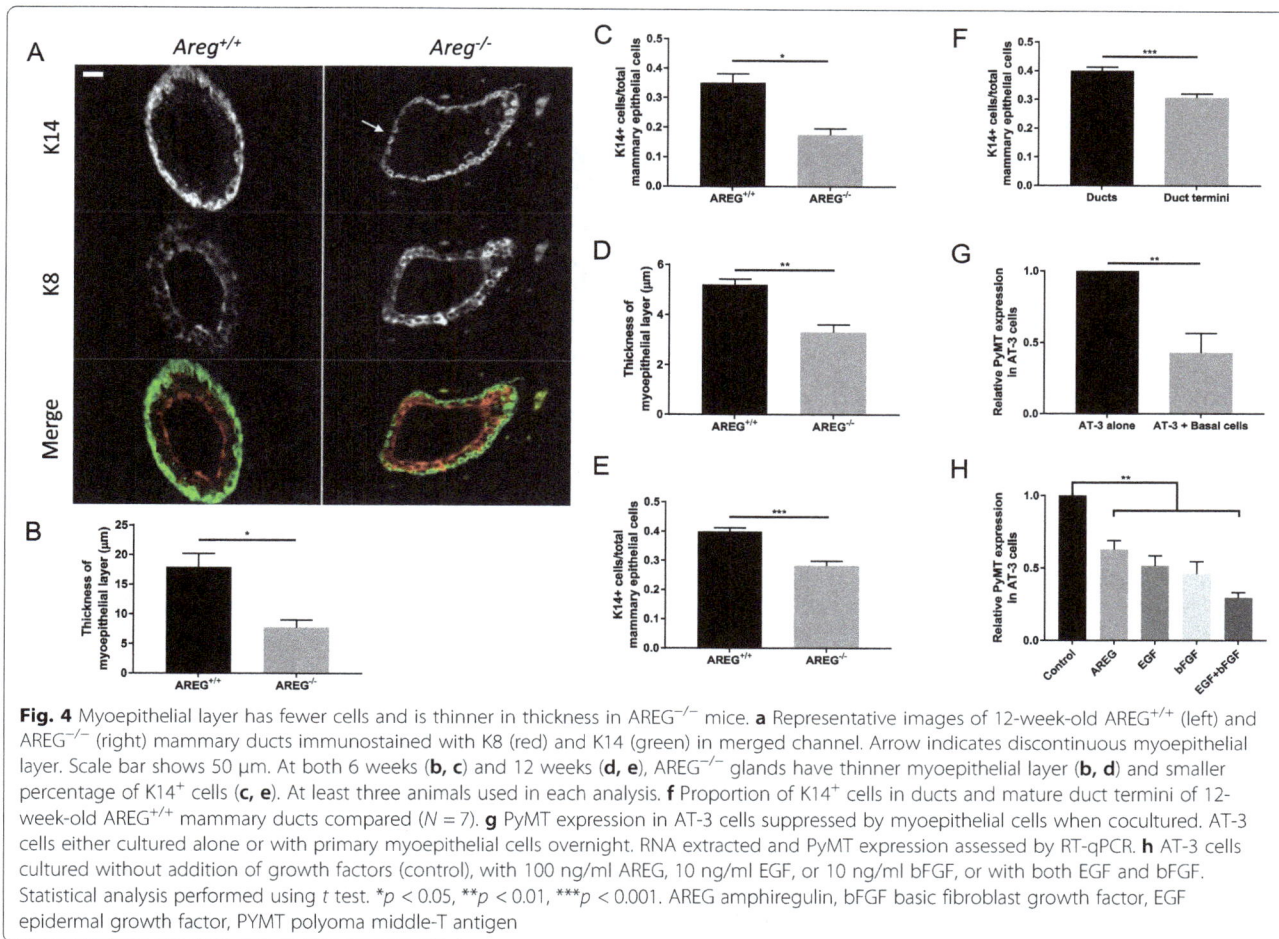

Fig. 4 Myoepithelial layer has fewer cells and is thinner in thickness in AREG$^{-/-}$ mice. **a** Representative images of 12-week-old AREG$^{+/+}$ (left) and AREG$^{-/-}$ (right) mammary ducts immunostained with K8 (red) and K14 (green) in merged channel. Arrow indicates discontinuous myoepithelial layer. Scale bar shows 50 μm. At both 6 weeks (**b, c**) and 12 weeks (**d, e**), AREG$^{-/-}$ glands have thinner myoepithelial layer (**b, d**) and smaller percentage of K14$^+$ cells (**c, e**). At least three animals used in each analysis. **f** Proportion of K14$^+$ cells in ducts and mature duct termini of 12-week-old AREG$^{+/+}$ mammary ducts compared ($N = 7$). **g** PyMT expression in AT-3 cells suppressed by myoepithelial cells when cocultured. AT-3 cells either cultured alone or with primary myoepithelial cells overnight. RNA extracted and PyMT expression assessed by RT-qPCR. **h** AT-3 cells cultured without addition of growth factors (control), with 100 ng/ml AREG, 10 ng/ml EGF, or 10 ng/ml bFGF, or with both EGF and bFGF. Statistical analysis performed using t test. *$p < 0.05$, **$p < 0.01$, ***$p < 0.001$. AREG amphiregulin, bFGF basic fibroblast growth factor, EGF epidermal growth factor, PYMT polyoma middle-T antigen

Late-stage AREG$^{-/-}$ tumors are histologically distinct from AREG$^{+/+}$ tumors

Late-stage (1-cm diameter as measured by caliper) AREG$^{+/+}$ PyMT tumors are characterized by solid sheets of cells with occasional ductal structures remaining at the periphery [15]. However, size-matched (1-cm diameter) AREG$^{-/-}$ PyMT tumors are more heterogeneous in their histology; they are often composed of both solid and papillary tumor areas (Fig. 5a). These papillary tumor regions are characterized by finger-like fronds that are composed of fibrovascular stalks lined by neoplastic epithelial cells [32]. When we compared the percentage of each tumor occupied by solid or papillary histology, we found that AREG$^{-/-}$ tumors had a significantly greater proportion of papillary tumor histology than AREG$^{+/+}$ tumors (Fig. 5b). We also noticed that many tumors, particularly AREG$^{-/-}$ tumors, are very cystic (Additional file 3: Figure S3). If a tumor had at least one cyst, we characterized that tumor as cystic. Our analysis revealed that while some AREG$^{+/+}$ tumors are cystic, all of the AREG$^{-/-}$ tumors had cysts (Fig. 5c). Thus, in addition to having more papillary features, the AREG$^{-/-}$ tumors are also more cystic.

To better understand the implications of histological differences on tumor growth, we assessed AREG$^{+/+}$ and AREG$^{-/-}$ tumors for the presence of necrosis (Fig. 6a, H&E images). In both types of tumors, there is considerable variability in the amount of necrosis, ranging from none at all to over 50% necrotic. Overall, AREG$^{-/-}$ tumors are less necrotic than the wildtype counterpart (Fig. 6b). When we compared necrotic areas between solid areas of AREG$^{+/+}$ tumors and AREG$^{-/-}$ tumors, a significant difference remains while the papillary areas have little to no necrosis regardless of AREG status (Additional file 4: Figure S4). This suggests that the differences in necrosis we have observed between AREG$^{+/+}$ and AREG$^{-/-}$ tumors are due to both an increased proportion of papillary tumor histology (which is not necrotic) as well as reduced necrosis in the solid tumor regions in the AREG$^{-/-}$ tumors.

We also immunostained these tissues for Ki67 (Fig. 6a, Ki67 images). We compared the Ki67$^+$ areas in solid and papillary regions and found that in both AREG$^{+/+}$ and AREG$^{-/-}$ tumors, papillary regions have less Ki67 staining (Fig. 6c, d). Since AREG$^{+/+}$ tumors are proportionally

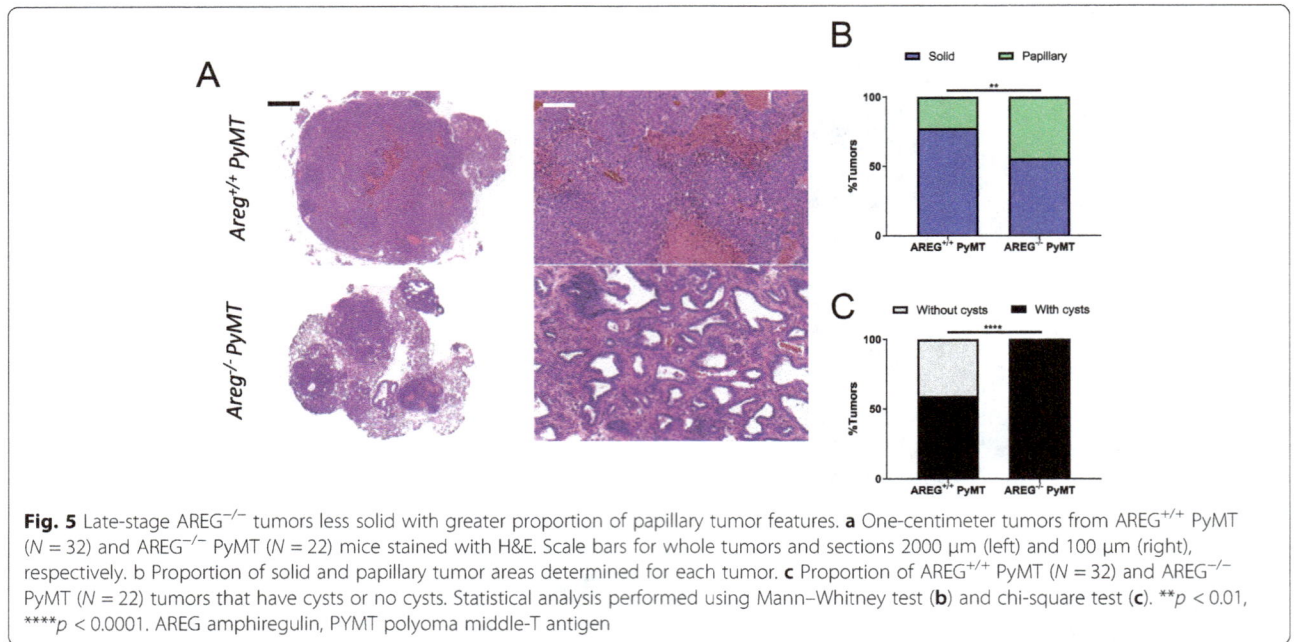

Fig. 5 Late-stage AREG$^{-/-}$ tumors less solid with greater proportion of papillary tumor features. **a** One-centimeter tumors from AREG$^{+/+}$ PyMT ($N = 32$) and AREG$^{-/-}$ PyMT ($N = 22$) mice stained with H&E. Scale bars for whole tumors and sections 2000 μm (left) and 100 μm (right), respectively. **b** Proportion of solid and papillary tumor areas determined for each tumor. **c** Proportion of AREG$^{+/+}$ PyMT ($N = 32$) and AREG$^{-/-}$ PyMT ($N = 22$) tumors that have cysts or no cysts. Statistical analysis performed using Mann–Whitney test (**b**) and chi-square test (**c**). **$p < 0.01$, ****$p < 0.0001$. AREG amphiregulin, PYMT polyoma middle-T antigen

more solid than AREG$^{-/-}$ tumors, this indicates that, as a whole, AREG$^{+/+}$ tumors are more proliferative than AREG$^{-/-}$ tumors. However, this may be counteracted by increased necrosis: in the solid areas where tumor proliferation is high, tumor cells far from the blood vessel do not receive enough oxygen and nutrients and become hypoxic [33–35]. Rapid growth of the tumor causes exhaustion of the nutrients and oxygen supplied by the nearby blood vessels and, as a result, forms necrotic zones. Conversely, in the papillary and cystic areas that are more

common in the AREG$^{-/-}$ tumors, there is slower growth, more stroma, and correspondingly less necrosis.

We used CD31 staining to compare the vasculature between AREG$^{+/+}$ and AREG$^{-/-}$ tumors (Additional file 5: Figure S5A). The vessel structures in AREG$^{+/+}$ tumors are thin and long while the vessels in AREG$^{-/-}$ tumors appear shorter and irregular in shape. These observations are complemented by quantification of CD31 signals, showing increased numbers of CD31$^+$ vessels in AREG$^{-/-}$ tumors (Additional file 5: Figure S5B).

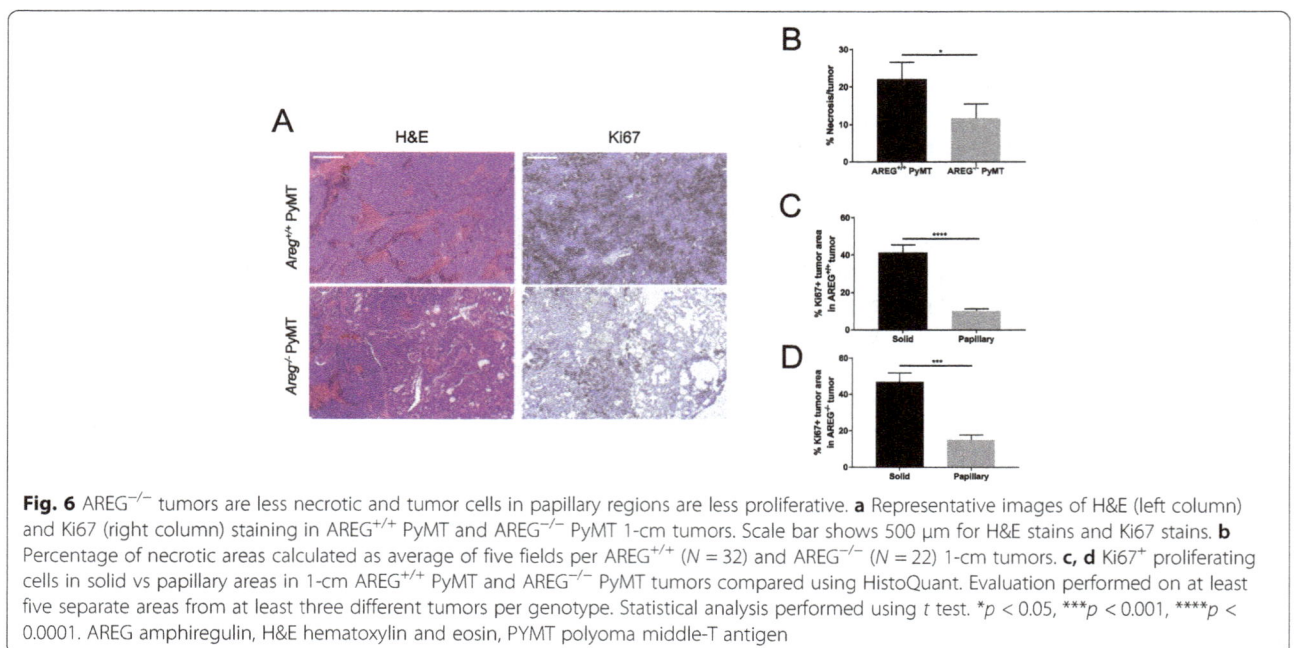

Fig. 6 AREG$^{-/-}$ tumors are less necrotic and tumor cells in papillary regions are less proliferative. **a** Representative images of H&E (left column) and Ki67 (right column) staining in AREG$^{+/+}$ PyMT and AREG$^{-/-}$ PyMT 1-cm tumors. Scale bar shows 500 μm for H&E stains and Ki67 stains. **b** Percentage of necrotic areas calculated as average of five fields per AREG$^{+/+}$ ($N = 32$) and AREG$^{-/-}$ ($N = 22$) 1-cm tumors. **c, d** Ki67$^+$ proliferating cells in solid vs papillary areas in 1-cm AREG$^{+/+}$ PyMT and AREG$^{-/-}$ PyMT tumors compared using HistoQuant. Evaluation performed on at least five separate areas from at least three different tumors per genotype. Statistical analysis performed using t test. *$p < 0.05$, ***$p < 0.001$, ****$p < 0.0001$. AREG amphiregulin, H&E hematoxylin and eosin, PYMT polyoma middle-T antigen

Lower AREG expression is associated with papillary breast cancer

From our results using the PyMT mouse model, we found that the absence of AREG changes the tumor histological growth pattern, with AREG$^{-/-}$ tumors developing with more papillary features. In human breast cancer, invasive papillary cancer (IPC) is a subtype of infiltrating ductal carcinoma (IDC). The genomic profile of the PyMT mouse model has been characterized as most similar to the luminal B molecular subtype [36]. Therefore, we examined The Cancer Genome Atlas (TCGA) for patient samples that have been identified as luminal B. Using the available pathological reports, the patient samples were separated into nonpapillary IDC versus IPC. We then evaluated the AREG expression of these tumors as provided in TCGA. Interestingly, we found that patients with IPC have a significantly lower AREG expression than those with nonpapillary IDC (Fig. 7), consistent with our results that AREG$^{-/-}$ tumors are more papillary.

Discussion

In our studies, we found that the loss of AREG resulted in accelerated expansion of PyMT-positive lesions in the PyMT mouse model of breast cancer. As early as 6 weeks of age, lesions in AREG$^{-/-}$ PyMT mice were increasing in size more quickly. Lesions in both AREG$^{+/+}$ PyMT mice and AREG$^{-/-}$ PyMT mice were PyMT-positive. However, it was unclear why there was a larger PyMT-positive area in the AREG$^{-/-}$ PyMT mice. When we compared the cellular composition of the mammary ducts in AREG$^{+/+}$ and AREG$^{-/-}$ pubertal and adult mice, we found that AREG$^{-/-}$ ducts had fewer myoepithelial cells and thinner myoepithelial cell layers than AREG$^{+/+}$ ducts. Interestingly, in AREG$^{+/+}$ PyMT MFPs, the PyMT-positive lesions do not express AREG. We cocultured primary myoepithelial cells with AT-3 cells, a breast tumor cell line derived from the MMTV-PyMT mouse model, and found a significant reduction in PyMT expression in the AT-3 cells. Furthermore, when we cultured AT-3 cells with EGFR ligands AREG and EGF, or FGFR ligand bFGF, PyMT expression was reduced. In late-stage AREG$^{-/-}$ tumors, we also found a striking difference in the tumor growth pattern. Most of the AREG$^{-/-}$ tumors presented with increased papillary histology, cysts, and number of intratumoral vessels. Finally, we compared the tumor histology and AREG expression of luminal B breast cancer patient samples in TCGA and found papillary breast cancer was associated with low AREG expression.

In the PyMT model, PyMT expression in the mammary gland is driven by the MMTV promoter [37]. Stimulation of the MMTV promoter is primarily controlled by binding of glucocorticoid-bound glucocorticoid receptor complexes to

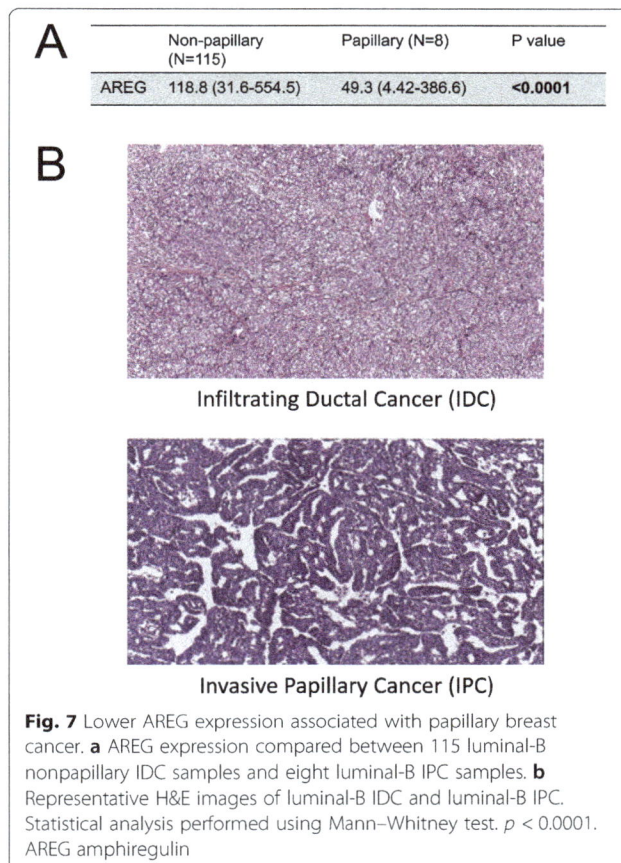

	Non-papillary (N=115)	Papillary (N=8)	P value
AREG	118.8 (31.6-554.5)	49.3 (4.42-386.6)	**<0.0001**

Infiltrating Ductal Cancer (IDC)

Invasive Papillary Cancer (IPC)

Fig. 7 Lower AREG expression associated with papillary breast cancer. **a** AREG expression compared between 115 luminal-B nonpapillary IDC samples and eight luminal-B IPC samples. **b** Representative H&E images of luminal-B IDC and luminal-B IPC. Statistical analysis performed using Mann–Whitney test. $p < 0.0001$. AREG amphiregulin

the hormone receptor element in the long terminal repeat (LTR) region of the MMTV promoter [38, 39]. Interestingly, EGF has been shown to stimulate tyrosine phosphorylation of the glucocorticoid receptor in breast epithelial HBL100 cells [40]. As a result of EGF stimulation, binding of dexamethasone to the glucocorticoid receptor is reduced [41]. Dexamethasone treatment inhibits proliferation of HBL100 cells. However, adding EGF to the dexamethasone treatment overcomes dexamethasone-mediated inhibition of cell proliferation. EGF has also been shown to increase the expression of *Egr2*, a gene that is inhibited by glucocorticoids [42, 43]. This suggests that activation of the EGFR signaling pathway can reduce GR signaling, which is important for MMTV promoter stimulation. Thus, EGF, and possibly AREG, may suppress PyMT expression through inhibition of glucocorticoids binding to its receptor.

It is also possible that loss of AREG alters the balance of proliferation between different cell types that can contribute to formation of a tumor. AREG expression might suppress the proliferation of cells with the capability of driving MMTV promoter activity, and then loss of AREG could lead to increased proliferation of such cells. Alternatively, AREG may bias differentiation. The cell fate of mammary epithelial progenitors has been shown to be partially dependent on EGFR signaling during development [14]. Under high levels of EGFR activation, progenitor cells preferentially differentiate into luminal epithelial cells. The common luminal progenitor gives rise to both ER-positive and ER-negative ductal cells as well as ER-negative alveolar cells [44]. Potentially, the loss of AREG could bias differentiation toward the alveolar cell phenotype, resulting in more cells that can express PyMT. Further studies will be needed to resolve these possibilities.

Furthermore, we have provided evidence that myoepithelial cells can also reduce PyMT expression. Although the mechanism is unknown, myoepithelial cells have a plethora of activities and functions, aside from the canonical mechanical contractile function. In particular, it has been shown that myoepithelial cells are tumor suppressors, involved in the inhibition of breast tumor cell proliferation in vitro and breast tumor growth in vivo, as well as angiogenesis [45, 46]. Myoepithelial cells also produce activin, a member of the TGF-β superfamily, which can also inhibit breast cancer cell proliferation by activating cell cycle arrest mediated by Smads [47, 48]. In other studies, TGF-β negatively regulates MMTV expression in a mammary tumor cell line [49]. Therefore, it is possible that myoepithelial cell-secreted factors may reduce PyMT expression via suppression of the MMTV promoter.

From our studies, we have developed a model that summarizes our key findings (Fig. 8). As key mediators of estrogen-induced mammary ductal development, epithelial AREG and stromal EGFR promote ductal elongation during puberty [11, 13]. Paracrine EGFR–FGFR signaling between mammary epithelial and neighboring stromal cells has been shown to be critical in proper ductal growth and branching [31]. In AREG$^{+/+}$ mice (Fig. 8a, top), AREG stimulates fibroblasts to produce FGFs, which bind to FGF receptors on the epithelial cells to stimulate ductal growth and branching. In AREG$^{-/-}$ mice (Fig. 8a, bottom), there is diminished paracrine signaling between mammary epithelial cells and stromal cells, and as a result the ductal tree fails to grow beyond the postnatal stage and myoepithelial cell coverage is reduced in the ducts. In the AREG$^{+/+}$ PyMT mice (Fig. 8b, top), PyMT expression may be suppressed in ducts and terminal end buds both by myoepithelial cells and growth factors such as AREG, EGF, and bFGF, or there is suppression of the generation of cells that can expression PyMT. We propose that in AREG$^{+/+}$ PyMT mice, tumors are initiated at mature duct termini where myoepithelial coverage is lower, giving rise to the observed multifocal initiation. On the other hand, in the AREG$^{-/-}$ PyMT mice, both myoepithelial coverage and growth factor expression are reduced, leading to broader PyMT expression resulting in increased lesion formation throughout the ductal tree. As a result, AREG$^{-/-}$ tumors form a wider range of tumor morphologies, including less aggressive papillary and cystic structures.

Currently, treatment of breast cancer with receptor tyrosine kinase (RTK) inhibitors that target EGFR, such as gefitinib, has been met with mixed success [4–6].

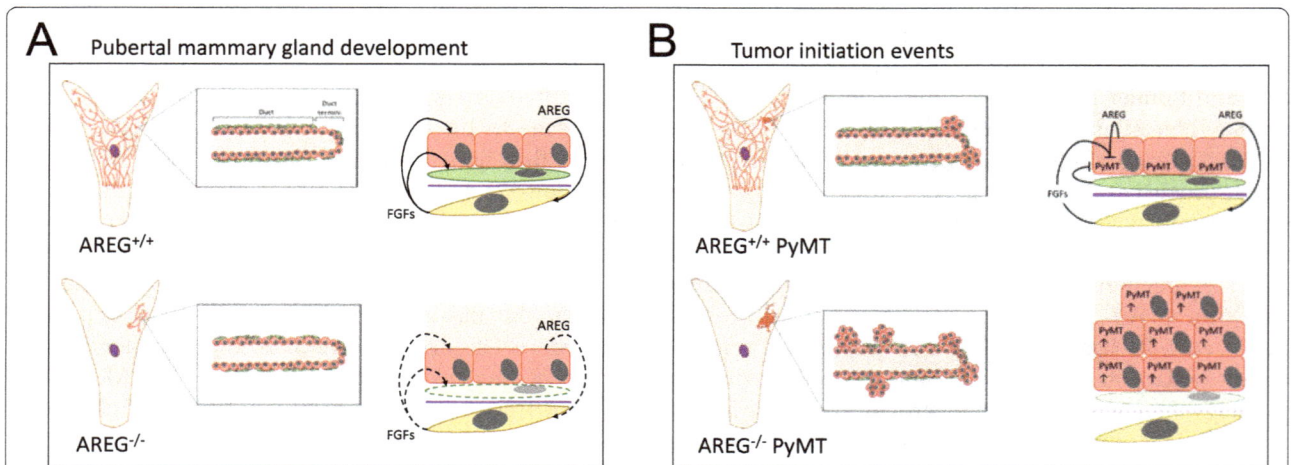

Fig. 8 Working model to explain increased tumor initiation and morphological changes in AREG$^{-/-}$ tumors. (**a**) In mammary duct in absence of PyMT (top), myoepithelial cells (green) form continuous layer around luminal epithelial cells. In mature duct termini, myoepithelial layer is discontinuous. Luminal epithelial cells secrete AREG that binds to EGFR on stromal cells (yellow). Stimulated stromal cells produce FGFR ligands that bind to FGFR luminal epithelial cells and myoepithelial cells [31, 56]. In absence of AREG (bottom), EGFR/FGFR paracrine loop is interrupted and impairs proper mammary ductal development. (**b**) In AREG$^{+/+}$ PyMT animals (top), PyMT initiates transformation of luminal epithelial cells in mature duct termini where there are fewer myoepithelial cells. Myoepithelial cells as well as secreted growth factors such as AREG and bFGF suppress PyMT expression in mammary duct. In AREG$^{-/-}$ PyMT mice (bottom), PyMT expression is more widespread. Due to global reduction in myoepithelial cells and reduced AREG and FGF expression, oncogenic transformation takes place more broadly in ductal tree. AREG amphiregulin, FGF basic fibroblast growth factor, PYMT polyoma middle-T antigen

Getfitnib treatment in patients with hormone receptor-positive or hormone receptor-negative metastatic breast cancer is associated with low clinical benefit rate (CBR). These treatments are also commonly associated with cutaneous, gastrointestinal, and hair-related toxicities [50, 51]. Therefore, EGFR-targeted therapies are not well tolerated and have low efficacy for some patients. AREG as a novel target for breast cancer therapy is attractive [52, 53], potentially reducing the side effects of broad EGFR inhibition while targeting breast tumor growth that is driven by AREG. One study using an antibody against AREG in ovarian cancer xenografts has successfully reduced tumor growth [54]. In our model, loss of AREG dramatically altered the histological morphology seen in late-stage tumors from a solid to a papillary structure. In human breast cancer, papillary carcinoma is associated with a higher survival rate than invasive ductal carcinoma [55]. AREG-targeted therapy could avoid negative side effects associated with broad EGFR inhibitors, but could also potentially direct tumor growth toward a less aggressive pattern.

Conclusions

Our studies demonstrate a novel role of AREG in myoepithelial cell coverage of mammary ducts during development. In the PyMT model of breast cancer, we have shown that myoepithelial cells and growth factors AREG, EGF, and bFGF suppress PyMT expression. These findings may explain the accelerated growth and progression of early-stage AREG$^{-/-}$ tumors in the MMTV-PyMT model. Interestingly, late-stage AREG$^{-/-}$ tumors are less proliferative and demonstrate increased areas of papillary and cystic features. In human breast cancer, luminal-B IPCs have lower AREG expression compared to IDCs. Together, our results provide new insight into the function of AREG in mammary gland biology, regulation of PyMT, and breast tumor growth.

Additional files

Additional file 1: Figure S1 Growth of AREG$^{+/+}$ PyMT and AREG$^{-/-}$ PyMT lesions. Volumes of palpable lesions that could be reproducibly detected in AREG$^{+/+}$ PyMT (**A**, $N = 32$) and AREG$^{-/-}$ PyMT (**B**, $N = 22$) mice were measured using a digital caliper. (**C**) Kaplan–Meier plot of percentage of mice with no palpable lesions. Statistical analysis performed using a log-rank test (PPTX 143 kb)

Additional file 2: Figure S2 Loss of AREG does not have a significant effect on tumor cell intravasation and metastasis. (**A**) Number of metastatic foci in lungs of AREG$^{+/+}$ PyMT ($N = 16$) and AREG$^{-/-}$ PyMT ($N = 9$) mice. (**B**) Total area of all metastatic foci in each lung calculated for AREG$^{+/+}$ PyMT ($N = 16$) and AREG$^{-/-}$ PyMT ($N = 9$) mice. (**C**) Blood collected from right atrium of AREG$^{+/+}$ PyMT ($N = 8$) and AREG$^{-/-}$ PyMT ($N = 8$) mice, and CTCs counted and number adjusted to 1 ml of blood. Statistical analysis performed using Mann–Whitney test. n.s. not significant (PPTX 124 kb)

Additional file 3: Figure S3 Cysts present in AREG$^{+/+}$ PyMT and AREG$^{-/-}$ PyMT tumors. H&E stains of AREG$^{+/+}$ PyMT and AREG$^{-/-}$ PyMT 1-cm tumors show presence of cysts. Scale bar shows 2000 μm (PPTX 2060 kb)

Additional file 4: Figure S4 Necrosis reduced in solid areas of AREG$^{-/-}$ PyMT tumors. Percentage necrosis in solid and papillary areas of AREG$^{+/+}$ PyMT ($N = 32$) and AREG$^{-/-}$ PyMT ($N = 22$) tumors assessed individually. Significant differences observed between solid areas of AREG$^{+/+}$ PyMT and AREG$^{-/-}$ PyMT tumors. In addition, papillary regions of both tumor genotypes have little to no necrosis. Statistical analysis performed using Mann–Whitney test. *$p < 0.05$, ***$p < 0.001$, ****$P < 0.0001$. n.s. not significant (PPTX 61 kb)

Additional file 5: Figure S5 Loss of AREG is associated with increased vascular density in late-stage mammary tumors. (**A**) Representative images of CD31 staining of AREG$^{+/+}$ PyMT and AREG$^{-/-}$ PyMT 1-cm tumors. (**B**) Compared to AREG$^{+/+}$ PyMT tumors, more CD31$^+$ vessels per field in AREG$^{-/-}$ PyMT tumors. Scale bar shows 100 μm. Statistical analyses performed using a t test. *$p < 0.05$, $N = 3$ (PPTX 182 kb)

Acknowledgements

The authors would like to thank the support and advice from present and past members of the Segall, Cox, Condeelis, and Hodgson laboratories. This work was facilitated by the use of the P250 high-capacity slide scanner that was purchased with funding from National Institutes of Health. The authors would also like to thank the Albert Einstein Cancer Center for assisting our work conducted through the Genomics and Flow Cytometry Core Facilities.

Funding

JES is the Betty and Sheldon Feinberg Senior Faculty Scholar in Cancer Research at the Albert Einstein College of Medicine. Funding was provided by National Institutes of Health grants CA100324 (JSC, JES), T32-GM007288 (SPHM, RMC), SIG grant 1S10OD019961-01, and the Albert Einstein Cancer Center (support grant P30CA013330). This work was also supported by the Integrated Imaging Program and the Gruss Lipper Biophotonics Center.

Authors' contributions

JES and SPHM provided the overall design of the experiments and writing of the manuscript, with SPHM contributing most of the experiments. MP contributed to the K14 analysis. RMC provided assistance with the in-vivo experiments. JRC and WG assisted with mammary epithelial cell isolation and FACS analysis. GSK and JSC helped with in-vivo transplant experiments. MHO performed early tumor staging and histological analysis of late-stage tumors. DMWZ provided the AREG$^{-/-}$ mice. SIA provided the AT-3 cell line. PAK provided intellectual discussion and ideas. All authors read and approved the final manuscript.

Competing interests

The authors declare that they have no competing interests.

Author details

^{1}Department of Anatomy and Structural Biology, Albert Einstein College of Medicine, 1301 Morris Park Avenue, Bronx, NY 10461, USA. ^{2}Department of Cell Biology, Albert Einstein College of Medicine, Bronx, NY 10461, USA. ^{3}Gruss Lipper Biophotonics Center, Albert Einstein College of Medicine, Bronx, NY 10461, USA. ^{4}Integrated Imaging Program, Albert Einstein College of Medicine, Bronx, NY 10461, USA. [5]Institute of Immunology and Infection Research, University of Edinburgh, Edinburgh, UK. [6]Department of Immunology, Roswell Park Comprehensive Cancer Center, Buffalo, NY 14263, USA. [7]Kabara Cancer Research Institute, Gundersen Medical Foundation, La Crosse, WI 54601, USA.

References

1. Siegel RL, Miller KD, Jemal A. Cancer statistics, 2018. CA Cancer J Clin. 2018; 68(1):7–30.
2. Sainsbury JR, et al. Epidermal-growth-factor receptor status as predictor of early recurrence of and death from breast cancer. Lancet. 1987;1(8547): 1398–402.
3. Masuda H, et al. Role of epidermal growth factor receptor in breast cancer. Breast Cancer Res Treat. 2012;136(2):331–45.
4. Butti R, et al. Receptor tyrosine kinases (RTKs) in breast cancer: signaling, therapeutic implications and challenges. Mol Cancer. 2018;17(1):34.
5. Green MD, et al. Gefitinib treatment in hormone-resistant and hormone receptor-negative advanced breast cancer. Ann Oncol. 2009;20(11):1813–7.
6. Osborne CK, et al. Gefitinib or placebo in combination with tamoxifen in patients with hormone receptor-positive metastatic breast cancer: a randomized phase II study. Clin Cancer Res. 2011;17(5):1147–59.
7. Peterson EA, et al. Amphiregulin Is a critical downstream effector of estrogen signaling in ERalpha-positive breast cancer. Cancer Res. 2015; 75(22):4830–8.
8. Willmarth NE, Ethier SP. Autocrine and juxtacrine effects of amphiregulin on the proliferative, invasive, and migratory properties of normal and neoplastic human mammary epithelial cells. J Biol Chem. 2006;281(49): 37728–37.
9. Willmarth NE, et al. Altered EGFR localization and degradation in human breast cancer cells with an amphiregulin/EGFR autocrine loop. Cell Signal. 2009;21(2):212–9.
10. Baillo A, Giroux C, Ethier SP. Knock-down of amphiregulin inhibits cellular invasion in inflammatory breast cancer. J Cell Physiol. 2011;226(10):2691–701.
11. Ciarloni L, Mallepell S, Brisken C. Amphiregulin is an essential mediator of estrogen receptor alpha function in mammary gland development. Proc Natl Acad Sci U S A. 2007;104(13):5455–60.
12. Sternlicht MD, Sunnarborg SW. The ADAM17-amphiregulin-EGFR axis in mammary development and cancer. J Mammary Gland Biol Neoplasia. 2008; 13(2):181–94.
13. Sternlicht MD, et al. Mammary ductal morphogenesis requires paracrine activation of stromal EGFR via ADAM17-dependent shedding of epithelial amphiregulin. Development. 2005;132(17):3923–33.
14. Pasic L, et al. Sustained activation of the HER1-ERK1/2-RSK signaling pathway controls myoepithelial cell fate in human mammary tissue. Genes Dev. 2011;25(15):1641–53.
15. Lin EY, et al. Progression to malignancy in the polyoma middle T oncoprotein mouse breast cancer model provides a reliable model for human diseases. Am J Pathol. 2003;163(5):2113–26.
16. Maglione JE, et al. Transgenic Polyoma middle-T mice model premalignant mammary disease. Cancer Res. 2001;61(22):8298–305.
17. Guy CT, et al. Activation of the c-Src tyrosine kinase is required for the induction of mammary tumors in transgenic mice. Genes Dev. 1994; 8(1):23–32.
18. Raptis L, et al. Cellular ras gene activity is required for full neoplastic transformation by polyomavirus. J Virol. 1991;65(10):5203–10.
19. Webster MA, et al. Requirement for both Shc and phosphatidylinositol 3′ kinase signaling pathways in polyomavirus middle T-mediated mammary tumorigenesis. Mol Cell Biol. 1998;18(4):2344–59.
20. Luetteke NC, et al. Targeted inactivation of the EGF and amphiregulin genes reveals distinct roles for EGF receptor ligands in mouse mammary gland development. Development. 1999;126(12):2739–50.
21. Wyckoff JB, et al. A critical step in metastasis: in vivo analysis of intravasation at the primary tumor. Cancer Res. 2000;60(9):2504–11.
22. Boimel PJ, et al. Contribution of CXCL12 secretion to invasion of breast cancer cells. Breast Cancer Res. 2012;14(1):R23.
23. Patsialou A, et al. Selective gene-expression profiling of migratory tumor cells in vivo predicts clinical outcome in breast cancer patients. Breast Cancer Res. 2012;14(5):R139.
24. Karagiannis GS, et al. Neoadjuvant chemotherapy induces breast cancer metastasis through a TMEM-mediated mechanism. Sci Transl Med. 2017;9(397).
25. Plante I, Stewart MK, Laird DW. Evaluation of mammary gland development and function in mouse models. J Vis Exp. 2011;(53).
26. Guo W, et al. Slug and Sox9 cooperatively determine the mammary stem cell state. Cell. 2012;148(5):1015–28.
27. Cerami E, et al. The cBio cancer genomics portal: an open platform for exploring multidimensional cancer genomics data. Cancer Discov. 2012; 2(5):401–4.
28. Gao J, et al. Integrative analysis of complex cancer genomics and clinical profiles using the cBioPortal. Sci Signal. 2013;6(269):pl1.
29. Sternlicht MD, et al. The human myoepithelial cell is a natural tumor suppressor. Clin Cancer Res. 1997;3(11):1949–58.
30. Stewart TJ, Abrams SI. Altered immune function during long-term host-tumor interactions can be modulated to retard autochthonous neoplastic growth. J Immunol. 2007;179(5):2851–9.
31. Koledova Z, et al. SPRY1 regulates mammary epithelial morphogenesis by modulating EGFR-dependent stromal paracrine signaling and ECM remodeling. Proc Natl Acad Sci U S A. 2016;113(39):E5731–40.
32. Pal SK, et al. Papillary carcinoma of the breast: an overview. Breast Cancer Res Treat. 2010;122(3):637–45.
33. Fenton BM, et al. Zonal image analysis of tumour vascular perfusion, hypoxia, and necrosis. Br J Cancer. 2002;86(11):1831–6.
34. Chung AS, Lee J, Ferrara N. Targeting the tumour vasculature: insights from physiological angiogenesis. Nat Rev Cancer. 2010;10(7):505–14.
35. Bordoli MR, et al. Prolyl-4-hydroxylase PHD2- and hypoxia-inducible factor 2-dependent regulation of amphiregulin contributes to breast tumorigenesis. Oncogene. 2011;30(5):548–60.
36. Hollern DP, Andrechek ER. A genomic analysis of mouse models of breast cancer reveals molecular features of mouse models and relationships to human breast cancer. Breast Cancer Res. 2014;16(3):R59.
37. Guy CT, Cardiff RD, Muller WJ. Induction of mammary tumors by expression of polyomavirus middle T oncogene: a transgenic mouse model for metastatic disease. Mol Cell Biol. 1992;12(3):954–61.
38. Yamamoto KR. Steroid receptor regulated transcription of specific genes and gene networks. Annu Rev Genet. 1985;19:209–52.
39. Buetti E, Diggelmann H. Glucocorticoid regulation of mouse mammary tumor virus: identification of a short essential DNA region. EMBO J. 1983; 2(8):1423–9.
40. Rao KV, Fox CF. Epidermal growth factor stimulates tyrosine phosphorylation of human glucocorticoid receptor in cultured cells. Biochem Biophys Res Commun. 1987;144(1):512–9.
41. Rao KV, Williams RE, Fox CF. Altered glucocorticoid binding and action in response to epidermal growth factor in HBL100 cells. Cancer Res. 1987; 47(22):5888–93.
42. Chandra A, et al. Epidermal growth factor receptor (EGFR) signaling promotes proliferation and survival in osteoprogenitors by increasing early growth response 2 (EGR2) expression. J Biol Chem. 2013;288(28):20488–98.
43. Leclerc N, et al. Gene expression profiling of glucocorticoid-inhibited osteoblasts. J Mol Endocrinol. 2004;33(1):175–93.
44. Visvader JE, Stingl J. Mammary stem cells and the differentiation hierarchy: current status and perspectives. Genes Dev. 2014;28(11):1143–58.
45. Farhanji B, et al. Tumor suppression effects of myoepithelial cells on mice breast cancer. Eur J Pharmacol. 2015;765:171–8.
46. Nguyen M, et al. The human myoepithelial cell displays a multifaceted anti-angiogenic phenotype. Oncogene. 2000;19(31):3449–59.
47. Deugnier MA, et al. The importance of being a myoepithelial cell. Breast Cancer Res. 2002;4(6):224–30.
48. Burdette JE, et al. Activin A mediates growth inhibition and cell cycle arrest through Smads in human breast cancer cells. Cancer Res. 2005;65(17):7968–75.
49. Cato AC, et al. The regulation of expression of mouse mammary tumor virus DNA by steroid hormones and growth factors. J Steroid Biochem. 1989;34(1–6):139–43.
50. Gutzmer R, et al. Cutaneous side effects of EGF-receptor inhibition and their management. Hautarzt. 2006;57(6):509–13.
51. Hartmann JT, et al. Tyrosine kinase inhibitors—a review on pharmacology, metabolism and side effects. Curr Drug Metab. 2009;10(5):470–81.
52. Willmarth NE, Ethier SP. Amphiregulin as a novel target for breast cancer therapy. J Mammary Gland Biol Neoplasia. 2008;13(2):171–9.
53. Xu Q, Chiao P, Sun Y. Amphiregulin in cancer: new insights for translational medicine. Trends Cancer. 2016;2(3):111–3.

54. Carvalho S, et al. An antibody to amphiregulin, an abundant growth factor in patients' fluids, inhibits ovarian tumors. Oncogene. 2016;35(4):438–47.

55. Zheng YZ, Hu X, Shao ZM. Clinicopathological characteristics and survival outcomes in invasive papillary carcinoma of the breast: a SEER population-based study. Sci Rep. 2016;6:24037.

56. Pond AC, et al. Fibroblast growth factor receptor signaling is essential for normal mammary gland development and stem cell function. Stem Cells. 2013;31(1):178–89.

20

Insulin-like growth factor receptor signaling in breast tumor epithelium protects cells from endoplasmic reticulum stress and regulates the tumor microenvironment

Alison E. Obr[1], Sushil Kumar[2], Yun-Juan Chang[3], Joseph J. Bulatowicz[1], Betsy J. Barnes[4], Raymond B. Birge[2], Deborah A. Lazzarino[2], Emily Gallagher[5], Derek LeRoith[5] and Teresa L. Wood[1]*[iD]

Abstract

Background: Early analyses of human breast cancer identified high expression of the insulin-like growth factor type 1 receptor (IGF-1R) correlated with hormone receptor positive breast cancer and associated with a favorable prognosis, whereas low expression of IGF-1R correlated with triple negative breast cancer (TNBC). We previously demonstrated that the IGF-1R acts as a tumor and metastasis suppressor in the Wnt1 mouse model of TNBC. The mechanisms for how reduced IGF-1R contributes to TNBC phenotypes is unknown.

Methods: We analyzed the METABRIC dataset to further stratify IGF-1R expression with patient survival and specific parameters of TNBC. To investigate molecular events associated with the loss of IGF-1R function in breast tumor cells, we inhibited IGF-1R in human cell lines using an IGF-1R blocking antibody and analyzed MMTV-Wnt1-mediated mouse tumors with reduced IGF-1R function through expression of a dominant-negative transgene.

Results: Our analysis of the Molecular Taxonomy of Breast Cancer International Consortium (METABRIC) dataset revealed association between low IGF-1R and reduced overall patient survival. IGF-1R expression was inversely correlated with patient survival even within hormone receptor-positive breast cancers, indicating reduced overall patient survival with low IGF-1R was not due simply to low IGF-1R expression within TNBCs. Inhibiting IGF-1R in either mouse or human tumor epithelial cells increased reactive oxygen species (ROS) production and activation of the endoplasmic reticulum stress response. IGF-1R inhibition in tumor epithelial cells elevated interleukin (IL)-6 and C-C motif chemokine ligand 2 (CCL2) expression, which was reversed by ROS scavenging. Moreover, the *Wnt1/dnIGF-1R* primary tumors displayed a tumor-promoting immune phenotype. The increased CCL2 promoted an influx of CD11b[+] monocytes into the primary tumor that also had increased matrix metalloproteinase (MMP)-2, MMP-3, and MMP-9 expression. Increased MMP activity in the tumor stroma was associated with enhanced matrix remodeling and collagen deposition. Further analysis of the METABRIC dataset revealed an increase in IL-6, CCL2, and MMP-9 expression in patients with low IGF-1R, consistent with our mouse tumor model and data in human breast cancer cell lines.

Conclusions: Our data support the hypothesis that reduction of IGF-1R function increases cellular stress and cytokine production to promote an aggressive tumor microenvironment through infiltration of immune cells and matrix remodeling.

Keywords: IGF-1R, IL-6, CCL2, Breast cancer, Wnt1, Cellular stress, MMP

* Correspondence: woodte@njms.rutgers.edu
[1]Department of Pharmacology, Physiology & Neuroscience, Rutgers-New Jersey
Medical School, Cancer Institute of New Jersey, Newark, NJ 07101, USA
Full list of author information is available at the end of the article

Background

Triple-negative breast cancers (TNBCs), classified as estrogen receptor (ER)-negative, progesterone receptor (PR)-negative and lacking human epidermal growth factor receptor 2 (HER2) amplification remain the most aggressive breast tumor subtype, and approximately 50% of TNBCs classify as basal-like [1]. While chemotherapy treatment for TNBC primary tumors is effective short-term, tumors ultimately recur and frequently metastasize [2, 3]. Hyperactivation of the Wnt pathway is common in breast carcinomas where it is often activated in the absence of downstream mutations [4], and Wnt1 overexpression in mammary epithelium is sufficient to form basal-like tumors in mice with low metastatic potential [5].

Signaling through the insulin-like growth factor type 1 receptor (IGF-1R) is complex, and defining its role in breast tumorigenesis has been controversial. Early studies reported that expression of the IGF-1R correlated with ER expression and predicted a favorable phenotype [6]. Numerous studies have further confirmed cross-talk between the ER and IGF-1R in breast cancer (for review, see [7]). Consistent with these data, loss of IGF-1R has been associated with breast tumor progression into a more undifferentiated phenotype [8], suggesting that IGF-1R is involved in tumor suppression. However, other findings have shown that IGF signaling is a positive mediator of breast cancer growth and survival (for reviews, see [9, 10]). Since IGF signaling promotes tumor cell proliferation and survival, various inhibitors have been developed to attenuate IGF signaling (for reviews, see [11, 12]). Despite early preclinical findings, the usefulness of disrupting IGF-1R signaling in clinical trials has been less than promising and, in some cases, inhibiting the pathway has led to worse outcomes [11, 12]. Collectively, these diverse results support the possibility that the IGF-1R has a dual function as both a tumor suppressor and an oncogene.

In our recent studies, we established a mouse line with transgenic expression of a kinase-dead, dominant-negative IGF-1R (*MMTV-dnIGF-1R*) in combination with *MMTV-Wnt1* expression to test how decreased IGF-1R signaling in the mammary epithelium impacts a well-established mouse model of basal-like breast cancer [5]. Attenuation of IGF-1R in this model resulted in decreased tumor latency, an enhanced basal phenotype, and potentiation of lung metastases (Additional file 1: Table S1, see also [1]). These results were surprising given that the *MMTV-Wnt1* tumors have low metastatic potential [5]. However, similar findings were reported from conditionally deleting IGF-1R in a prostate cancer mouse model [13]. These data are also consistent with new reports that have correlated high IGF-1R and ERα expression in luminal B breast tumors with a better prognosis [14]. Recent

queries of the Cancer Genome Atlas (TCGA) database for IGF-1R expression identified higher IGF-1R expression in luminal A and luminal B breast tumors and lower expression in HER2-like and triple-negative tumors [15]. Taken together, these data suggest the function of IGF-1R is dependent on the tumor type and signaling context.

Several studies have established that IGF signaling is important for maintaining cellular stress homeostasis such that modifications in IGF signaling result in alterations in stress signaling. Endoplasmic reticulum (EnR) stress is a consequence of increased misfolded proteins and results in the production of reactive oxygen species (ROS) and ultimately cell death (for reviews, see [16, 17]. Reduction-of-function mutations in the IGF signaling pathway in *Caenorhabditis elegans* result in activation of the unfolded protein response (UPR) leading to an enhanced EnR stress response [18]. Furthermore, activation of IGF-1 signaling in breast cancer and neuronal cells protects from EnR-stress-induced apoptosis by enhancing EnR stress responses to promote cellular adaptability for cell survival maintenance [19, 20]. Moreover, the inhibition of IGF signaling in breast cancer cells results in activation of EnR stress to induce autophagy and protect from apoptosis [21]. These results suggest the IGF pathway protects cells from EnR stress, and that perturbation of the IGF pathway leads to enhanced overall EnR stress.

In the present study, we tested the hypothesis that attenuated IGF-1R function promotes tumor epithelial cell stress resulting in tumor stromal environment alterations to establish an aggressive phenotype in breast tumors. We determined that IGF-1R is essential in tumor suppression in breast tumorigenesis. We demonstrate that attenuated IGF-1R signaling in the *MMTV-Wnt1* mouse mammary tumor model and in human breast cancer cell lines increases tumor epithelial cellular stress, resulting in upregulation of cytokine production. These changes result in altered migration and infiltration of tumor immune cells and dramatic alterations in the tumor microenvironment associated with promoting primary tumor epithelial cell extravasation.

Methods
Antibodies and reagents
Rabbit monoclonal anti-phospho-eIF2a (D9G8), rabbit monoclonal anti-eukaryotic initiation factor 2-alpha (eIF2a) (D7D3), rabbit monoclonal anti-protein disulfide isomerase (PDI) (C81H6), mouse monoclonal anti-C/EBP homologous protein (CHOP) (L63F7), rabbit monoclonal anti-phospho-Akt (Ser473) (D9E), rabbit monoclonal anti-Akt (11E7), rabbit monoclonal anti-phospho-IGF-1R/IR (D6D5L), and rabbit monoclonal anti-IGF-1R (D23H3) antibodies were purchased from Cell Signaling. Rabbit polyclonal anti-matrix metalloproteinase (MMP)-2 (ab37150) and anti-MMP-9 (ab38898) antibodies were

purchased from Abcam. Mouse monoclonal anti-β-actin (A5441) was purchased from Sigma Aldrich. IMC-A12 (10 mg/ml), a monoclonal antibody against IGF-1R, was provided by ImClone Systems, a wholly owned subsidiary of Eli Lilly and Co. Human IgG antibody (31154; 11.3 mg/ml), a monoclonal antibody used as a control, was purchased from Invitrogen. N-acetyl-L-cysteine (A9165) was purchased from Sigma Aldrich.

Animal models

All animal protocols were approved by the Rutgers University Institutional Animal Care and Use Committee (Newark, NJ, USA). All experiments were managed in accord with the National Institutes of Health (NIH) guidelines for the care and use of laboratory animals. The *MMTV-Wnt1* line on an FVB background (FVB.Cg-Tg(Wnt1)1Hev/J) was obtained as a gift from Dr Yi Li. The *MMTV-Wnt1//MMTV-dnIgf1r* line was described previously [1]. Female littermates (*MMTV-Wnt1/dnIGF-1R*; homozygous for *dnIGF-1R* versus *MMTV-Wnt1*) were used for experiments. Tumors were harvested when they reached 1.5 cm^3.

Cell lines

The human MCF7 breast cancer cell line was provided by Dr Robert Wieder (Rutgers University-NJMS) and validated with the human short tandem repeat (STR) profiling cell authentication service (American Type Culture Collection (ATCC)). The RAW264.7 mouse monocyte cell line was purchased from ATCC. All cells were maintained at 37 °C and 5% CO_2 and in either MEM (MCF7) or DMEM (RAW264.7) medium supplemented with 10% FBS (Sigma Aldrich) and 100 U/ml of penicillin and streptomycin.

Detection of reactive oxygen species and cellular stress

Fresh tumors were drop-fixed in methacarn (60% methanol, 30% chloroform, 10% glacial ascetic acid) overnight at 4 °C, embedded in paraffin, and sectioned at 7 μm. Tumor sections were processed for OxyIHC™ with antigen retrieval, chemical derivatization of protein carbonyl groups with 2,4-dinitrophenylhydrazine (DNPH), and incubation with dinitrophenyl (DNP) moiety-specific primary antibody (1:100) overnight at 4 °C according to the manufacturer's protocol (Millipore, S7450). Negative controls for each tumor section were processed without primary antibody and with derivatization control solution. Positive detection of protein oxidation was obtained using 3,3′ diaminobenzidine (DAB) and counterstained with hematoxylin.

MCF7 cells were stained with 2′,7′-dichlorofluorescin diacetate (DCFDA) reagent (20 μM, Abcam) according to the manufacturer's protocol, washed, and treated with human IgG or IMC-A12 (100 nM) at varying time points in 1X Supplemental Buffer. MCF7 cells were treated with Tert-Butyl Hydrogen Peroxide (TBHP) (100 μM) for 4 h

as a positive control. DCFDA levels were measured with the Perkin Elmer Victory3V plate reader using the Excitation 485/Emission 535 filter.

To inhibit ROS production, MCF7 cells were treated with N-acetyl cysteine (NAC, 5 mM) for 1 h before treatment with either human IgG or A12 (100 nM). Cells were harvested after 24 h in TRI Reagent (Sigma Aldrich) for RNA isolation and qRT-PCR analysis.

Protein isolation, immunoblotting, and ELISA detection

Snap-frozen tumor pieces were pulverized using liquid nitrogen. Pulverized tumor pieces and cells from cell lines were lysed with radioimmunoprecipitation assay (RIPA) buffer. Lysates containing equal amounts of total protein were boiled in 2X Laemmli buffer (BioRad) and electrophoresed on 4–12% polyacrylamide sodium dodecyl sulfate (SDS) gels (Invitrogen). Separated proteins were transferred to nitrocellulose membranes, incubated with anti-phospho-eIF2a (1:1000), anti-eIF2a (1:1000), and anti-ß-actin (1:5000) for cell-line lysates or anti-CHOP (1:1000), anti-PDI (1:1000), and anti-ß-actin (1:5000) for whole-tumor lysates, and antibody binding to protein bands was detected by enhanced chemiluminescence (Amersham).

Whole tumor lysates in RIPA buffer were incubated with the human IL-6 Quantikine ELISA kit (R&D Systems) according to the manufacturer's protocol. Levels of IL-6 were detected using the Perkin Elmer Victory3V plate reader at an absorbance of 450 nm.

RNA isolation and quantitative real-time PCR by targeted pathway arrays

Whole tumor RNA was extracted using TRI Reagent (Sigma Aldrich) according to manufacturer's protocol. For the cytokine/chemokine targeted array provided by Dr Sophia Ran, RNA from five tumors was reverse transcribed separately and the cytokine/chemokine array was performed and analyzed using the ΔΔ cycle threshold (Ct) method as previously described [22] to determine expression of *MMTV-Wnt1/dnIGF-1R* compared to *MMTV-Wnt1* tumors by fold change. For the Wnt signaling pathway targeted array (Qiagen RT^2 Profiler Array, PAMM-043Z), 1 μg of RNA from five tumors was pooled and reverse transcribed using the RT2 easy first strand synthesis kit (Qiagen) per manufacturer's protocol. The array was performed using the BioRad CFX96 real-time PCR machine and the RT2 SYBR Green qPCR mastermix (Qiagen) per manufacturer's protocol. Analysis was performed using the ΔΔCt method with the RT^2 Profiler PCR Array Data Analysis Suite (Qiagen).

Analysis of tumor immune cells by flow cytometry

Tumor immune cells isolated as described above were resuspended at 10^6 cells/100 μl in FACS buffer (2% BSA, 2% goat serum in PBS). Cells were immunolabeled with the following fluorochrome-conjugated cell surface antibodies: anti-CD45 PE/Cy5 (0.25 μg/100 μl), anti-CD11b PerCP (0.25 μg/100 μl), anti-CD4 FITC (0.25 μg/100 μl), anti-CD8 PE (0.25 μg/100 μl), anti-CD25 PE/Cy7 (0.5 μg/100 μl), and anti-FOXP3 Alexa Fluor 647 (5 μl/100 μl) all purchased from BioLegend. Single cells were prepared for flow cytometry as previously described [23] or according to the manufacturer's protocol (BioLegend, for FOXP3). Cell-associated fluorescence was acquired and analyzed using the BD LSR II cytometer and TreeStar Inc. FlowJo software, respectively.

Mammary epithelial cell dissociation for flow sorting and flow cytometry

Mammary tumor epithelial cells (MECs) were isolated from MMTV-Wnt1 or MMTV-Wnt1/dnIGF-1R mice similarly to our prior study [1]. Whole tumors were excised and dissociated with the gentleMACs tissue dissociator (130–093-235, protocol m_TDK2) and mouse specific tumor dissociation kit (Miltenyi, 130–096-730). Organoids that retain basement membrane attachments were trypsinized (0.05% Trypsin-EDTA, Gibco) and filtered with a 40-μm cell strainer (BD Biosciences) to isolate a single cell suspension of dissociated tumor MECs. Isolated tumor MECs were counted using a hemocytometer prior to flow cytometry or sorting.

Mammary tumor immune cells were isolated from tumors as described previously [23]. Whole tumors were excised, minced, and digested with Collagenase-I (10 U/ml), Collagenase-IV (400 U/ml; Worthington), and DNase-1 (30 mg/ml; Sigma Aldrich) for 25 min at 37 °C. Cells from digested tumors were filtered with a 70-μm cell strainer (BD Biosciences) and pelleted. Red blood cells were lysed with an erythrocyte lysis buffer (150 mM Ammonium chloride, 1 mM Potassium bicarbonate, 130 μM EDTA, pH 7.2) for 2 min, filtered with a 70-μm cell strainer (BD Biosciences) and pelleted. Isolated immune cells were counted using a hemocytometer prior to flow cytometry or magnetic bead sorting.

Sorting of mammary tumor epithelial and immune cells

Tumor MECs from either MMTV-Wnt1 or MMTV-Wnt1/dnIGF-1R mice (n = 5) were isolated for single cells as described above and resuspended at 10⁶ cells/ml in FACS buffer (2% BSA, 2% goat serum in PBS). Cells were immunolabeled with fluorochrome-conjugated cell surface antibodies as described in our previous studies [1]. Single cells were prepared for FACS as previously described [24] and sorted at 70 psi using a 70-um nozzle on the Beckton Dickenson FACS Vantage directly into RLT Buffer (Qiagen, 79216) for RNA isolation and qRT-PCR analysis.

Tumor immune cells from individual tumors (n = 4 per genotype) were isolated for single cells as described above and resuspended at 10⁷ cells in MACS BSA Stock Solution according to the manufacturer's protocol (Miltenyi,

130–091-376). Cells were immunolabeled with rat monoclonal anti-CD11b antibody conjugated to magnetic microbeads (Miltenyi, 130–049-601). Immuno-labeled cells were run through a magnetic column according to the manufacturer's protocol (Miltenyi); both CD11b negative and positive flow-through were collected. Cells were resuspended in RLT Buffer (Qiagen) for RNA isolation and qRT-PCR analysis.

RNA isolation and real-time quantitative PCR

For sorted tumor epithelial and immune cells, RNA was extracted and purified according to the manufacturer's protocol (Qiagen). Whole tumor and human cell line RNA was extracted using TRI Reagent (Sigma Aldrich) according to the manufacturer's protocol. RNA concentration and quality were assayed by absorbance (A_{230}, A_{260}, A_{280}) with the NanoDrop ND-1000 (Thermo Scientific). Complementary DNA (cDNA) was transcribed according to the manufacturer's protocol using SuperScript II (Invitrogen) from total RNA (200 ng sorted cells, 1000 ng whole tumor and cell lines). Samples were run in technical triplicate to determine relative gene expression by real-time quantitative PCR (qRT-PCR) detected with SsoAdvanced Universal SYBR Green Supermix (BioRad) using the BioRad CFX96 real-time PCR machine according to the manufacturer's instructions. Transcript levels were normalized to glyceraldehyde-3-phosphate dehydrogenase (GAPDH, for mouse) or ß-actin (for human), and data were analyzed using the Q-Gene software (BioTechniques Software Library) [25]. Primer oligonucleotide pairs for qRT-PCR are provided in Additional file 2: Table S2.

Knockdown of IL-6 and CCL2 expression by small interfering RNA (siRNA)

SMARTpool ON-TARGET plus siRNA for IL-6 (L-043739-00-005) and CCL2 (L-042243-00-0005) and for scramble siGENOME Control Pool Non-Targeting #2 (Scr, D-001206-14-05) were resuspended (5 μM) using 1X siRNA buffer as described by the manufacturer's protocol (Dharmacon). MCF7 cells treated with human IgG or IMC-A12 (100 nM) for 24 h were transfected with Scr, IL-6, or CCL2 siRNA (25 ng) using transfection reagent DharmaFECT 1 per manufacturer's protocol (Dharmacon). Cells were harvested after 24 h with Accutase (Sigma Aldrich) for monocyte migration assays or in TRI Reagent (Sigma Aldrich) for RNA isolation and qRT-PCR analysis.

Measurement of monocyte migration in real time

Cell migration of a monocyte cell line (RAW264.7) was performed using a real-time, label-free monitoring system (xCELLigence RTCA DP, Acea Biologicals) that measures micro-impedance of electrical current. MCF7 cells were seeded in the lower chamber of a CIM-16 plate (Acea Biologicals) at 20,000 cells/180 μl in MEM supplemented with 10% FBS and treated with human IgG or IMC-A12 (100 nM) for 24 h. RAW264.7 monocytes were serum-starved (DMEM supplemented with 0.1% FBS) overnight and seeded in the CIM-16 plate upper chamber at 40,000 cells/100 μl after a medium-only baseline reading was taken. The migration rate is plotted as delta cell index (electrical impendence change) over 48 h (data point every 10 min).

MCF7 cells treated with human IgG or IMC-A12 (100 nM) for 24 h and transfected with siScr control, siIL-6, or siCCL2 and seeded in the lower chamber of a CIM-16 plate (Acea Biosciences) as described above. Serum-starved (DMEM supplemented with 0.1% FBS overnight) RAW264.7 monocytes were seeded in the CIM-16 plate upper chamber and a baseline reading was taken as described above. The impedance data were acquired and plotted as described above.

Histology and immunofluorescence

Tumor tissues ($n = 4$ per genotype) were drop-fixed in 4% paraformaldehyde (PFA), embedded in paraffin, and sectioned at 7 μm. Tumor sections were used for hematoxylin and eosin or Masson's Trichrome staining, or further processed for antigen retrieval for immunofluorescence (IF) as described previously [26]. Masson's Trichrome staining was performed according to the manufacturer's protocol (Abcam). Tissue sections were immunostained with primary antibodies - MMP-2 (1:50) or MMP-9 (1:50) - and with species-specific fluorochrome-conjugated secondary antibodies (1:500, Invitrogen). All IF sections were stained with 4',6-diamidino-2-phenylindole (DAPI) (1:10,000) to visualize cell nuclei.

Tissue *in situ* zymography

In situ zymography was performed as described previously [27]. Tumor tissues ($n = 4$ per genotype) were drop-fixed in IHC Zinc Fixative (BD Pharmingen) for 24 h at 4 °C, embedded in paraffin, and sectioned at 8 μm. The DQ gelatin substrate (Invitrogen) was incubated with tissue sections as previously described [27].

Image capture

An Olympus Provis AX70 brightfield/fluorescent microscope attached to the QIClick QImaging camera with iVision Mac scientific imaging processing software (4.0.16, BioVision Technologies) was used to capture images from histological and immunofluorescence staining. At least five individual fields were captured from tumor sections at × 10 or × 20 magnification ($n = 4$ per genotype).

Molecular Taxonomy of Breast Cancer International Consortium (METABRIC) dataset analysis

METABRIC data [28] downloaded from cBioPortal [29, 30] were used for the analysis, with expression values and associated clinical data generated from 1982 patients. The z scores comprised 299 patients with TNBC and 990 patients with ER+/PR+ breast cancer. Gene expression levels in individual patients were identified from the METABRIC dataset using the z scores identified from cBioPortal. Selected gene expression values of patients with TNBC or ER+/PR+ cancer, and different prediction analysis of microarray 50 (PAM50) identified subtypes were analyzed using the independent two-sample t test. Logistic regression was used to examine the distribution of expression values between each cancer type group and to estimate the probability of one subtype versus another subtype based on observed expression values. The Kaplan–Meier survival curve generated from the METABRIC dataset was plotted using the Package "survival" within the R environment. The log-rank test was performed to test the statistical difference between survival functions of the sub-grouped patients. All these calculations were conducted within the R environment, R version 3.3.2.

Statistics

All graphical data were expressed as the mean ± SEM. Statistical comparisons were carried out using GraphPad Prism6 software. Student's t test was used for two-group comparisons. One-way analysis of variance (ANOVA) with Bonferroni's post-hoc test was used for multiple treatment comparisons. Specific comparisons are described in the figure legends when necessary. Power calculations were performed based on pilot data to determine the number of tumor samples necessary. For immune flow cytometry, a standard deviation of 27% and an approximate normal distribution of the data were assumed. Using the two-sample, two-sided t test to detect a significant difference with $\alpha = 0.025$ and 80% power, suggested nine animals per group were needed. For qRT-PCR, a two-sided hypothesis test and $\alpha = 0.0025$ and 80% power, indicated four animals per group for detectable differences.

Results

Low IGF-1R expression is associated with triple-negative, basal-like breast cancer and reduced overall survival

Recent analysis of TCGA database for IGF-1R expression demonstrated IGF-1R expression levels are reduced in TNBC [15]. To further stratify the expression level of IGF-1R in breast cancers, we queried the METABRIC dataset that includes a larger patient sample size. Similar to Farabaugh et al. [15], IGF-1R expression was significantly lower in TNBC compared to ER+/PR+ breast cancer (Fig. 1a). Moreover, IGF-1R expression was lower in poorly differentiated, more aggressive basal-like breast cancers compared to the differentiated luminal A and luminal B subtypes as defined by PAM50 analysis (Fig. 1b). Importantly, analysis from the METABRIC dataset of patient overall survival in both ER+/PR+ breast cancer and

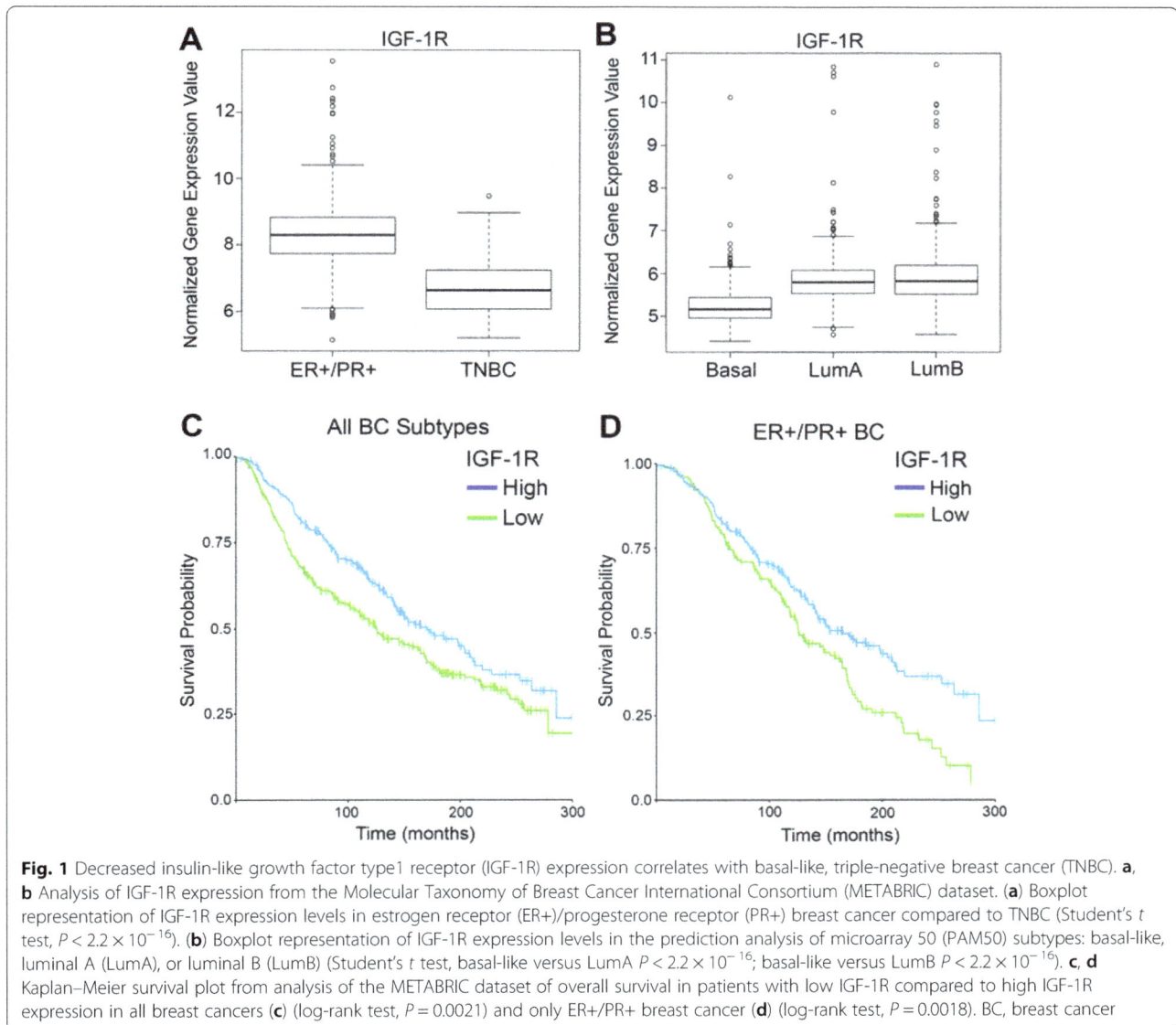

Fig. 1 Decreased insulin-like growth factor type1 receptor (IGF-1R) expression correlates with basal-like, triple-negative breast cancer (TNBC). **a**, **b** Analysis of IGF-1R expression from the Molecular Taxonomy of Breast Cancer International Consortium (METABRIC) dataset. (**a**) Boxplot representation of IGF-1R expression levels in estrogen receptor (ER+)/progesterone receptor (PR+) breast cancer compared to TNBC (Student's t test, $P < 2.2 \times 10^{-16}$). (**b**) Boxplot representation of IGF-1R expression levels in the prediction analysis of microarray 50 (PAM50) subtypes: basal-like, luminal A (LumA), or luminal B (LumB) (Student's t test, basal-like versus LumA $P < 2.2 \times 10^{-16}$; basal-like versus LumB $P < 2.2 \times 10^{-16}$). **c**, **d** Kaplan–Meier survival plot from analysis of the METABRIC dataset of overall survival in patients with low IGF-1R compared to high IGF-1R expression in all breast cancers (**c**) (log-rank test, $P = 0.0021$) and only ER+/PR+ breast cancer (**d**) (log-rank test, $P = 0.0018$). BC, breast cancer

TNBC revealed low expression of IGF-1R significantly correlates with worse overall survival compared to high expression of IGF-1R (Fig. 1c). Further stratification of ER+/PR+ patients confirmed worse overall survival correlates with low IGF-1R compared to high IGF-1R expression, even within this breast cancer subtype (Fig. 1d). Taken together, these data support the hypothesis that IGF-1R functions as a tumor suppressor in human breast cancer, and that reduced IGF-1R expression is detrimental to patient outcome.

Tumor epithelial cell stress is activated by loss of IGF signaling

The IGF signaling pathway plays an important role in maintaining cellular stress homeostasis for cell proliferation and survival [19, 31, 32]. Previous studies from

Novosyadlyy, et al. [19] established that activation of the IGF signaling pathway maintains EnR stress homeostasis by augmenting the adaptive capacity of the EnR and protecting against EnR-stress-induced apoptosis in MCF7 cells. Previous studies demonstrated activation of EnR stress signaling by increased generation of reactive oxygen species (ROS), which can be produced directly from the EnR through protein disulfide isomerase (PDI) [17]. Based on these and other studies linking EnR stress with tumorigenesis [18, 21, 33], we tested whether loss of IGF signaling in tumor epithelium increases EnR stress in breast tumor epithelial cells. Accumulation of ROS results in the addition of carboxyl groups to newly translated proteins [34]. We detected increased immunostaining for carboxyl groups in *MMTV-Wnt1/dnIGF-1R* compared to *MMTV-Wnt1* tumors (Fig. 2a–c). We further measured

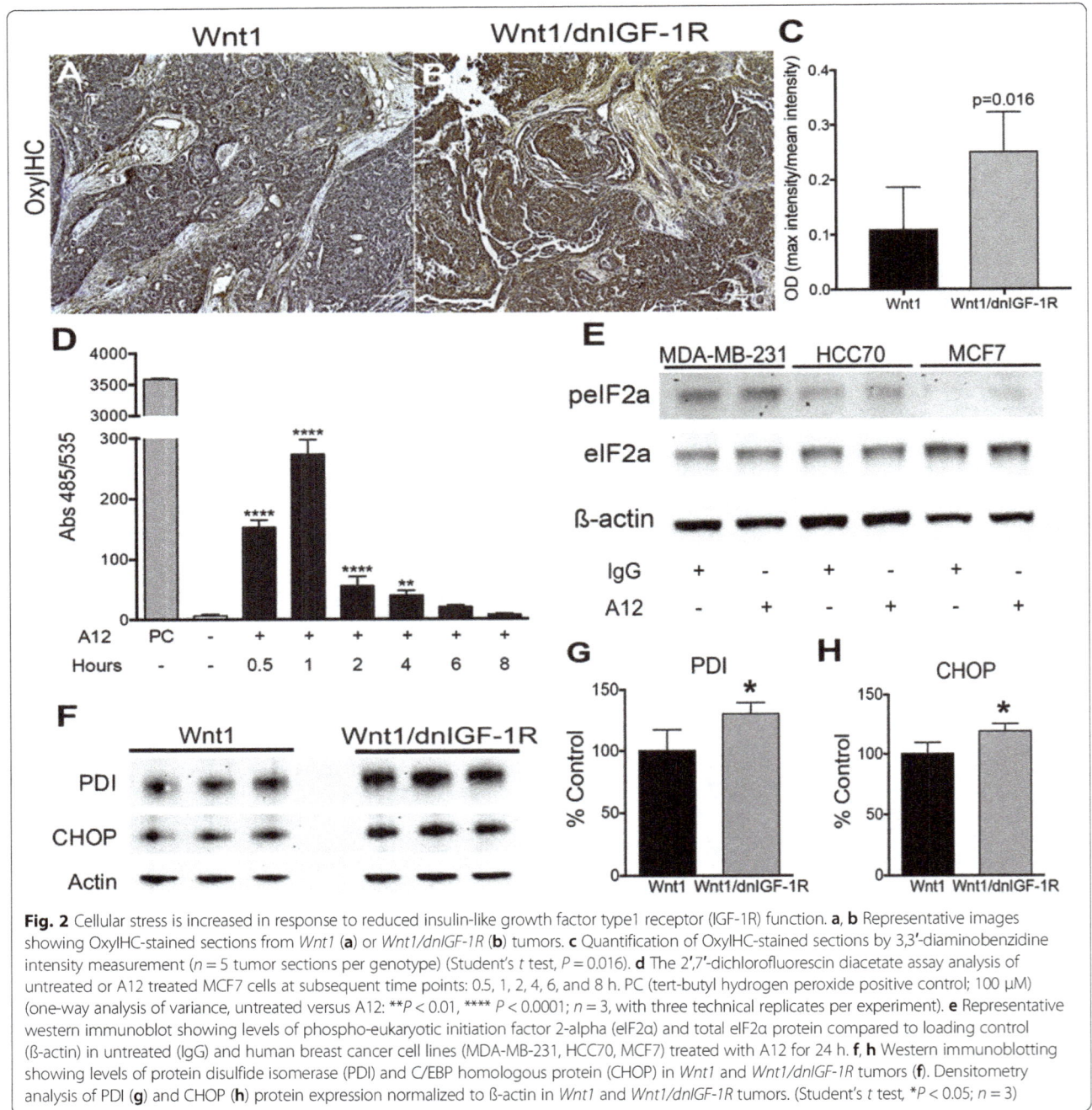

Fig. 2 Cellular stress is increased in response to reduced insulin-like growth factor type1 receptor (IGF-1R) function. **a, b** Representative images showing OxyIHC-stained sections from *Wnt1* (**a**) or *Wnt1/dnIGF-1R* (**b**) tumors. **c** Quantification of OxyIHC-stained sections by 3,3'-diaminobenzidine intensity measurement ($n = 5$ tumor sections per genotype) (Student's t test, $P = 0.016$). **d** The 2',7'-dichlorofluorescin diacetate assay analysis of untreated or A12 treated MCF7 cells at subsequent time points: 0.5, 1, 2, 4, 6, and 8 h. PC (tert-butyl hydrogen peroxide positive control; 100 µM) (one-way analysis of variance, untreated versus A12: **$P < 0.01$, **** $P < 0.0001$; $n = 3$, with three technical replicates per experiment). **e** Representative western immunoblot showing levels of phospho-eukaryotic initiation factor 2-alpha (eIF2α) and total eIF2α protein compared to loading control (ß-actin) in untreated (IgG) and human breast cancer cell lines (MDA-MB-231, HCC70, MCF7) treated with A12 for 24 h. **f, h** Western immunoblotting showing levels of protein disulfide isomerase (PDI) and C/EBP homologous protein (CHOP) in *Wnt1* and *Wnt1/dnIGF-1R* tumors (**f**). Densitometry analysis of PDI (**g**) and CHOP (**h**) protein expression normalized to ß-actin in *Wnt1* and *Wnt1/dnIGF-1R* tumors. (Student's t test, *$P < 0.05$; $n = 3$)

changes in ROS production with the DCFDA assay in MCF7 cells and observed increased fluorescence from 30 min to 4 h after IGF-1R inhibition with an IGF-1R blocking antibody, IMC-A12 (A12) (Fig. 2d). MCF7, a luminal human breast cancer cell line, has high levels of IGF-1R whereas HCC70, a basal-like breast cancer cell line, has intermediate levels of IGF-1R, and MDA-MB-231, a mesenchymal-like TNBC line, has low levels of IGF-1R relative to each other [35, 36]. Blocking IGF-1R in MCF7 cells with a monoclonal inhibiting antibody (A12) results in

reduced Akt and IGF-1R phosphorylation after IGF-1 treatment as well as reduced total IGF-1R as expected due to receptor internalization and degradation (Additional file 3: Figure S1) [37]. Phosphorylation of eIF2α, a downstream effector of the EnR stress response, was increased in human breast cancer cell lines, HCC70 and MCF7, but not MDA-MB-231 after IGF-1R inhibition (Fig. 2e), while total eIF2α was unchanged, suggesting inhibition of IGF signaling activates EnR stress signaling in breast cell lines with low basal EnR stress. Moreover, PDI and CHOP, downstream targets of eIF2α activation, were increased in *MMTV-Wnt1/dnIGF-1R* tumors (Fig. 2f-h). Taken together, these data demonstrate that reduction of IGF signaling in tumor epithelial cells both in vivo and in vitro results in enhanced cellular stress through production of ROS and activation of the EnR stress pathway.

Cellular stress with reduced IGF-1R signaling induces cytokine and chemokine expression

Activation of cellular stress results in an epithelial inflammatory response by production of cytokines and chemokines [38, 39]. Thus, we measured cytokine and chemokine gene expression in our mouse tumors with reduced IGF-1R activity by employing a targeted qRT-PCR array specifically designed for known altered cytokines and chemokines in solid tumors [22]. By measuring expression in the whole tumor, we found alterations in 20 cytokines and chemokines in *MMTV-Wnt1/dnIGF-1R* compared to *MMTV-Wnt1* tumors (Additional file 4: Table S3). Specifically, we observed an increase in C-C motif chemokine ligand 2 (CCL2), interleukin-10 (IL-10), and interleukin-6 (IL-6) whereas tumor necrosis factor-alpha (TNF-α) was decreased in *MMTV-Wnt1/dnIGF-1R* tumors (Fig. 3a). Alterations in these cytokines/chemokines suggest a tumor-promoting immune cell microenvironment [40, 41].

Previous studies have shown IL-6 is expressed in tumor epithelial cells resulting in tumor cell growth [42]. We investigated whether the loss of IGF-1R function altered IL-6 expression in the tumor epithelial cell population by measuring IL-6 expression in the CD24⁺/CD29^lo (luminal) and CD24⁺/CD29^hi (basal) cell populations. Interestingly, IL-6 messenger RNA (mRNA) expression was significantly increased in both CD24⁺/CD29^lo and CD24⁺/CD29^hi epithelial cells (Fig. 3b). Furthermore, previous studies have shown both IL-6 and CCL2 are expressed in human breast cancer cell lines and enhance tumor growth, migration, and immune cell recruitment [43, 44]. MCF7 cells with IGF-1R inhibition had increased IL-6 and CCL2 gene expression (Fig. 3c) and IL-6 protein expression (Additional file 5: Figure S2), further supporting the conclusion that attenuation of IGF-1R increases epithelial specific cytokine and chemokine expression.

We further tested whether increased IL-6 and CCL2 expression in tumor epithelial cells is a direct result of increased cellular stress in response to IGF-1R inhibition. To demonstrate that increased cellular stress activated through the loss of IGF-1R directly results in altered IL-6 and CCL2 expression, we blocked ROS production using a ROS scavenger, N-acetyl-L-cysteine (NAC) in MCF7 cells treated with the IGF-1R blocking antibody. Scavenging of ROS by NAC resulted in

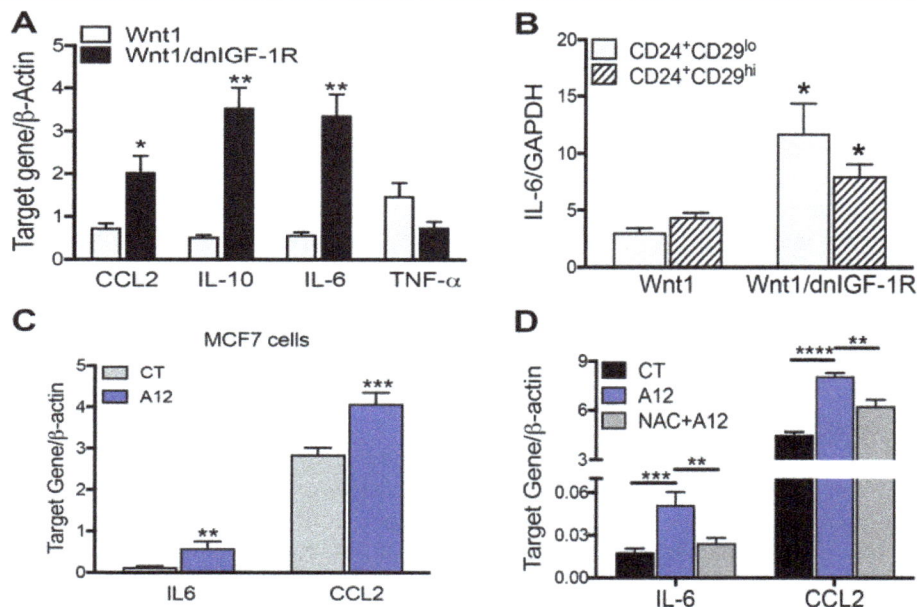

Fig. 3 Reduced insulin-like growth factor type1 receptor (IGF-1R) alters cytokine and chemokine production in tumor epithelia. **a** RT-PCR analysis of CCL2, IL-10, IL-6, and TNF-α in *Wnt1/dnIGF-1R* versus *Wnt1* tumors (Student's *t* test *$P < 0.05$, **$P < 0.01$; $n = 5$). **b** RT-PCR analysis of IL-6 in CD24⁺CD29^lo, Lin⁻ (CD45, CD31, Gr-1, Ter-119) luminal cells and CD24⁺CD29^hi, Lin⁻ (CD45, CD31, Gr-1, Ter-119) basal cells from *Wnt1/dnIGF-1R* versus *Wnt1* tumors (Student's *t* test *$P < 0.05$; $n = 4$, 3 technical replicates per sample). **c** RT-PCR analysis of IL-6 and CCL2 in human IgG (IgG) or IMC-A12 (A12) treated MCF7 cells (Student's *t* test **$P < 0.01$, ***$P < 0.001$; $n = 3$, with three biological replicates per experiment). **d** RT-PCR analysis of IL-6 and CCL2 in MCF7 cells treated with IgG, A12, or A12 + N-acetyl-L-cysteine (NAC) (one-way analysis of variance compared to A12, **$P < 0.01$, ***$P < 0.001$, ****$P < 0.0001$; $n = 3$, with three biological replicates per experiment)

decreased IL-6 and CCL2 gene expression (Fig. 3d) suggesting direct regulation of cytokine production through cellular stress activation driven by attenuated IGF-1R function.

Attenuated IGF-1R enhances tumor immune cell invasion

Alterations in cytokine and chemokine production in the tumor epithelium as a result of attenuated IGF-1R signaling suggests changes in immune cell recruitment to the primary tumor. The immune microenvironment is a major component of the primary tumor critical for maintaining either a tumorigenic or tumor cytotoxic environment dependent on the primary tumor immune cell profile and cytokine/chemokine production [45, 46]. Immune cell profiling by flow cytometry revealed an increase in total leukocytes stained for CD45 (Fig. 4a, b) in *MMTV-Wnt1/ dnIGF-1R* compared to *MMTV-Wnt1* tumors. Surprisingly, helper/regulatory CD4$^+$ T cells (CD4$^+$, CD45$^+$), known to promote tumor growth, were unchanged (Fig. 4c, d), and additional flow cytometry analysis by CD25 and FOXP3 staining showed no change in regulatory T cells (Additional file 6: Figure S3). Cytotoxic T cells (CD8$^+$, CD45$^+$), however, were significantly decreased in *MMTV-Wnt1/ dnIGF-1R* tumors (Fig. 4e, f) suggesting a reduced tumor cytotoxic immune microenvironment. We also observed an increase in CD11b$^+$, CD45$^+$ monocytes (Fig. 4g, h) in *MMTV-Wnt1/dnIGF-1R* tumors indicating an influx of immune cells with potential to differentiate into tumor-associated macrophages (TAMs). Taken together, these data indicate that reduced epithelial IGF-1R function in *MMTV-Wnt1* tumors results in an influx of immune cells that enhance tumor growth and contribute to an aggressive tumor microenvironment.

Production of IL-6/CCL2 due to attenuation of IGF-1R promotes tumor monocyte migration

To test whether attenuated IGF-1R function in human breast tumor cells directly alters the recruitment of monocytes, we modeled migration in vitro with the xCELLigence RTCA DP real-time migration assay using the MCF7 breast cancer cell line. RAW264.7 monocyte migration increased towards MCF7 cells treated with A12, compared to the control-untreated or IgG-antibody-treated MCF7 cells (Fig. 5a, b). Prior studies demonstrated production of CCL2 and IL-6 in breast epithelial cells is responsible for monocyte recruitment to solid tumors [47, 48]. To test whether CCL2 or IL-6 production due to attenuated IGF-1R function directly alters the recruitment of monocytes, we again modeled migration in vitro. RAW264.7 monocyte migration increased towards MCF7 cells with IGF-1R inhibition (Fig. 5a-b, e) which was decreased with CCL2 knockdown (Fig. 5d, e), but not with IL-6 knockdown (Fig. 5c, e) suggesting production of CCL2 through IGF-1R inhibition enhances monocyte migration.

Previously, it was shown that TAMs produce matrix metalloproteinases (MMPs) to degrade tumor matrix and promote tumor cell extravasation [49]. To test for MMP production in the monocyte specific population of *MMTV-Wnt1/dnIGF-1R* tumors we analyzed *MMP* gene expression in isolated CD11b$^+$ monocytes. *MMP-2*, *MMP-3*, and *MMP-9* levels were significantly increased in CD11b$^+$ monocytes from *MMTV-Wnt1/dnIGF-1R* tumors (Fig. 5f). These data suggest the increased accumulation of monocytes in *MMTV-Wnt1/dnIGF-1R* tumors promotes tumorigenesis through production of MMPs [49].

Reduced IGF-1R signaling in Wnt1-driven mammary tumors promotes an aggressive tumor microenvironment

Breakdown of the tumor basement membrane and surrounding matrix is critical for tumor cell extravasation and restructuring of the tumor microenvironment. MMPs are overexpressed and actively secreted in primary tumors that maintain an aggressive tumor microenvironment [50]. The accumulation of monocytes in *MMTV-Wnt1/ dnIGF-1R* tumors that produce MMPs suggests potential for secretory activity and matrix remodeling. Immunostaining revealed increased MMP2 and MMP9 in the stromal compartment of *MMTV-Wnt1/dnIGF-1R* tumors (Fig. 6a-d). Using in situ zymography, we further determined that the increased MMP expression correlated with increased MMP activity within the stroma of tumors with reduced IGF-1R signaling (Fig. 6e, f).

Increased MMP secretion and activity in tumors with attenuated IGF-1R suggests there is active tumor stroma matrix remodeling. With hematoxylin and eosin staining, we observed morphological alterations in the tumor stroma with attenuated IGF signaling (*MMTV-Wnt1/ dnIGF-1R*) (Fig. 6g, h). Further analysis by Masson's Trichrome staining revealed increased collagen in tumors with IGF-1R inhibition (Fig. 6i, j), which is associated with increased risk of metastasis [51]. These data suggest the primary tumor actively remodels the matrix in response to reduced IGF-1R function in the tumor epithelium.

Low IGF-1R expression inversely correlates with cytokine and MMP expression in humans

Previous analysis of the human patient gene expression datasets revealed IL-6, CCL2, and MMP9 expression are upregulated in TNBC compared to ER+/PR+ breast cancer [42, 48]. Our analysis of the METABRIC dataset confirmed increased expression of IL-6, CCL2, and MMP9 in TNBC (Additional file 7: Figure S4). Further analysis revealed IL-6, CCL2, and MMP9 were upregulated in breast tumors with low compared to high IGF-1R (Fig. 7a-c). Moreover, CHOP and MMP2 expression were upregulated in tumors with low IGF-1R, whereas expression was unchanged in TNBC compared to ER+/PR+ breast cancer (Additional file 7: Figure S4) revealing CHOP and MMP2

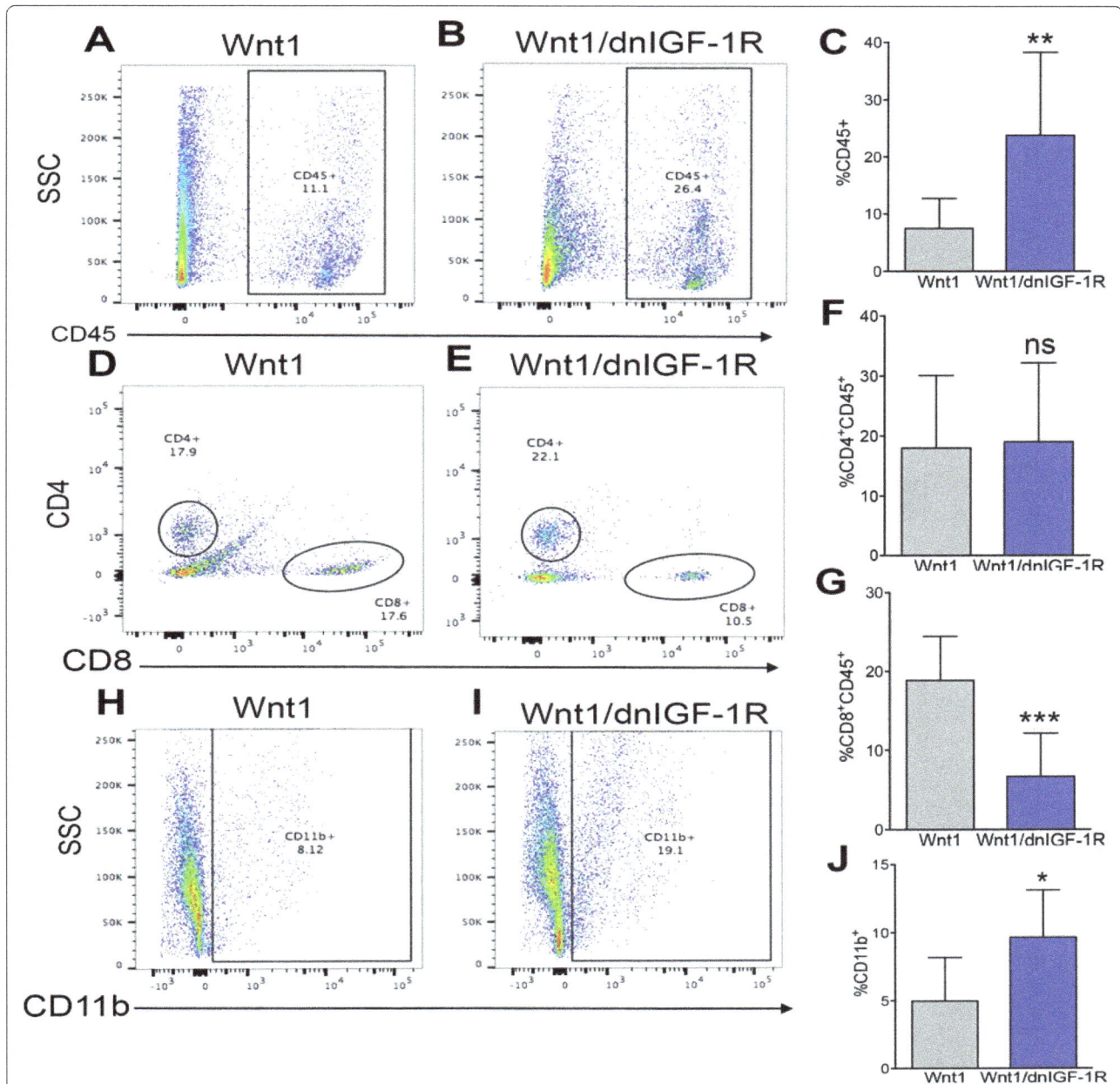

Fig. 4 *MMTV-Wnt1/dnIGF-1R* tumors have altered immune cell infiltration. **a, b** Representative dot plot derived from flow cytometry measuring leukocyte marker CD45-PE/Cy5 of purified immune cells from *Wnt1* (**a**) and *Wnt1/dnIGF-1R* (**b**) tumors. **c** Quantification of flow cytometry of CD45$^+$ leukocytes in *Wnt1* versus *Wnt1/dnIGF-1R* tumors (*Wnt1/dnIGF-1R* versus *Wnt1* **$P < 0.01$; $n = 20$ each group). **d, e** representative dot plot of flow cytometry using cell surface markers to select for helper/regulatory T cells (CD4$^+$CD45$^+$) or cytotoxic T cells (CD8$^+$CD45$^+$) in *Wnt1* (**d**) or *Wnt1/dnIGF-1R* (**e**) tumors. **f, g** Quantification of flow cytometry of CD4$^+$CD45$^+$-stained T cells (**f**) or CD8$^+$CD45$^+$-stained cytotoxic T cells (**g**) in *Wnt1* versus *Wnt1/dnIGF-1R* tumors (CD4$^+$CD45$^+$ *Wnt1/dnIGF-1R* cells versus *Wnt1* cells $P > 0.05$ (ns, not significant); CD8$^+$CD45$^+$ *Wnt1/dnIGF-1R* cells versus *Wnt1* cells ***$P < 0.001$; $n = 20$ each group). **h, i** representative dot plot of flow cytometry using monocyte marker CD11b-PerCP of purified immune cells from *Wnt1* (**h**) and *Wnt1/dnIGF-1R* (**i**) tumors. **j** Quantification of flow cytometry of CD11b$^+$ monocytes in *Wnt1* versus *Wnt1/dnIGF-1R* tumors (*Wnt1/dnIGF-1R* versus *Wnt1* *$P < 0.05$; $n = 20$ each group)

are more correlated with IGF-1R levels than with hormone receptor status. Taken together, we determined that IL-6, CCL2, MMP9, MMP2, and CHOP expression are all inversely correlated with IGF-1R expression in human breast cancer.

Discussion

Historically, IGF-1R was proposed to have oncogenic effects in breast tumorigenesis, where overexpression or hyperactivation leads to increased tumor cell proliferation and survival [6, 9, 10]. However, recent reports have

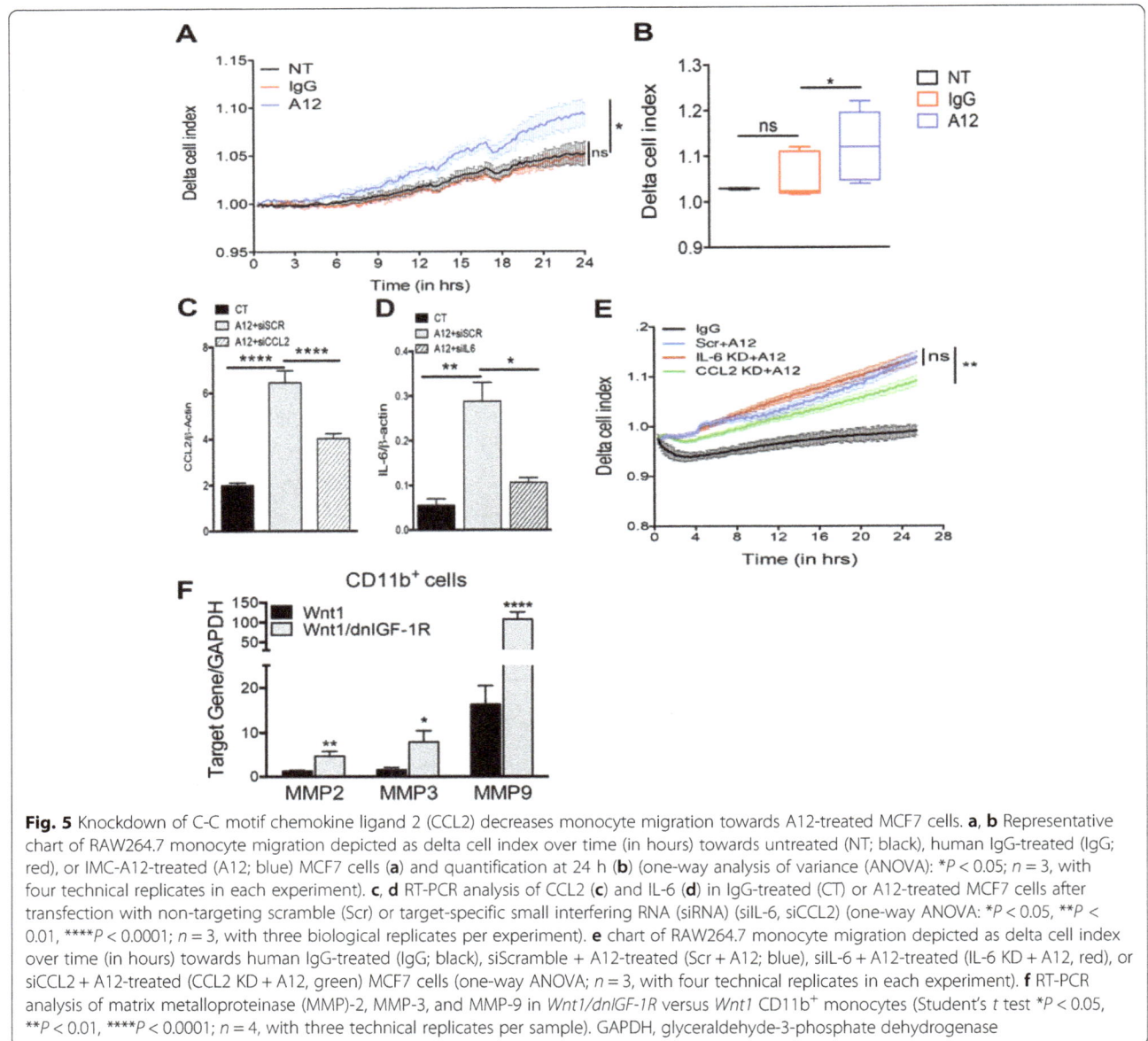

Fig. 5 Knockdown of C-C motif chemokine ligand 2 (CCL2) decreases monocyte migration towards A12-treated MCF7 cells. **a**, **b** Representative chart of RAW264.7 monocyte migration depicted as delta cell index over time (in hours) towards untreated (NT; black), human IgG-treated (IgG; red), or IMC-A12-treated (A12; blue) MCF7 cells (**a**) and quantification at 24 h (**b**) (one-way analysis of variance (ANOVA): *$P < 0.05$; $n = 3$, with four technical replicates in each experiment). **c**, **d** RT-PCR analysis of CCL2 (**c**) and IL-6 (**d**) in IgG-treated (CT) or A12-treated MCF7 cells after transfection with non-targeting scramble (Scr) or target-specific small interfering RNA (siRNA) (siIL-6, siCCL2) (one-way ANOVA: *$P < 0.05$, **$P < 0.01$, ****$P < 0.0001$; $n = 3$, with three biological replicates per experiment). **e** chart of RAW264.7 monocyte migration depicted as delta cell index over time (in hours) towards human IgG-treated (IgG; black), siScramble + A12-treated (Scr + A12; blue), siIL-6 + A12-treated (IL-6 KD + A12, red), or siCCL2 + A12-treated (CCL2 KD + A12, green) MCF7 cells (one-way ANOVA; $n = 3$, with four technical replicates in each experiment). **f** RT-PCR analysis of matrix metalloproteinase (MMP)-2, MMP-3, and MMP-9 in *Wnt1/dnIGF-1R* versus *Wnt1* CD11b[+] monocytes (Student's *t* test *$P < 0.05$, **$P < 0.01$, ****$P < 0.0001$; $n = 4$, with three technical replicates per sample). GAPDH, glyceraldehyde-3-phosphate dehydrogenase

suggested that overexpression of IGF-1R in ER+/PR+ breast cancers results in a favorable prognosis [6, 15], and low expression of IGF-1R leads to a more undifferentiated tumor phenotype and worse overall survival [8, 13] (Fig. 1). Consistent with these reports, we previously demonstrated that expression of a dominant-negative IGF-1R in a basal-like breast cancer tumor mouse model driven by the Wnt1 oncogene resulted in a more undifferentiated tumor and metastatic phenotype [1]. Interestingly, inhibitors of IGF-1R have been unsuccessful in the clinic, and the cause for this is still not understood [11, 12]. The exacerbated phenotype in the dominant-negative IGF-1R tumors raises the question of whether IGF-1R and the Wnt pathway

interact in breast tumorigenesis. METABRIC analysis of several Wnt signaling targets overexpressed in breast cancer revealed that Wnt2 and Frizzled 9 (Fzd9) were inversely correlated with IGF-1R expression in humans (Additional file 8: Figure S5). Interestingly, unbiased analysis with a targeted Wnt signaling array identified Wnt2 and Fzd9 as upregulated (9.3-fold, 2.3-fold) in *MMTV-Wnt1/dnIGF-1R* compared to *MMTV-Wnt1* tumors (Additional file 8: Figure S5), further linking the bigenic mouse model with human disease. Previous studies have shown upregulated Wnt2 in the primary breast tumor is linked to metastatic disease [52], and more recently, Wnt2 was identified as a regulator of tumor initiation in a

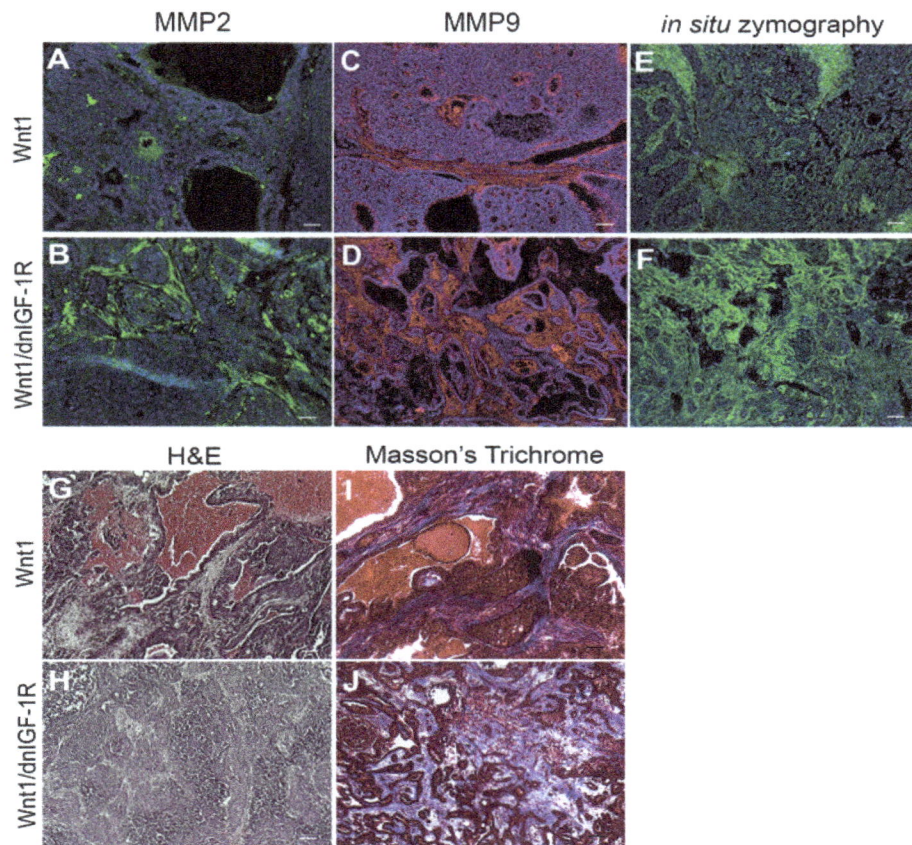

Fig. 6 Increased aggressive tumor microenvironment in *MMTV-Wnt1/dnIGF-1R* compared to *MMTV-Wnt1* tumors. **a-d** Representative photomicrographs showing immunofluorescence staining of matrix metalloproteinase (MMP)2 (green) and MMP9 (red) in *Wnt1* (**a, c**) and *Wnt1/dnIGF-1R* (**b, d**) tumor sections. **e, f** Representative photomicrographs depicting active MMPs through *in situ* zymography (green) in *Wnt1* (**e**) and *Wnt1/dnIGF-1R* (**f**). **g, h** Representative H&E-stained tissue sections from *MMTV-Wnt1 (Wnt1)* (**g**) and *MMTV-Wnt1/dnIGF-1R (Wnt1/dnIGF-1R)* (**h**) tumors. **i, j** Representative Masson's Trichrome-stained tissue sections for collagen (blue) in *Wnt1* (**i**) and *Wnt1/dnIGF-1R* (**j**). Sections (**a-f**) were stained with 4',6-diamidino-2-phenylindole to detect nuclei (blue). Scale bar = 100 μm

basal-like breast cancer model [53]. Moreover, Wnt2 is the only Wnt ligand that activates Fzd9, subsequently activating the canonical Wnt signaling pathway [54].

The mechanisms by which decreased IGF-1R function might contribute to an aggressive, invasive tumor phenotype have not been identified. In this study, we revealed a novel role for IGF-1R as a suppressor of tumorigenesis by regulating the tumor microenvironment through protecting tumor epithelial cells from EnR stress. Previously, it was found that a reduction in IGF signaling increased cellular stress and production of ROS in vascular smooth muscle cells, 3T3-L1 adipocytes, and MCF7 cells [21, 55–57]. Moreover, IGF-1 stimulation protects against thapsagargin-induced EnR stress activity in MCF7 cells suggesting the IGF-1 signaling pathway augments the adaptability of breast tumor cells to EnR stress [19]. Increased oxidative stress results in production of cytokines in tumor epithelium [38, 58] and a pro-inflammatory

response in a number of tissues [59]. In our study, cellular oxidative stress was increased as a result of attenuating IGF-1R directly resulting in cytokine production, specifically IL-6 and CCL2 (Figs. 2, 3). Previous studies have also shown increased production of ROS activates the EnR stress pathway; this subsequent activation increases the production of ROS through PDI resulting in a positive feedback loop [16, 17]. We showed that inhibition of IGF-1R in tumor epithelium results in activation of the EnR stress pathway and upregulation of PDI suggesting that the increased ROS production may be through amplified EnR stress.

Both IL-6 and CCL2 play a major role in promoting tumorigenesis by altering the primary tumor immune microenvironment and enhancing a more aggressive primary tumor phenotype [43, 44, 60]. Importantly, IL-6 and CCL2 production in mouse and human tumor epithelial cells is elevated with reduced IGF-1R function (Fig. 3). As

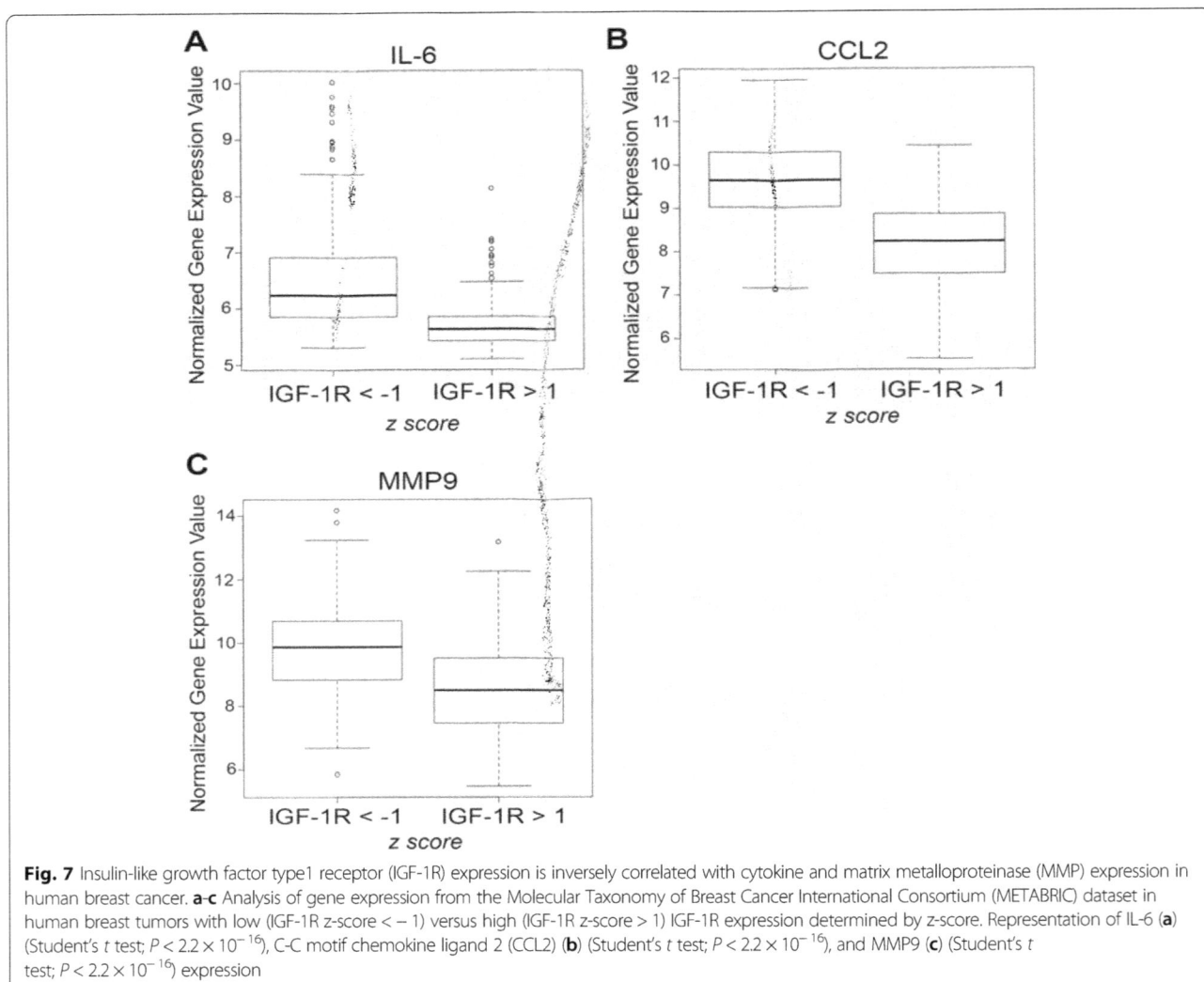

Fig. 7 Insulin-like growth factor type1 receptor (IGF-1R) expression is inversely correlated with cytokine and matrix metalloproteinase (MMP) expression in human breast cancer. **a-c** Analysis of gene expression from the Molecular Taxonomy of Breast Cancer International Consortium (METABRIC) dataset in human breast tumors with low (IGF-1R z-score < − 1) versus high (IGF-1R z-score > 1) IGF-1R expression determined by z-score. Representation of IL-6 (**a**) (Student's t test; $P < 2.2 \times 10^{-16}$), C-C motif chemokine ligand 2 (CCL2) (**b**) (Student's t test; $P < 2.2 \times 10^{-16}$), and MMP9 (**c**) (Student's t test; $P < 2.2 \times 10^{-16}$) expression

a result of altered cytokine production within the primary tumor epithelium, we observed altered immune cell invasion in *MMTV-Wnt1/dnIGF-1R* tumors. The decrease in CD8[+] cytotoxic T cells indicates fewer immune cells responsible for tumor degradation present within the primary tumors lacking IGF-1R function. Furthermore, we observed an increased influx of CD11b[+] monocytes that have potential to polarize into tumor-associated macrophages (TAMs) dependent on surrounding signals from the tumor (Fig. 4). Moreover, consistent with previous reports we showed that CCL2 is necessary for macrophage migration [47]. Although IL-6 is not necessary for macrophage recruitment in our model, the upregulation of IL-6 in tumor epithelium may be important for other functions such as tumor initiation, growth, and metastasis [42, 43, 61] (Fig. 5). Although monocyte recruitment is increased in tumors with attenuated IGF-1R signaling, it is still unclear whether these monocytes become tumor-degrading or

tumor-promoting macrophages. TAMs involved in tumorigenesis are known to produce matrix metalloproteinases (MMPs) [49]. The increased production of MMPs within the monocytes from *MMTV-Wnt1/dnIGF-1R* tumors suggests an enrichment of tumor-promoting TAMs (Fig. 5). Therefore, the composition of the immune microenvironment in *MMTV-Wnt1/dnIGF-1R* primary tumors favors tumor growth and extravasation.

Prior studies have shown that increased expression of key tumor microenvironment components such as collagen and MMP2/MMP9 are necessary for tumor epithelial extravasation [50, 51, 62, 63]. Secretion of active MMP2 and MMP9 into the stroma of primary tumors allows for break-down of the surrounding tumor matrix and matrix remodeling to promote epithelial cell invasion [64]. Here, we observed increased MMP activity within the stroma of *MMTV-Wnt1/dnIGF-1R* tumors that corresponded with the increased MMP2 and

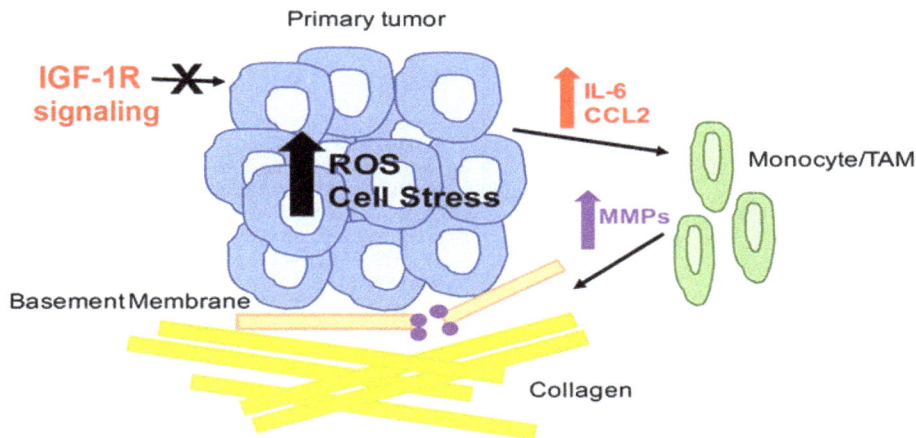

Fig. 8 Model for insulin-like growth factortype 1 receptor (IGF-1R) regulation of primary tumor cellular stress and enhancement of an aggressive tumor microenvironment. Reduced or inhibited IGF-1R function results in increased reactive oxygen species (ROS) accumulation and primary tumor epithelial endoplasmic reticulum (EnR) stress leading to increased production of IL-6 and C-C motif chemokine ligand 2 (CCL2) by the primary tumor epithelium. Secretion of IL-6 and CCL2 signals for monocyte infiltration and differentiation to tumor-associated macrophages (TAM). This differentiation increases MMP expression and secretion resulting in active tumor basement membrane breakdown allowing for increased collagen deposition to provide an environment for tumor cell extravasation

MMP9 expression (Fig. 6). De novo collagen deposition is necessary during tumor matrix remodeling and increased collagen is correlated with metastatic tumors [65, 66]. Increased collagen levels measured by Masson's Trichrome staining revealed that tumors lacking a functional IGF-1R have a significantly altered tumor microenvironment that is consistent with promoting tumor cell invasion (Fig. 6).

It is well-known that IL-6, CCL2, and MMP9 expression are increased in TNBC compared to ER+/PR+ breast cancer [42, 48, 67]. Consistent with our mouse tumor model with reduced IGF-1R signaling, low IGF-1R is inversely correlated with IL-6, CCL2, and MMP9 expression in human tumors (Fig. 7). Interestingly, MMP2 and CHOP were also upregulated in human tumors with low IGF-1R, similar to our mouse model, whereas these two genes were unchanged in TNBC compared to ER+/PR+ breast cancer. Taken together, our data suggest this set of genes is specifically correlated with human tumors that have low levels of IGF-1R.

Conclusions

We have defined IGF-1R as a negative regulator of cytokine production by protecting epithelial cells from oxidative stress, resulting in maintenance of a tumor microenvironment that suppresses tumor cell invasion (Fig. 8). Taken together, these data support a protective function of the IGF-1R in breast epithelial cells and suggest that reduction of IGF-1R signaling in the epithelial cells leads to increased ROS production and EnR stress, altered cytokine production, and as a result, tumor

microenvironment remodeling to promote cellular invasion and metastasis.

Additional files

Additional file 1: Table S1. *MMTV-Wnt1* tumor phenotype is altered with reduced IGF-1R [1]. (DOCX 16 kb)

Additional file 2: Table S2. qRT-PCR primer list. (DOCX 14 kb)

Additional file 3: Figure S1. IMC-A12 blocks activation of IGF-1R signaling. Western blot analysis of pAkt (473) and pIGF-1R in IgG or A12 treated MCF7 cells with or without IGF-1. (TIF 339 kb)

Additional file 4: Table S3. Cytokine and chemokine profile is altered in *MMTV-Wnt1* tumors with attenuated IGF-1R. Gene expression fold change measured by the $\Delta\Delta$Ct method comparing *MMTV-Wnt1* and *MMTV-Wnt1/dnIGF-1R* tumors. Student's *t* test was performed to determine the corresponding *p* values. (DOCX 25 kb)

Additional file 5: Figure S2. IL-6 protein expression is increased in tumor cells with reduced IGF signaling. ELISA analysis of IL-6 in IgG or A12 treated MCF7 cells (Student's *t* test *P* < 0.05, *n* = 3; 3 biological replicates per experiment). (TIF 57 kb)

Additional file 6: Figure S3. Reduced IGF-1R in primary tumors does not alter the active T cell population. (A, B) Quantification of flow cytometry of CD3$^+$ T cells (A) and activated regulatory T cells positive for FOXP3 and CD25 (B) in *Wnt1* versus *Wnt1/dnIGF-1R* tumors (*Wnt1/dnIGF-1R* versus *Wnt1* **P* < 0.01; *n* = 20 each group). (TIF 70 kb)

Additional file 7: Figure S4. Cytokine and MMP expression in human breast cancer patients. Analysis of gene expression from the METABRIC dataset. (A-C) Boxplot representation of IL-6 (A) (Student's *t* test, *P* < 2.2 × 10^{-16}), CCL2 (B) (Student's *t* test, *P* < 2.2 × 10^{-16}), and MMP9 (C) (Student's *t* test, *P* < 2.2 × 10^{-16}) expression levels in ER+/PR+ breast cancer compared to triple-negative breast cancer (TNBC). (D-G) Boxplot representation of MMP2 and CHOP (D, F) expression levels in ER+/PR+ breast cancer compared to TNBC (MMP2: Student's *t* test, *P* < 2.2 × 10^{-16}; CHOP: *P* < 2.2 × 10^{-16}). Boxplot representation of MMP2 and CHOP (E, G) expression in human breast tumors with low (IGF-1R z-score < − 1) versus high (IGF-1R z-score > 1) IGF-1R expression (Student's *t* test, MMP2, *P* < 6.864 × 10^{-10}; CHOP, *P* < 3.172 × 10^{-10}). (TIF 253 kb)

> **Additional file 8: Figure S5.** Wnt2 and Frizzled9 expression are inversely correlated with IGF-1R expression in breast cancer. (A, B) Analysis of gene expression from the METABRIC dataset. Boxplot representation of Wnt2 (A) (Student's t test, $P < 2.2 \times 10^{-16}$) and Fzd9 (Frizzled9) (B) (Student's t test, $P < 2.2 \times 10^{-16}$) in human breast tumors with low (IGF-1R z-score < -1) versus high (IGF-1R z score > 1) IGF-1R expression. (C, D). qRT-PCR analysis of Wnt2 (C) and Fzd9 (D) in *MMTV-Wnt1* compared to *MMTV-Wnt1/dnIGF-1R* tumors ($n = 4$). (TIF 232 kb)

Abbreviations

ANOVA: Analysis of variance; ATCC: American Type Culture Collection; BSA: Bovine serum albumin; CCL2: C-C motif chemokine ligand 2; CHOP: C/EBP homologous protein; DAB: 3,3'-Diaminobenzidine; DCFDA: 2',7'-Dichlorofluorescin diacetate; DMEM: Dulbecco's modified Eagle's medium; eIF2-α: Eukaryotic initiation factor 2-alpha; ELISA: Enzyme-linked immunosorbent assay; EnR: Endoplasmic reticulum; ER+/PR+: Estrogen receptor/progesterone receptor-positive; FACS: Fluorescence-activated cell sorting; FBS: Fetal bovine serum; GAPDH: Glyceraldehyde-3-phosphate dehydrogenase; HR: Hormone receptor; IGF-1: Insulin-like growth factor-1; IGF-1R: Insulin-like growth factortype 1 receptor; IHC: Immunohistochemistry; IL-10: Interleukin-10; IL-6: Interleukin-6; LumA: Luminal A; LumB: Luminal B; MEC: Mammary tumor epithelial cell; MEM: Minimum essential medium; METABRIC: Molecular Taxonomy of Breast Cancer International Consortium; MMP: Matrix metalloproteinase; NAC: N-acetyl cysteine; PAM50: Prediction analysis of microarray 50; PBS: Phosphate-buffered saline; PDI: Protein disulfide isomerase; qRT-PCR: Quantitative real-time polymerase chain reaction; RIPA: Radioimmunoprecipitation assay; ROS: Reactive oxygen species; Scr: Scramble; siRNA: Small interfering RNA; TAM: Tumor-associated macrophage; TCGA: The Cancer Genome Atlas; TNBC: Triple-negative breast cancer; TNF-α: Tumor necrosis factor-alpha; UPR: Unfolded protein response

Acknowledgements

We thank Dr Sukhwinder Singh of the NJMS Flow Cytometry and Immunology Core Laboratory for the assistance with flow cytometry analysis and sorting, the Office of Advanced Research Computing (OARC) at Rutgers University under NIH 1S10OD012346-01A1 for the critical work made possible through access to the Perceval Linux cluster, Quan Shang for technical assistance, Dr Sophia Ran for assistance with the cytokine and chemokine targeted array, Dr Yi Li for providing the *MMTV-Wnt1* mice, Dr Edouard Azzam and Dr Nicholas Colangelo for assistance with the zymography assays, and Dr Amy Davidow for assistance with biostatistical analysis.

Funding

This work was supported by Public Health Service National Institutes of Health grants NCI R01CA204312 (TLW) and NCI R01165077 (RBB), New Jersey Commission on Cancer Research Postdoctoral Fellowship DFHS15PPC039 and American Cancer Society-Fairfield County Roast Postdoctoral Fellowship 130455-PF-17-244-01-CSM (AEO), and New Jersey Health Foundation grant (RBB).

Authors' contributions

AEO performed the majority of the experiments and statistical analyses and participated in the study design and writing the draft manuscript. SK performed the migration assays and analysis. Y-JC performed the METABRIC analysis. JJB performed the peIF2a western blots. BJB, RBB, DAL, EG, and DL contributed to study design, results interpretation, and manuscript editing. TLW is the principal investigator for this project. All authors read and approved the final manuscript.

Competing interests

The authors declare that they have no competing interests.

Author details

[1]Department of Pharmacology, Physiology & Neuroscience, Rutgers-New Jersey Medical School, Cancer Institute of New Jersey, Newark, NJ 07101, USA. [2]Department of Microbiology, Biochemistry & Molecular Genetics, Rutgers-New Jersey Medical School, Cancer Institute of New Jersey, Newark, NJ 07101, USA. [3]Office of Advance Research Computing, Rutgers-New Jersey Medical School, Newark, NJ 07102, USA. [4]Feinstein Institute for Medical Research, Northwell Health, Manhasset, NY 11030, USA. [5]Division of Endocrinology, Diabetes and Bone Diseases, The Samuel Bronfman Department of Medicine, Icahn Sinai School of Medicine at Mt. Sinai, New York, NY 10029, USA.

References

1. Rota LM, Albanito L, Shin ME, Goyeneche CL, Shushanov S, Gallagher EJ, et al. IGF1R inhibition in mammary epithelia promotes canonical Wnt signaling and Wnt1-driven tumors. Cancer Res. 2014;74(19):5668–79.
2. Mimeault M, Batra SK. Molecular biomarkers of cancer stem/progenitor cells associated with progression, metastases, and treatment resistance of aggressive cancers. Cancer Epidemiol Biomark Prev. 2014;23(2):234–54.
3. Yau C, Esserman L, Moore DH, Waldman F, Sninsky J, Benz CC. A multigene predictor of metastatic outcome in early stage hormone receptor-negative and triple-negative breast cancer. Breast Cancer Res. 2010;12(5):R85.
4. Howe LR, Brown AM. Wnt signaling and breast cancer. Cancer Biol Ther. 2004;3(1):36–41.
5. Li Y, Hively WP, Varmus HE. Use of MMTV-Wnt-1 transgenic mice for studying the genetic basis of breast cancer. Oncogene. 2000;19(8):1002–9.
6. Papa V, Gliozzo B, Clark GM, McGuire WL, Moore D, Fujita-Yamaguchi Y, et al. Insulin-like growth factor-I receptors are overexpressed and predict a low risk in human breast cancer. Cancer Res. 1993;53(16):3736–40.
7. Bartella V, De Marco P, Malaguarnera R, Belfiore A, Maggiolini M. New advances on the functional cross-talk between insulin-like growth factor-I and estrogen signaling in cancer. Cell Signal. 2012;24(8):1515–21.
8. Schnarr B, Strunz K, Ohsam J, Benner A, Wacker J, Mayer D. Down-regulation of insulin-like growth factor-I receptor and insulin receptor substrate-1 expression in advanced human breast cancer. Int J Cancer. 2000;89(6):506–13.
9. Pollak M. Insulin and insulin-like growth factor signalling in neoplasia. Nat Rev Cancer. 2008;8(12):915–28.
10. Lann D, LeRoith D. The role of endocrine insulin-like growth factor-I and insulin in breast cancer. J Mammary Gland Biol Neoplasia. 2008;13(4):371–9.
11. Yang Y, Yee D. Targeting insulin and insulin-like growth factor signaling in breast cancer. J Mammary Gland Biol Neoplasia. 2012;17(3–4):251–61.
12. Boone DN, Lee AV. Targeting the insulin-like growth factor receptor: developing biomarkers from gene expression profiling. Crit Rev Oncog. 2012;17(2):161–73.
13. Sutherland BW, Knoblaugh SE, Kaplan-Lefko PJ, Wang F, Holzenberger M, Greenberg NM. Conditional deletion of insulin-like growth factor-I receptor in prostate epithelium. Cancer Res. 2008;68(9):3495–504.
14. Yerushalmi R, Gelmon KA, Leung S, Gao D, Cheang M, Pollak M, et al. Insulin-like growth factor receptor (IGF-1R) in breast cancer subtypes. Breast Cancer Res Treat. 2012;132(1):131–42.
15. Farabaugh SM, Boone DN, Lee AV. Role of IGF1R in breast cancer subtypes, stemness, and lineage differentiation. Front Endocrinol. 2015;6:59.
16. Hetz C. The unfolded protein response: controlling cell fate decisions under ER stress and beyond. Nat Rev Mol Cell Biol. 2012;13(2):89–102.
17. Cao SS, Kaufman RJ. Endoplasmic reticulum stress and oxidative stress in cell fate decision and human disease. Antioxid Redox Signal. 2014;21(3):396–413.
18. Henis-Korenblit S, Zhang P, Hansen M, McCormick M, Lee SJ, Cary M, et al. Insulin/IGF-1 signaling mutants reprogram ER stress response regulators to promote longevity. Proc Natl Acad Sci U S A. 2010;107(21):9730–5.

19. Novosyadlyy R, Kurshan N, Lann D, Vijayakumar A, Yakar S, LeRoith D. Insulin-like growth factor-I protects cells from ER stress-induced apoptosis via enhancement of the adaptive capacity of endoplasmic reticulum. Cell Death Differ. 2008;15(8):1304–17.

20. Zou CG, Cao XZ, Zhao YS, Gao SY, Li SD, Liu XY, et al. The molecular mechanism of endoplasmic reticulum stress-induced apoptosis in PC-12 neuronal cells: the protective effect of insulin-like growth factor I. Endocrinology. 2009;150(1):277–85.

21. Zhou Y, Liang X, Chang H, Shu F, Wu Y, Zhang T, et al. Ampelopsin-induced autophagy protects breast cancer cells from apoptosis through Akt-mTOR pathway via endoplasmic reticulum stress. Cancer Sci. 2014;105(10):1279–87.

22. Pimenta EM, De S, Weiss R, Feng D, Hall K, Kilic S, et al. IRF5 is a novel regulator of CXCL13 expression in breast cancer that regulates CXCR5(+) B- and T-cell trafficking to tumor-conditioned media. Immunol Cell Biol. 2015; 93(5):486–99.

23. Pachynski RK, Scholz A, Monnier J, Butcher EC, Zabel BA. Evaluation of tumor-infiltrating leukocyte subsets in a subcutaneous tumor model. J Vis Exp. 2015;98(e52657):1–10.

24. Smalley MJ, Kendrick H, Sheridan JM, Regan JL, Prater MD, Lindeman GJ, et al. Isolation of mouse mammary epithelial subpopulations: a comparison of leading methods. J Mammary Gland Biol Neoplasia. 2012;17(2):91–7.

25. Muller PY, Janovjak H, Miserez AR, Dobbie Z. Processing of gene expression data generated by quantitative real-time RT-PCR. BioTechniques. 2002;32(6): 1372–4 6, 8-9.

26. Sun Z, Shushanov S, LeRoith D, Wood TL. Decreased IGF type 1 receptor signaling in mammary epithelium during pregnancy leads to reduced proliferation, alveolar differentiation, and expression of insulin receptor substrate (IRS)-1 and IRS-2. Endocrinology. 2011;152(8):3233–45.

27. Hadler-Olsen E, Kanapathippillai P, Berg E, Svineng G, Winberg JO, Uhlin-Hansen L. Gelatin in situ zymography on fixed, paraffin-embedded tissue: zinc and ethanol fixation preserve enzyme activity. J Histochem Cytochem. 2010;58(1):29–39.

28. Curtis C, Shah SP, Chin SF, Turashvili G, Rueda OM, Dunning MJ, et al. The genomic and transcriptomic architecture of 2,000 breast tumours reveals novel subgroups. Nature. 2012;486(7403):346–52.

29. Gao J, Aksoy BA, Dogrusoz U, Dresdner G, Gross B, Sumer SO, et al. Integrative analysis of complex cancer genomics and clinical profiles using the cBioPortal. Sci Signal. 2013;6(269):pl1.

30. Cerami E, Gao J, Dogrusoz U, Gross BE, Sumer SO, Aksoy BA, et al. The cBio cancer genomics portal: an open platform for exploring multidimensional cancer genomics data. Cancer Discov. 2012;2(5):401–4.

31. Lyons A, Coleman M, Riis S, Favre C, O'Flanagan CH, Zhdanov AV, et al. Insulin-like growth factor 1 signaling is essential for mitochondrial biogenesis and mitophagy in cancer cells. J Biol Chem. 2017;292(41):16983–98.

32. Favre C, Zhdanov A, Leahy M, Papkovsky D, O'Connor R. Mitochondrial pyrimidine nucleotide carrier (PNC1) regulates mitochondrial biogenesis and the invasive phenotype of cancer cells. Oncogene. 2010;29(27):3964–76.

33. Endo H, Murata K, Mukai M, Ishikawa O, Inoue M. Activation of insulin-like growth factor signaling induces apoptotic cell death under prolonged hypoxia by enhancing endoplasmic reticulum stress response. Cancer Res. 2007;67(17):8095–103.

34. Berlett BS, Stadtman ER. Protein oxidation in aging, disease, and oxidative stress. J Biol Chem. 1997;272(33):20313–6.

35. Mukohara T, Shimada H, Ogasawara N, Wanikawa R, Shimomura M, Nakatsura T, et al. Sensitivity of breast cancer cell lines to the novel insulin-like growth factor-1 receptor (IGF-1R) inhibitor NVP-AEW541 is dependent on the level of IRS-1 expression. Cancer Lett. 2009;282(1):14–24.

36. Zhang H, Pelzer AM, Kiang DT, Yee D. Down-regulation of type I insulin-like growth factor receptor increases sensitivity of breast cancer cells to insulin. Cancer Res. 2007;67(1):391–7.

37. Burtrum D, Zhu Z, Lu D, Anderson DM, Prewett M, Pereira DS, et al. A fully human monoclonal antibody to the insulin-like growth factor I receptor blocks ligand-dependent signaling and inhibits human tumor growth in vivo. Cancer Res. 2003;63(24):8912–21.

38. Bao B, Ahmad A, Kong D, Ali S, Azmi AS, Li Y, et al. Hypoxia induced aggressiveness of prostate cancer cells is linked with deregulated expression of VEGF, IL-6 and miRNAs that are attenuated by CDF. PLoS One. 2012;7(8):e43726.

39. Potula HS, Wang D, Quyen DV, Singh NK, Kundumani-Sridharan V, Karpurapu M, et al. Src-dependent STAT-3-mediated expression of monocyte chemoattractant protein-1 is required for 15(S)-hydroxyeicosatetraenoic acid-induced vascular smooth muscle cell migration. J Biol Chem. 2009;284(45):31142–55.

40. Allavena P, Sica A, Solinas G, Porta C, Mantovani A. The inflammatory micro-environment in tumor progression: the role of tumor-associated macrophages. Crit Rev Oncol Hematol. 2008;66(1):1–9.

41. Farajzadeh Valilou S, Keshavarz-Fathi M, Silvestris N, Argentiero A, Rezaei N. The role of inflammatory cytokines and tumor associated macrophages (TAMs) in microenvironment of pancreatic cancer. Cytokine Growth Factor Rev. 2018;39:46–61.

42. Hartman ZC, Poage GM, den Hollander P, Tsimelzon A, Hill J, Panupinthu N, et al. Growth of triple-negative breast cancer cells relies upon coordinate autocrine expression of the proinflammatory cytokines IL-6 and IL-8. Cancer Res. 2013;73(11):3470–80.

43. Sullivan NJ, Sasser AK, Axel AE, Vesuna F, Raman V, Ramirez N, et al. Interleukin-6 induces an epithelial-mesenchymal transition phenotype in human breast cancer cells. Oncogene. 2009;28(33):2940–7.

44. Tsuyada A, Chow A, Wu J, Somlo G, Chu P, Loera S, et al. CCL2 mediates cross-talk between cancer cells and stromal fibroblasts that regulates breast cancer stem cells. Cancer Res. 2012;72(11):2768–79.

45. Grivennikov SI, Greten FR, Karin M. Immunity, inflammation, and cancer. Cell. 2010;140(6):883–99.

46. Esquivel-Velazquez M, Ostoa-Saloma P, Palacios-Arreola MI, Nava-Castro KE, Castro JI, Morales-Montor J. The role of cytokines in breast cancer development and progression. J Interf Cytokine Res. 2015;35(1):1–16.

47. Qian BZ, Li J, Zhang H, Kitamura T, Zhang J, Campion LR, et al. CCL2 recruits inflammatory monocytes to facilitate breast-tumour metastasis. Nature. 2011;475(7355):222–5.

48. Bonapace L, Coissieux MM, Wyckoff J, Mertz KD, Varga Z, Junt T, et al. Cessation of CCL2 inhibition accelerates breast cancer metastasis by promoting angiogenesis. Nature. 2014;515(7525):130–3.

49. Qian BZ, Pollard JW. Macrophage diversity enhances tumor progression and metastasis. Cell. 2010;141(1):39–51.

50. Kessenbrock K, Wang CY, Werb Z. Matrix metalloproteinases in stem cell regulation and cancer. Matrix Biol. 2015;44–46:184–90.

51. Takai K, Le A, Weaver VM, Werb Z. Targeting the cancer-associated fibroblasts as a treatment in triple-negative breast cancer. Oncotarget. 2016; 7(50):82889–901.

52. Ellsworth RE, Seebach J, Field LA, Heckman C, Kane J, Hooke JA, et al. A gene expression signature that defines breast cancer metastases. Clin Exp Metastasis. 2009;26(3):205–13.

53. Zhang M, Tsimelzon A, Chang CH, Fan C, Wolff A, Perou CM, et al. Intratumoral heterogeneity in a Trp53-null mouse model of human breast cancer. Cancer Discov. 2015;5(5):520–33.

54. Karasawa T, Yokokura H, Kitajewski J, Lombroso PJ. Frizzled-9 is activated by Wnt-2 and functions in Wnt/beta -catenin signaling. J Biol Chem. 2002; 277(40):37479–86.

55. Meng Q, Qin Y, Deshpande M, Kashiwabuchi F, Rodrigues M, Lu Q, et al. Hypoxia-inducible factor-dependent expression of angiopoietin-like 4 by conjunctival epithelial cells promotes the angiogenic phenotype of pterygia. Invest Ophthalmol Vis Sci. 2017;58(11):4514–23.

56. Su C, Chen M, Huang H, Lin J. Testosterone enhances lipopolysaccharide-induced interleukin-6 and macrophage chemotactic protein-1 expression by activating the extracellular signal-regulated kinase 1/2/nuclear factor-kappaB signalling pathways in 3T3-L1 adipocytes. Mol Med Rep. 2015;12(1):696–704.

57. Lin C, Liao W, Jian Y, Peng Y, Zhang X, Ye L, et al. CGI-99 promotes breast cancer metastasis via autocrine interleukin-6 signaling. Oncogene. 2017; 36(26):3695–705.

58. Mimeault M, Batra SK. Hypoxia-inducing factors as master regulators of stemness properties and altered metabolism of cancer- and metastasis-initiating cells. J Cell Mol Med. 2013;17(1):30–54.

59. Zhang K, Kaufman RJ. From endoplasmic-reticulum stress to the inflammatory response. Nature. 2008;454(7203):455–62.

60. Wellenstein MD, de Visser KE. Cancer-cell-intrinsic mechanisms shaping the tumor Immune landscape. Immunity. 2018;48(3):399–416.

61. Dethlefsen C, Hojfeldt G, Hojman P. The role of intratumoral and systemic IL-6 in breast cancer. Breast Cancer Res Treat. 2013;138(3):657–64.

62. Ye X, Weinberg RA. Epithelial-mesenchymal plasticity: a central regulator of cancer progression. Trends Cell Biol. 2015;25(11):675–86.

63. Blot E, Chen W, Vasse M, Paysant J, Denoyelle C, Pille JY, et al. Cooperation between monocytes and breast cancer cells promotes factors involved in cancer aggressiveness. Br J Cancer. 2003;88(8):1207–12.
64. Egeblad M, Werb Z. New functions for the matrix metalloproteinases in cancer progression. Nat Rev Cancer. 2002;2(3):161–74.
65. Acerbi I, Cassereau L, Dean I, Shi Q, Au A, Park C, et al. Human breast cancer invasion and aggression correlates with ECM stiffening and immune cell infiltration. Integr Biol (Camb). 2015;7(10):1120–34.
66. Lu P, Weaver VM, Werb Z. The extracellular matrix: a dynamic niche in cancer progression. J Cell Biol. 2012;196(4):395–406.
67. Mehner C, Hockla A, Miller E, Ran S, Radisky DC, Radisky ES. Tumor cell-produced matrix metalloproteinase 9 (MMP-9) drives malignant progression and metastasis of basal-like triple negative breast cancer. Oncotarget. 2014; 5(9):2736–49.

21

Denosumab treatment is associated with the absence of circulating tumor cells in patients with breast cancer

Marcus Vetter[1,2†], Julia Landin[2†], Barbara Maria Szczerba[3†], Francesc Castro-Giner[3,4†], Sofia Gkountela[3], Cinzia Donato[3], Ilona Krol[3], Ramona Scherrer[3], Catharina Balmelli[2], Alexandra Malinovska[2], Alfred Zippelius[2], Christian Kurzeder[1,5], Viola Heinzelmann-Schwarz[1], Walter Paul Weber[5], Christoph Rochlitz[2] and Nicola Aceto[3*] [iD]

Abstract

Background: The presence of circulating tumor cells (CTCs) in patients with breast cancer correlates to a bad prognosis. Yet, CTCs are detectable in only a minority of patients with progressive breast cancer, and factors that influence the abundance of CTCs remain elusive.

Methods: We conducted CTC isolation and enumeration in a selected group of 73 consecutive patients characterized by progressive invasive breast cancer, high tumor load and treatment discontinuation at the time of CTC isolation. CTCs were quantified with the Parsortix microfluidic device. Clinicopathological variables, blood counts at the time of CTC isolation and detailed treatment history prior to blood sampling were evaluated for each patient.

Results: Among 73 patients, we detected at least one CTC per 7.5 ml of blood in 34 (46%). Of these, 22 (65%) had single CTCs only, whereas 12 (35%) featured both single CTCs and CTC clusters. Treatment with the monoclonal antibody denosumab correlated with the absence of CTCs, both when considering all patients and when considering only those with bone metastasis. We also found that low red blood cell count was associated with the presence of CTCs, whereas high CA 15-3 tumor marker, high mean corpuscular volume, high white blood cell count and high mean platelet volume associated specifically with CTC clusters.

Conclusions: In addition to blood count correlatives to single and clustered CTCs, we found that denosumab treatment associates with most patients lacking CTCs from their peripheral circulation. Prospective studies will be needed to validate the involvement of denosumab in the prevention of CTC generation.

Keywords: Circulating tumor cells, Circulating tumor cell clusters, Denosumab, Breast cancer, Metastasis

Background

Circulating tumor cells (CTCs) are derivatives of solid tumor lesions that detach from the tumor and enter the bloodstream [1]. In patients with breast cancer, CTCs have been shown to be predictive of a shorter disease-free survival and overall survival [2, 3], with a worse prognosis in patients who present with a count of at least five CTCs per 7.5 ml of blood [2, 3]. Generally,

high CTC counts have been associated with a poor prognosis in multiple settings, including those patients that are newly diagnosed with metastatic breast cancer and about to start a therapy [3, 4]. At the morphological level, breast CTCs occur in the blood of patients as single CTCs or as CTC clusters, with the latter being associated with a shorter metastasis-free survival than in patients in whom only single CTCs are found [5].

Although the association between CTCs and bad prognosis is well established in breast cancer, CTCs are detectable only in a subset (~ 20–40%) of patients [2, 5]. To date, no parameters have been found that could explain CTC abundance in patients, leading to difficulties in enabling patient stratification prior to CTC-related

* Correspondence: nicola.aceto@unibas.ch
†Marcus Vetter, Julia Landin, Barbara Maria Szczerba and Francesc Castro-Giner contributed equally to this work.
3Department of Biomedicine, Cancer Metastasis Laboratory, University of Basel and University Hospital Basel, Mattenstrasse 28, CH-4058 Basel, Switzerland
Full list of author information is available at the end of the article

investigations [6, 7], as well as limiting our understanding of those factors that may influence the spread of cancer.

In this study, we aimed to investigate a number of clinicopathological variables, blood counts at the time of CTC isolation and detailed treatment history prior to blood sampling in a cohort of 73 consecutive patients with invasive breast cancer characterized by progressive disease, high tumor load and treatment discontinuation (or without any pretreatment) at the time of CTC isolation, before the next line of therapy. Additionally, we not only investigated parameters that are associated with the presence of CTCs but also specifically interrogated our datasets to identify features that are associated with CTC clusters. The rationale of our study was therefore to identify, in an unbiased manner (i.e., not driven by preexisting hypotheses), clinical parameters that correlate with CTC presence in patients with progressive breast cancer.

Methods
Patient selection
Seventy-three consecutive patients with invasive breast cancer, progressive disease, high tumor load, treatment discontinuation at the time of CTC isolation (before the next line of therapy) and no preselection for breast cancer subtype or specific metastatic sites were enrolled in the study. Eligible patients were > 18 years old with any menopausal status and had an Eastern Cooperative Oncology Group performance status of 0–3. Disease had to be measurable by Response Evaluation Criteria in Solid Tumors (RECIST) version 1.1 or nonmeasurable bone-only disease. Tumor load was defined by either the size of the primary tumor or the number and size of metastatic lymph nodes or distant sites, and patients with higher tumor load were prioritized. All subjects donated 7.5–15 ml of blood in ethylenediaminetetraacetic acid (EDTA) vacutainers at least once, and each signed an informed consent before joining the study. The study was performed under the protocols EKNZ BASEC 2016-00067 and EK 321/10, which received ethical and institutional review board approvals before study initiation (Ethics Committee northwest/central Switzerland [EKNZ]). This study was performed in compliance with the Declaration of Helsinki.

CTC isolation and enumeration strategy
Patient-derived CTCs were captured on the microfluidic Parsortix Cell Separation Cassette (GEN3D6.5; ANGLE, Guildford, UK) within 1 h of blood draw, directly from unmanipulated blood samples. Next, in-cassette staining was performed with an antibody cocktail comprising antibodies against epithelial cell adhesion molecule (EpCAM)-Alexa Fluor 488 (AF488) (#CST5198; Cell Signaling Technology, Danvers, MA, USA), human epidermal growth factor

receptor 2 (HER2)-AF488 (#324410; BioLegend, San Diego, CA, USA), epidermal growth factor receptor (EGFR)-fluorescein isothiocyanate (FITC) (#GTX11400; GeneTex, Irvine, CA, USA) and CD45-BV605 (#304042; BioLegend). CTCs were characterized as AF488/FITC-positive and BV605-negative and enumerated manually by two independent operators under a fluorescence microscope at 20× magnification.

Clinical parameter assessment
Primary tumor samples were collected at the initial diagnosis, and IHC was performed for estrogen receptor (ER), progesterone receptor (PR), HER2 and Ki-67. If the patient had primary metastatic disease, a biopsy from the metastatic site was obtained when possible, including marker assessment: ER, PR and HER2. Histopathological diagnosis was conducted by two independent pathologists from the breast cancer unit at the University Hospital Basel. All patients were treated at the Breast Cancer Unit University Hospital Basel according to local standard operating procedures and National Comprehensive Cancer Network and European Society for Medical Oncology guidelines by senior breast oncologists. If a patient had a progression within new distant sites, a new biopsy from that site was taken, when possible, to determine ER, PR and HER2. Patients under systemic treatment had tumor assessment at least every 12 weeks with computed tomographic scans or earlier if tumor progression was anticipated. CTC collection was performed at progression and prior to the next line of therapy or before any treatment was conducted. The patients' data was retrieved by detailed retrospective chart review. Data collection included demographics and disease-specific and treatment-specific data including age, gender, primary stage, histologic subtype, ER/PR/HER2 status, grading, Ki-67, date of primary diagnosis and relapse, type of relapse (localized, metastatic), site of distant disease, bone-modifying agents (bisphosphonates, denosumab), palliative irradiation, and type of systemic treatment, including time on treatment and time to next subsequent treatment. Data was correlated with CTC counts.

Blood parameter assessment
Complete blood counts were measured with the ADVIA 120 Hematology Analyzer (Siemens Healthcare Diagnostics, Tarrytown, NY, USA) using Multispecies version 5.9.0-MS software (Bayer Diagnostics, Tarrytown, NY, USA). Blood samples were taken before each new therapy cycle or at least every month, including cancer antigen 15-3 (CA 15-3), alkaline phosphatase, Ca^{2+}, C-reactive protein, lactate dehydrogenase, red blood cells (RBC), hemoglobin, hematocrit, mean corpuscular volume (MCV), mean corpuscular hemoglobin concentration, white blood cells

(WBC), neutrophils, lymphocytes, monocytes, eosinophils, basophils, large unstained cells, platelets and mean platelet volume (MPV). In the vast majority of cases, blood samples were taken simultaneously with the CTC sample or within 7 days after CTCs were taken. Eight of 73 patients had only partial data available, whereas no blood counts were reported at the time of CTC detection for nine of 73 patients.

Statistical analysis

We first screened our data to exclude variables and patients with high content of missing information, as well as observations with implausible values. Cancer therapies were simplified into three main nonexclusive categories (targeted therapy, chemotherapy and hormone therapy) (Additional file 1: Table S1). Some patients had undergone multiple lines of therapy. For this reason, we assessed the effects of accumulated therapies and the therapy at CTC evaluation separately.

We investigated the association between the different variables of interest and the presence of CTCs using Fisher's exact test for categorical variables, two-sided Wilcoxon rank-sum test for continuous variables (e.g., complete blood counts) and Kruskal-Wallis test for ordinal variables with more than two levels (e.g., stage at diagnosis). A list of the statistical tests used for each variable can be found in Additional file 2: Table S2. For each test, we present the nominal P value. An estimate and 95% CI are also provided for continuous and two-level categorical variables. The estimate corresponds to the OR in Fisher's exact test and to the estimated median of the difference between samples from both groups in the Wilcoxon rank-sum test. To account for potential confounding variables, logistic regression analysis was conducted, adjusting by age at primary diagnosis, tumor stage at diagnosis, tumor grade and histologic subtype. Adjusted P values were calculated following the Benjamini-Hochberg method, combining all tests performed in this work. Associations with an adjusted P value ≤ 0.05 are highlighted in the text. We conducted the data wrangling and statistical analysis in R (version 3.4.0; R Foundation for Statistical Computing, Vienna, Austria).

Results

Patient characteristics

Given previously reported correlations between number of CTCs and tumor load [8], as well as the findings that CTC counts predict poor prognosis in breast cancer [3, 4, 9], we focused on a group of 73 consecutive patients with invasive breast cancer with the following characteristics: high tumor load, detailed treatment history available, progressive disease associated with treatment discontinuation at the time of CTC isolation (before the next line of therapy), and availability of comprehensive blood counts performed at CTC collection. Selected patients ranged from 36 to 85 years of age and carried

either invasive ductal, lobular or inflammatory carcinoma, with a broad expression range of ER, PR, HER2 and Ki-67 protein levels, as well as tumor grade varying from 1 to 3. Detailed characteristics of patients, therapies and statistical tests used for the analysis are listed in Additional file 1: Table S1, Additional file 2: Table S2, and Additional file 3: Table S3.

CTC isolation and enumeration

Blood samples were drawn in EDTA vacutainers and processed directly with the Parsortix microfluidic device [10], with a dedicated protocol enabling the isolation of > 99% of breast CTCs from unlabeled blood samples (Additional file 4: Figure S1A). Upon enrichment, CTCs were stained with an antibody cocktail against EpCAM, EGFR and HER2 and counterstained for the WBC marker CD45 (Additional file 4: Figure S1A and B). With this approach, we detected at least one CTC per 7.5 ml of peripheral blood in 34 (46.6%) patients. Among these, we observed that 22 (64.7%) patients were characterized by the presence of single CTCs and that 12 (35.3%) patients had both single CTCs and CTC clusters (Additional file 4: Figure S1C).

Features of patients with CTCs

We investigated a number of clinicopathological variables to identify features associated with patients in whom either single CTCs or CTC clusters were found, compared with patients with no detectable CTCs. We first observed that previous treatments with targeted therapy (including but not limited to hormonal, anti-HER2, anti-CDK4/6 treatments), chemotherapy or radiotherapy did not correlate with the presence of CTCs (Additional file 5: Table S4). Yet, we found that treatment with the anti-bone resorption antibody denosumab (received by 21 of 73 patients) was associated with the absence of CTCs (OR, 0.25; 95% CI, 0.06–0.86; $P = 0.019$). Namely, the prevalence of CTCs was 14.7% (5 of 21) among patients treated with denosumab and 55.8% (29 of 52) among nontreated patients (Table 1). Further, when considering only those patients in whom CTCs were detected, the average CTC number was 9.8 for patients treated with denosumab ($n = 5$) versus 24.79 for nontreated patients ($n = 29$). Despite their role as anti-bone resorption agents, the same association was not seen for bisphosphonates ($P = 0.784$). Importantly, anti-bone resorption treatment with either denosumab or bisphosphonates was decided on the basis of treatment initiation date (denosumab was approved in Switzerland in December 2011 and given as the preferred treatment option to eligible patients after that date), whereas patients who started receiving bisphosphonates (i.e., prior to December 2011) continued receiving bisphosphonates unless major side effects

Table 1 Clinical features of patients with circulating tumor cells

	No CTC (n = 39)	CTC (n = 34)	P value	Estimate (95% CI)
Age at primary diagnosis, years, mean (SD)	58.38 (11.85)	55.1 (11.04)	0.444	− 2.76 (− 8.49, 2.84)
Age at first CTC evaluation, years, mean (SD)	63.53 (11.69)	59.58 (10.7)	0.163	− 4.11 (− 9.27, 1.63)
Stage at diagnosis, n (%)			0.679	–
I	4 (10.53%)	5 (14.71%)		
IA	1 (2.63%)	0 (0%)		
II	5 (13.16%)	4 (11.76%)		
IIA	1 (2.63%)	4 (11.76%)		
III	11 (28.95%)	7 (20.59%)		
IIIA	2 (5.26%)	0 (0%)		
IIIC	0 (0%)	2 (5.88%)		
IV	14 (36.84%)	11 (32.35%)		
Lymphocyte node involvement, n (%)			0.881	–
N0	11 (31.43%)	8 (25.81%)		
N1	11 (31.43%)	14 (45.16%)		
N2	6 (17.14%)	0 (0%)		
N3	6 (17.14%)	9 (29.03%)		
Histologic subtype, n (%)			0.964	–
Invasive lobular	6 (15.38%)	4 (11.76%)		
Invasive ductal	31 (79.49%)	29 (85.29%)		
Inflammatory invasive lobular	1 (2.56%)	1 (2.94%)		
Inflammatory	2 (5.13%)	2 (5.88%)		
% of ER$^+$ cells, mean (SD)	65.82 (42.48)	59.79 (40.93)	0.386	0 (− 10, 0)
% of PR$^+$ cells, mean (SD)	38.97 (40.04)	26.35 (33.78)	0.171	− 4 (− 20, 0)
% of Ki-67$^+$ cells, mean (SD)	27.08 (17.13)	31.59 (21.55)	0.514	5 (− 5, 10)
HER2$^+$	7 (17.95%)	7 (22.58%)	0.766	1.33 (0.35–5.11)
Triple-negative	4 (10.81%)	3 (9.68%)	1.000	0.89 (0.12–5.73)
Tumor grade			0.985	–
1	4 (10.53%)	4 (12.12%)		
2	17 (44.74%)	14 (42.42%)		
3	17 (44.74%)	15 (45.45%)		
Bisphosphonates	9 (23.68%)	7 (20.59%)	0.784	0.84 (0.23–2.94)
Denosumab	16 (41.03%)	5 (14.71%)	0.019	0.25 (0.06–0.86)
Radiotherapy	22 (56.41%)	13 (38.24%)	0.160	0.48 (0.17–1.35)
Relapse				
Any	31 (79.49%)	25 (73.53%)	0.589	0.72 (0.21–2.45)
Local	3 (7.69%)	4 (11.76%)	0.698	1.59 (0.25–11.72)
Metastasis	26 (66.67%)	19 (55.88%)	0.470	0.64 (0.22–1.82)
Days between primary diagnosis and relapse, mean (SD)	1954.08 (2042.25)	1893.48 (1853.86)	0.966	− 9.37 (− 1000, 756)
Established metastatic disease at CTC evaluation	35 (89.74%)	30 (88.24%)	1.000	0.86 (0.15–5.04)
Number of metastatic sites, mean (SD)	2.09 (1.01)	1.9 (0.94)	0.473	0 (− 1, 0)
Metastasis site, n (%)				
Bone	27 (69.23%)	17 (51.52%)	0.150	0.45 (0.15–1.28)
Liver	10 (25.64%)	12 (36.36%)	0.447	1.57 (0.51–4.9)
Lymph node	9 (23.08%)	10 (30.3%)	0.599	1.38 (0.43–4.54)

Table 1 Clinical features of patients with circulating tumor cells *(Continued)*

	No CTC (n = 39)	CTC (n = 34)	P value	Estimate (95% CI)
Pleural	7 (17.95%)	2 (6.06%)	0.162	0.29 (0.03–1.68)
Peritoneal	3 (7.69%)	4 (12.12%)	0.698	1.59 (0.25–11.72)
Lung	4 (10.26%)	4 (12.12%)	1.000	1.16 (0.2–6.83)
Skin	3 (7.69%)	0 (0%)	0.243	0 (0–2.74)
Brain	2 (5.13%)	2 (6.06%)	1.000	1.15 (0.08–16.76)
Uterus	1 (2.56%)	1 (3.03%)	1.000	1.15 (0.01–92.67)
Muscular	1 (2.56%)	2 (6.06%)	0.595	2.35 (0.12–143.61)

Abbreviations: ER Estrogen receptor, *HER2* Human epidermal growth factor receptor 2, *PR* Progesterone receptor
The table shows clinical features of patients with and without circulating tumor cells (CTCs)

occurred (Additional file 6: Table S5). When we restricted the analysis to the 44 patients with bone metastasis, denosumab was administered to 20 of 44 of them, and it also correlated with a reduction in CTC numbers compared with the remaining 24 patients with bone metastasis but no denosumab treatment (OR, 0.22; 95% CI, 0.04–0.96; $P = 0.03$) (Table 2). These results were confirmed using logistic regression adjusting by age at primary diagnosis, tumor stage at diagnosis, tumor grade and histologic subtype (OR, 0.25; 95% CI, 0.06–0.82; $P = 0.03$). When comparing clinicopathological variables in patients who were treated or not with denosumab, as expected, we observed a correlation with bone metastasis (OR, 22.53; 95% CI, 3.14–995.64; $P = 5.6e$-05; adjusted $P = 0.01$) (Additional file 7: Table S6), but no effect on progression-free survival was seen (Additional file 8: Figure S2). Together, our data show that denosumab treatment is associated with a marked reduction of CTC counts in patients with breast cancer.

Features of patients with CTC clusters

We further asked whether any clinicopathological variables might be associated specifically with the presence of CTC clusters, compared with patients in whom CTC clusters were not found (i.e., having either single CTCs or no CTCs). We found that both younger age at primary diagnosis and younger age at first CTC evaluation were associated with the presence of CTC clusters (Table 3). Particularly, we observed average ages at primary diagnosis of 50.63 years (SD, 12.60) for patients with CTC clusters and 58.08 years (SD, 10.99) for patients with no CTC clusters ($P = 0.033$), as well as average ages at first CTC evaluation of 54.87 years (SD,

12.14) for patients with CTC clusters and 63.03 years (SD, 10.77) for patients with no CTC clusters ($P = 0.025$). We also observed that although HER2 was expressed in 22% (13 of 61) of patients with no CTC clusters (7 of 39) (i.e., 17.95% of patients with no CTCs and 6 of 22 [30%] of patients with single CTCs only), it was expressed in only 1 patient (9.09%) with CTC clusters (OR, 0.36; 95% CI, 0.01–2.97; $P = 0.44$), even though the relationship between HER2 negativity and CTC clusters did not reach statistical significance (Table 3).

When considering only patients with CTCs and comparing those with CTC clusters versus those with single CTCs, we found that also in this context younger age at primary diagnosis ($P = 0.044$) and younger age at first CTC evaluation ($P = 0.058$) were associated with the presence of CTC clusters (Additional file 9: Table S7).

Blood parameters associated with CTCs

In addition to investigating the clinical parameters summarized above, for each patient, we also evaluated comprehensive blood counts performed at CTC collection. We first asked whether blood-related parameters were associated with the presence of CTCs (either single or clustered), compared with patients in whom CTCs were not detected. We observed that patients with detectable CTCs had a lower RBC count (OR, – 0.42; 95% CI, – 0.8 – -0.08; $P = 0.019$) than patients with no CTCs (Table 4).

Blood parameters associated with CTC clusters

We then asked whether specific blood-related parameters could be associated with the presence of CTC clusters, compared with patients with no CTC clusters (i.e., having either no CTCs or single CTCs only). In this

Table 2 Circulating tumor cells detection according to denosumab treatment and bone metastasis

	Number of samples	No CTCs	CTCs	P value	Estimate (95% CI)	P value	Estimate (95% CI)
Reference	28	12 (43%)	16 (57%)	Reference		–	–
Bone metastasis	24	11 (46%)	13 (54%)	1.000	0.89 (0.26–3.05)	Reference	
Bone metastasis and denosumab	20	16 (80%)	4 (20%)	0.017	0.19 (0.04–0.81)	0.030	0.22 (0.04–0.96)

The table shows the number of patients with and without circulating tumor cells (CTCs) among individuals with bone metastasis who were treated or not with denosumab

Table 3 Clinical features of patients with circulating tumor cell clusters

	No CTC clusters (n = 61)	CTC clusters (n = 12)	P value	Estimate (95% CI)
Age at primary diagnosis, years, mean (SD)	58.08 (10.99)	50.63 (12.6)	0.033	− 8.26 (− 15.3, − 0.44)
Age at first CTC evaluation, years, mean (SD)	63.03 (10.77)	54.87 (12.14)	0.025	− 8.3 (− 16.06, − 1.04)
Stage at diagnosis, n (%)			0.726	–
I	7 (11.67%)	2 (16.67%)		
IA	1 (1.67%)	0 (0%)		
II	7 (11.67%)	2 (16.67%)		
IIA	4 (6.67%)	1 (8.33%)		
III	16 (26.67%)	2 (16.67%)		
IIIA	2 (3.33%)	0 (0%)		
IIIC	1 (1.67%)	1 (8.33%)		
IV	21 (35%)	4 (33.33%)		
Lymphocyte node involvement, n (%)			0.855	–
N0	15 (27.27%)	4 (36.36%)		
N1	22 (40%)	3 (27.27%)		
N2	6 (10.91%)	0 (0%)		
N3	11 (20%)	4 (36.36%)		
Histologic subtype, n (%)			0.679	–
Invasive lobular	9 (14.75%)	1 (8.33%)		
Invasive ductal	49 (80.33%)	11 (91.67%)		
Inflammatory invasive lobular	1 (1.64%)	1 (8.33%)		
Inflammatory	3 (4.92%)	1 (8.33%)		
% of ER$^+$ cells, mean (SD)	62.34 (41.8)	66.42 (42.1)	0.675	0 (− 10, 20)
% of PR$^+$ cells, mean (SD)	32.71 (37.79)	34 (37.3)	0.888	0 (− 10, 20)
% of Ki-67$^+$ cells, mean (SD)	30 (19.65)	23 (16.43)	0.384	− 5 (− 20, − 10)
HER2$^+$, n (%)	13 (22.03%)	1 (9.09%)	0.442	0.36 (0.01–2.97)
Triple-negative, n (%)	7 (12.28%)	0 (0%)	0.588	0 (0–3.7)
Tumor grade, n (%)			0.093	–
1	5 (8.33%)	3 (27.27%)		
2	26 (43.33%)	5 (45.45%)		
3	29 (48.33%)	3 (27.27%)		
Bisphosphonates, n (%)	14 (23.33%)	2 (16.67%)	1.000	0.66 (0.06–3.68)
Denosumab, n (%)	19 (31.15%)	2 (16.67%)	0.489	0.45 (0.04–2.41)
Radiotherapy, n (%)	30 (49.18%)	5 (41.67%)	0.756	0.74 (0.17–3.06)
Relapse, n (%)				
Any	47 (77.05%)	9 (75%)	1.000	0.9 (0.19–5.83)
Local	4 (6.56%)	3 (25%)	0.082	4.61 (0.58–32.62)
Metastasis	40 (65.57%)	5 (41.67%)	0.193	0.38 (0.08–1.59)
Days between primary diagnosis and relapse, mean (SD)	1969.49 (2003.96)	1636.67 (1538.48)	0.633	− 236.86 (− 1643, 1203)
Established metastatic disease at CTC evaluation, n (%)	54 (88.52%)	11 (91.67%)	1.000	1.42 (0.15–70.01)
Number of metastatic sites, mean (SD)	1.96 (0.98)	2.18 (0.98)	0.452	0 (0–1)
Metastasis site, n (%)				
Bone	37 (61.67%)	7 (58.33%)	1.000	0.91 (0.22–4.08)
Liver	19 (31.67%)	3 (25%)	1.000	0.74 (0.12–3.42)
Lymph node	15 (25%)	4 (33.33%)	0.497	1.52 (0.29–6.74)

Table 3 Clinical features of patients with circulating tumor cell clusters *(Continued)*

	No CTC clusters (n = 61)	CTC clusters (n = 12)	P value	Estimate (95% CI)
Pleural	9 (15%)	0 (0%)	0.339	0 (0–2.57)
Peritoneal	5 (8.33%)	2 (16.67%)	0.323	2.21 (0.19–16.05)
Lung	7 (11.67%)	1 (8.33%)	1.000	0.7 (0.01–6.47)
Skin	3 (5%)	0 (0%)	1.000	0 (0–12.81)
Brain	3 (5%)	1 (8.33%)	0.521	1.74 (0.03–24.14)
Uterus	1 (1.67%)	1 (8.33%)	0.304	5.27 (0.06–433.34)
Muscular	2 (3.33%)	1 (8.33%)	0.421	2.63 (0.04–54.78)

Abbreviations: ER Estrogen receptor, *HER2* Human epidermal growth factor receptor 2, *PR* Progesterone receptor
The table shows clinical features of patients with and without circulating tumor cell clusters (CTC clusters)

case, we found that patients with CTC clusters have 14-fold higher levels of the CA 15-3 tumor marker ($P = 0.021$), higher MCV ($P = 0.033$), higher WBC ($P = 0.03$) and higher MPV ($P = 0.032$) than patients in whom CTC clusters were not found (Table 5). We also restricted this analysis to patients with CTCs and compared patients with CTC clusters with patients with only single CTCs. In this setting, we further confirmed that patients with CTC clusters have 38-fold higher CA 15-3 tumor antigen ($P = 0.0089$), as well as nearly twofold higher total

WBC counts ($P = 0.0045$) and higher neutrophil counts ($P = 0.03$) (Additional file 10: Table S8).

Discussion

In a selected cohort of 73 patients with progressive invasive breast cancer, we provide a detailed description of a number of clinicopathological parameters and blood counts at the time of CTC isolation that correlate with the presence of single CTCs and CTC clusters. Interestingly, we observed that treatment with the monoclonal

Table 4 Complete blood counts in patients with circulating tumor cells

	No CTC (n = 39)	CTC (n = 34)	P value	Estimate (95% CI)
CA 15-3, mean (SD)	223.71 (384.68)	1084.15 (4136.87)	0.658	6.7 (− 19.2, 87.6)
Alkaline phosphatase, mean (SD)	105.47 (103.98)	198.15 (365.58)	0.401	6 (− 12, 27)
Calcium (korr), mean (SD)	2.34 (0.15)	2.32 (0.25)	0.145	− 0.06 (− 0.13, 0.02)
CRP, mean (SD)	31.92 (47.56)	26.87 (47.69)	0.982	0 (− 8.8, 3.8)
LDH, mean (SD)	281.61 (118.18)	300.15 (228.57)	0.772	− 5 (− 36, 23)
RBC, 10^{12}/L, mean (SD)	4.37 (0.56)	3.85 (0.77)	0.019	− 0.42 (− 0.8, − 0.08)
HGB, g/L, mean (SD)	130.14 (19.85)	118.15 (24.11)	0.051	− 11 (− 21, 0)
HCT, L/L, mean (SD)	0.38 (0.06)	0.35 (0.06)	0.053	− 0.03 (− 0.06, 0)
MCV, fl, mean (SD)	87.46 (5.68)	89.73 (5.26)	0.227	2 (− 1, 4)
MCH, pg, mean (SD)	29.62 (2.52)	30.66 (1.96)	0.157	0.8 (− 0.3, 1.8)
MCHC, g/L, mean (SD)	339.03 (13.98)	341.19 (12.79)	0.667	2 (− 6, 8)
WBC, 10^9/L, mean (SD)	7.35 (2.13)	7.24 (3.53)	0.334	− 0.6 (− 1.88, 0.81)
Neutrophils, 10^9/L, mean (SD)	5.33 (1.87)	5.12 (2.87)	0.239	− 0.63 (− 1.65, 0.56)
Lymphocytes, 10^9/L, mean (SD)	1.37 (0.67)	1.41 (0.85)	0.941	− 0.02 (− 0.38, 0.38)
Monocytes, 10^9/L, mean (SD)	0.42 (0.12)	0.44 (0.2)	0.843	− 0.01 (− 0.08, 0.07)
Eosinophils, 10^9/L, mean (SD)	0.16 (0.18)	0.17 (0.12)	0.423	0.02 (− 0.03, 0.09)
Basophils, 10^9/L, mean (SD)	0.04 (0.07)	0.04 (0.03)	0.256	0.01 (− 0.01, 0.02)
LUC, 10^9/L, mean (SD)	0.15 (0.22)	0.12 (0.08)	0.912	0 (− 0.03, 0.02)
PLT, 10^9/L, mean (SD)	289.92 (139.86)	249.93 (91.52)	0.277	− 30 (− 84, 24)
MPV, fl, mean (SD)	8.2 (1.51)	8.68 (1.52)	0.109	0 (0–1)

Abbreviations: CA 15-3 Cancer antigen 15-3, *CRP* C-reactive protein, *HCT* Hematocrit, *HGB* Hemoglobin, *LDH* Lactate dehydrogenase, *LUC* Large unstained cells, *MCH* Mean corpuscular hemoglobin, *MCHC* Mean corpuscular hemoglobin concentration, *MCV* Mean corpuscular volume, *MPV* Mean platelet volume, *PLT* Platelets, *RBC* Red blood cells, *WBC* White blood cells
The table shows complete blood counts in patients with and without circulating tumor cells (CTCs).

Table 5 Complete blood counts in patients with circulating tumor cell clusters

	No CTC clusters (n = 61)	CTC clusters (n = 12)	P value	Estimate (95% CI)
CA 15-3, mean (SD)	172.5 (324.45)	2554.6 (6387.64)	0.021	204.16 (9.7–515)
Alkaline phosphatase, mean (SD)	106.4 (104.27)	310.25 (525.57)	0.301	10 (− 12, 74.58)
Calcium (korr), mean (SD)	2.33 (0.14)	2.36 (0.35)	0.698	− 0.02 (− 0.16, 0.14)
CRP, mean (SD)	27.76 (44.47)	37.25 (58.6)	0.279	2.9 (− 4, 21.4)
LDH, mean (SD)	271 (102.59)	363.33 (329.24)	0.463	17 (− 26, 76)
RBC, 10^{12}/L, mean (SD)	4.26 (0.6)	3.66 (0.93)	0.078	− 0.51 (− 1.16, 0.06)
HGB, g/L, mean (SD)	127.52 (20.18)	114.18 (29.19)	0.183	− 12 (− 30, 6)
HCT, L/L, mean (SD)	0.38 (0.05)	0.34 (0.08)	0.159	− 0.03 (− 0.09, 0.01)
MCV, fl, mean (SD)	87.7 (5.58)	91.73 (4.41)	0.033	4 (0–7)
MCH, pg, mean (SD)	29.8 (2.42)	31.24 (1.51)	0.064	1.1 (0–2.3)
MCHC, g/L, mean (SD)	339.8 (13.38)	340.64 (14.25)	0.646	2 (− 10, 10)
WBC, 10^9/L, mean (SD)	6.87 (2.25)	9.38 (3.99)	0.030	2.54 (0.26–4.68)
Neutrophils, 10^9/L, mean (SD)	4.94 (1.87)	6.65 (3.6)	0.177	1.22 (− 0.52, 3.68)
Lymphocytes, 10^9/L, mean (SD)	1.38 (0.69)	1.42 (1)	0.756	− 0.11 (− 0.62, 0.6)
Monocytes, 10^9/L, mean (SD)	0.41 (0.13)	0.5 (0.24)	0.336	0.06 (− 0.08, 0.26)
Eosinophils, 10^9/L, mean (SD)	0.16 (0.16)	0.17 (0.14)	0.974	0 (− 0.07, 0.1)
Basophils, 10^9/L, mean (SD)	0.04 (0.06)	0.04 (0.04)	0.983	0 (− 0.02, 0.02)
LUC, 10^9/L, mean (SD)	0.14 (0.19)	0.12 (0.11)	0.471	− 0.01 (− 0.05, 0.02)
PLT, 10^9/L, mean (SD)	278.02 (125.8)	251.5 (109.99)	0.667	− 15.84 (− 94, 47)
MPV, fl, mean (SD)	8.32 (1.62)	8.82 (0.87)	0.032	1 (0–1)

Abbreviations: CA 15-3 Cancer antigen 15-3, *CRP* C-reactive protein, *HCT* Hematocrit, *HGB* Hemoglobin, *LDH* Lactate dehydrogenase, *LUC* Large unstained cells, *MCH* Mean corpuscular hemoglobin, *MCHC* Mean corpuscular hemoglobin concentration, *MCV* Mean corpuscular volume, *MPV* Mean platelet volume, *PLT* Platelets, *RBC* Red blood cells, *WBC* White blood cells
The table shows complete blood counts in patients with and without circulating tumor cell clusters (CTC clusters)

antibody denosumab in patients with bone metastasis strongly correlated with the absence of CTCs from their peripheral circulation, suggesting a scenario in which the treatment itself might influence CTC spread from the bone tissue. Importantly, this correlation is not seen regarding treatment with the anti-bone resorption drug bisphosphonate, possibly because of different administration routes or dosing schedules [11] or, alternatively, potential off-target binding of denosumab to proteins other than receptor activator of nuclear factor κB ligand (RANKL).

Although its focus was on clinical parameters, our study did not provide molecular insights into the mechanism of action of denosumab in the context of its role in inhibiting CTC generation. Yet, considering that most denosumab-treated patients are characterized by bone metastatic disease but no primary breast tumor (which has been surgically removed prior to denosumab treatment), CTCs represent derivatives of their bone metastatic lesions. In this setting, we speculate that the effect of denosumab in suppressing CTC generation could be a result of RANKL inhibition within the bone, preventing the maturation of preosteoclasts into osteoclasts [12] and protecting the bone from degradation, leading to a

lower likelihood of a bone metastatic lesion to shed CTCs. However, we cannot exclude an action of denosumab on breast cancer cells themselves, which have previously been shown to express high receptor activator of nuclear factor κB (RANK) levels [13, 14] and may be susceptible to its inhibition. Prospective studies and molecular assays will be needed to specifically dissect the role and mechanism of action of denosumab in CTC generation.

Recently, a phase 3 clinical trial designed to determine the long-term effects of denosumab treatment (D-CARE; ClinicalTrials.gov, NCT01077154) showed no benefits in metastasis-free survival and overall survival of patients with breast cancer. Importantly, individuals within this study were mainly patients with early breast cancer (i.e., stage IIB to IIIC), while our patient cohort was largely dominated by patients with stage IV disease. Although we are not aware of CTC enumeration data being evaluated within the D-CARE study, it is possible that denosumab might play a different role in the intravasation of bone metastasis-derived CTCs (as seen in our study) as opposed to primary tumor-derived CTCs (D-CARE).

Among other correlations, we observed an intriguing association between the absence of HER2 expression in the primary tumor and the presence of CTC clusters.

Although this result did not reach statistical significance, our observation regarding HER2 does not seem to be influenced by the metastatic tropism of HER2-positive breast cancers, and it might reveal important insights into the signaling networks involving CTC cluster formation, also considering HER2 expression fluctuations in CTCs and breast cancer metastasis [15, 16]. In other words, we speculate that HER2 signaling might influence cancer cells to intravasate as single CTCs, whereas its absence might point them toward collective invasion into the bloodstream. This hypothesis will require experimental testing.

We also found that CTC clusters, but not CTCs in general, are more prevalent in younger patients. Both CTC clusters and younger age have been associated with worse prognosis and reduced survival rates [2, 5, 17–20]. In this case, it is unlikely that younger age represents an independent risk factor for CTC cluster formation, but rather it may reflect an association with tumor aggressiveness [21].

Last, blood counts at the time of CTC collection provide evidence for applying well-established, cost-effective and widespread blood-testing strategies to stratify patients with higher likelihood to present with detectable CTCs. For instance, we find that lower RBC count has good correlation with the presence of CTCs. Additionally, CA 15-3 tumor antigen is highly increased in patients with CTC clusters, possibly reflecting a higher tumor load but also tumors that are characterized by an elevated shedding of mucin 1 (MUC-1)-containing cells into the bloodstream [22]. A functional relationship between MUC-1 and CTC clusters remains to be investigated. We also observed that higher MCV, higher MPV and higher WBC counts correlate with the presence of CTC clusters. We envision these parameters to be used to stratify patient populations to conduct CTC-related studies in the setting of advanced breast cancer.

Altogether, our study is meant as an exploratory analysis to evaluate the association of multiple clinical predictors with the presence of CTCs. Given the high number of hypotheses tested and the relatively low number of patient samples in the study ($n = 73$), none of the associations reported show a P value less than 0.05 after adjustment for multiple comparisons, with the exception of the correlation between denosumab treatment and the presence of bone metastasis (adjusted $P = 0.01$). For this reason, subsequent prospective and experimental studies should be conducted to validate the associations that are presented in this work, including the role of denosumab in CTC shedding.

Conclusions

Our data provide evidence of the association between treatment with the monoclonal antibody denosumab and the absence of CTCs from the peripheral circulation of patients with breast cancer. This finding suggests that denosumab treatment may be beneficial to reduce cancer spread in patients who are diagnosed with bone metastasis.

Although factors such as limited blood volume and diverse CTC isolation technologies may influence CTC detection rate in patients with cancer, the identification of a set of clinical correlatives to CTCs in breast cancer is likely to facilitate the identification of those patients who would benefit the most from CTC analysis, including genetic profile assessment for patient stratification [6, 23] and testing of drug susceptibility [7]. As an added benefit to this analysis, the identification of denosumab treatment as a strategy to reduce CTC intravasation warrants further investigation.

Additional files

Additional file 1: Table S1. Drug classification. The table shows the drug classification used for the analysis, grouping drugs into targeted therapy, chemotherapy, hormone therapy and immunotherapy. *Abbreviations: cbx6* Chromobox 6, *CDK4* Cyclin-dependent kinase 4, *CDK6* Cyclin-dependent kinase 6, *EGFR* Epidermal growth factor receptor, *Her2* Human epidermal growth factor receptor 2, *mTOR* Mechanistic target of rapamycin, *PD-L1* Programmed cell death 1 ligand 1, *VEGF* Vascular endothelial growth factor. (XLSX 10 kb)

Additional file 2: Table S2. Variable classification and statistical test applied. The table shows the type of variable and statistical test used for the analysis of individual clinicopathological parameters. *Abbreviations: ER,* Estrogen receptor, *HER2,* Human epidermal growth factor receptor 2, *PR* Progesterone receptor. (XLSX 10 kb)

Additional file 3: Table S3. Patient characteristics. The table shows the characteristics of the 73 patients included in the study. *Abbreviations: ER* Estrogen receptor, *HER2* Human epidermal growth factor receptor 2, *ID* Invasive ductal, *IL* Invasive lobular, *NA* Not available, *PR* Progesterone receptor, *ECOG* Eastern Cooperative Oncology Group (as defined by Oken et al. [24]). (XLSX 14 kb)

Additional file 4: Figure S1. Circulating tumor cell (CTC) capture strategy. (**a**) Schematic drawing showing the size-based capturing principle of the Parsortix microfluidic device (*left*). Plot showing the capture efficiency of the Parsortix microfluidic device for MCF7 cells spiked in healthy blood samples (*right*). Representative images of a captured MCF7 single cell, a cell cluster (*green*) and a contaminant white blood cell (WBC; red) in the Parsortix microfluidic cassette (*bottom*). (**b**) Representative images of a captured single CTC, a CTC cluster (*green*) and a contaminant WBC (*red*) from a breast cancer patient sample. (**c**) Bar graph showing the number of patients in whom no CTCs, single CTCs or CTC clusters were found. (PDF 245 kb)

Additional file 5: Table S4. Therapy evaluation in patients with circulating tumor cells. The table shows the types of therapy that patients with and without circulating tumor cells (CTCs) underwent. (XLSX 9 kb)

Additional file 6: Table S5. Bisphosphonates or denosumab treatment. The table shows whether bisphosphonates or denosumab was administered to each of the patients included in the study. (XLSX 10 kb)

Additional file 7: Table S6. Clinical features of patients who were treated or not with denosumab. The table shows clinical features of patients who were treated or not with denosumab. *Abbreviations: ER* Estrogen receptor, *HER2* Human epidermal growth factor receptor 2, *PR* Progesterone receptor. (XLSX 11 kb)

Additional file 8: Figure S2. Progression-free survival of patients who were treated or not with denosumab. Kaplan-Meier curve showing the progression-free survival probability of patients who were treated (*red*) or not (*green*) with denosumab (*top*). $P = 0.95$ by pairwise log-rank test. The table shows the number of patients at each time point (*bottom*). (PDF 188 kb)

Additional file 9: Table S7. Clinical features of patients with single circulating tumor cell and circulating tumor cell clusters. The table shows clinical features of patients in whom only single circulating tumor cells (CTC single cell) or also clustered circulating tumor cells (CTC clusters) were found. *Abbreviations: ER* Estrogen receptor, *HER2* Human epidermal growth factor receptor 2, *PR* Progesterone receptor. (XLSX 11 kb)

Additional file 10: Table S8. Complete blood counts in patients with single circulating tumor cells and circulating tumor cell clusters. The table shows complete blood counts in patients in whom only single circulating tumor cells (single CTC) or also clustered circulating tumor cells (CTC clusters) were found. *Abbreviations: CA 15-3* Cancer antigen 15-3, *CRP* C-reactive protein, *HCT* Hematocrit, *HGB* Hemoglobin, *LDH* Lactate dehydrogenase, *LUC* Large unstained cells, *MCH* Mean corpuscular hemoglobin, *MCHC* Mean corpuscular hemoglobin concentration, *MCV* Mean corpuscular volume, *MPV* Mean platelet volume, *PLT* Platelets, *RBC* Red blood cells, *WBC* White blood cells. (XLSX 10 kb)

Abbreviations

AF488: Alexa Fluor 488; CA 15-3: Cancer antigen 15-3; CRP: C-reactive protein; CTC: Circulating tumor cell; EDTA: Ethylenediaminetetraacetic acid; EGFR: Epidermal growth factor receptor; EpCAM: Epithelial cell adhesion molecule; ER: Estrogen receptor; FITC: Fluorescein isothiocyanate; HCT: Hematocrit; HER2: Human epidermal growth factor receptor 2; HGB: Hemoglobin; LDH: Lactate dehydrogenase; LUC: Large unstained cells; MCH: Mean corpuscular hemoglobin; MCHC: Mean corpuscular hemoglobin concentration; MCV: Mean corpuscular volume; MPV: Mean platelet volume; MUC-1: Mucin 1; PLT: Platelets; PR: Progesterone receptor; RANK: Receptor activator of nuclear factor κB; RANKL: Receptor activator of nuclear factor κB ligand; RBC: Red blood cells; WBC: White blood cells

Acknowledgements

We thank all the patients who participated in the study, all involved clinicians and study nurses, and all members of the Aceto laboratory for feedback and discussions. We also thank Julia Gutzwiller for data collection.

Funding

Research in the Aceto laboratory is supported by the European Research Council, the Swiss National Science Foundation, the Swiss Cancer League, the Basel Cancer League, the two cantons of Basel through the ETH Zürich, and the University of Basel.

Authors' contributions

MV, JL, CB, AM, AZ, CK, VHS, WPW and CR consented all study patients, collected patient samples, interpreted the data and provided clinical input. BMS, SG, CD, IK and RS performed microfluidic CTC isolation and enumeration, data interpretation and troubleshooting. FCG. performed statistical analysis. NA supervised the study and drafted the manuscript. All authors read and approved the final version of the manuscript.

Competing interests

NA, BMS and FCG are listed as inventors in a patent application filed by the University of Basel, entitled "Inhibitors of bone resorption for treatment of metastasis" (#EP18161098). The other authors declare that they have no competing interests.

Author details

[1]Gynecologic Cancer Center, University Hospital Basel, 4056 Basel, Switzerland. [2]Department of Medical Oncology, University Hospital Basel, 4056 Basel, Switzerland. [3]Department of Biomedicine, Cancer Metastasis Laboratory, University of Basel and University Hospital Basel, Mattenstrasse 28, CH-4058 Basel, Switzerland. [4]SIB Swiss Institute of Bioinformatics, 1015 Lausanne, Switzerland. [5]Breast Center, University Hospital Basel, 4056 Basel, Switzerland.

References

1. Aceto N, Toner M, Maheswaran S, Haber DA. En route to metastasis: circulating tumor cell clusters and epithelial-to-mesenchymal transition. Trends Cancer. 2015;1:44–52.
2. Rack B, Schindlbeck C, Jückstock J, Andergassen U, Hepp P, Zwingers T, et al. Circulating tumor cells predict survival in early average-to-high risk breast cancer patients. J Natl Cancer Inst. 2014;106:dju066.
3. Cristofanilli M, Budd GT, Ellis MJ, Stopeck A, Matera J, Miller MC, et al. Circulating tumor cells, disease progression, and survival in metastatic breast cancer. N Engl J Med. 2004;351:781–91.
4. Giuliano M, Giordano A, Jackson S, Hess KR, De Giorgi U, Mego M, et al. Circulating tumor cells as prognostic and predictive markers in metastatic breast cancer patients receiving first-line systemic treatment. Breast Cancer Res. 2011;13:R67.
5. Aceto N, Bardia A, Miyamoto DT, Donaldson MC, Wittner BS, Spencer JA, et al. Circulating tumor cell clusters are oligoclonal precursors of breast cancer metastasis. Cell. 2014;158:1110–22.
6. Carter L, Rothwell DG, Mesquita B, Smowton C, Leong HS, Fernandez-Gutierrez F, et al. Molecular analysis of circulating tumor cells identifies distinct copy-number profiles in patients with chemosensitive and chemorefractory small-cell lung cancer. Nat Med. 2017;23:114–9.
7. Yu M, Bardia A, Aceto N, Bersani F, Madden MW, Donaldson MC, et al. Cancer therapy: ex vivo culture of circulating breast tumor cells for individualized testing of drug susceptibility. Science. 2014;345:216–20.
8. Kaifi JT, Kunkel M, Dicker DT, Joude J, Allen JE, Das A, et al. Circulating tumor cell levels are elevated in colorectal cancer patients with high tumor burden in the liver. Cancer Biol Ther. 2015;16:690–8.
9. Cristofanilli M, Broglio KR, Guarneri V, Jackson S, Fritsche HA, Islam R, et al. Circulating tumor cells in metastatic breast cancer: biologic staging beyond tumor burden. Clin Breast Cancer. 2007;7:471–9.
10. Xu L, Mao X, Imrali A, Syed F, Mutsvangwa K, Berney D, et al. Optimization and evaluation of a novel size based circulating tumor cell isolation system. PLoS One. 2015;10:e0138032.
11. Whitaker M, Guo J, Kehoe T, Benson G. Bisphosphonates for osteoporosis—where do we go from here? N Engl J Med. 2012;366:2048–51.
12. Hanley DA, Adachi JD, Bell A, Brown V. Denosumab: mechanism of action and clinical outcomes. Int J Clin Pract. 2012;66:1139–46.
13. Blake ML, Tometsko M, Miller R, Jones JC, Dougall WC. RANK expression on breast cancer cells promotes skeletal metastasis. Clin Exp Metastasis. 2014; 31:233–45.
14. Pfitzner BM, Branstetter D, Loibl S, Denkert C, Lederer B, Schmitt WD, et al. RANK expression as a prognostic and predictive marker in breast cancer. Breast Cancer Res Treat. 2014;145:307–15.
15. Jordan NV, Bardia A, Wittner BS, Benes C, Ligorio M, Zheng Y, et al. HER2 expression identifies dynamic functional states within circulating breast cancer cells. Nature. 2016;537:102–6.
16. Houssami N, Macaskill P, Balleine RL, Bilous M, Pegram MD. HER2 discordance between primary breast cancer and its paired metastasis: tumor biology or test artefact? Insights through meta-analysis. Breast Cancer Res Treat. 2011;129:659–74.
17. Anderson WF, Pfeiffer RM, Dores GM, Sherman ME. Comparison of age distribution patterns for different histopathologic types of breast carcinoma. Cancer Epidemiol Biomark Prev. 2006;15:1899–905.
18. Adami HO, Malker B, Holmberg L, Persson I, Stone B. The relation between survival and age at diagnosis in breast cancer. N Engl J Med. 1986;315:559–63.

19. Fredholm H, Magnusson K, Lindstrom LS, Garmo H, Falt SE, Lindman H, et al. Long-term outcome in young women with breast cancer: a population-based study. Breast Cancer Res Treat. 2016;160:131–43.

20. Bleyer A, Barr R, Hayes-Lattin B, Thomas D, Ellis C, Anderson B, et al. The distinctive biology of cancer in adolescents and young adults. Nat Rev Cancer. 2008;8:288–98.

21. Koleckova M, Kolar Z, Ehrmann J, Korinkova G, Trojanec R. Age-associated prognostic and predictive biomarkers in patients with breast cancer. Oncol Lett. 2017;13:4201–7.

22. Duffy MJCA. 15-3 and related mucins as circulating markers in breast cancer. Ann Clin Biochem. 1999;36(Pt 5):579–86.

23. Lohr JG, Adalsteinsson VA, Cibulskis K, Choudhury AD, Rosenberg M, Cruz-Gordillo P, et al. Whole-exome sequencing of circulating tumor cells provides a window into metastatic prostate cancer. Nat Biotechnol. 2014;32:479–84.

24. Oken MM, Creech RH, Tormey DC, Horton J, Davis TE, McFadden ET, Carbone PP. Toxicity and response criteria of the Eastern Cooperative Oncology Group. Am J Clin Oncol. 1982;5(6):649–55.

Permissions

Contributors

Johanna O. P. Wanders and Carla H. van Gils
Julius Center for Health Sciences and Primary Care, University Medical Center Utrecht, 3508 GA Utrecht, The Netherlands

Petra H. M. Peeters
Julius Center for Health Sciences and Primary Care, University Medical Center Utrecht, 3508 GA Utrecht, The Netherlands MRC-PHE Centre for Environment and Health, Department of Epidemiology and Biostatistics, School of Public Health, Imperial College London, St. Mary's Campus, Norfolk Place W2 1PG, London, UK

Nico Karssemeijer and Katharina Holland
Department of Radiology and Nuclear Medicine, Radboud University Medical Center, Geert Grooteplein 10, 6525 GA Nijmegen, The Netherlands

Michiel Kallenberg, Mads Nielsen and Martin Lillholm
Department of Computer Science, University of Copenhagen, Universitetsparken 5, DK-2100 Copenhagen, Denmark
Biomediq A/S, Fruebjergvej 3, 2100 Copenhagen, Denmark

Wei Xu
Department of Laboratory Medicine, The First Hospital of Jilin University, Changchun 130021, Jilin Province, China

Hui Zhang
Department of Laboratory Medicine, The First Hospital of Jilin University, Changchun 130021, Jilin Province, China
UK Markey Cancer Center, University of Kentucky, Lexington, KY 40536, USA

Gaofeng Xiong and Yifei Qi
UK Markey Cancer Center, University of Kentucky, Lexington, KY 40536, USA

Ren Xu
UK Markey Cancer Center, University of Kentucky, Lexington, KY 40536, USA
Department of Pharmacology and Nutritional Sciences, University of Kentucky, Lexington, KY 40536, USA

Tricia Fredericks
Division of Gynecologic Oncology, Department of Obstetrics and Gynecology, University of Kentucky, Lexington, KY 40504, USA

Piotr G. Rychahou
Department of Surgery, College of Medicine, University of Kentucky, Lexington, KY 40504, USA

Jia-Da Li
Center for Medical Genetics, School of Life Sciences, Central South University, Changsha 410078, Hunan Province, China

Taina Pihlajaniemi
Center for Cell-Matrix Research and Biocenter Oulu, Faculty of Biochemistry and Molecular Medicine, University of Oulu, 90014 Oulu, Finland

Mandy Dumortier, Isabelle Damour, Nathalie Marchand, Yvan de Launoit and David Tulasne
University of Lille, CNRS, Institut Pasteur de Lille, UMR 8161 - M3T – Mechanisms of Tumorigenesis and Targeted Therapies, F-59000 Lille, France

Anne Chotteau-Lelièvre
University of Lille, CNRS, Institut Pasteur de Lille, UMR 8161 - M3T – Mechanisms of Tumorigenesis and Targeted Therapies, F-59000 Lille, France

CNRS UMR 8161, Institut de Biologie de Lille - Institut Pasteur de Lille, 1 Rue Pr Calmette, BP447, 59021 Lille, France

Franck Ladam
Department of Biochemistry and Molecular Pharmacology, University of Massachusetts Medical School, Worcester, MA 01605-2324, USA

Sophie Vacher and Ivan Bièche
Unit of Pharmacogenomics, Department of Genetics, Institut Curie, Paris, France

Judith Penkert, Gunnar Schmidt, Winfried Hofmann, Stephanie Schubert, Maximilian Schieck, Bernd Auber, Tim Ripperger, Thomas Illig, Brigitte Schlegelberger and Doris Steinemann
Department of Human Genetics, Hannover Medical School, Carl-Neuberg-Strasse 1, 30625 Hannover, Germany

Karl Hackmann
Institute for Clinical Genetics, Faculty of Medicine Carl Gustav Carus, TU Dresden, Dresden, Germany
German Cancer Research Center (DKFZ), Heidelberg, Germany
National Center for Tumor Diseases (NCT) Partner Site Dresden, Dresden, Germany

Marc Sturm
Institute of Medical Genetics and Applied Genomics, University of Tübingen, Tübingen, Germany

Holger Prokisch
Institute of Human Genetics, Helmholtz Zentrum München, Neuherberg, Germany

Ursula Hille-Betz
Department of Gynecology and Obstetrics, Hannover Medical School, Hannover, Germany

Dorothea Mark
Department of Internal Medicine, Hematology/Oncology, University Hospital Frankfurt, Frankfurt, Germany

Yuzhi Wang, Lele Wu, Xue Gong, Yan Liu and Liming Chen
The Key Laboratory of Developmental Genes and Human Disease, Ministry of Education, Institute of Life Science, Southeast University, Nanjing 210096, People's Republic of China
Jiangsu Key Laboratory for Molecular and Medical Biotechnology, College of Life Science, Nanjing Normal University, Nanjing 210023, People's Republic of China

Zhifang Ma, Fei Ma, Jun Zhang, Weiguang Liu and Guanyun Wei
Jiangsu Key Laboratory for Molecular and Medical Biotechnology, College of Life Science, Nanjing Normal University, Nanjing 210023, People's Republic of China

Jean Paul Thiery
Cancer Science Institute, National University of Singapore, 14 Medical Drive, Singapore, Singapore
Institute of Molecular and Cell Biology, A*STAR, 61 Biopolis Drive, Singapore, Singapore
Department of Biochemistry, Yong Loo Lin School of Medicine, National University of Singapore, 8 Medical Drive, Singapore, Singapore

Carrie B. Hruska, Tiffinee N. Swanson, Alyssa N. Mammel, David S. Lake, Armando Manduca, Amy Lynn Conners, Dana H. Whaley and Michael K. O'Connor
Department of Physiology and Biomedical Engineering, Mayo Clinic, 200 First Street SW, Rochester, MN 55905, USA

Jennifer R. Geske, Christopher G. Scott, Rickey E. Carter and Celine M. Vachon
Department of Health Sciences Research, Mayo Clinic, 200 First Street SW, Rochester, MN 55905, USA

Deborah J. Rhodes
Department Medicine, Mayo Clinic, 200 First Street SW, Rochester, MN 55905, USA

Mustapha Abubakar, Ruth M. Pfeiffer and Xiaohong R. Yang
Integrative Tumor Epidemiology Branch, Division of Cancer Epidemiology and Genetics, National Cancer Institute (NCI), National Institutes of Health, 9609 Medical Center Drive, Rockville, MD 20850, USA

Hyuna Sung
Integrative Tumor Epidemiology Branch, Division of Cancer Epidemiology and Genetics, National Cancer Institute (NCI), National Institutes of Health, 9609 Medical Center Drive, Rockville, MD 20850, USA
Surveillance and Health Services Research, American Cancer Society, 250 Williams Street NW, Atlanta, GA 30303, USA

Devi BCR and Tieng Swee Tang
Department of Radiotherapy, Oncology and Palliative Care, Sarawak General Hospital, Kuching, Sarawak, Malaysia

Jennifer Guida
Division of Cancer Control and Population Sciences, National Cancer Institute, National Institutes of Health, Rockville, MD, USA

Carolina Ortega-Olvera, Claudia Elena González-Acevedo and Ma. de Lourdes Hernández-Blanco
Universidad Autónoma de San Luis Potosí, Facultad de Enfermería y Nutrición, Niño Artillero #130, Zona Universitaria, C.P. 78240 San Luis Potosí, S.L.P., México

Alfredo Ulloa-Aguirre
Red de Apoyo a la Investigación, Universidad Nacional Autónoma de México-Instituto Nacional de Ciencias Médicas y Nutrición Salvador Zubirán, calle Vasco de Quiroga No. 15, Col. Belisario Domínguez Sección XVI, Del. Tlalpan, C.P. 14080 Ciudad de México, México

Angélica Ángeles-Llerenas
Centro de Investigación en Salud Poblacional, Instituto Nacional de Salud Pública, Av. Universidad No. 655, Col. Santa María Ahuacatitlán, Cuernavaca C.P. 62100, Morelos, México

Gabriela Torres-Mejía
Centro de Investigación en Salud Poblacional, Instituto Nacional de Salud Pública, Av. Universidad No. 655, Col. Santa María Ahuacatitlán, Cuernavaca C.P. 62100, Morelos, México
Instituto Nacional de Salud Pública, Centro de Investigación en Salud Poblacional, Avenida Universidad 655, Col. Santa María Ahuacatitlán, C.P. 62100 Cuernavaca, Morelos, México

Fernando Enrique Mainero-Ratchelous
Hospital de Ginecología y Obstetricia No. 4 Luis Castelazo Ayala, Instituto Mexicano del Seguro Social, Avenida Río Magdalena No. 289, Col. Tizapán, San Angel, Ciudad de México C.P. 01090, México

Elad Ziv
Department of Medicine, Division of General Internal Medicine, Institute for Human Genetics, Helen Diller Family Comprehensive Cancer Center, University of California, San Francisco, 1450 3rd St, San Francisco, CA 94143, USA
Department of Epidemiology and Biostatistics, Helen Diller Family Comprehensive Cancer Center, University of California, San Francisco, 1450 3rd St, San Francisco, CA 94143, USA

Larissa Avilés-Santa
National Heart, Lung, and Blood Institute at the National Institutes of Health, 6701 Rockledge, Room 10188, Bethesda, MD 20892, USA

Edelmiro Pérez-Rodríguez
Hospital Universitario "Dr José Eleuterio González". Madero y Dr. Aguirre Pequeño, Col. Mitras, C.P. 64460 Monterrey, N.L., México

Qiong Gao
The Breast Cancer Now Toby Robins
Research Centre at the Institute of
Cancer Research, 237 Fulham Road,
London SW3 6JB, UK

Richard Buus and Mitch Dowsett
The Breast Cancer Now Toby Robins
Research Centre at the Institute of
Cancer Research, 237 Fulham Road,
London SW3 6JB, UK
Ralph Lauren Centre for Breast
Cancer Research, Royal Marsden
Hospital, London, UK

Belinda Yeo
Olivia Newton-John Cancer Research
Institute, Melbourne, Australia
Austin Health, Melbourne, Australia

**Jack Cuzick, Ivana Sestak and Adam
R. Brentnall**
Centre for Cancer Prevention,
Wolfson Institute of Preventive
Medicine, Queen Mary University of
London, London, UK

Marie Klintman
Lund University, Skane University
Hospital, Faculty of Medicine,
Department of Clinical Sciences
Lund, Oncology and Pathology,
Lund, Sweden.

Maggie Chon U. Cheang
Clinical Trials and Statistic Unit, The
Institute of Cancer Research, London,
UK

Komel Khabra
Research Data Management and
Statistics Unit, Royal Marsden
Hospital, London, UK

**Chara Papadaki, Maria Spiliotaki
and Georgios Mastrostamatis**
Laboratory of Translational Oncology,
School of Medicine, University of
Crete, Heraklion, 71003 Heraklion,
Crete, Greece

**Dimitrios Mavroudis and Sofia
Agelaki**
Laboratory of Translational Oncology,
School of Medicine, University of
Crete, Heraklion, 71003 Heraklion,
Crete, Greece

Department of Medical Oncology,
University General Hospital of
Heraklion, 1352 Heraklion, Crete,
Greece

Michalis tratigos
Department of Medical Oncology,
University General Hospital of
Heraklion, 1352 Heraklion, Crete,
Greece

Georgios Markakis
Department of Agricultural, Technological Education Institute of Heraklion,
72100 Heraklion, Crete, Greece

Christoforos Nikolaou
Computational Genomics Group,
Department of Biology, University of
Crete, 70013 Heraklion, Greece
Institute of Molecular Biology and
Biotechnology, Foundation for
Research and Technology, 70013
Heraklion, Crete, Greece

**Yan Zuo, Arzu Ulu and Jeffrey A.
Frost**
Department of Integrative Biology
and Pharmacology, University of
Texas Health Science Center at
Houston, 6431 Fannin St, Houston,
TX 77030, USA

Jeffrey T. Chang
Department of Integrative Biology
and Pharmacology, University of
Texas Health Science Center at
Houston, 6431 Fannin St, Houston,
TX 77030, USA
School of Biomedical Informatics,
University of Texas Health Science
Center at Houston, 6431 Fannin St,
Houston, TX 77030, USA

**Nathalie Sami, Kyuwan Lee, Frank
C Sweeney and Christina Stewart**
Division of Biokinesiology and
Physical Therapy, University of
Southern California (USC), |1540 E.
Alcazar St., CHP 155, Los Angeles,
CA 90089, USA

Christina M Dieli-Conwright
Division of Biokinesiology and
Physical Therapy, University of
Southern California (USC), |1540 E.
Alcazar St., CHP 155, Los Angeles,
CA 90089, USA

Department of Medicine, Keck School
of Medicine, University of Southern
California, Los Angeles, CA 90033,
USA

Kerry S Courneya
Faculty of Kinesiology, Sport, and
Recreation, University of Alberta,
Edmonton, AB T6G 2H9, Canada

Wendy Demark-Wahnefried
Department of Nutrition Sciences,
University of Alabama at
Birmingham, Birmingham, AL 35294,
USA

Thomas A Buchanan
Division of Endocrinology and
Diabetes, Keck School of Medicine,
USC, Los Angeles, CA 90033, USA

Darcy Spicer
Department of Medicine, Keck School
of Medicine, University of Southern
California, Los Angeles, CA 90033,
USA

Debu Tripathy
Department of Breast Medical
Oncology, The University of Texas
MD Anderson Cancer Center,
Houston, TX 77030, USA

Leslie Bernstein
Division of Biomarkers of Early
Detection and Prevention, Beckman
Research Institute, City of Hope
(COH), Duarte, CA 91010, USA

Joanne E Mortimer
Division of Medical Oncology and
Experimental Therapeutics, COH,
Duarte, CA 91010, USA

Xu Liang
Department of Breast Oncology, Key
Laboratory of Carcinogenesis and
Translational Research (Ministry of
Education), Peking University Cancer
Hospital and Institute, Beijing, China
Pharmacogenomic Unit, Department
of Genetics, Curie Institute, PSL
Research University, 26 rue d'Ulm,
75005 Paris, France

Sophie Vacher, Anais Boulai and Céline Callens
Pharmacogenomic Unit, Department of Genetics, Curie Institute, PSL Research University, 26 rue d'Ulm, 75005 Paris, France

Ivan Bièche
Pharmacogenomic Unit, Department of Genetics, Curie Institute, PSL Research University, 26 rue d'Ulm, 75005 Paris, France
EA7331, Paris Descartes University, Sorbonne Paris Cité, Faculty of Pharmaceutical and Biological Sciences, Paris, France

Virginie Bernard
Clinic bioinformatic Unit, Department of Biopathology, Curie Institute, PSL Research University, Paris, France

Sylvain Baulande and Mylene Bohec
Institut Curie Genomics of Excellence (ICGex) Platform, Curie Institute, PSL Research University, Paris, France

Florence Lerebours
Department of Medical Oncology, Curie Institute, René Huguenin Hospital, Saint-Cloud, France

Chao Wang, Adam R. Brentnall and Jack Cuzick
Centre for Cancer Prevention, Wolfson Institute of Preventive Medicine, Queen Mary University of London, Charterhouse Square, London EC1M 6BQ, UK

Elaine F. Harkness and Susan Astley
Centre for Imaging Science, School of Health Sciences, University of Manchester, Stopford Building, Oxford Road, Manchester M13 9PT, UK

D. Gareth Evans
Department of Genomic Medicine, University of Manchester, St Mary's Hospital, M13 9WL, Manchester, UK

Jana Biermann, Toshima Z. Parris, Anna Danielsson, Hanna Engqvist, Per Karlsson and Khalil Helou
Department of Oncology, Institute of Clinical Sciences, Sahlgrenska Cancer Center, Sahlgrenska Academy at University of Gothenburg, SE-405 30 Gothenburg, Sweden

Elisabeth Werner Rönnerman
Department of Oncology, Institute of Clinical Sciences, Sahlgrenska Cancer Center, Sahlgrenska Academy at University of Gothenburg, SE-405 30 Gothenburg, Sweden Department of Clinical Pathology and Genetics, Sahlgrenska University Hospital, 413 45 Gothenburg, Sweden

Szilárd Nemes
Swedish Hip Arthroplasty Register, 405 30 Gothenburg, Sweden

Anikó Kovács
Department of Clinical Pathology and Genetics, Sahlgrenska University Hospital, 413 45 Gothenburg, Sweden

Eva Forssell-Aronsson
Department of Radiation Physics, Institute of Clinical Sciences, Sahlgrenska Cancer Center, Sahlgrenska Academy at University of Gothenburg, 405 30 Gothenburg, Sweden

Carla L. Alves, Daniel Elias and Maria B. Lyng
Department of Cancer and Inflammation Research, Institute of Molecular Medicine, University of Southern Denmark, J.B. Winsløwsvej 25, 5000 Odense C, Denmark

Henrik J. Ditzel
Department of Cancer and Inflammation Research, Institute of Molecular Medicine, University of Southern Denmark, J.B. Winsløwsvej 25, 5000 Odense C, Denmark
Department of Oncology, Odense University Hospital, 5000 Odense, Denmark
Academy of Geriatric Cancer Research (AgeCare), Odense University Hospital, 5000 Odense, Denmark

Martin Bak
Department of Pathology, Odense University Hospital, 5000 Odense, Denmark

Brooke N. McKnight and Nerissa T. Viola-Villegas
Department of Oncology, Karmanos Cancer Institute, 4100 John R Street, Detroit, MI 48201, USA

Thomas Hardiman
Cancer Bioinformatics, King's College London, Innovation Hub, Cancer Centre at Guy's Hospital, Great Maze Pond, London SE1 9RT, UK
School of Cancer and Pharmaceutical Sciences, CRUK King's Health Partners Centre, King's College London, Innovation Hub, Comprehensive Cancer Centre at Guy's Hospital, Great Maze Pond, London SE1 9RT, UK

Gaurav Chatterjee and Trupti Pai
Cancer Bioinformatics, King's College London, Innovation Hub, Cancer Centre at Guy's Hospital, Great Maze Pond, London SE1 9RT, UK
School of Cancer and Pharmaceutical Sciences, CRUK King's Health Partners Centre, King's College London, Innovation Hub, Comprehensive Cancer Centre at Guy's Hospital, Great Maze Pond, London SE1 9RT, UK
Department of Pathology, Tata Memorial Centre, 8th Floor, Annexe Building, Mumbai, India

Anita Grigoriadis
Cancer Bioinformatics, King's College London, Innovation Hub, Cancer Centre at Guy's Hospital, Great Maze Pond, London SE1 9RT, UK
School of Cancer and Pharmaceutical Sciences, CRUK King's Health Partners Centre, King's College London, Innovation Hub, Comprehensive Cancer Centre at Guy's Hospital, Great Maze Pond, London SE1 9RT, UK
Breast Cancer Now Research Unit, Innovation Hub, Cancer Centre at Guy's Hospital, King's College London, Faculty of Life Sciences and Medicine, London SE1 9RT, UK

Sarah E. Pinder
School of Cancer and Pharmaceutical Sciences, CRUK King's Health Partners Centre, King's College London, Innovation Hub, Comprehensive Cancer Centre at Guy's Hospital, Great Maze Pond, London SE1 9RT, UK

Kelly Avery-Kiejda, Rodney J. Scott
Priority Research Centre for Cancer, School of Biomedical Sciences and Pharmacy, Faculty of Health, University of Newcastle, Newcastle, NSW 2308, Australia

Jo Spencer
Peter Gorer Department of Immunobiology, King's College London, Guy's Hospital, 2nd Floor, Borough Wing, London SE1 9RT, UK

Serena P. H. Mao, Minji Park and Ramon M. Cabrera
Department of Anatomy and Structural Biology, Albert Einstein College of Medicine, 1301 Morris Park Avenue, Bronx, NY 10461, USA

Jeffrey E. Segall
Department of Anatomy and Structural Biology, Albert Einstein College of Medicine, 1301 Morris Park Avenue, Bronx, NY 10461, USA
Gruss Lipper Biophotonics Center, Albert Einstein College of Medicine, Bronx, NY 10461, USA

George S. Karagiannis, Maja H. Oktay and John S. Condeelis
Department of Anatomy and Structural Biology, Albert Einstein College of Medicine, 1301 Morris Park Avenue, Bronx, NY 10461, USA
Gruss Lipper Biophotonics Center, Albert Einstein College of Medicine, Bronx, NY 10461, USA
Integrated Imaging Program, Albert Einstein College of Medicine, Bronx, NY 10461, USA

Wenjun Guo and John R. Christin
Department of Cell Biology, Albert Einstein College of Medicine, Bronx, NY 10461, USA

Dietmar M. W. Zaiss
Institute of Immunology and Infection Research, University of Edinburgh, Edinburgh, UK

Scott I. Abrams
Department of Immunology, Roswell Park Comprehensive Cancer Center, Buffalo, NY 14263, USA

Paraic A. Kenny
Kabara Cancer Research Institute, Gundersen Medical Foundation, La Crosse, WI 54601, USA

Alison E. Obr, Joseph J. Bulatowicz and Teresa L. Wood
Department of Pharmacology, Physiology and Neuroscience, Rutgers-New Jersey Medical School, Cancer Institute of New Jersey, Newark, NJ 07101, USA

Sushil Kumar, Raymond B. Birge and Deborah A. Lazzarino
Department of Microbiology, Biochemistry and Molecular Genetics, Rutgers-New Jersey Medical School, Cancer Institute of New Jersey, Newark, NJ 07101, USA

Yun-Juan Chang
Office of Advance Research Computing, Rutgers-New Jersey Medical School, Newark, NJ 07102, USA

Betsy J. Barnes
Feinstein Institute for Medical Research, Northwell Health, Manhasset, NY 11030, USA

Emily Gallagher and Derek LeRoith
Division of Endocrinology, Diabetes and Bone Diseases, The Samuel Bronfman Department of Medicine, Icahn Sinai School of Medicine at Mt. Sinai, New York, NY 10029, USA

Viola Heinzelmann-Schwarz
Gynecologic Cancer Center, University Hospital Basel, 4056 Basel, Switzerland

Marcus Vetter
Gynecologic Cancer Center, University Hospital Basel, 4056 Basel, Switzerland
Department of Medical Oncology, University Hospital Basel, 4056 Basel, Switzerland

Christian Kurzeder
Gynecologic Cancer Center, University Hospital Basel, 4056 Basel, Switzerland

Breast Center, University Hospital Basel, 4056 Basel, Switzerland

Julia Landin, Catharina Balmelli, Alexandra Malinovska, Alfred Zippelius and Christoph Rochlitz
Department of Medical Oncology, University Hospital Basel, 4056 Basel, Switzerland

Nicola Aceto, Sofia Gkountela, Cinzia Donato, Ilona Krol, Ramona Scherrer and Barbara Maria Szczerba
Department of Biomedicine, Cancer Metastasis Laboratory, University of Basel and University Hospital Basel, Mattenstrasse 28, CH-4058 Basel, Switzerland

Francesc Castro-Giner
Department of Biomedicine, Cancer Metastasis Laboratory, University of Basel and University Hospital Basel, Mattenstrasse 28, CH-4058 Basel, Switzerland
SIB Swiss Institute of Bioinformatics, 1015 Lausanne, Switzerland

Walter Paul Weber
Breast Center, University Hospital Basel, 4056 Basel, Switzerland

Index